Rickettsial Diseases

INFECTIOUS DISEASE AND THERAPY

Series Editor

Burke A. Cunha

Winthrop-University Hospital
Mineola, and
State University of New York School of Medicine
Stony Brook, New York

1. Parasitic Infections in the Compromised Host, *edited by Peter D. Walzer and Robert M. Genta*
2. Nucleic Acid and Monoclonal Antibody Probes: Applications in Diagnostic Methodology, *edited by Bala Swaminathan and Gyan Prakash*
3. Opportunistic Infections in Patients with the Acquired Immunodeficiency Syndrome, *edited by Gifford Leoung and John Mills*
4. Acyclovir Therapy for Herpesvirus Infections, *edited by David A. Baker*
5. The New Generation of Quinolones, *edited by Clifford Siporin, Carl L. Heifetz, and John M. Domagala*
6. Methicillin-Resistant *Staphylococcus aureus*: Clinical Management and Laboratory Aspects, *edited by Mary T. Cafferkey*
7. Hepatitis B Vaccines in Clinical Practice, *edited by Ronald W. Ellis*
8. The New Macrolides, Azalides, and Streptogramins: Pharmacology and Clinical Applications, *edited by Harold C. Neu, Lowell S. Young, and Stephen H. Zinner*
9. Antimicrobial Therapy in the Elderly Patient, *edited by Thomas T. Yoshikawa and Dean C. Norman*
10. Viral Infections of the Gastrointestinal Tract: Second Edition, Revised and Expanded, *edited by Albert Z. Kapikian*
11. Development and Clinical Uses of *Haemophilus b* Conjugate Vaccines, *edited by Ronald W. Ellis and Dan M. Granoff*
12. *Pseudomonas aeruginosa* Infections and Treatment, *edited by Aldona L. Baltch and Raymond P. Smith*
13. Herpesvirus Infections, *edited by Ronald Glaser and James F. Jones*
14. Chronic Fatigue Syndrome, *edited by Stephen E. Straus*
15. Immunotherapy of Infections, *edited by K. Noel Masihi*
16. Diagnosis and Management of Bone Infections, *edited by Luis E. Jauregui*
17. Drug Transport in Antimicrobial and Anticancer Chemotherapy, *edited by Nafsika H. Georgopapadakou*
18. New Macrolides, Azalides, and Streptogramins in Clinical Practice, *edited by Harold C. Neu, Lowell S. Young, Stephen H. Zinner, and Jacques F. Acar*
19. Novel Therapeutic Strategies in the Treatment of Sepsis, *edited by David C. Morrison and John L. Ryan*

20. Catheter-Related Infections, *edited by Harald Seifert, Bernd Jansen, and Barry M. Farr*
21. Expanding Indications for the New Macrolides, Azalides, and Streptogramins, *edited by Stephen H. Zinner, Lowell S. Young, Jacques F. Acar, and Harold C. Neu*
22. Infectious Diseases in Critical Care Medicine, *edited by Burke A. Cunha*
23. New Considerations for Macrolides, Azalides, Streptogramins, and Ketolides, *edited by Stephen H. Zinner, Lowell S. Young, Jacques F. Acar, and Carmen Ortiz-Neu*
24. Tickborne Infectious Diseases: Diagnosis and Management, *edited by Burke A. Cunha*
25. Protease Inhibitors in AIDS Therapy, *edited by Richard C. Ogden and Charles W. Flexner*
26. Laboratory Diagnosis of Bacterial Infections, *edited by Nevio Cimolai*
27. Chemokine Receptors and AIDS, *edited by Thomas R. O'Brien*
28. Antimicrobial Pharmacodynamics in Theory and Clinical Practice, *edited by Charles H. Nightingale, Takeo Murakawa, and Paul G. Ambrose*
29. Pediatric Anaerobic Infections: Diagnosis and Management, Third Edition, Revised and Expanded, *Itzhak Brook*
30. Viral Infections and Treatment, *edited by Helga Ruebsamen-Waigmann, Karl Deres, Guy Hewlett, and Reinhold Welker*
31. Community-Aquired Respiratory Infections, *edited by Charles H. Nightingale, Paul G. Ambrose, and Thomas M. File*
32. Catheter-Related Infections: Second Edition, *Harald Seifert, Bernd Jansen and Barry Farr*
33. Antibiotic Optimization: Concepts and Strategies in Clinical Practice (PBK), *edited by Robert C. Owens, Jr., Charles H. Nightingale and Paul G. Ambrose*
34. Fungal Infections in the Immunocompromised Patient, *edited by John R. Wingard and Elias J. Anaissie*
35. Sinusitis: From Microbiology To Management, *edited by Itzhak Brook*
36. Herpes Simplex Viruses, *edited by Marie Studahl, Paola Cinque and Tomas Bergström*
37. Antiviral Agents, Vaccines, and Immunotherapies, *Stephen K. Tyring*
38. Epstein-Barr Virus, *Alex Tselis and Hal B. Jenson*
39. Infection Management for Geriatrics in Long-Term Care Facilities, Second Edition, *edited by Thomas T. Yoshikawa and Joseph G. Ouslander*
40. Infectious Diseases in Critical Care Medicine, Second Edition, *edited by Burke A. Cunha*
41. Infective Endocarditis: Management in the Era of Intravascular Devices, *edited by John L. Brusch*
42. Fever of Unknown Origin, *edited by Burke A. Cunha*
43. Rickettsial Diseases, *edited by Didier Raoult and Philippe Parola*

Rickettsial Diseases

edited by

Didier Raoult
Unité des Rickettsies
Université de la Méditerranée
Marseille, France

Philippe Parola
Unité des Rickettsies
Université de la Méditerranée
Marseille, France

informa
healthcare

New York   London

Informa Healthcare USA, Inc.
52 Vanderbilt Avenue
New York, NY 10017

© 2007 by Informa Healthcare USA, Inc.
Informa Healthcare is an Informa business

No claim to original U.S. Government works
Printed in the United States of America on acid-free paper
10 9 8 7 6 5 4 3 2 1

International Standard Book Number-10: 0-8493-7611-4 (Hardcover)
International Standard Book Number-13: 978-0-8493-7611-5 (Hardcover)

This book contains information obtained from authentic and highly regarded sources. Reprinted material is quoted with permission, and sources are indicated. A wide variety of references are listed. Reasonable efforts have been made to publish reliable data and information, but the author and the publisher cannot assume responsibility for the validity of all materials or for the consequences of their use.

No part of this book may be reprinted, reproduced, transmitted, or utilized in any form by any electronic, mechanical, or other means, now known or hereafter invented, including photocopying, microfilming, and recording, or in any information storage or retrieval system, without written permission from the publishers.

For permission to photocopy or use material electronically from this work, please access www.copyright.com (http://www.copyright.com/) or contact the Copyright Clearance Center, Inc. (CCC) 222 Rosewood Drive, Danvers, MA 01923, 978-750-8400. CCC is a not-for-profit organization that provides licenses and registration for a variety of users. For organizations that have been granted a photocopy license by the CCC, a separate system of payment has been arranged.

Trademark Notice: Product or corporate names may be trademarks or registered trademarks, and are used only for identification and explanation without intent to infringe.

Library of Congress Cataloging-in-Publication Data

Rickettsial diseases / edited by Didier Raoult, Philippe Parola.
　　p. ; cm. -- (Infectious disease and therapy ; v. 43)
　Includes bibliographical references.
　ISBN-13: 978-0-8493-7611-5 (hardcover : alk. paper)
　ISBN-10: 0-8493-7611-4 (hardcover : alk. paper)
　1. Rickettsial diseases. I. Raoult, Didier. II. Parola, Philippe. III. Series.
　　[DNLM: 1. Rickettsia Infections--physiopathology. 2. Rickettsia Infections--microbiology. 3. Rickettsia Infections--therapy. W1 IN406HMN v.43 2007 / WC 600 R53877 2007]

RC114.7.R58 2007
616.9'22--dc22
　　　　　　　　　　　　　　　　　　　　　　　　　　　　　　　　　　　　　2006101892

Visit the Informa Web site at
www.informa.com

and the Informa Healthcare Web site at
www.informahealthcare.com

*To my wife Natacha, my children Magali, Sacha and Lola, and
my granchild César*
—*Didier Raoult*

To my wife, Géraldine, and my parents, Marie-Claire and Jean-Pierre
—*Philippe Parola*

Preface

In the last 20 years, the rickettsial field has undergone significant evolution at the epidemiological, microbiological, and molecular levels. Between 1984 and 2004 alone, at least nine additional rickettsial species or subspecies were identified as causes of tick-borne rickettsioses around the world. Of these agents, six were initially isolated from ticks, often years or decades before a definitive association with human disease was established. Also, outbreaks of the louse-borne epidemic typhus re-emerged in Africa, with the most recent outbreak (and the largest since World War II) observed in Burundi in the 1990s, during their civil war. Fleas, which have been historically associated with the transmission of murine typhus, have been involved in the cycle of *Rickettsia felis*, an emerging pathogen belonging to the spotted-fever group of *Rickettsia*. Furthermore, about one million cases of scrub typhus due to *Orientia tsutsugamushi* have been estimated to occur each year around the world and as many as one billion people may be exposed, particularly in rural locations.

Recent developments in molecular taxonomic methods have resulted in the reclassification of the rickettsiae. For example, the *Rochalimaea*, united within the genus *Bartonella*, and *Coxiella* were removed from the order Rickettsiales and the classification of this order continues to be modified as new data becomes available. Because Q fever caused by *Coxiella burnetii* is still considered as a "rickettsiosis" and remains in the field of rickettsiologists, it will be largely described in this book.

The rickettsial field has recently entered the genome area. In 2001, the first genome of a tick-transmitted rickettsia (*R. conorii* strain Seven) was fully sequenced and revealed several unique characteristics among bacterial genomes, including long palindromic repeat fragments irregularly distributed throughout the genome. Further, comparison of the *R. conorii* genome with that of *R. prowazekii* (the agent of epidemic typhus and included in the typhus group of the genus *Rickettsia*), provided additional data on the evolution of rickettsial genomes, the latter appearing to be a subset of the first. Recently, the genomes of *R. sibirica*, *R. rickettsii*, *R. akari*, *R. felis*, and *R. typhi* have been reported. Those of *R. belli*, *R. massiliae*, *R. africae*, and *R. slovaca* are currently being sequenced. These data will certainly provide insights into the mechanism of rickettsial pathogenicity and will provide new molecular diagnostic targets and new tools for phylogenetic and taxonomic studies as well as new treatment measures.

We anticipate that this book will appeal to physicians specializing in infectious diseases, dermatology, or even travel medicine, as well as clinical laboratory personnel and epidemiologists. Not only physicians and scientists in Europe and the United States will find this book useful, but also those from tropical regions in Africa, Asia, Australia, and the Americas, where numerous emerging diseases have been described in recent years and where rickettsial diseases constitute a differential diagnosis in febrile patients.

Didier Raoult
Philippe Parola

Contents

Preface v
Contributors. . . . ix

Section I: *Rickettsia* and Human Rickettsioses

1. Bacteriology, Taxonomy, and Phylogeny of *Rickettsia*   1
   Pierre-Edouard Fournier and Didier Raoult

2. Pathogenesis, Immunity, Pathology, and Pathophysiology in Rickettsial Diseases   15
   David H. Walker, Nahed Ismail, Juan P. Olano, Gustavo Valbuena, and Jere McBride

3. Arthropods and Rickettsiae   27
   Sam R. Telford III and Philippe Parola

4. Murine Typhus   37
   Yanis Tselentis and Achilleas Gikas

5. Louse-Borne Epidemic Typhus   51
   Linda Houhamdi and Didier Raoult

6. Rickettsialpox   63
   Christopher D. Paddock and Marina E. Eremeeva

7. Flea-Borne Spotted Fever   87
   Abir Znazen and Didier Raoult

Section II: Tick-Borne Rickettsioses

8. Rocky Mountain Spotted Fever   97
   James E. Childs and Christopher D. Paddock

9. African Tick-Bite Fever   117
   Mogens Jensenius, Lucy Ndip, and Bjørn Myrvang

10. *Rickettsia conorii* Infections (Mediterranean Spotted Fever, Israeli Spotted Fever, Indian Tick Typhus, Astrakhan Fever)   125
    Clarisse Rovery and Didier Raoult

11. Other Tick-Borne Rickettsioses   139
    Oleg Mediannikov, Philippe Parola, and Didier Raoult

12. Other Rickettsiae of Possible or Undetermined Pathogenicity   163
    Oleg Mediannikov, Christopher D. Paddock, and Philippe Parola

Section III: Anaplasmataceae and Human Anaplasmosis and Ehrlichioses

13. Bacteriology and Phylogeny of Anaplasmataceae 179
    Philippe Brouqui and Kotaro Matsumoto

14. Vectors and Reservoir Hosts of Anaplasmataceae 199
    Hisashi Inokuma

15. Human Ehrlichioses 213
    Juan P. Olano

16. Anaplasmosis in Humans 223
    Anna Grzeszczuk, Nicole C. Barat, Johan S. Bakken, and J. Stephen Dumler

Section IV: *Orientia tsutsugamushi* and Scrub Typhus

17. *Orientia tsutsugamushi* and Scrub Typhus 237
    George Watt and Pacharee Kantipong

Section V: *Coxiella burnetii* and Q Fever

18. Bacteriology of *Coxiella* 257
    Katja Mertens and James E. Samuel

19. Immune Response to Q Fever 271
    Jean-Louis Mege

20. Epidemiology of Q Fever 281
    Thomas J. Marrie

21. Clinical Aspects, Diagnosis, and Treatment of Q Fever 291
    Hervé Tissot-Dupont and Didier Raoult

Section VI: *Wolbachia*

22. *Wolbachia* and Filarial Nematode Diseases in Humans 303
    Kelly L. Johnston and Mark J. Taylor

Section VII: Diagnostic Strategy of Rickettsial Diseases in Humans

23. Diagnostic Strategy of Rickettsioses and Ehrlichioses 315
    Florence Fenollar, Pierre-Edouard Fournier, and Didier Raoult

Section VIII: Rickettsial Diseases of Domestic Animals

24. Rickettsial Diseases of Domestic Animals 331
    Patrick J. Kelly

Section IX: Genomics of Rickettsial Agents

25. Genomics of Rickettsial Agents 345
    Hiroyuki Ogata and Patricia Renesto

Section X: Antimicrobial Susceptibility of Rickettsial Agents

26. Antimicrobial Susceptibility of Rickettsial Agents 361
    Jean-Marc Rolain

Index 371

Contributors

Johan S. Bakken Department of Family Medicine, School of Medicine, University of Minnesota at Duluth and St. Luke's Infectious Disease Associates, St. Luke's Hospital, Duluth, Minnesota, U.S.A.

Nicole C. Barat Division of Medical Microbiology, Department of Pathology, The Johns Hopkins University School of Medicine, Baltimore, Maryland, U.S.A.

Philippe Brouqui Faculté de Médecine, Unité des Rickettsies, Université de la Méditerranée, Marseille, France

James E. Childs Department of Epidemiology and Public Health, Yale University School of Medicine, New Haven, Connecticut, U.S.A.

J. Stephen Dumler Division of Medical Microbiology, Department of Pathology, The Johns Hopkins University School of Medicine, Baltimore, Maryland, U.S.A.

Marina E. Eremeeva Rickettsial Zoonoses Branch, Division of Viral and Rickettsial Diseases, Centers for Disease Control and Prevention, Atlanta, Georgia, U.S.A.

Florence Fenollar Faculté de Médecine, Unité des Rickettsies, Université de la Méditerranée, Marseille, France

Pierre-Edouard Fournier Faculté de Médecine, Unité des Rickettsies, Université de la Méditerranée, Marseille, France

Achilleas Gikas Laboratory of Clinical Bacteriology, Parasitology, Zoonoses, and Geographical Medicine, University of Crete, Crete, Greece

Anna Grzeszczuk Department of Infectious Diseases, Medical University of Bialystok, Bialystok, Poland

Linda Houhamdi Faculté de Médecine, Unité des Rickettsies, Institut Fédératif de Recherche 48, Centre National de Recherche Scientifique, Université de la Méditerranée, Marseille, France

Hisashi Inokuma Department of Clinical Veterinary Science, Obihiro University of Agriculture and Veterinary Medicine, Obihiro, Japan

Nahed Ismail Department of Pathology, University of Texas Medical Branch, Galveston, Texas, U.S.A.

Mogens Jensenius Department of Infectious Diseases, Ullevål University Hospital, Oslo, Norway

Kelly L. Johnston Filariasis Research Laboratory, Molecular and Biochemical Parasitology, Liverpool School of Tropical Medicine, Pembroke Place, U.K.

Pacharee Kantipong Department of Internal Medicine, Chiangrai Regional Hospital, Chiangrai, Thailand

Patrick J. Kelly Ross University School of Veterinary Medicine, Basseterre, St. Kitts, West Indies

Thomas J. Marrie Faculty of Medicine and Dentistry, University of Alberta, Edmonton, Alberta, Canada

Kotaro Matsumoto Faculté de Médecine, Unité des Rickettsies, Université de la Méditerranée, Marseille, France

Jere McBride Department of Pathology, University of Texas Medical Branch, Galveston, Texas, U.S.A.

Oleg Mediannikov Unité des Rickettsies, Université de la Méditerranée, Marseille, France and Laboratory of Rickettsial Ecology, Gamaleya Institute of Epidemiology and Microbiology, Moscow, Russia

Jean-Louis Mege Unité des Rickettsies, Université de la Méditerranée, Marseille, France

Katja Mertens Department of Microbial and Molecular Pathogenesis, Texas A&M University System Health Science Center, College Station, Texas, U.S.A.

Bjørn Myrvang Department of Infectious Diseases and Center for Imported and Tropical Diseases, Ullevål University Hospital, Oslo, Norway

Lucy Ndip Department of Biochemistry and Microbiology, University of Buea, Buea, Cameroon

Hiroyuki Ogata Structural and Genomic Information Laboratory, Parc Scientifique de Luminy, Marseille, France

Juan P. Olano Department of Pathology, University of Texas Medical Branch, Galveston, Texas, U.S.A.

Christopher D. Paddock Infectious Disease Pathology Activity, Division of Viral and Rickettsial Diseases, Centers for Disease Control and Prevention, Atlanta, Georgia, U.S.A.

Philippe Parola Faculté de Médecine, Unité des Rickettsies, Université de la Méditerranée, Marseille, France

Didier Raoult Faculté de Médecine, Unité des Rickettsies, Université de la Méditerranée, Marseille, France

Patricia Renesto Faculté de Médecine, Unité des Rickettsies, Marseille, France

Jean-Marc Rolain Faculté de Médecine et de Pharmacie, Unité des Rickettsies, Université de la Méditerranée, Marseille, France

Clarisse Rovery Faculté de Médecine, Unité des Rickettsies, Université de la Méditerranée, Marseille, France

James E. Samuel Department of Microbial and Molecular Pathogenesis, Texas A&M University System Health Science Center, College Station, Texas, U.S.A.

Mark J. Taylor Filariasis Research Laboratory, Molecular and Biochemical Parasitology, Liverpool School of Tropical Medicine, Pembroke Place, U.K.

Sam R. Telford III Division of Infectious Diseases, Cummings School of Veterinary Medicine, Tufts University, North Grafton, Massachusetts, U.S.A.

Hervé Tissot-Dupont Faculté de Médecine, Unité des Rickettsies, Centre National de Référence, Marseille, France

Contributors

Yanis Tselentis   Laboratory of Clinical Bacteriology, Parasitology, Zoonoses, and Geographical Medicine, University of Crete, Crete, Greece

Gustavo Valbuena   Department of Pathology, University of Texas Medical Branch, Galveston, Texas, U.S.A.

David H. Walker   Department of Pathology, University of Texas Medical Branch, Galveston, Texas, U.S.A.

George Watt   Family Health International, Asia-Pacific Regional Office, Bangkok, Thailand

Abir Znazen   Laboratoire de Microbiologie, Centre Hospitalo-Universitaire, Habib Bourguiba Sfax, Tunisie

Section I: *RICKETTSIA* AND HUMAN RICKETTSIOSES

1 | Bacteriology, Taxonomy, and Phylogeny of *Rickettsia*

Pierre-Edouard Fournier and Didier Raoult
Faculté de Médecine, Unité des Rickettsies, Université de la Méditerranée, Marseille, France

INTRODUCTION

Traditional identification methods used in bacteriology cannot be routinely applied to rickettsiae because of the few phenotypic characters expressed by these strictly intracellular organisms. As a consequence, "*Rickettsia*" has long been used as a generic term for many small bacteria that could not be cultivated and were not otherwise identified. However, taxonomic progress made over the last 35 years has deeply modified the definition of "rickettsia." In particular, the introduction of molecular techniques has revolutionized the study of gene and genome evolution and has allowed new approaches to phylogenetic and taxonomic inferences. As a result of deep taxonomic changes, the term "rickettsia" currently only applies to arthropod-borne bacteria belonging to the genus *Rickettsia* within the family Rickettsiaceae in the order Rickettsiales, α-Proteobacteria. The *Rickettsia* genus is currently made of 24 recognized species, and also contains several dozens of as-yet uncharacterized strains or tick amplicons. Most of these bacteria are associated with ticks, which are their vectors and reservoirs, but some are vectorized by lice, fleas, or mites. In contrast with louse- and flea-borne rickettsioses, tick-borne rickettsioses have specific geographic distributions, directly depending on the distribution of their vectors. *Rickettsia* species cause rickettsioses, which are among the oldest known arthropod-borne diseases (1). Currently, 16 rickettsioses are recognized. Among these, several are caused by rickettsiae that were initially isolated from ticks and subsequently considered as nonpathogenic. A priori, it is difficult to predict which rickettsiae are potential human pathogens. It should be considered that rickettsiae found in arthropods capable of biting humans are potential human pathogens.

In this chapter, we will describe the bacteriology, taxonomy, and phylogeny of members of the genus *Rickettsia*.

BACTERIOLOGY

Bacteria within the genus *Rickettsia* are obligate intracellular short rods, 0.3 to 0.5 × 0.8 to 2.0 μm^2. The cytoplasm of these bacteria contains ribosomes and strands of DNA and is limited by a typical Gram-negative trilamellar structure made of a bilayer inner membrane, a peptidoglycan layer, and a bilayer outer membrane. Within host cells, rickettsiae are surrounded by an electron-lucent slime layer. Rickettsiae are not stained by the Gram method, but retain basic fuschin when stained using the Gimenez method (2). Using this method, they appear bright red, whereas the background is stained in pale blue with the malachite green counterstain.

Members of the genus *Rickettsia* are divided into two main groups: the spotted fever group (SFG) and typhus group (TG), depending on several characters: (*i*) SFG rickettsiae are mainly associated with ticks, but also with fleas (*Rickettsia felis*) and mites (*R. akari*), have an optimal growth temperature of 32°C, have a G + C content between 32 and 33, can polymerize actin and thus move into the nuclei of host cells (3–5), and cause spotted fevers in humans; (*ii*) TG rickettsiae are associated with human body lice (*R. prowazekii*) or fleas (*R. typhi*), have an optimal growth temperature of 35°C, have a G + C content of 29, cannot polymerize actin and thus cannot enter the nuclei of host cells and are only found in the cytoplasm of host cells (3,5), and cause typhus in humans (Table 1). Within ticks, transovarial and trans-stadial

(Text continues on p. 6)

TABLE 1 Main Features of the Currently Validated Species of the Genera *Rickettsia* and *Orientia*

Variables	Geographic distribution[a]	Vector[b]	Optimal culture temperature		Intracellular localization		Pathogenicity for rodents		G + C content		Antibiotic susceptibility		Deposit in official culture collection
			32–34°C	35°C	Cytoplasm	Nucleus	Mice	Guinea pigs	29–30%	32–33%	Erythromycin	Rifampin	
Validated *Rickettsia* species of recognized pathogenicity													
Spotted fever group													
R. rickettsii	6, 7	*D. andersoni, D. variabilis, R. sanguineus, Am. cajennense, Am. aureolatum*	+		+		+	−	+	−		+	+
R. sibirica subsp. *sibirica*	3	*D. marginatus, D. nutallii, D. silvarum, D. pictus, D. sinicus, D. auratus, Ha. concinna, Ha. wellingtoni, Ha. yeni*	+	+	+		+	−	+	−	+	+	+
"*R. sibirica* subsp. *mongolotimonae*"	1, 2, 3	*Hy. asiaticum, Hy. Truncatum*	+		+		+				+		+
R. conorii													
"*R. conorii* subsp. *conorii*"	1, 2, 3	*R. sanguineus, Ha. leachii*		+							+	+	+
"*R. conorii* subsp. *indica*"	3	*R. sanguineus, B. microplus, Ha. leachii*		+			+				+		+
"*R. conorii* subsp. *caspia*"	1, 2, 3	*R. sanguineus, R. pumilio*									+		+
"*R. conorii* subsp. *israelensis*"	1, 2	*R. sanguineus*	+		+		+	−	+	−	+	+	+
R. parkeri	6, 7	*Am. maculatum, Am. americanum, Am. triste*									+		+

Species	Biogroup	Vectors	C1	C2	C3	C4	C5	C6	C7	C8
R. massliae	1, 2	R. turanicus, R. sanguineus, R. mushamae, R. lunulatus, R. sulcatus	+	+				+	−	+
R. africae	2, 6	Am. hebraeum, Am. variegatum, R. appendiculatus	+	+	+		−	+	−	+
R. honei	3, 4, 6	Ap. hydrosauri, Am. cajennense, I. granulomatis	+	+	+				+	+
R. slovaca	1, 3	D. marginatus, D. reticulatus	+	+	+			+	+	+
R. aeschlimannii	1, 2, 3	Hy. m. marginatum, Hy. m. rufipes, R. appendiculatus, Ha. punctata	+	+	+			+	−	+
R. heilongjiangensis	3	D. silvarum	+	+	+					+
R. japonica	3	I. ovatus, D. taiwanensis, Ha. longicornis, Ha. flava	+	+	+			+	+	+
R. australis	4	I. holocyclus, I. tasmani, I. cornuatus	+	+	+	+			+	+
R. akari	8	Al. sanguineus	+[c]	+	+	+	+	+	+	+
R. felis	8	C. felis, Arc. erinacei	+[c]	+	+	+	+	+	+	+
Typhus group										
R. prowazekii	8	P. humanus humanus	+	+		+	−	+	+	+
R. typhi	8	X. cheopis, C. felis, L. segnis	+	+		+	+	+	+	+
Scrub typhus group										
O. tsutsugamushi	3, 4	Leptotrombidium sp.	+	+	+	+			?	+

(Continued)

TABLE 1 Main Features of the Currently Validated Species of the Genera *Rickettsia* and *Orientia* (*Continued*)

Variables	Geographic distribution[a]	Vector[b]	Optimal culture temperature		Intracellular localization		Pathogenicity for rodents		G + C content		Antibiotic susceptibility		Deposit in official culture collection
			32–34°C	35°C	Cytoplasm	Nucleus	Mice	Guinea pigs	29–30%	32–33%	Erythromycin	Rifampin	
Spotted fever group													
R. montanensis	6	*D. variabilis,* *D. andersoni*	+	+	+		−	−		−	−	−	+
R. rhipicephali	1, 2, 6	*R. sanguineus,* *D. occidentalis,* *D. andersoni*	+	+	+		−	−		−	−	−	+
R. asiatica	3	*I. ovatus*	+	+	+								+
R. tamurae	3	*Am. testudinarium*	+	+	+								+
R. helvetica	1, 3	*I. ricinus,* *I. ovatus,* *I. persulcatus,* *I. monospinosus*	+	+	+					−		+		+
R. peacockii	6	*D. andersoni*	+	+	+							+		−
"Ancestral" group													
R. canadensis	6	*Ha. leporispalustris*	+	+	+		−	−	+	−		+		+
R. bellii	6, 7	*D. variabilis,* *D. occidentalis,* *D. albopictus,* *Ha. lepopalustris,* *O. concanensis,* *Arg. cooleyi,* *Am. cooperi*	+	+	+		−	−	+	−		+		+

Validated *Rickettsia* species of uncertain or unknown pathogenicity

As-yet unvalidated species with proposed names

Species	Restricted area[a]	Vector[b]				
Candidatus R. andeana	7	*I. boliviensis*				−
Candidatus R. principis	3	*Ha. japonica*				−
Candidatus R. tarasevichiae	3	*I. persulcatus*				−
R. amblyommii	6, 7	*Am. americanum, Am. cajennense, Am. coelebs*				−
R. marmionii	4	Not described				−
R. monacensis	1	*I. ricinus*	+			−
R. moreli	1	*I. ricinus*		+		−
R. raoultii	1, 3	*R. pumilio, D. reticulatus, D. niveus, D. marginatus, D. nutallii*	+	+	+	+
Rickettsia sp. AB bacterium	1	*Adalia bipunctata*				−
R. texiana	6	*Am. americanum*				−
R. thailandii	3	*I. granulomatis*				−

+, presence of the character; −, absence of the character.
[a]Restricted areas are as follows: 1, Europe; 2, Africa and the Middle East; 3, Asia and Japan; 4, Australia, Tasmania, and Oceania; 5, Africa; 6, North America and the West Indies; 7, South America.
[b]*Al., Allodermanyssus; Am., Amblyomma; Ap., Aponoma; Arc., Archeopsylla; Arg., Argas; C., Ctenocephalides; D., Dermacentor; Ha., Haemaphysalis; Hy., Hyalomma; I., Ixodes; L., Leptopsylla; O., Ornithodoros; P., Pediculus; R. Rhipicephalus; X., Xenopsylla.*
[c]*R. felis* is also able to grow at 28°C in XTC-2 cells (23).

transmissions are essential mechanisms for the maintenance of spotted fever rickettsiae. In contrast, flea- or louse-borne rickettsiae are not transmitted transovarially and thus these bacteria have mammal reservoirs (humans for *R. prowazekii*, rodents for *R. typhi*, and cats for *R. felis*). Rickettsiae are unstable when separated from host components, except for highly stable forms found in the feces of arthropod hosts, as observed for *R. prowazekii* and *R. typhi* which are able to survive within louse feces for several weeks (7,8). Rickettsiae are rapidly inactivated at 56°C.

Until 2001, the genome size of rickettsiae was estimated by pulse field gel electrophoresis and ranged from 1.1 to 1.6 Mb. Since 1998, genome sequences from four *Rickettsia* species have been determined and published, including *R. conorii* (9), *R. felis* (10), *R. prowazekii* (11), and *R. typhi* (12). The analysis of the obtained sequences has highlighted unique characteristics among bacterial genomes: a genome size <1.4 Mb; the presence of a large number of 95- to 150-nucleotide long palindromic repeat fragments (13), including some inserted into protein-coding genes but compatible with the encoded protein's three-dimensional fold and functions; an ongoing degradation process of genes, from complete transcribed genes to split transcribed genes and then to split untranscribed genes (9). In addition, genome sequencing provided the first evidence of a conjugative plasmid in an intracellular bacterium, in *R. felis* (10). This finding suggested that conjugation could play a role in the evolution of rickettsial genomes.

Rickettsiae grow in association with eukaryotic cells within which they live free and divide by binary fission in the cytoplasm (4,14). As a consequence, rickettsiae must be cultivated in tissue culture or yolk sac of developing chicken embryos. L929 and Vero cells are used most frequently. Rickettsial growth in cell monolayers is monitored by the development of plaques that represent the disruption of massively infected cells. SFG rickettsiae form plaques with a diameter of 2 to 3 mm after five to eight days, whereas TG rickettsiae form smaller plaques (1 mm) after 8 to 10 days. Rickettsiae have a membrane-bound adenosine diphosphate/adenosine triphosphate (ADP/ATP) translocase that mediates exchange of ATP and ADP. Five copies of this gene are present in *R. conorii* and *R. prowazekii* genomes (9,15). The exchange of extracellular ATP for intracellular ADP is regulated by the concentration of phosphate in the host. Rickettsiae possess genes encoding all enzymes of the tricarboxylic acid cycle. They do not utilize glucose, but metabolize glutamate as their main source of energy. They do not synthesize or degrade nucleoside monophosphates. They produce endotoxins whose role is uncompletely understood.

Rickettsiae possess major antigens such as lipopolysaccharide, lipoprotein, outer membrane proteins of the surface cell antigen (SCA) family, and heat shock proteins. The Weil-Felix test, initially developed as a diagnostic test for rickettsioses, was based on the antigenic cross-reactions among rickettsial antigens, mostly lipopolysaccharide (LPS), and *Proteus vulgaris* strains OX19 and OX2, and *Proteus mirabilis* OXK (16). Other antigens have been characterized in *Rickettsia* species, including a 17-kDa lipoprotein (17) and members of the autotransporter protein family SCA. These include the 120-kDa S-layer protein (OmpB or Sca5) (18), OmpA, present only in SFG rickettsiae (19), and Sca4 (20). Additional 14 genes putatively encoding SCA proteins were identified in sequenced rickettsial genomes (21), one of which, *sca1*, was present in all species (22).

PHYLOGENY

Initially, phylogenetic studies of rickettsiae, as for other prokaryotes, were based on the comparison of morphological, antigenic, and metabolic characters. The order *Rickettsiales*, within which bacteria of the genus *Rickettsia* were classified, historically contained small, rod-shaped Gram-negative organisms that retained basic fuschin when stained by the method of Gimenez (2), divided by binary fission, could be cultivated in living tissues and could cause diseases in invertebrate hosts (which acted as vectors and reservoirs) or vertebrate hosts which were infected through arthropod bites (23). However, phylogenetic relationships based on these criteria were highly unreliable. The advent of molecular methods allowed phylogenic relationships among intracellular bacteria to be reliably estimated. The phylogenetic study based on the comparison of 16S rRNA gene sequences showed that several of the bacteria classified in the order *Rickettsiales* did not belong to the α-subclass of the *Proteobacteria* phylum. As a consequence, *Coxiella burnetii* and *Rickettsiella grylli* were reclassified within *Legionellaceae* (24,25),

Eperythrozoon sp. and *Haemobartonella* sp. within *Mycoplasmataceae* (26), *Wolbachia persica* within the γ-subdivision of *Proteobacteria* close to *Francisella* sp. (25), *Wolbachia melophagi* within *Bartonellaceae* (Birtles and Molyneux, GenBank Accession No. X89110), and *Bartonella* sp., *Rochalimaea* sp., and *Grahamella* sp. within *Bartonellaceae* (27,28). In addition, within the genus *Rickettsia*, taxonomic changes also occurred. *Rickettsia tsutsugamushi*, the agent of scrub typhus, was found to be distinct enough by 16S rRNA gene sequence comparison to warrant transfer into the genus *Orientia* which includes a single species, *Orientia tsutsugamushi* (29).

Within the genus *Rickettsia*, prior to gene sequencing, polymerase chain reaction (PCR) coupled with restriction fragment length polymorphism (RFLP) applied to the *gltA* and *ompA* genes showed that *R. canadensis* and *R. bellii* occupied an intermediate position between the typhus and SFGs (30), that three clusters were identified within the SFG (*R. rickettsii* and *R. slovaca*; *R. rhipicephali* and *R. montanensis*; *R. sibirica*, *R. honei*, and *R. conorii*), and that the *R. conorii* species was heterogeneous (31).

However, it was not until gene sequencing that phylogenic relationships among *Rickettsia* species could reliably be estimated. The first gene to be used for phylogenic purposes was the 16S rDNA (32,33). A specific sequence was obtained for each serotype, but high sequence similarity between 99.9 and 97.2 was observed. These studies confirmed the evolutionary unity of the genus (Fig. 1), but as the sequences were almost identical, significant inferences about intragenus phylogeny were not possible. *R. felis* was closely related to *R. akari* and *R. australis*, but not related to the TG as deduced from serologic criteria. *R. canadensis* was shown to be outside the TG. Within the SFG, a cluster including *R. massiliae*, *R. rhipicephali*, *R. amblyommii*, and

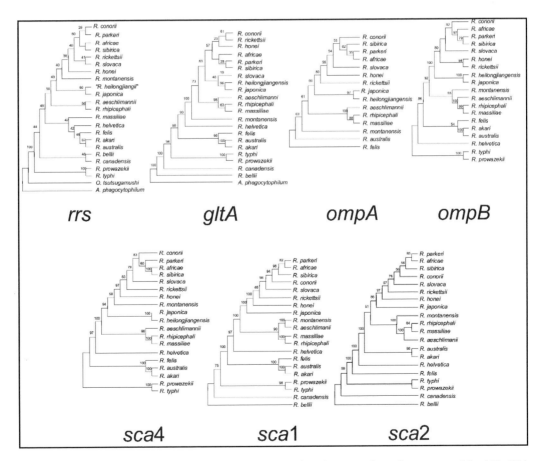

FIGURE 1 Phylogenic organization of *Rickettsia* species based on the comparison of sequences of the 16S rDNA, *gltA*, *ompA*, *ompB*, *sca*4, *sca*1, and *sca*2 genes, using the Maximum Parsimony method.

R. montanensis was described. It was proposed that *R. bellii* and *R. canadensis* diverged prior to the schism between the SFG and the TG (33).

Subsequently, phylogenic studies were inferred from sequences from more divergent genes that included *gltA* (34), the gene encoding the 17-kDa protein (35), and genes from the autotransporter family *sca*: *ompA* (19), *ompB* (36), *sca*4 (20), *sca*1 (22), and *sca*2 (37). Phylogenetic analysis inferred from sequences of the 17-kDa protein-encoding gene provided nonsignificant bootstrap values for most of the nodes (35). Phylogenic relationships inferred from sequences of the *gltA* gene were supported by significant bootstrap values for all the nodes except those within groups in the SFG (Fig. 1) (34). The *R. rickettsii* group included: *R. conorii, R. honei, R. rickettsii, R. africae, R. parkeri, R. sibirica, R. slovaca,* and *R. japonica.* The *R. massiliae* group was made of *R. massiliae, R. rhipicephali, R. aeschlimannii,* and *R. montanensis.* The coherence of the latter group was reinforced by the resistance to erythromycin and rifampin of the species it contained (38). *R. canadensis*, AB bacterium, and *R. bellii* clustered neither in the TG nor in the SFG and were shown to be the most outlying rickettsiae. *R. helvetica, R. akari,* and *R. australis* clustered between the *R. massiliae* group and the TG. Using *ompA* sequence comparison, the phylogenetic organization in the *R. rickettsii* group was well established (19). Different clusters were determined. The *R. conorii* complex included the different strains closely related to *R. conorii* (Malish, Moroccan, Indian, Israeli, and Astrakhan). A second cluster included *R. sibirica, R. africae,* and *R. parkeri. R. rickettsii, R. slovaca, R. honei,* and *R. japonica* were found alone in different branches. Significant bootstrap values were found for all the nodes except for *R. honei*. However, the *ompA* gene could not be amplified from all *Rickettsia* species (19). Phylogenetic analysis inferred from the sequences of the *ompB* gene confirmed the groups identified by *ompA* sequencing (36) (Fig. 1). Bootstrap values were significant for most of the nodes with the exception of those inside the cluster including *R. parkeri* and *R. africae.* The phylogenetic positions of *R. helvetica, R. akari, R. australis, R. typhi,* and *R. prowazekii* were the same that those determined by *gltA* sequence comparison. *Sca*4 sequence comparison identified five well-supported phylogenetic groups (Fig. 1). These included: the previously described *R. massiliae* and *R. rickettsii* groups as well as the TG; the *R. helvetica* group that contained only *R. helvetica*; and the *R. akari* group including *R. australis, R. akari,* and *R. felis.* Finally, the phylogenetic organization of *Rickettsia* species inferred from the comparison of sequences of the *sca*1 and *sca*2 genes were similar to those obtained from the analyses of *ompA, ompB,* and *sca*4 (22,37). In addition to the previously described groups, it was proposed that *R. bellii, R. canadensis,* and *Rickettsia* sp. strain AB bacterium, being the outlayers of the *Rickettsia* species, be grouped into an "ancestral" group (33). However, the consistency of this group has later been discussed on the basis of genetic criteria (39).

TAXONOMY

Because phenotypic methods used to classify axenically cultivable bacteria were not applicable to intracellular bacteria, most bacteria obligately associated with eukaryotic cells were initially included in the order *Rickettsiales*. The order *Rickettsiales* was initially divided into the families *Rickettsiaceae, Bartonellaceae,* and *Anaplasmataceae.* Within the family *Rickettsiaceae,* the tribe *Rickettsiae* was composed of the genera *Rickettsia, Coxiella,* and *Rochalimaea.* The development of PCR and nucleotide sequencing, particularly the study of 16S rRNA or rDNA, has considerably modified the taxonomic classification of bacteria, in particular, intracellular bacteria that express few phenotypic criteria commonly used for identification and classification. Following the reclassification of several genera, as described above, the order *Rickettsiales* is currently comprised the genera *Anaplasma, Ehrlichia, Neorickettsia, Orientia, Rickettsia,* and *Wolbachia* (29,40).

Currently, a *Rickettsia* is a strictly intracellular bacillus of 0.3 to 0.5 mm in diameter and 0.8 to 2.0 mm in length, with a Gram-negative-type membrane, and Gimenez stain positive (2). The target cells of *Rickettsia* sp. in humans are endothelial cells within which they multiply in the cytoplasm. In addition, *Rickettsia* strains share a high degree of 16S rDNA nucleotide sequence similarity (41) and are phylogenetically close. As a matter of fact, due to the lack of official rules, defining a species within the *Rickettsia* genus has long been a matter of debate. The guidelines established for extracellular bacteria do not fit well with the strictly intracellular nature of these bacteria. In particular, their initial differentiation relied on a combination of few phenotypic and genomic parameters. Rickettsial isolates have initially been classified within three groups: the SFG, TG, and the scrub typhus group (STG), on the basis of the following characteristics: (*i*) the intracellular position in the nucleus and cytoplasm for SFG rickettsiae and *R. canadensis*, which are able to polymerize cellular actin (42), but only in the cytoplasm for others which cannot polymerize actin; (*ii*) an optimal growth temperature of 32°C for the SFG and 35°C for the TG and STG; and (*iii*) the cross-reaction of sera from a patient with rickettsial infection with the somatic antigen of strains of *Proteus vulgaris*, OX19 for the TG and *R. rickettsii*, OX2 for the SFG, and OXK for the STG. Subsequently, the STG was deleted following reclassification of *R. tsutsugamushi* within the genus *Orientia* (29). Other criteria have also been used to describe *Rickettsia* species, including the geographical distribution of strains; their arthropod vector; pathogenicity for humans, mice, and guinea pigs; size; optimal culture temperature; time for plaque formation; hemolytic activity (23); cross-immunity and vaccine protection tests in guinea pigs (43); complement fixation (44); and toxin neutralization (45). However, since 1978, the immunofluorescent antibody assay with acute-phase mouse sera has been used as a reference method for the identification of new SFG rickettsiae (46). This test detects species-specific epitopes of the surface-exposed S-layer proteins (rOmpA and rOmpB), as well as the Sca4 (PS-120) protein, of rickettsiae. Using this method, a species corresponds to a serotype, with a rickettsial isolate being assumed to belong to a species if both strains exhibit a specificity difference of <3 (46). Although useful, mouse immunization suffers drawbacks such as a lack of reproducibility and the necessity to compare each new isolate to all previously described species. Other phenotypic methods such as the use of monoclonal antibodies (47,48) and sodium dodecyl sulfate–polyacrylamide gel electrophoresis did not bring any determinant progress to rickettsial taxonomy.

In addition, the official molecular criteria used for the identification of bacterial species, that is, the DNA G + C content (32–33% for the SFG and 29% for the TG), and DNA–DNA reassociation (49) [degrees of DNA–DNA hybridization of 94%, 74%, and 73% between *R. rickettsii* and *R. conorii*, *R. sibirica* and *R. montanensis*, respectively (50), and of 70–77% between *R. prowazekii* and *R. typhi* (51)] are not adequate for rickettsiae. Likewise, the average nucleotide identity (ANI) method (52), designed as an alternative of DNA–DNA hybridization for the delineation of bacterial species, is not suitable for rickettsiae as well. Using this criterion, *R. conorii*, *R. rickettsii*, and *R. sibirica*, with ANI values of >94%, belong to the same species, as do *R. typhi* and *R. prowazekii*. Pulsed field gel electrophoresis is useful for differentiating rickettsiae, but it suffers from the absence of any database allowing the comparison of PFGE profiles, and the lack of reproducibility. Over the last 15 years, a number of genes including those encoding 16S rRNA (16S rDNA), citrate synthase (*glt*A), the 17-kDa common antigen, surface-exposed, high-molecular-weight antigenic proteins of the *sca* family (*omp*A, *omp*B, *sca*4, *sca*1, and *sca*2) have been used to rapidly and reliably differentiate members of the genus *Rickettsia* either by analysis of PCR–RFLP or by direct sequence determination (19,20,22,32,34–37). To facilitate the classification of bacterial isolates as rickettsiae at the genus, group, and species levels, genetic criteria based on a multi-locus sequence typing (MLST) method were proposed (39). The MLST-based criteria used sequences of the 16SrDNA, *glt*A, *omp*A, *omp*B, and *sca*4 genes (Fig. 2), and were established using a panel of 20 uncontested *Rickettsia* species previously officially validated using mouse serotyping (*R. prowazekii*, *R. typhi*, *R. rickettsii*, *R. conorii*, *R. africae*, *R. sibirica*, *R. slovaca*, *R. honei*, *R. japonica*, *R. australis*, *R. akari*, *R. felis*, *R. aeschlimannii*, *R. helvetica*, *R. massiliae*, *R. rhipicephali*, *R. montanensis*, and *R. parkeri*). To incorporate these genetic criteria into the definition of a *Rickettsia* species, an international committee of expert rickettsiologists recently proposed guidelines to classify rickettsial isolates at various taxonomic levels (Fig. 2) and to clarify the nomenclature within the genus *Rickettsia* (53). In addition, the subspecies taxonomic rank was created for members of the *Rickettsia* genus to classify isolates of a species that exhibited specific phenotypic characteristics (54,55). The guidelines recommended the use of a polyphasic approach that incorporated phenotypic, genotypic, and phylogenic criteria (Fig. 2). This polyphasic approach enabled classification of rickettsial isolates of uncertain taxonomic rank (*R. mongolotimonae* within the *R. sibirica* species; *Rickettsia* sp. strain S within the *R. africae* species; *Rickettsia* sp. strain Bar29 within the *R. massiliae* species; *Rickettsia* sp. strain BJ-90 within the *R. sibirica* species; Indian tick typhus rickettsia, Astrakhan fever rickettsia, and Israeli spotted fever rickettsia within the *R. conorii* species). These criteria

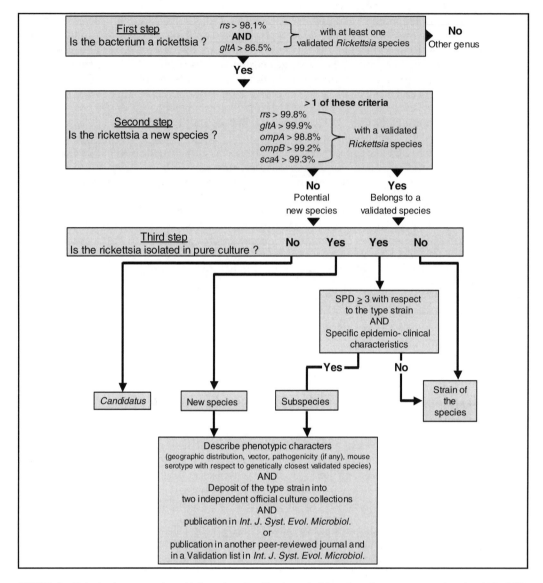

FIGURE 2 Polyphasic taxonomic guidelines for classification of rickettsiae. Genes: rrs encodes the 16S rDNA; gltA encodes the citrate synthase; *ompA* encodes rOmpA; *ompB* encodes rOmpB; *sca4* encodes Sca4 (5PS-120). *Abbreviation*: SPD, specificity difference in mouse serotyping.

also allowed the creation of the new species *R. heilongjiangensis* (13). Finally, a sensitive method was developed to discriminate among isolates of a single *Rickettsia* species. This method, named multi-spacer typing (MST), was based on the assumption that intergenic spacers, being noncoding sequences, undergo less evolutionary pressure than coding sequences such as genes, and thus are more variable between strains of a bacterium. MST identified 27 genotypes among 39 *R. conorii* strains (56), four genotypes among 15 *R. prowazekii* strains (57), and thus demonstrated to be valuable for the discrimination of rickettsiae at the strain level.

CONCLUSIONS

Owing to the improved diagnostic methods and increased interest, the number of representatives of the genus *Rickettsia* has increased dramatically over the past 20 years, with 24 currently validated species and several dozens of as-yet unclassified isolates or genotypes. These arthropod-associated intracellular bacteria are now recognized in all parts of the world. The comparison of the phylogenic organizations obtained from the study of several genes with different functions provided basis to establish a reliable taxonomy of the bacteria included in the genus *Rickettsia*. These data were incorporated into polyphasic consensus guidelines that provide clear recommendations for the taxonomic classification and nomenclature of rickettsiae and rickettsial diseases. These guidelines may later be updated by the introduction of additional genetic or phenotypic characteristics and of new *Rickettsia* species.

REFERENCES

1. Maxey EE. Some observations of the so-called spotted fever of Idaho. Med Sentinel 1899; 10:433–438.
2. Gimenez DF. Staining rickettsiae in yolk-sac cultures. Stain Technol 1964; 39:135–140.
3. Heinzen RA, Hayes SF, Peacock MG, Hackstad T. Directional actin polymerization associated with spotted fever group rickettsia infection of Vero cells. Infect Immun 1993; 61:1926–1935.
4. Teysseire N, Boudier JA, Raoult D. *Rickettsia conorii* entry into Vero cells. Infect Immun 1995; 63:366–374.
5. Teysseire N, Chiche-Portiche C, Raoult D. Intracellular movements of *Rickettsia conorii* and *R. typhi* based on actin polymerization. Res Microbiol 1992; 143:821–829.
6. La Scola B, Meconi S, Fenollar F, Rolain JM, Roux V, Raoult D. Emended description of *Rickettsia felis* (Bouyer et al. 2001): a temperature-dependant cultured bacterium. Int J Syst Evol Microbiol 2002; 52:2035–2041.
7. Houhamdi L, Fournier P-E, Fang R, Lepidi H, Raoult D. An experimental model of human body louse infection with *Rickettsia prowazekii*. J Infect Dis 2002; 186:1639–1646.
8. Houhamdi L, Fournier P-E, Fang R, Raoult D. An experimental model of human body louse infection with *Rickettsia typhi*. Ann NY Acad Sci 2003; 990:617–627.
9. Ogata H, Audic S, Renesto-Audiffren P, et al. Mechanisms of evolution in *Rickettsia conorii* and *R. prowazekii*. Science 2001; 293:2093–2098.
10. Ogata H, Renesto P, Audic S, et al. The genome sequence of *Rickettsia felis* identifies the first putative conjugative plasmid in an obligate intracellular parasite. PLoS Biol 2005; 3:e248.
11. Andersson SGE, Zomorodipour A, Andersson JO, et al. The genome sequence of *Rickettsia prowazekii* and the origin of mitochondria. Nature 1998; 396:133–140.
12. McLeod MP, Qin X, Karpathy SE, et al. Complete genome sequence of *Rickettsia typhi* and comparison with sequences of other rickettsiae. J Bacteriol 2004; 186:5842–5855.
13. Ogata H, Audic S, Abergel C, Fournier P-E, Claverie JM. Protein coding palindromes are a unique but recurrent feature in *Rickettsia*. Genome Res 2002; 12:808–816.
14. Burgdorfer W, Anacker RL, Bird RG, Bertram DS. Intranuclear growth of *Rickettsia rickettsii*. J Bacteriol 1968; 96:1415–1418.
15. Winkler HH. Rickettsial permeability: an ADP–ATP transport system. J Biol Chem 1976; 251:389–396.
16. Amano KI, Williams JC, Dasch GA. Structural properties of lipopolysaccharides from *Rickettsia typhi* and *Rickettsia prowasekii* and their chemical similarity to the lipopolysaccharide from proteus vulgaris OX19 used in the Weil-Felix test. Infect Immun 1998; 66:923–926.
17. Anderson BE, MacDonald GA, Jones DC, Regnery RL. A protective protein antigen of *Rickettsia rickettsii* has tandemly repeated, hear-identical sequences. Infect Immun 1990; 58:2760–2769.
18. Ching WM, Dasch GA, Carl M, Dobson ME. Structural analyses of the 120-kDa serotype protein antigens of typhus group rickettsiae: comparison with other S-layer proteins. Ann NY Acad Sci 1990; 590:334–351.
19. Fournier P-E, Roux V, Raoult D. Phylogenetic analysis of spotted fever group rickettsiae by study of the outer surface protein rOmpA. Int J Syst Bacteriol 1998; 48:839–849.
20. Sekeyova Z, Roux V, Raoult D. Phylogeny of *Rickettsia* spp. inferred by comparing sequences of 'gene D,' which encodes an intracytoplasmic protein. Int J Syst Evol Microbiol 2001; 51:1353–1360.
21. Blanc G, Ngwamidiba M, Ogata H, Fournier P-E, Claverie JM, Raoult D. Molecular evolution of rickettsia surface antigens: evidence of positive selection. Mol Biol Evol 2005; 22:2073–2083.
22. Ngwamidiba M, Blanc G, Raoult D, Fournier P-E. *Sca*1, a previously undescribed paralog from autotransporter protein-encoding genes that may serve as identification and phylogenetic tool in *Rickettsia* species. BMC Microbiol 2006; 6:12.
23. Weiss E, Moulder JW. Order I *Rickettsiales*, Gieszczkiewicz 1939. In: Krieg NR, Holt JG, eds. Bergey's Manual of Systematic Bacteriology. Baltimore, MD: Williams & Wilkins, 1984:687–703.
24. Roux V, Bergoin M, Lamaze N, Raoult D. Reassessment of the taxonomic position of *Rickettsiella grylli*. Int J Syst Bacteriol 1997; 47:1255–1257.
25. Weisburg WG, Dobson ME, Samuel JE, et al. Phylogenetic diversity of the rickettsiae. J Bacteriol 1989; 171:4202–4206.

26. Neimark H, Johansson KE, Rikihisa Y, Tully JG. Proposal to transfer some members of the genera *Haemobartonella* and *Eperythrozoon* to the genus *Mycoplasma* with descriptions of 'Candidatus Mycoplasma haemofelis,' 'Candidatus Mycoplasma haemomuris,' 'Candidatus Mycoplasma haemosuis' and 'Candidatus Mycoplasma wenyonii.' Int J Syst Evol Microbiol 2001; 51:891–899.
27. Birtles RJ, Harrison TG, Saunders NA, Molyneux DH. Proposals to unify the genera *Grahamella* and B*artonella*, with descriptions of *Bartonella talpae* comb. nov., *Bartonella peromysci* comb. nov., and three new species, *Bartonella grahamii* sp. nov., *Bartonella taylorii* sp. nov., and *Bartonella doshiae* sp. nov. Int J Syst Bacteriol 1995; 45:1–8.
28. Brenner DJ, O'Connor SP, Winkler HH, Steigerwalt AG. Proposals to unify the genera *Bartonella* and *Rochalimaea*, with descriptions of *Bartonella quintana* comb. nov., *Bartonella vinsonii* comb. nov., *Bartonella henselae* comb. nov., and *Bartonella elizabethae* comb. nov., and to remove the family Bartonellaceae from the order Rickettsiales. Int J Syst Bacteriol 1993; 43:777–786.
29. Tamura A, Ohashi N, Urakami H, Miyamura S. Classification of *Rickettsia tsutsugamushi* in a new genus, *Orientia* gen nov, as *Orientia tsutsugamushi* comb. nov. Int J Syst Bacteriol 1995; 45:589–591.
30. Eremeeva ME, Yu X, Raoult D. Differentiation among spotted fever group rickettsiae species by analysis of restriction fragment length polymorphism of PCR-amplified DNA. J Clin Microbiol 1994; 32:803–810.
31. Roux V, Fournier P-E, Raoult D. Differentiation of spotted fever group rickettsiae by sequencing and analysis of restriction fragment length polymorphism of PCR amplified DNA of the gene encoding the protein rOmpA. J Clin Microbiol 1996; 34:2058–2065.
32. Roux V, Raoult D. Phylogenetic analysis of the genus *Rickettsia* by 16S rDNA sequencing. Res Microbiol 1995; 146:385–396.
33. Stothard DR, Clark JB, Fuerst PA. Ancestral divergence of *Rickettsia bellii* from the spotted fever and typhus groups of *Rickettsia* and antiquity of the genus *Rickettsia*. Int J Syst Bacteriol 1994; 44:798–804.
34. Roux V, Rydkina E, Eremeeva M, Raoult D. Citrate synthase gene comparison, a new tool for phylogenetic analysis, and its application for the rickettsiae. Int J Syst Bacteriol 1997; 47:252–261.
35. Anderson BE, Tzianabos T. Comparative sequence analysis of a genus—common rickettsial antigen gene. J Bacteriol 1989; 171:5199–5201.
36. Roux V, Raoult D. Phylogenetic analysis of members of the genus *Rickettsia* using the gene encoding the outer-membrane protein rOmpB (ompB). Int J Syst Evol Microbiol 2000; 50:1449–1455.
37. Ngwamidiba M, Blanc G, Ogata H, Raoult D, Fournier P-E. Phylogenetic study of *Rickettsia* species using sequences of the autotransporter protein-encoding gene sca2. Ann NY Acad Sci 2005; 1063:94–99.
38. Rolain JM, Maurin M, Vestris G, Raoult D. In vitro susceptibilities of 27 rickettsiae to 13 antimicrobials. Antimicrob Agents Chemother 1998; 42:1537–1541.
39. Fournier P-E, Dumler JS, Greub G, Zhang J, Yimin W, Raoult D. Gene sequence-based criteria for the identification of new *Rickettsia* isolates and description of *Rickettsia heilongjiangensis* sp. nov. J Clin Microbiol 2003; 41:5456–5465.
40. Dumler JS, Barbet AF, Bekker CPJ, et al. Reorganisation of genera in the families *Rickettsiaceae* and *Anaplasmataceae* in the order *Rickettsiales*: unification of some species of *Ehrlichia* with *Anaplasma*, *Cowdria* with *Ehrlichia* and *Ehrlichia* with *Neorickettsia*, descriptions of six new species combinations and designation of *Ehrlichia equi* and 'HGE agent' as subjective synonyms of *Ehrlichia phagocytophila*. Int J Syst Evol Microbiol 2001; 51:2145–2165.
41. Weisburg WG, Barns SM, Pelletier DA, Lane DJ. 16S ribosomal DNA amplification for phylogenetic study. J Bacteriol 1991; 173:697–703.
42. Gouin E, Egile C, Dehoux P, et al. The RickA protein of *Rickettsia conorii* activates the Arp2/3 complex. Nature 2004; 427:457–461.
43. Pijper A. Etude expérimentale comparée de la Fièvre boutonneuse et de la Tick-Bite-Fever. Arch Inst Pasteur Tunis 1936; 25:388–401.
44. Plotz H, Reagan RL, Wertman K. Differentiation between "Fièvre boutonneuse" and Rocky Mountain spotted fever by means of complement fixation. Proc Soc Exp Biol Med 1944; 55:173–176.
45. Bell EJ, Stoenner HG. Immunologic relationships among the spotted fever group of rickettsias determined by toxin neutralisation tests in mice with convalescent animal serums. J Immunol 1960; 84:171–182.
46. Philip RN, Casper EA, Burgdorfer W, Gerloff RK, Hugues LE, Bell EJ. Serologic typing of rickettsiae of the spotted fever group by micro-immunofluorescence. J Immunol 1978; 121:1961–1968.
47. Walker DH, Liu QH, Yu XJ, Li H, Taylor C, Feng HM. Antigenic diversity of *Rickettsia conorii*. Am J Trop Med Hyg 1992; 47:78–86.
48. Xu WB, Raoult D. Taxonomic relationships among spotted fever group Rickettsiae as revealed by antigenic analysis with monoclonal antibodies. J Clin Microbiol 1998; 36:887–896.
49. Wayne LG, Brenner DJ, Colwell RR, et al. Report of the Ad hoc committee on reconciliation of approaches to bacterial systematics. Int J Syst Bacteriol 1987; 37:463–464.
50. Myers WF, Wisseman CL Jr. The taxonomic relationship of *Rickettsia canada* to the typhus and spotted fever groups of the genus Rickettsia. In: Burgdorfer W, Anacker RL, eds. Rickettsiae and Rickettsial Diseases. New York: Academic Press, 1981:313–325.

51. Myers WF, Wisseman CL Jr. Genetic relatedness among the typhus group of rickettsiae. Int J Syst Bacteriol 1980; 30:143–150.
52. Konstantinidis KT, Tiedje JM. Genomic insights that advance the species definition for prokaryotes. Proc Natl Acad Sci USA 2005; 102:2567–2572.
53. Raoult D, Fournier P-E, Eremeeva M, et al. Naming of rickettsiae and rickettsial diseases. Ann NY Acad Sci 2005; 1063:1–12.
54. Fournier P-E, Zhu Y, Yu X, Raoult D. Proposal to create subspecies of *Rickettsia sibirica* and an emended description of *Rickettsia sibirica*. Ann NY Acad Sci 2006; 1078:597–606.
55. Zhu Y, Fournier P-E, Eremeeva M, Raoult D. Proposal to create subspecies of *Rickettsia conorii* based on multi-locus sequence typing and an emended description of *Rickettsia conorii*. BMC Microbiol 2005; 5:11.
56. Fournier P-E, Zhu Y, Ogata H, Raoult D. Use of highly variable intergenic spacer sequences for multispacer typing of *Rickettsia conorii* strains. J Clin Microbiol 2004; 42:5757–5766.
57. Zhu Y, Fournier P-E, Ogata H, Raoult D. Multispacer typing of *Rickettsia prowazekii* enabling epidemiological studies of epidemic typhus. J Clin Microbiol 2005; 43:4708–4712.

2 | Pathogenesis, Immunity, Pathology, and Pathophysiology in Rickettsial Diseases

David H. Walker, Nahed Ismail, Juan P. Olano, Gustavo Valbuena, and Jere McBride
Department of Pathology, University of Texas Medical Branch, Galveston, Texas, U.S.A.

INTRODUCTION

The pathogenesis of diseases caused by *Rickettsia*, *Orientia*, *Ehrlichia*, *Anaplasma*, *Neorickettsia*, and *Coxiella* differ greatly owing to differences in target cells, bacterial genomes, and cell wall structure, and bacteria–host cell interactions including subcellular location, immune responses stimulated during the infection, pathogenic mechanisms, and pathologic lesions (1,2). This chapter focuses on infections with *Rickettsia*. The concept *pathogenesis* comprises three components: the sequence of events from transmission until immune clearance of the agent, the host–pathogen interaction ranging from the whole patient to the cellular level, and the pathogenic mechanisms of cellular and tissue injury.

SEQUENCE OF EVENTS IN RICKETTSIAL INFECTIONS
Transmission

All *Rickettsia* have an arthropod host which serves as the biologic vector that transmits the pathogens to humans. Tick- and mite-borne *Rickettsia* are inoculated into the skin of the host from the arthropod's saliva during its blood meal. Typhus group *Rickettsia* are mainly transmitted in the feces of the louse (*Pediculus humanus corporis*) for epidemic typhus or flea for murine typhus. It is widely believed that the infected insect feces are autoinoculated into the skin of the patient by scratching the pruritic bite site. Interestingly, extracellular *Rickettsia prowazekii* in louse feces and *R. typhi* in flea feces are stably infectious for months if not longer. The possibilities of inoculation via rubbing the mucous membranes (e.g., conjunctiva) or via inhalation of aerosols of infectious *R. prowazekii* or *R. typhi* organisms should not be discounted, and the latter has occurred in the research laboratory. A small fraction of cases of murine typhus are transmitted by flea bite. Furthermore, some cases of tick-borne rickettsioses are transmitted by transfer of rickettsiae to the conjunctiva by fingers contaminated with infectious tick hemolymph or organs after crushing a tick that has been removed from a person or animal. Aerosol transmission has been demonstrated experimentally to be very efficient, requiring 1000-fold fewer inhaled rickettsial organisms than anthrax spores.

Routes of Spread in the Body

The occurrence of prominent lymphadenopathy in the region draining the rickettsial portal of entry at the eschar in *R. africae*, *R. slovaca*, and *R. parkeri* infections supports the hypothesis that rickettsiae spread from the site of tick feeding to the regional lymph node via lymphatic vessels. Dissemination throughout the body occurs via the bloodstream. Rickettsial infection involves every organ, but spread beyond the lymphatic and blood vessels does not occur.

Target Cells and Organs

The initial target cells of *Rickettsia* at the site of inoculation in the skin have not been identified. Because rickettsiae are obligately intracellular organisms and do not replicate extracellularly, it is highly likely that rickettsiae rapidly enter cells in the skin. *Rickettsia* are capable of infecting any type of nucleated cells; thus, their initial target is not necessarily endothelium. Among the possible dermal target cells are fibroblasts, macrophages, dermal dendritic cells, and lymphatic endothelium. It is proposed that infected dendritic cells migrate to regional lymph nodes where innate and adaptive immunity are stimulated.

The main target cells of rickettsiosis are endothelial cells, most likely the result of vascular location and hematogenous dissemination of rickettsiae rather than interaction between a rickettsial adhesin and a special receptor expressed only on endothelial cells.

Rickettsiae are also engulfed by fixed mononuclear phagocytes during their spread through the blood stream. Thus, macrophages, especially in the spleen and liver, are minor target cells. *Rickettsia rickettsii* is the only organism in the genus that invades beyond the blood vessel lining endothelium; they invade adjacent vascular smooth muscle cells, particularly in arterioles.

Although *Rickettsia* infects all organs, the lungs and brain are the critical targets determining the lethality of rickettsioses. The events that are visible in the skin—silent seeding of the dermal blood vessels, vasodilatation (macular rash), perivascular edema (maculopapular rash), disruption of vascular integrity (petechial maculopapular rash), and resolution in survivors—occur throughout the organs of the body.

Injury Associated with Rickettsial Infection

Rickettsial infection is multifocal occurring in networks of contiguous cells, and organ and tissue injury occurs in these foci. The hundreds of maculopapules in the skin of a patient with Rocky Mountain spotted fever or epidemic louse-borne typhus are representative of only a small fraction of the visceral involvement. When endothelial cells infected with *R. prowazekii* or *R. typhi* are filled to capacity with replicating organisms, they burst by releasing the bacteria that infect other endothelial cells. Death of the burst endothelial cells allows red blood cells to hemorrhage into the surrounding tissue and exposes the basement membrane to platelets and clotting factors.

Spotted fever group rickettsiae spread from cell to cell by host actin-based mobility, do not accumulate in large numbers in endothelial cells, and injure the cells by damaging their membranes. Infection of endothelial cells stimulates them to produce reactive oxygen species that cause lipid peroxidation of the cellular membranes (3–5). Water leaks into the cells with injured membranes and is sequestered in the endoplasmic reticulum. Injured endothelial cells may die and/or detach and be swept away in the blood stream, allowing hemorrhage to occur, or endothelium may be activated by the immune system to kill the intracellular rickettsiae (6).

The pathogenic mechanism of oxidative stress associated with *R. rickettsii* injury to endothelial cells has been investigated extensively in cell culture, and oxidative stress occurs in experimentally infected animals. However, it has not been demonstrated how important this mechanism is in the pathogenesis of the disease in animals or humans (7). Other potential pathogenic mechanisms have not been investigated except for the determination that rickettsial lipopolysaccharide does not have significant endotoxin activity. The potential role of oxidative stress in the pathogenesis of typhus rickettsioses has not been investigated.

Rickettsial infection of human endothelial cells in vitro leads to the development of interendothelial gaps indicative of discontinuities in the adherens junctions (8). Formation of the gaps coincides with change in endothelial cells from small polygonal to large spindle shape with development of stress fibers.

The pathophysiologic event that is most important in rickettsial infections is increased permeability of the microcirculation, possibly due to the presence of gaps between infected endothelial cells (8–10). Changes in junctional proteins after infection include p120 in adherens junctions with β-catenin and occludin. Specifically, the location of p120 moves away from the adherens junction after rickettsial infection of murine and human microvascular endothelial cells, and β-catenin changes from a linear to a granular arrangement in infected cells. Likewise, the location of occludin is altered in primary brain murine microvascular endothelial cells.

Immune Clearance of Rickettsiae

Recovery from rickettsial infection is associated with strong immunity against reinfection. Studies of experimentally infected animals have revealed reduction of the rickettsial load below the limits of detection in association with recovery from the infection. However, convalescence from human infection with R. prowazekii is followed by asymptomatic latent carriage of the rickettsiae in an unknown location in the body. When undefined host events presumed to be related to altered immunity occur, there is reactivation of latent R. prowazekii infection, an illness known as recrudescent typhus or Brill-Zinsser disease. Although reactivation of other rickettsioses has not been observed, R. rickettsii has been isolated from lymph nodes of patients who had recovered from Rocky Mountain spotted fever a year or more previously.

THE *RICKETTSIA*–HOST CELL INTERACTION
Entry of Rickettsiae into the Host Cell

In order to survive, obligately intracellular bacteria such as *Rickettsia* must enter a cell in the vertebrate or arthropod host. Two major surface proteins of spotted fever group rickettsiae, outer membrane proteins A (OmpA) and B (OmpB), are rickettsial ligands for host cells (11,12). OmpB binds to Ku70, a host cell protein that spans the cell membrane (12,13). This adhesion results in recruitment of more Ku70 to the cell membrane for binding to highly abundant OmpB molecules and in recruitment of ubiquitin ligase to the nascent rickettsial entry site (12). The Ku70 molecules are ubiquitinated, and signal transduction events lead to phagocytosis of the adherent rickettsia associated with Arp2/3 complex recruitment to the entry focus. The small GTPase, Cdc 42, protein tyrosine kinase, phosphoinositide 3-kinase, and Src-family kinases activate the Arp2/3 complex to direct changes in the cytoskeletal actin at the entry site resulting in focal-induced phagocytosis of the rickettsia by the so-called zipper mechanism (14). Rickettsial entry into the host cell is rapid, generally occurring in about 15 minutes.

Rickettsial Escape from the Phagosome

Rickettsia are highly adapted to living in the host cell cytosol where they acquire the necessary nutrients, adenosine triphosphate, and nucleotides and amino acids for replication. The phagosome in which they enter is a potential death trap if lysosomal fusion occurs, but they escape rapidly by lysing the phagosomal membrane. The rickettsial proteins that can digest the host cell phagosomal membrane are phospholipase D and hemolysin C (TlyC) (15,16).

Spread of Rickettsiae to Other Cells

All investigated spotted fever group rickettsiae except R. peacockii activate polymerization of host cell actin at one pole of the bacterium. The continuous conversion of globular actin to filamentous actin propels the rickettsia forward through the cytosol until it collides with the host cell membrane (17,18). Some rickettsia carom off the inner surface of the cell membrane like a billiard ball. Other rickettsia deform the membrane, and a filopodium develops into which the polymerized actin pushes the rickettsia. If the endothelial cell membrane at the site of the filopodium abuts an adjacent endothelial cell and the membranes of both cells are breached, the rickettsia enters the second endothelial cell without exposure to the constituents of the extracellular fluid. If the rickettsia exits a luminal filopodium, it enters the blood stream. If R. rickettsii exits the basal endothelial cell membrane, it can spread to an adjacent vascular smooth muscle cell.

Actin-based mobility of R. conorii and other spotted fever group rickettsiae is initiated by a rickettsial protein RickA that is expressed on the rickettsial cell wall (19,20). The carboxy terminal domain of RickA is similar to particular domains of WASP-family proteins that activate Arp2/3, and indeed Arp2/3 is activated by RickA. The Arp2/3 complex is recruited to the rickettsial surface where it acts as a nucleator of actin polymerization. Unlike actin tails that move other organisms, the tails of *Rickettsia* do not contain Arp2/3. Consistent with the importance of RickA in rickettsial actin-based mobility, R. prowazekii and R. typhi lack the gene *rickA*, and *rickA* of R. peacockii is inactivated by transposon insertion. Thus, R. prowazekii and R. peacockii do not have actin tails and do not spread from cell to cell. The burst release of R. prowazekii is the result. R. typhi has erratic actin-based mobility that must rely upon a *rickA*-independent molecular mechanism.

HOST DEFENSES AGAINST RICKETTSIAE

The development of excellent models of disseminated rickettsial infections of endothelium in inbred strains of mice has enabled the identification of the effectors of protective immunity. Whether these effector mechanisms are important in human rickettsioses still remains to be determined. The early immune events occurring in the skin and draining lymph nodes, including the potential immunomodulatory effects of arthropod saliva, also remain to be elucidated.

Innate Immunity

Rickettsial infection activates natural killer cell activity, which dampens rickettsial establishment of infection and rickettsial growth early in infection in association with the production of gamma interferon (IFN-γ) (21). Rickettsial infection also stimulates the production of type I interferon (IFN-α and IFN-β), which independently has no protective effect. However, IFN-α and IFN-β enhance activation of natural killer cells, maturation of dendritic cells, and production of interleukin-12, which is a cytokine that favors T helper type 1 cellular immunity and is produced early in rickettsial infection. Indeed, the levels of IL-12 are increased in the sera of C3H/HeN mice early in the course of R. conorii infection.

Rickettsia-infected endothelial cells produce IL-6, IL-8, and MCP-1, and rickettsia-infected macrophages secrete tumor necrosis factor (TNF-α) (22). Moreover, the concentration of IL-6 is elevated in the sera of C3H/HeN mice infected with R. conorii, and IL-1 and TNF-α are increased in the sera of C57Bl/6 mice infected with R. australis. IL-1 and IL-6 are proinflammatory cytokines that play a role in the activation of innate immune cells and induction of the specific acquired immune response. Rickettsial infection is associated with an acute-phase response. However, the roles, if any, of acute-phase proteins such as C-reactive protein, complement components, C3 and C4, and fibrinogen as host defenses against rickettsiae are not known.

Macrophages and polymorphonuclear leukocytes are professional phagocytic cells that are essential components of innate immunity against many bacteria. Rickettsiae avoid killing by macrophages during primary rickettsial infection by escaping from phagosomes into the cytosol, avoiding the rickettsicidal effect of phagolysosomal fusion. Neutrophils are an insignificant population in the sites of rickettsial infections.

Rickettsial infection of endothelial cells also activates NF-κB, an important transcription factor that mediates the production of proinflammatory cytokines and chemokines. NF-κB activation occurs downstream of rickettsial activation of the IκB kinase complex which phosphorylates IκBa and IκBb (inhibitors of NF-κB) leading to their subsequent degradation by the 26S proteasome (23). The degradation of IκBa and IκBb activates NF-κB dimers, which are translocated into the nucleus, bind to NF-κB enhancer sequences via the DNA-binding domain, and regulate the transcription of specific cytokine and chemokine genes. Another effect of NF-κB activation is inhibition of apoptosis of *Rickettsia*-infected target cells by preventing activation of upstream caspases-8 and -9 and the effector caspase-3. The prevention of apoptosis enhances survival of endothelial cells in which further rickettsial growth can occur. NF-κB alterations have been documented in vitro. In vivo, this mechanism could conceivably play an important role early in the infectious process when rickettsiae are invading their initial targets until the infection is established. However, later in the infectious process when both innate and adaptive immunity are fully activated, NF-κB signals are most likely overridden by the CD8 cytotoxic T-lymphocytes, which induce apoptosis of rickettsia-infected endothelial cells.

Adaptive Immunity
Role of Endothelial Cells and Other Target Cells in Killing Intracellular Rickettsiae

Activation of murine endothelial cells by IFN-γ and TNF-α results in synthesis of rickettsicidal nitric oxide (6). These cytokines act synergistically to stimulate expression of inducible nitric oxide synthetase. Neutralization of IFN-γ or TNF-α or gene knockout of IFN-γ results in an overwhelming infection after a low-dose rickettsial challenge (24,25). Cytokine-activated rickettsial killing by endothelial cells is associated with autophagy and rickettsial digestion within an autophagolysosome (26). It is hypothesized that healthy rickettsiae have evolved mechanisms to inhibit autophagy, the cell's second line of defense, but injured or host defense-inhibited rickettsiae lose this immune evasive activity.

Human endothelial cells activated by IFN-γ, TNF-α, IL-1β, and RANTES (CCL5) also kill intracellular rickettsiae (27). Some activated human endothelial cells have been demonstrated to produce rickettsicidal nitric oxide in vitro. All cytokine-activated human endothelial cells are capable of killing intracellular rickettsiae by producing hydrogen peroxide. The formation of both nitric oxide and reactive oxygen species could lead to the formation of peroxynitrite that also has potent rickettsicidal activity.

In human rickettsial diseases, macrophages are a minor target cell of rickettsial infection, and hepatocytes are a suspected minor target based on pathologic lesions in hepatic biopsies and observations early in the course of experimental animal infections (28). Human macrophages activated by IFN-γ, TNF-α, and IL-1β kill intracellular rickettsiae by production of hydrogen peroxide and tryptophan starvation of rickettsiae via indoleamine-2,3-dioxygenase-mediated degradation of tryptophan (27). In contrast, a human hepatocyte cell line (AKN-1) kills intracellular *R. rickettsii* through synthesis of nitric oxide after activation by IFN-γ, TNF-α, IL-1β, and RANTES.

The mRNA of inducible nitric oxide synthase, IFN-γ, CCL5, and indoleamine-2,3-dioxygenase is expressed in biopsies of skin lesions from patients with Mediterranean spotted fever. These data suggest that nitric oxide production and tryptophan degradation occur at the sites of immunity to rickettsiae in humans. The cells that express these rickettsicidal effector mechanisms and mediators are thought to be the endothelium, perivascular lymphocytes, dendritic cells, and macrophages.

Roles of Lymphocytes in Immunity to Rickettsiae

Both CD4 and CD8 T-lymphocytes contribute to the control of rickettsial growth and killing and to the host's survival of rickettsial infection, most likely by secreting IFN-γ and TNF-α (6). C3H/HeN mice depleted of CD4 T-lymphocytes have the same course of illness and recovery from experimental infection with *R. conorii* as sham-depleted mice. In contrast, mice depleted of CD8 lymphocytes die or remain persistently infected when they are inoculated with the same dose of *R. conorii* that results in the survival of wild-type mice. Cytotoxic activity of CD8 T-lymphocytes is crucial to the clearance of rickettsial infection (25). Perforin gene knockout mice are 1000-fold more susceptible to death from *R. australis* infection than wild-type C57BL/6 mice. The LD_{50} for *R. australis* in major histocompatibility class (MHC) I gene knockout mice is 0.5 plaque-forming units; one organism is sufficient to initiate an infection that cannot be controlled without MHC-I molecule presentation of *R. australis* antigen to CD8 cytotoxic T-lymphocytes.

Mechanisms of Homing of Natural Killer Cells, Immune CD4 and CD8 Lymphocytes, and Macrophages to Sites of Rickettsia-Infected Endothelium

An important phenomenon is the interaction of *Rickettsia*-infected endothelium with cells of the immune system. The histopathologically visible result is perivascular infiltration of CD4 and CD8 T-lymphocytes and macrophages around the networks of contiguous infected endothelial cells of the microcirculation. It is presumed that the initial, and sometimes only, interaction of the endothelium with circulating lymphocytes and monocytes is at the luminal interface.

Among the chemokines that can play a role in directing T-lymphocytes to adhere to endothelium, CXCL9 (Mig), CXCL10 (IP-10), and CX3CL1 (fractalkine) are expressed at high levels in the endothelium of *R. conorii*-infected mice, and CXCL9 and CXCL10 are expressed in endothelium of the brain in fatal human cases of Rocky Mountain spotted fever (29). However, treatment of mice with antibodies to CXCL9 and CXCL10 does not alter the survival, and *R. conorii* infection of mice with gene knockout for the receptor of these chemokines does not affect survival or T-lymphocyte infiltration (30). The only evidence that CXCR3 gene knockout has any effect on host defense is a higher rickettsial burden in the lungs of these mice than in wild-type mice on day six of infection. Thus, these chemokines are not required for clearance of rickettsial infection. Even if they are active in the process, there are sufficient other redundant systems to mediate host immune cell chemotaxis.

Expression of intercellular adhesion molecule-1 and vascular cell adhesion molecule-1 on endothelium of all organs beginning on day two of experimental rickettsial infection of mice suggests that these adhesion molecules, in conjunction with the effects of antigen presentation by endothelial cell MHC molecules to T-cell receptors, could initiate the signals for activation of the effector mechanisms of T-lymphocytes.

The early elevation of expression of fractalkine in endothelium of infected mice correlates with the kinetics of perivascular infiltration by macrophages, the target of fractalkine in mice (31).

Role of Antibodies in Rickettsial Immunity

The importance of cell-mediated immunity in recovery from infection with obligately intracellular *Rickettsia* and the rationale that antibodies had no access to cytosolic rickettsiae resulted in the neglect of the study of humoral immunity to rickettsiae. Historically, rabbit anti-*R. rickettsii* serum had been used to treat humans with Rocky Mountain spotted fever in the preantibiotic era with the apparent effect of reduction in the case fatality rate. Dose-dependent protection by immune serum was also demonstrated in experimentally infected monkeys and guinea pigs.

Mice lacking both T- and B-lymphocyte components of the immune system are protected against a lethal dose of *R. conorii* by passive transfer of polyclonal immune serum or monoclonal antibodies to OmpA or OmpB before infection, but antibodies to rickettsial lipopolysaccharide (LPS) are not protective (32). Protection requires opsonization; Fab and F(ab)$_2$ fragments of effective antibodies do not protect mice. Polyclonal antibodies to *R. conorii* and a monoclonal antibody to OmpB prevent rickettsial escape from the phagosome, resulting in rickettsial death in phagolysosomes. Antibodies to *R. conorii* administered as late as four or five days after infection reduce the bacterial load and prolong the life of the animal substantially.

During primary sublethal infection with *R. conorii*, mice develop antibodies to LPS on day six, but antibodies against OmpA and OmpB are not detected until day 12 at which point the rickettsial infection is already controlled. These observations indicate that antibodies play little or no role in clearance of a primary rickettsial infection, but that circulating antibodies or a prompt anamnestic antibody response prevents disease caused by a reinfection.

In vitro opsonized rickettsiae enter murine endothelial cells and macrophages where they are killed by nitric oxide, superoxide, and other reactive oxygen species, and by tryptophan starvation (33).

Downregulation of the Immune Response

Interleukin-10 (IL-10) plays an antiinflammatory role in controlling the strongly activated immune response following clearance of rickettsial infection. The serum concentration of IL-10 in C3H/HeN mice is elevated on day 10 after inoculation of *R. typhi*, but not at the peak of the bacterial load on day five or in convalescence on day 15 (34). On day 10, the rickettsial load is below the limit of detection, having been controlled by the immune response. Continued activation of antirickettsial, cell-mediated immunity after bacterial clearance could be more harmful than beneficial. The observed effects of immune regulation by high IL-10 levels include decreased IL-12 concentration and transient immunosuppression of T-cell responses between days 10 and 15. Stimulation of spleen cells collected from *R. typhi*-infected mice with concanavalin A during this period yields lower production of IL-2 and IL-12 than those of naïve mice (34). Similarly, serum IL-10 concentrations are increased in the sera of patients with Mediterranean spotted fever, and rickettsial antigen-stimulated peripheral blood mononuclear cells from patients with this rickettsiosis also produce increased amounts of IL-10 (35).

Prospects for Vaccines Against Rickettsial Diseases

After recovery from a spotted fever or typhus rickettsiosis, patients and experimental animals develop solid immunity that prevents reinfection. Historically, killed whole rickettsial vaccines have ameliorated the outcome of rickettsial infection. A live attenuated vaccine against epidemic typhus effectively prevented the illness, but unfortunately was prone to reversion to virulence. Thus, past experience indicates that stimulation of protective immunity is entirely feasible.

Subunit vaccine development has focused on the major antigens recognized by the humoral immune response, namely OmpA and OmpB (36,37). They stimulate immunity that is usually only partially protective. Recent studies of cross-protective immunity between spotted fever and typhus group rickettsiae have demonstrated that cross-protection is mediated by T-lymphocytes in the absence of cross-reactive antibodies (38). A challenge will be to identify the shared rickettsial proteins that stimulate the components of the immune system, both cellular and humoral, that confer protection. OmpA and OmpB would very likely be components of an ideal subunit vaccine as would other undetermined, but conserved rickettsial proteins.

PATHOLOGY OF RICKETTSIAL DISEASES

Traditionally, pathology is inappropriately often considered to be synonymous with histopathology; however, by definition pathology encompasses all the disease-associated events as detected by all available methods. Characterizing events such as edema by histopathology is limited owing to the shrinkage of tissue by formaldehyde fixation. Therefore, many other techniques are utilized to provide a comprehensive interpretation of disease pathology.

Vascular Inflammation

The earliest change in tissue is most easily visible in the living patient, active vasodilation such as occurs in the macular rash of rickettsioses. Subsequently, increased vascular permeability results in perivascular edema followed by perivascular accumulation of CD4 and CD8 T-lymphocytes and macrophages in the foci of microcirculation that are infected by rickettsiae (39). Increased vascular permeability, endothelial injury, and the lymphohistiocytic cellular response are often referred to as a vasculitis. The definition of the term "vasculitis" varies greatly. Many clinicians' concept is vague, meaning an often serious systemic illness with fever, rash, difficult-to-determine cause, ominous prognosis, and no real implications of blood vessel pathology. Pathologists expect vasculitis to be a disease with blood vessels nearly obliterated by infiltration of polymorphonuclear leukocytes, many of which have undergone cell death. Neither of these concepts applies to rickettsial vasculitis.

The idea of inflammation held by many immunologists that includes activation of NF-κB and the presence of proinflammatory cytokines bears more truth in the pathogenesis of rickettsial vasculitis, but is not visible microscopically. The perivascular T-lymphocytes and macrophages are extremely likely to represent the components of the immune response that controls the infection. That the cytokines secreted by these cells may play a role in causing the fever and other symptoms and that the timing of action of cytotoxic T-lymphocytes against rickettsia-infected endothelium would be detrimental if the target was too large and dispersed are evidence that the immune system could also be pathogenic. On balance, however, the immune response to rickettsiae is beneficial.

A perivascular lymphohistiocytic infiltrate is observed in the brain, lung, heart, kidneys, skin, gastrointestinal tract, pancreas, gallbladder, skeletal muscle, testes, and other organs during rickettsial infection. In the brain, the infiltration of the neuropil by lymphocytes and macrophages has the special name, glial nodule. There are other diseases that cause a similar lesion, and patients who die before day 10 of illness may not have developed glial nodules.

Hemostasis and Thrombosis

Disseminated multifocal rickettsial infection of endothelial cells injures the endothelium with consequences ranging from impairment of its normal anticoagulant function to denuding of the endothelial monolayer exposing the basement membrane and collagen to plasma clotting factors, von Willebrand factor, and platelets. Meticulous searches for fibrin-platelet thrombi in vascular lesions of rickettsial diseases reveal that they are rare, both in biopsies of living patients and in autopsies. Hemostatic plugs of platelets and fibrin are observed only in foci of severe vascular injury. The hemostatic plugs seldom occlude the blood vessel. Studies in experimentally infected dogs by retinal fluorescein angiography have shown that there are numerous foci of increased vascular permeability and only rare foci of occlusive thrombosis (9). Even in patients with fulminant Rocky Mountain spotted fever (defined by Parker as fatal in five days or less of illness) in which severe coagulopathy and more extensive thrombi occur, the thrombi are located only in foci of severe rickettsial infection and injury of endothelium, an expected physiological response (40). The vast regions of the circulation with uninfected endothelium contain no thrombosis. Generalized activation of thrombosis as a pathogenic mechanism does not occur even in this most severe form of the most pathogenic rickettsiosis. The histopathology of disseminated intervascular coagulation (e.g., many renal glomerular capillaries occluded by fibrin) is rarely observed in the organs of rickettsial diseases (41).

Patients with fatal rickettsial infection frequently suffer hypotensive shock and the pathologic sequelae including acute tubular necrosis of the kidneys due to poor perfusion. However, infarcts of the organs are seldom observed, consistent with the paucity of occlusive thrombi. That infarction does occur occasionally is documented in the brain where infarcts have been described in the white matter of some patients. Cutaneous necrosis including gangrene occurs in 4% of fatal cases of Rocky Mountain spotted fever (42). The histopathology of the gangrene shows that tissue necrosis is caused primarily by vascular injury at the level of the microcirculation. Eschars of patients with Mediterranean spotted fever contain vascular injury, inflammation, and edema, but only very limited thrombosis (43). Thus, although intuitive armchair consideration of rickettsial pathogenesis has led to proposal of hypotheses based on a central role for infarcts associated with thrombosis, the pathology and experimental evidence indicate that such hypotheses are incorrect.

PATHOPHYSIOLOGY OF RICKETTSIAL INFECTIONS
Edema, Hypovolemia, and Sequelae

Alterations in normal physiology of the body associated with rickettsioses ensue from multifocal injury to the microcirculation and possibly the systemic effects of cytokines. Increased microvascular permeability leads to edema, hypovolemia, and hypotension (10). In severe cases, hypotensive shock results in ischemia.

At the early stage of hypovolemia, perfusion of the brain is maintained by decreased perfusion of other organs. Reduced perfusion of the kidneys results in reduction in the glomerular filtration rate, oliguria, and increased blood urea concentration (41). This prerenal azotemia can be corrected by administration of fluids that restore the blood volume and renal blood flow. Without treatment of the underlying disease, microvascular endothelial injury continues. If the patient's condition progresses to the development of hypotensive shock, severe renal ischemia may cause acute tubular necrosis and anuric acute renal failure.

Another sequela of hypovolemia is hyponatremia. The response of the anterior pituitary gland to the low blood volume is secretion of antidiuretic hormone (ADH), which causes increased renal resorption of water (44). The resorbed water dilutes the intravascular sodium concentration to less than 132 mEq/l in 56% of patients with Rocky Mountain spotted fever. This sequence of events is an appropriate secretion of ADH and is not the syndrome of inappropriate secretion of ADH.

The composition of the edema fluid in rickettsial diseases has not been determined, but the development of hypoalbuminemia in 12% to 30% of patients with Rocky Mountain spotted fever suggests that plasma proteins and ions including albumin and sodium likely leak out of the damaged microcirculation into the tissues (42,45).

Cardiopulmonary Dynamics

The pulmonary microcirculation is heavily infected by rickettsiae in severely ill patients. The effect is noncardiogenic pulmonary edema. Interstitial pneumonitis, alveolar edema, and adult respiratory distress syndrome are the most severe manifestations (46). Despite the presence of perivascular lymphocytes and macrophages in the interstitium of the myocardium, the cardiac myocytes appear to be normal, and echocardiography reveals normal myocardial function. The principal pathophysiologic manifestation of *R. rickettsii* in the heart is arrhythmia, which is observed in 7% to 16% of patients, presumably secondary to vascular lesions adjacent to the cardiac conduction system (42,45).

Neurologic Involvement in Rickettsial Diseases

The name typhus originated from the Greek word *typhos*, which means smoky and refers to the cloudy sensorium of patients with typhus and other life-threatening rickettsioses. Rickettsial encephalitis in Rocky Mountain spotted fever generally manifests first as confusion or lethargy in 26% to 28% of cases (42,45). As the disease progresses, stupor or delirium is observed in 21% to 26% of cases, ataxia in 18%, coma in 9% to 10%, and seizures in 8%. The same number of neurologic signs have been reported as there are foci in the nervous system for rickettsial lesions to damage. Involvement of blood vessels contiguous to the cerebrospinal fluid leads to pleocytosis in 34% to 38% of patients, usually 10 to 100 cells/μl with predominance of lymphocytes and macrophages. However, occasionally more than 100 cells/μl with polymorphonuclear predominance are observed. The occurrence of coma or seizures is highly associated with a fatal outcome. The relative importance of the various potential, pathological conditions including hypoxemia, ischemia, cerebral edema, and inflammation in cerebral pathophysiology has not been determined. Because of the importance of rickettsial meningoencephalitis in the outcome of infection, the neuropathogenesis and neuropathophysiology of rickettsial diseases merits careful investigation.

Hepatic Involvement in Rickettsial Diseases

Hepatic infection and lesions occur in the life-threatening rickettsioses, but the hepatic rickettsial burden and pathology are minor. Focal hepatocellular necrosis results in mild-to-moderate increases in serum concentrations of alanine aminotransferase and aspartate aminotransferase. Focal vascular infection and lesions are observed in the portal triads. Hyperbilirubinemia occurs in 18% to 30% of patients with Rocky Mountain spotted fever, and jaundice is observed in 8% to 9% (42,45). The cause of hyperbilirubinemia is hemolysis in a small portion of patients. Hepatic failure does not occur as a result of rickettsial infection.

Coagulation and Bleeding

Patients with Rocky Mountain spotted fever and Mediterranean spotted fever develop a procoagulant state associated with endothelial injury, release of procoagulant factors, activation of the coagulation cascade resulting in generation of thrombin, platelet activation, increased fibrinolytic factors, and consumption of natural anticoagulants (47,48). Thrombocytopenia develops in 32% to 52% of patients with Rocky Mountain spotted fever and 35% of those with Mediterranean spotted fever, probably caused in part by platelet adhesion to infected endothelial cells and consumption in hemostatic plugs at sites of endothelial denudation. Increased plasma levels of β-thromboglobulin and decreased concentrations of platelet factor 4 suggest that platelet activation occurs in patients with Rocky Mountain spotted fever (48). Normal concentrations of factors XII, XI, X, IX, and II suggest that activation of kallikrein does not surpass capacity of plasma kallikrein inhibitor to prevent systemic effects. Increased plasma fibrinopeptide A and prothrombin fragments 1 + 2 suggest thrombin generation, but elevated levels of plasma fibrinogen indicate that disseminated intravascular coagulation rarely occurs. The high fibrinogen concentration is a result of the acute-phase response.

Activation of the fibrinolytic system in Rocky Mountain spotted fever and Mediterranean spotted fever is demonstrated by increased concentrations of fibrin and fibrinogen degradation products. The reduction in plasma levels of plasminogen and α2-antiplasmin and increased α2-antiplasmin–plasmin complexes and tissue plasminogen activator also suggest activation of the fibrinolytic system. Higher levels of plasminogen activator inhibitors than tissue plasminogen activator would favor a hypercoagulable antifibrinolytic state. Decreased antithrombin III levels in Rocky Mountain spotted fever and evidence for activation of the protein C pathway in Mediterranean spotted fever likely reflect the homeostatic mechanisms that prevent local pathologic thrombosis.

Kinetic evaluation of a large battery of coagulation factors in mice lethally infected with *R. conorii* demonstrated the effects of multifocal severe endothelial injury, namely increased thrombin generation, decreased factor VIII, increased factor V procoagulant activity, decreased prekallikrein levels, decreased tissue plasminogen activator activity, and increased plasminogen activator inhibitor activity (49). Disseminated intravascular coagulation did not occur. Sublethal infection was characterized by acute-phase reaction (e.g., elevated fibrinogen and factor VIII), release of endothelial cell components, but no major activation of the coagulation system. There was significant inhibition of endothelial cell-driven fibrinolysis. These and the human infection data indicate that the coagulation and fibrinolytic systems maintain homeostasis and do not activate uncontrolled pathological thrombosis or consumption of clotting factors. However, the role of certain byproducts of the coagulation/fibrinolytic system such as activated protein C and thrombin in microvascular permeability merits further investigation.

Anemia develops in 30% of patients with Rocky Mountain spotted fever, and blood transfusions are required in 11%. Seldom is there significant overt bleeding. In 10% of patients, blood is detected in stool or vomitus, but massive upper gastrointestinal hemorrhage leading to death or gastrointestinal surgery is rare. Thus, sufficient hemostatic function is generally maintained.

HOST RISK FACTORS FOR SEVERITY OF ILLNESS

Age is the most consistent host factor for severity of illness in rickettsial infections (50,51). In the preantibiotic era, the case fatality rate for Rocky Mountain spotted fever was 7.6% for patients younger than 16 years of age, compared with 25% for patients 16 years of age or older. The case fatality rate continues to be substantially higher in older persons currently with increased lethality in each older decade of life.

Higher case fatality rates for males that was documented for Rocky Mountain spotted fever and typhus historically has equalized between males and females infected with Rocky Mountain spotted fever in recent studies. That gender is likely to play a role is supported by higher fatalities among adult male guinea pigs infected with *R. rickettsii* than adult females, and a lower dose of *R. conorii* that kills adult male C3H/HeN mice than adult females. The basis for this difference in susceptibility/resistance is not known.

Host factors related to underlying diseases and enhanced oxidative stress also appear to determine severity of rickettsioses. Patients with diabetes mellitus have an increased risk of a fatal outcome with Mediterranean spotted fever. Anecdotal descriptions suggest that alcohol abuse and cardiovascular disease may be risk factors for severity of rickettsial illness.

Sulfonamide treatment exacerbates the severity of illness caused by rickettsial infection. It is possible that sulfonamides increase oxidative stress, a pathogenic mechanism of cell injury in *R. rickettsii* infection in vitro. Glucose-6-phosphate dehydrogenase deficiency is associated with the occurrence of fulminant Rocky Mountain spotted fever in African-American males and has been reported in unusually severe cases of murine typhus and Mediterranean spotted fever. Glucose-6-phosphate dehydrogenase is a component of the antioxidant protective mechanisms, and its deficiency could result in increased damage secondary to oxidative stress. Fulminant Rocky Mountain spotted fever is associated with hemolysis whether or not the patient is deficient in glucose-6-phosphate dehydrogenase. The release of iron-containing hemoglobin from erythrocytes could exacerbate the reactions involving free radicals of oxygen that are hypothesized to play a role in tissue injury in spotted fever rickettsiosis.

CONCLUSIONS

Despite the more than a century of biomedical studies of rickettsial infections, our knowledge of the pathogenic mechanisms of tissue injury and increased microvascular permeability is woefully incomplete. Optimal treatment and clinical management require better knowledge of the diseases. Prospective, comprehensive, pathophysiologic clinical studies of rickettsial diseases have been too few. The case fatality rates for rickettsial diseases, such as 50% for Rocky Mountain spotted fever in Brazil and 4% for Mediterranean spotted fever in Portugal, emphasize that, in addition to earlier diagnosis and antimicrobial treatment, better knowledge of pathogenesis and pathophysiology is needed.

REFERENCES

1. Ogata H, Audic S, Renesto-Audiffren P. Mechanisms of evolution in *Rickettsia conorii* and *R. prowazekii*. Science 2001; 293:2093–2098.
2. McLeod MP, Qin X, Karpathy SE, et al. Complete genome sequence of *Rickettsia typhi* and comparison with sequences of other rickettsiae. J Bacteriol 2004; 186:5842–5855.
3. Eremeeva ME, Dasch GA, Silverman DJ. Quantitative analyses of variations in the injury of endothelial cells elicited by 11 isolates of *Rickettsia rickettsii*. Clin Diagn Lab Immunol 2001; 8:788–795.
4. Eremeeva ME, Silverman DJ. Effects of the antioxidant α-lipoic acid on human umbilical vein endothelial cells infected with *Rickettsia rickettsii*. Infect Immun 1998; 66:2290–2299.
5. Santucci LA, Gutierrez PL, Silverman DJ. *Rickettsia rickettsii* induces superoxide radical and superoxide dismutase in human endothelial cells. Infect Immun 1992; 60:5113–5118.
6. Valbuena G, Feng HM, Walker DH. Mechanisms of immunity against rickettsiae: new perspectives and opportunities offered by unusual intracellular parasite. Microbes Infect 2002; 4:625–633.
7. Rydkina E, Sahni SK, Santucci LA, et al. Selective modulation of antioxidant enzyme activities in host tissues during *Rickettsia conorii* infection. Microb Pathog 2004; 36:293–301.
8. Valbuena G, Walker DH. Changes in the adherens junctions of human endothelial cells infected with spotted fever group rickettsiae. Virchows Arch 2005; 446:379–382.
9. Davidson MG, Breitschwerdt ED, Walker DH, et al. Vascular permeability and coagulation during *Rickettsia rickettsii* infection in dogs. Am J Vet Res 1990; 51:165–170.
10. Harrell GT, Aikawa JF. Pathogenesis of circulatory failure in Rocky Mountain spotted fever: alterations in the blood volume and the thiocyanate space at various stages of the disease. Arch Intern Med 1949; 83:331–347.
11. Li H, Walker DH. rOmpA is a critical protein for the adhesion of *Rickettsia rickettsii* to host cells. Microb Pathog 1998; 24:289–298.
12. Uchiyama T. Adherence to and invasion of Vero cells by recombinant *Escherichia coli* expressing the outer membrane protein rOmpB of *Rickettsia japonica*. Ann NY Acad Sci 2003; 990:585–590.
13. Martinez JJ, Seveau S, Veiga E, et al. Ku70, a component of DNA-dependent protein kinase, is a mammalian receptor for *Rickettsia conorii*. Cell 2005; 123:1013–1023.
14. Martinez JJ, Cossart P. Early signaling events involved in the entry of *Rickettsia conorii* into mammalian cells. Cell 2004; 117:5097–5106.
15. Whitworth T, Popov VL, Yu XJ, et al. Expression of the *Rickettsia prowazekii pld* or *tlyC* gene in *Salmonella enterica* serovar typhimurium mediates phagosomal escape. Infect Immun 2005; 73:668–673.
16. Renesto P, Dehoux P, Gouin E, et al. Identification and characterization of a phospholipase D-superfamily gene in rickettsiae. J Infect Dis 2003; 188:1276–1283.
17. Heinzen RA, Grieshaber SS, Van Kirk LS, et al. Dynamics of actin-based movement of *Rickettsia rickettsii* in Vero cells. Infect Immun 1999; 67:4201–4207.
18. Teysseire N, Chiche-Portiche C, Raoult D. Intracellular movements of *Rickettsia conorii* and *R. typhi* based on actin polymerization. Res Microbiol 1992; 143:821–829.
19. Gouin E, Egile C, Dehoux P, et al. The RickA protein of *Rickettsia conorii* activates the Arp2/3 complex. Nature 2004; 427:457–461.
20. Jeng RL, Goley ED, D'Alessio, et al. A *Rickettsia* WASP-like protein activates the Arp2/3 complex and mediates actin-based motility. Cell Microbiol 2004; 6(8):761–769.
21. Billings AN, Feng HM, Olano JP, et al. Rickettsial infection in murine models activates an early anti-rickettsial effect mediated by NK cells and associated with production of gamma interferon. Am J Trop Med Hyg 2001; 65:52–56.
22. Kaplanski G, Teysseire N, Farnarier C, et al. IL-6 and IL-8 production from cultured human endothelial cells stimulated by infection with *Rickettsia conorii* via a cell-associated IL-1 alpha-dependent pathway. J Clin Invest 1995; 96:2839–2844.
23. Clifton DR, Rydkina E, Freeman RS, et al. NF-κB activation during *Rickettsia rickettsii* infection of endothelial cells involves the activation of catalytic IκB kinases IKKα and IKKβ and phosphorylation-proteolysis of the inhibitor protein IκBα. Infect Immun 2005; 73:155–165.
24. Feng H-M, Popov VL, Walker DH. Depletion of gamma interferon and tumor necrosis factor alpha in mice with *Rickettsia conorii*-infected endothelium: impairment of rickettsicidal nitric oxide production resulting in fatal, overwhelming rickettsial disease. Infect Immun 1994; 62:1952–1960.
25. Walker DH, Olano JP, Feng H-M. Critical role of cytotoxic T lymphocytes in immune clearance of rickettsial infection. Infect Immun 2001; 69:1841–1846.
26. Walker DH, Popov VL, Crocquet-Valdes PA, et al. Cytokine-induced, nitric oxide-dependent, intracellular antirickettsial activity of mouse endothelial cells. Lab Invest 1997; 76:129–138.
27. Feng HM, Walker DH. Mechanisms of intracellular killing of *Rickettsia conorii* in infected human endothelial cells, hepatocytes, and macrophages. Infect Immun 2000; 68:6729–6736.
28. Walker DH, Staiti A, Mansueto S, et al. Frequent occurrence of hepatic lesions in boutonneuse fever. Acta Trop 1986; 43:175–181.

29. Valbuena G, Bradford W, Walker DH. Expression analysis of the T-cell-targeting chemokines CXCL9 and CXCL10 in mice and humans with endothelial infections caused by rickettsiae of the spotted fever group. Am J Pathol 2003; 163:1357–1369.
30. Valbuena G, Walker DH. Effect of blocking the CXCL9/10-CXCR3 chemokine system in the outcome of endothelial-target rickettsial infections. Am J Trop Med Hyg 2004; 71(4):393–399.
31. Valbuena G, Walker DH. Expression of CX3CL1 (fractalkine) in mice with endothelial-target rickettsial infection of the spotted-fever group. Virchows Arch 2004; 446:21–27.
32. Feng HM, Whitworth T, Olano JP, et al. Fc-dependent polyclonal antibodies and antibodies to outer membrane proteins A and B, but not to lipopolysaccharide, protect SCID mice against fatal *Rickettsia conorii* infection. Infect Immun 2003; 72:2222–2228.
33. Feng HM, Whitworth T, Popov V, et al. Effect of antibody on the rickettsia–host cell interaction. Infect Immun 2004; 22:3524–3530.
34. Walker DH, Popov VL, Feng HM. Establishment of a novel endothelial target mouse model of a typhus group rickettsiosis: evidence for critical roles for gamma interferon and CD8 T lymphocytes. Lab Invest 2000; 80:1361–1372.
35. Vitale G, Mansueto S, Gambino G, et al. The acute phase response in Sicilian patients with boutonneuse fever admitted to hospitals in Palermo, 1992–1997. J Infect 2001; 42:33–39.
36. Sumner JW, Sims KG, Jones DC, et al. Protection of guinea pigs from experimental Rocky Mountain spotted fever by immunization with baculovirus-expressed *Rickettsia rickettsii* rOmpA protein. Vaccine 1995; 13:29.
37. Diaz CM, Feng HM, Crocquet-Valdes P, Walker DH. Identification of protective components of two major outer membrane proteins of spotted fever group rickettsiae. Am J Trop Med Hyg 2001; 65:371–378.
38. Valbuena G, Jordan JM, Walker DH. T cells mediate cross-protective immunity between spotted fever group rickettsiae and typhus group rickettsiae. J Infect Dis 2004; 190:1221–1227.
39. Herrero-Herrero JI, Walker DH, Ruiz-Beltran R. Immunohistochemical evaluation of the cellular immune response to *Rickettsia conorii* in taches noires. J Infect Dis 1987; 155:802–805.
40. Walker DH, Hawkins HK, Hudson P. Fulminant Rocky Mountain spotted fever: its pathologic characteristics associated with glucose-6-phosphate dehydrogenase deficiency. Arch Pathol Lab Med 1983; 107:121–125.
41. Walker DH, Mattern WD. Acute renal failure in Rocky Mountain spotted fever. Arch Intern Med 1980; 139:443–448.
42. Kaplowitz LG, Fischer JJ, Sparling PF. Rocky Mountain spotted fever: a clinical dilemma. In: Remington JS, Swartz MN, eds. Current Clinical Topics in Infectious Disease. Vol. 2. New York: McGraw-Hill, 1981:89–108.
43. Walker DH, Occhino C, Tringali GR, et al. Pathogenesis of rickettsial eschars: the tache noire of boutonneuse fever. Hum Pathol 1988; 19:1449–1454.
44. Kaplowitz LG, Robertson GL. Hyponatremia in Rocky Mountain spotted fever: role of antidiuretic hormone. Ann Intern Med 1983; 98:334–335.
45. Helmick CG, Bernard KW, D'Angelo LJ. Rocky Mountain spotted fever: clinical, laboratory, and epidemiological features of 262 cases. J Infect Dis 1984; 150:480–488.
46. Walker DH, Crawford CG, Cain BG. Rickettsial infection of the pulmonary microcirculation: the basis for interstitial pneumonitis in Rocky Mountain spotted fever. Hum Pathol 1980; 11:263–272.
47. Elghetany TM, Walker DH. Hemostatic changes in Rocky Mountain spotted fever and Mediterranean spotted fever. Am J Clin Pathol 1999; 112:159–168.
48. Rao AK, Schapira M, Clements ML, et al. A prospective study of platelets and plasma proteolytic systems during the early stages of Rocky Mountain spotted fever. N Engl J Med 1988; 318:1021–1028.
49. Schmaier AH, Srikanth S, Elghetany MT, et al. Hemostatic/fibrinolytic protein changes in C3H/HeN mice infected with *Rickettsia conorii*—a model for Rocky Mountain spotted fever. Thromb Haemost 2001; 86:871–879.
50. Walker DH, Fishbein DB. Epidemiology of rickettsial diseases. Eur J Epidemiol 1991; 7:237–245.
51. Holman RC, Paddock CD, Curns AT, et al. Analysis of risk factors for fatal Rocky Mountain spotted fever: evidence for superiority of tetracyclines for therapy. J Infect Dis 2001; 184:1437–1444.

3 | Arthropods and Rickettsiae

Sam R. Telford III
Division of Infectious Diseases, Cummings School of Veterinary Medicine, Tufts University, North Grafton, Massachusetts, U.S.A.

Philippe Parola
Faculté de Médecine, Unité des Rickettsies, Université de la Méditerranée, Marseille, France

INTRODUCTION

In 2006, we celebrate the centenary of Howard Taylor Ricketts's seminal work establishing that *Dermacentor* ticks serve as vectors for the agent of Rocky Mountain spotted fever (RMSF) (1). Since that work, the vector–pathogen relationships of the rickettsioses have been increasingly better defined through intensive studies of RMSF, murine typhus, and epidemic typhus. The mite-borne rickettsioses (scrub typhus, rickettsialpox), however, remain understudied. We review herein the major features of the vector–pathogen relationships of the infections that serve as the main rickettsial clades, focusing on the evidence that serves as the basis for our interpretations, and suggest fruitful avenues of future inquiry.

The available evidence suggests that there is a general paradigm (with variations on the theme for specific species) for the vector aspects of rickettsial life cycles as there are for piroplasms within ticks, or malarial parasites within diptera. Such a paradigm for the rickettsial life cycle has implications for the evolution of the rickettsioses. Rickettsia-like agents are commonly found in arthropods (2), suggesting adaptive radiation concomitant with arthropod speciation over tens of millions of years. The description of organisms within spiders (3) and leeches (4) that are closely related to the rickettsial pathogens that are the focus of this book further underscores the antiquity and diversity of the relationship between these bacteria and invertebrates. The basic elements of rickettsial vector competence comprise a minimum infectious dose to initiate infection in the vector (5); a generalized infection of virtually all tissues; a "resting place" or main tissue reservoir such as the salivary gland or hindgut (6); the phenomenon of reactivation (7); a salivarian or stercorarian mode of inoculation; and capacity for transovarial transmission (TOT). Factors influencing rickettsial vectorial capacity (which is the sum of vector competence, a physiological trait, and ecological–behavioral aspects such as vector longevity and host range) that may be largely influenced by the agents themselves include effects on vector fitness and the nature of vector specificity. One test of the idea of a general rickettsial paradigm would be to determine whether rickettsiae infecting primitive hematophagous invertebrates such as leeches undergo reactivation.

Rickettsiae that are currently recognized as pathogenic for vertebrate hosts seem restricted to only a few species within a few kinds of hematophagous arthropods. The one exception to this statement is the group of related metastriate tick-transmitted infections causing variants of spotted fever or tick typhus, of which there are now a dozen recognized entities (8). Such an observation suggests that we have yet to discover a multitude of potential pathogens within the bloodsucking diptera or hemiptera, as well as in the fleas and mites. The finding that *Rickettsia parkeri* causes spotted fever in humans (9) suggests that some of the many "endosymbiotic" rickettsiae may indeed be pathogenic under the right circumstances. Surveys of hematophagous arthropods using polymerase chain reaction (PCR) sequencing are yielding many new entities, but their capacity to cause pathology remains speculative until they are isolated from diseased humans or animals. The limited diversity of the pathogenic rickettsiae may, alternatively, be evidence for the rarity of successful host-shifts with respect to the vertebrate. The caricature of such a process is the classic hypothesis of the origins of the agent of epidemic typhus from that of murine typhus wherein a rat-maintained infection became one maintained by humans (10). It may also be that natural selection tends to eliminate those rickettsiae that are pathogenic for their hosts, but the apparent lethality of infection by typhus or spotted-fever rickettsiae for their louse and tick hosts, respectively, would argue against this hypothesis because these infections are ecologically successful.

TICK-BORNE RICKETTSIAE

Ticks are prolific vectors, with more recognized transmitted agents than any arthropod other than mosquitoes. All of the nearly 900 known species of ticks require blood for their development and reproduction. Clinically relevant ticks belong to either the Ixodidae (the hard ticks) or the Argasidae (the soft ticks); a third family, the Nuttallielidae, comprises a monotypic genus of soft ticks found in southern Africa and for which an association with a pathogenic agent has yet to be described. The hard ticks are the main vectors for the spotted fever group (SFG) rickettsiae, with two exceptions (rickettsialpox, which is mite-transmitted, and *R. felis*, which is transmitted by fleas).

The biology of RMSF, including the vector–pathogen relationships, has been intensively studied since the early 1900s and serves as the foundation for understanding the transmission of the tick-maintained rickettsiae. Ricketts (11), Wolbach (12), and Spencer and Parker (7) elucidated most of the major features of the vector cycle by studying *Dermacentor andersoni* and *D. variabilis*, which are responsible for virtually all American cases of RMSF.

In addition to *Dermacentor* spp., other ticks found in the Uinted States have been shown to be naturally infected with *R. rickettsii* (usually by grinding up ticks, inoculating the homogenate into guinea pigs, describing a fever reaction or orchitis, and confirming homologous immunity using a challenge with a lab strain of *R. rickettsii*) or have been demonstrated as potential vectors of the pathogen in the laboratory. These include *Haemaphysalis leporispalustris*, *Ixodes dentatus*, *Dermacentor occidentalis*, *D. parumapertus*, *Amblyomma americanum*, *Rhipicephalus sanguineus*, and a soft tick, *Ornithodoros parkeri* (13–17). Some of these tick species seldom bite humans (e.g., *H. leporispalustris* and *D. parumapertus*), and for others contemporary evidence incriminating the tick as an important vector of RMSF is lacking (e.g., *O. parkeri* and *A. americanum*) (18). It is likely that several of these tick species are involved in maintaining and disseminating *R. rickettsii* in nature (19).

In the vertebrate host, rickettsemias that allow noninfected ticks to become infected only occur in selected animals. Meadow voles, golden-mantled ground squirrels, and chipmunks develop rickettsemias of sufficient magnitude and duration to infect laboratory-reared ticks (20), and this probably reflects what happens in nature. However, other wild and domesticated animals susceptible to infection with *R. rickettsii*, including dogs, cotton rats, and wood rats produce rickettsemias too low or too transient to routinely infect ticks (21,22).

Ticks may also acquire and maintain rickettsiae through inheritance or TOT. Because hard ticks feed only once at each life stage (23), rickettsiae acquired during a blood meal from a rickettsemic host or through transovarial route can only be transmitted to another host when the tick has molted to its next developmental stage and takes its next blood meal. Transstadial passage (transfer of bacteria from stage to stage) is a necessary component for the vector competence of the ticks. When rickettsiae are transmitted efficiently both transstadially and transovarially in a tick species, this tick will serve as a reservoir of the bacteria, and the distribution of the rickettsiosis will be identical to that of its tick host (23). For example, *R. slovaca* multiplies in almost all organs and fluids of its tick host, particularly in the salivary glands and ovaries, which enables transmission of rickettsiae during feeding and transovarially, respectively (24).

Ticks may acquire rickettsiae in two other ways. Sexual transmission of *R. rickettsii* from infected males to noninfected female ticks has been described, but this process is unlikely to significantly propagate the infection in tick lineages, as venereally infected females do not appear to transmit rickettsiae transovarially (25). A second suggested method of acquisition of rickettsiae by ticks is the process of cofeeding, which occurs as several ticks feed in proximity on the host. In this circumstance, direct spread of bacteria from an infected tick to an uninfected tick may occur during feeding at closely situated bite sites, as demonstrated with *R. rickettsii* and *D. andersoni* (26).

The vector–pathogen interface for most species of the tick-borne rickettsiae remains incompletely described, including their mode of perpetuation in nature. Although TOT is thought to be a generality, it has been demonstrated only for some SFG rickettsia including human pathogens such as *R. rickettsii, R. slovaca, R. sibirica* (27), *R. africae* (28), *R. helvetica* (29), *R. parkeri* (30), and *R. massiliae* (31). In some instances, TOT of a particular *Rickettsia* sp. may occur in a particular tick, but cannot be sustained for more than one generation (32).

The proportion of infected eggs (filial infection rate) obtained from females of the same tick species infected with the same rickettsial strain may vary for as yet unknown reasons (33,34). For some rickettsia–tick relationships, such as *R. montanensis* in *D. variabilis* (32), *R. slovaca* in *D. marginatus* (24), and *R. massiliae* in *Rh. sanguineus* group ticks (31), maintenance of rickettsiae via TOT may reach 100% and have no effect on the reproductive fitness and viability of the tick host. In contrast, TOT of *R. rickettsii* in *D. andersoni* diminishes survival and reproductive capacity of progeny (34). Recent experiments have shown that *R. rickettsii* is lethal for the majority of experimentally and transovarially infected *D. andersoni*. In one study, most nymphs infected as larvae by feeding on rickettsemic guinea pigs died during the molt into adults, and most of adult female ticks infected as nymphs died prior to feeding. Rickettsiae were vertically transmitted to 39% of offspring, and significantly fewer larvae developed from infected ticks (35). The lethal effect of *R. rickettsii* on its acarine host, coupled with the competitive interactions among different rickettsiae that inhabit the tick microenvironment, may influence the low prevalence of ticks infected with *R. rickettsii* in nature and affect its enzootic maintenance (35).

Basic questions remain about the vector–pathogen relationship for Mediterranean Spotted Fever (MSF), one of the oldest recognized tick-borne rickettsioses. We are unaware of any well-documented demonstration of TOT of *R. conorii* in its vector *Rh. sanguineus*. Interesting data were obtained when pioneers in rickettsiology studied this association (36). At that time, all stages (larvae, nymphs, and adults) were shown to be able to transmit the agent. Furthermore, unfed males and females were shown to be able to transmit the agent over winter. It was also shown that when eggs or larvae obtained from infected *Rh. sanguineus* females were crushed and inoculated to humans, MSF resulted. These data suggest that TOT of the MSF agent occurs in ticks and that reactivation is not required because infection occurred without prefeeding or heating the ticks prior to inoculation. However, neither the TOT rate (the proportion of infected females giving rise to at least one positive egg or larva) or the filial infection rate (FIR) (proportion of infected eggs or larvae obtained from an infected female) have been estimated. It is not known if TOT of *R. conorii* is maintained from generation to generation of *Rh. sanguineus*. Recently, Matsumoto et al. (37) studied the best way to infect *Rh. sanguineus* group ticks with *R. conorii*. Interestingly, a high mortality of the ticks infected with *R. conorii* was observed regardless of the method used. The harmful effect of *R. conorii* on *Rh. sanguineus* had been previously suggested by others (38). In the experiment of Matsumoto et al., the geographic origin of the ticks, which had been collected in Thailand before having been maintained in the laboratory, and the difficulty of specifically identifying ticks within this species complex—therefore allowing for the possibility that the ticks were not *R. Sanguineus* species complex—may partially explain the high mortality of the ticks. It is also possible that a greater pathogen load acquired during laboratory experiments than would be in a natural infection would influence estimates of infection-related morbidity and mortality in experimental ticks. However, subsequent experiments using local ticks and monitoring the pathogen load that had been ingested gave similar results (39). Thus, most aspects of the vector–pathogen relationship in MSF appear similar to those of RMSF.

No animal reservoir of *R. conorii* has been definitely identified in nature, and the role of dogs is controversial (40). Early rickettsiologists such as D. Olmer and J. Olmer in southern France or Blanc and Caminopetros in Greece have shown that foci of MSF are usually small with low propensity to diffusion. For instance, several cases have been observed in one town over several years, whereas no cases were observed in a neighboring town only 2 km away (36). This suggests that some ticks within the same species are able to maintain the rickettsia without any negative fitness effect, due to coadaptation at the population levels.

Questions regarding the specificity of associations among rickettsiae and a particular tick species are unresolved, in part because molecular phylogenetic methods have only been routinely used for a decade to definitively study rickettsial relationships. Consequently, it is difficult to determine how long a tick species has been associated with a rickettsial species if coevolution has occurred. It may be that there is much plasticity in vector–rickettsial interactions: lice appear to support experimental infection by virtually all the main clades of rickettsiae (41,42). *R. rickettsii* is associated with several different tick vectors from several different genera. In addition to the tick species known to be vectors in the United States and in Central and South America, natural infections with *R. rickettsii* have been identified in *Amblyomma cajennense* and in *A. aureolatum*. Moreover, *Rh. sanguineus* was recently rediscovered as a potential vector of *R. rickettsii* (43). This contrasts with other rickettsiae, such as *R. conorii*, which appear to be associated with only one tick vector, *Rh. sanguineus* (but not everywhere, i.e., *R. conorii* is absent from the New World) (44) or *R. helvetica* with *I. ricinus* (45). Between these extremes, there are certain rickettsiae that are associated with several species within the same genus, such as *R. africae* and *R. slovaca* with various *Amblyomma* spp. and *Dermacentor* spp., respectively (23). All these data are limited by the extent of the surveys that have been conducted and the number of ticks that have been assayed for rickettsial infections. In addition, reports of rickettsial isolations from ticks that had been removed from hosts (as opposed to those collected as host-seeking, unfed ticks) must be interpreted with caution because of the possibility that the host was rickettsemic. Finally, there is some evidence to indicate that not only SFG rickettsiae, but also some typhus group rickettsiae, particularly *Rickettsia prowazekii*, may, in certain circumstances, be associated with ticks (46,47). The relationship between soft ticks (Argasidae) and rickettsias is poorly known. Argasids do not seem to be associated with rickettsia, but it is likely that few ticks of this family have been screened for such agents.

Similarly, the effect of a *Rickettsia* sp. on its tick host and potential interactions with other rickettsiae associated with the same tick species require more study. In the 1980s, Burgdorfer et al. (48) demonstrated that ticks infected with the nonpathogenic SFG rickettsia *R. peacockii* were refractory to infection with and maintenance of *R. rickettsii*. Recent study of interspecies competition between different rickettsiae in the same tick, using cohorts of *R. montanensis*- and *R. rhipicephali*-infected *D. variabilis*, have demonstrated similar inhibitory effects between rickettsiae in that infected ticks exposed to the other rickettsial species by capillary feeding were incapable of maintaining both rickettsial species transovarially. Rickettsial infection of ovaries appears to alter the molecular expression of oocyte proteins such that secondary infections are blocked (32). The process of rickettsial "interference," that is, one species of SFG rickettsia successfully outcompeting another for the microenvironment inside the tick, may have profound implications regarding the distribution and frequency of various pathogenic rickettsiae and the specific diseases they cause (49).

The long-recognized phenomenon known as reactivation remains poorly understood (49). Reactivation may be a universal adaptation of tick-borne agents to the long periods of metabolic inactivity by their acarine hosts (50). By becoming dormant during the long transstadial phase and during host-seeking, the agent does not utilize scarce stored resources and reduces any effect on fitness. Female *D. andersoni* ticks infected with *R. rickettsii* and incubated at 4°C demonstrate lower mortality than infected ticks at 21°C (35). Once the tick attaches, the change in temperature and physiology of the tick host induces the agent to emerge from dormancy and attain infectivity. In nature, stress conditions encountered by rickettsiae within the tick include starvation and temperature shifts. In the laboratory, *R. rickettsii* in *D. andersoni* ticks loses its virulence for guinea pigs when the ticks are subjected to low environmental temperature or starvation. However, subsequent exposure of these same ticks to 37°C for 24 to 48 hours or the acquisition of a blood meal may restore the original virulence of the bacteria. During tick blood-feeding, rickettsiae undergo various physiological changes and proliferate intensively during reactivation (34,51,52).

The precise molecular mechanisms responsible for the adaptation of rickettsiae to different host conditions and for reactivation of virulence are unknown. Distinctive microcapsular and slime layers are observed by electron microscopy on reactivated rickettsiae (53). Early biochemical studies suggested that there are metabolic changes involving nicotinamide adenine dinucleotide (NAD), coenzyme A, adenosine triphosphate, and glutathione; virulent *R. rickettsii* could be rendered avirulent by para-aminobenzoic acid (54). However, the stress adaptation in some gram-negative bacteria, also called stringent response, has been shown to be mediated by the nucleotide guanosine-3,5(bis)pyrophosphate(ppGpp), which is modulated by *spoT* genes.

Interestingly, annotation of *R. conorii* genome reveals five *spoT* paralogs, and environmental stress conditions are accompanied by a variable *spoT1* transcription in *R. conorii* (55). This phenomenon could play a role in adaptation of rickettsiae to ticks and during the process of reactivation. It has also been hypothesized that changes in outer surface proteins occur during alternating infection in ticks and in mammals (55). Further studies of the molecular dynamics between rickettsiae and ticks, similar to work on molecular interactions at the tick ovary–rickettsia interface recently published by Mulenga et al. (56), will be needed to better understand these processes.

INSECT-PERPETUATED RICKETTSIAE

There are 2000 or so recognized flea species, but only two rickettsial infections (murine typhus, *R. felis*) associated with these insects. Similarly, there are 3000 species of lice (sucking as well as chewing), but only one rickettsial infection (*R. prowazekii*) known from these insects. If rickettsial diversification depends on cospeciation with the reservoir arthropod, we would expect to find many more rickettsiae within fleas or lice, as well as infections in the vertebrate hosts that serve as their blood-meal sources. Three possible hypotheses may be suggested to explain the apparent paradox: (*i*) The vast majority of flea and louse species are from rodents and have varying degrees of host specificity. Both of these insects are generally nest parasites, and cannot travel long distances in the absence of a vertebrate host. The probability of a host-shift or a recombination-like event to generate diversity would seem less than for a vector arthropod that was highly mobile or more promiscuous with respect to blood-meal sources. Even if there was opportunity for a host-shift event, unknown factors appear to inhibit the development of new vector–rickettsial associations. The head louse is conspecific with the body louse and is competent for *R. prowazekii* in laboratory experiments (57,58), but head lice have not been epidemiologically associated with epidemic typhus. Similarly, *R. typhi* replicates normally within body lice (59), but lice have not been associated with cases of murine typhus. (*ii*) The available life cycle evidence suggests that many bartonellae are maintained by fleas or lice (60,61). It may be that the "rule of the incumbent" (in politics, the current occupant of an office is difficult to depose; this seems to be a generality for the history of life) applies in that the very diverse and ubiquitous bartonellae (62) competitively exclude rickettsiae. At the individual vector level, such exclusion may comprise a negative fitness effect by two bacteria parasitizing one insect. On the other hand, the human body louse serves as the main vector for not only *R. prowazekii*, but also for *Bartonella quintana*, the agent of trench fever. (*iii*) Flea and louse species have not been actively surveyed for the presence of rickettsiae, other than peridomestic fleas for *R. typhi*. Although diverse fleas have been intensively surveyed for plague studies, assays such as mouse inoculation may not have allowed detection of rickettsiae that may have been present because most laboratory mouse strains usually respond subtly to rickettsial infection.

Rats (*Rattus* spp.) may be rickettsemic for as long as two weeks (63) and under experimental conditions, *Xenopsylla cheopis*, the main vector for *R. typhi*, may become infected even during the end of the rickettsemic period, suggesting a low minimum infectious dose. Ingested rickettsiae enter gut epithelial cells and replicate there. Sloughed epithelial cells or free rickettsiae emitted from burst cells are excreted in the flea feces. Fleas appear to be infected for the duration of their life, without effects on their fitness (63,64). Infection does not seem to escape the gut barrier and thus hemocoelic tissues are not infected (65). TOT has been demonstrated for *R. typhi* within *X. cheopis* (64).

Rickettsiae had long been noted within diverse fleas, including the common cat flea, *Ctenocephalides felis* (66). During the late 1980s, colonies of cat fleas maintained on specific pathogen-free blood were noted to have rickettsia-like bodies within their hemocoel (67). The significance of the "ELB agent" (named for EL Laboratory, which maintained one of the original sources of infected fleas) was demonstrated in 1994 when its DNA was detected in the blood of murine typhus-like cases in Texas (68). A new rickettsial species, *R. felis*, was subsequently isolated and described (69). *R. felis* appears to be stably maintained by TOT, with as many as 12 generations of persistence documented (70). In that study, horizontal transmission to and from cats was not detected, nor did uninfected fleas become infected by being placed with infected fleas. Thus, mammalian reservoirs may not be required for perpetuation. On the other hand, the failure to transmit by bite may reflect a stercorarian mode of transmission that is difficult to simulate in the laboratory.

DNA of *R. felis* has been detected in cat fleas from Thailand (71,72) and many other countries in Africa and Eurasia, suggesting that it has a global distribution. Of interest are recent reports where the agent was detected by PCR in *Xenopsylla* and *Archeopsylla* fleas from rodents and hedgehogs, and from *Anomiopsyllus* spp. (73,74), which demonstrate that *R. felis* may also be maintained by fleas other than those that are very common in cats or humans. Routine use of molecular methods to detect *R. felis* in fleas may lead to the discovery of heretofore unrecognized rickettsial diversity in these vector arthropods.

Transmission of epidemic typhus by the human body louse was demonstrated by Charles Nicolle, who received the Nobel Prize for this discovery (75). The louse acquires *R. prowazekii* after feeding on a bacteremic human, with 60% to 80% of lice becoming infected during a single blood meal from an acute typhus case (76). In contrast, infection rates were less than 5% for lice feeding on patients with recrudescent (Brill-Zinsser) typhus (57). In the louse, when the obligate intracellular *R. prowazekii* are ingested within monocytes with the infected blood meal, they only infect the epithelial cells of the anterior gut where they multiply (6). As a result of overreplication, infected epithelial cells enlarge and eventually burst five days postinfection, releasing the rickettsiae into the gut lumen, and massive quantities of rickettsiae are discharged in the feces starting from the fifth day postinfection. Infected lice often turn red, due to the release of ingested blood remnants into the hemocoel. Inasmuch as ruptured epithelial cells are not replaced, infection with *R. prowazekii* may lead to the death of the louse, although the frequency of such a phenomenon is dose- and temperature-dependent (77).

Transmission of *R. prowazekii* from the louse to the human occurs by contamination of the bite site with feces containing rickettsiae or by contamination of conjunctivae or mucous membranes with the crushed bodies or feces of infected lice. Infection through aerosols of feces-infected dust has been reported and provides the main risk of typhus exposure for healthcare providers who are in contact with the patients infested with the infected lice (6). The threat of typhus as a biological weapon lies in its stability in the dried louse feces, with viability and infectivity greater than 100 days (77) and the possibility of infection by inhalation of an aerosol. Unlike all other rickettsiae, *R. prowazekii* does not appear to be perpetuated by TOT (78), although one report suggests otherwise (79) for lice that were concurrently infected by relapsing fever spirochetes. Interestingly, concurrent infection with agents that mechanically disrupt the gut barrier alters vector competence for certain arboviruses within mosquitoes (80) suggesting the possibility that *R. prowazekii* may be inherited under unusual circumstances.

One of the greatest enigmas in the field of disease ecology is the natural presence of *R. prowazekii* in populations of eastern North American flying squirrels (81). These animals range from southern Canada into Mexico. Is epidemic typhus an infection that originated in the New World as a zoonosis from flying squirrels, and was exported to the Old World during colonial exploration? Or did epidemic typhus evolve as an anthroponosis in the Old World and imported into the New World during exploration by the Spanish conquistadors, somehow becoming established among flying squirrels and their fleas and lice?

MITE-PERPETUATED RICKETTSIAE

Mites are one of the most common groups of animals, with 45,000 recognized species. They are among the oldest terrestrial animals, dating in the fossil record to the Devonian (nearly 400 million years ago), and are found in every habitat on earth. There are two major orders of the acarines: the Acariformes and the Parasitiformes. In the former, there are two main groups, the Sarcoptiformes (astigmata) and the Trombidiformes (prostigmata), both of which contain species of clinical significance. The latter comprises three orders: the Holothyrida, the Ixodida, and the Mesostigmata. Of these, only the latter two are clinically significant; the holothyrids consist of about 20 species that are found only in Australasia and some neotropical forests. The mesostigmata (also known as gamasida or dermanyssoida) include some that infest birds or rodents that under certain circumstances will infest humans and cause itch. The ixodida consist of the ticks, which are essentially very large mites.

The house mouse mite (*Liponyssoides sanguineus*) is the vector for rickettsialpox due to infection by *Rickettsia akari*. The relatively mild disease, characterized by fever and exanthema, was first described in the neighborhood of Kew Gardens in the Bronx, New York, during the

1940s (82). Although this infection is widely distributed from Russia to South Africa to the United States, probably by transport with house mice (*Mus musculus*) and its mites, its biology remains poorly studied. The protonymph, deutonymph, and adult (but oddly, not the larva) of this mite feed on blood, suggesting that *R. akari* may also be transmitted by multiple life stages (83), unlike the mites that maintain the agent of scrub typhus. TOT has been documented (84), but the relative contribution of horizontal and vertical transmission to perpetuation remains undescribed. Whether reactivation occurs with *R. akari* also remains speculative.

The prostigmatid trombiculid mites (chiggers) are the vectors for the agent of scrub typhus (*Orientia tsutsugamushi*), a rickettsiosis of Eurasia and northeastern Australia. Nearly three billion people live in countries that are endemic for scrub typhus. Scrub typhus is acquired from infestation by tiny (0.2 mm) larval trombiculid mites such as *Leptotrombidium deliense* or *L. akamushi*. The nymphal and adult stages of this mite feed on detritus or other arthropods and do not take vertebrate blood. Therefore, *O. tsutsugamushi* relies mainly on transovarial or vertical transmission (passage through the egg) for perpetuation, with FIRs as great as 100% (85). Transmission can be very efficient: 75% of more than 4000 attempts to transmit to mice using experimentally infected mites were successful (86), but the capacity of laboratory colony matrilineages of mites to transmit apparently declines with each generation. Infected rodent hosts may infect larvae (87,88) and cofeeding with infected mites will infect clean larvae (89). TOT for more than one generation after feeding on infected rodents, however, was not demonstrated and it is not known how frequently horizontal amplification via rodent hosts serves to generate new matrilineages of infected chiggers in nature. Although there have been few studies of the life cycle of *O. tsutsugamushi* within chiggers (possibly because of the difficulty of keeping trombidiid mite colonies and manipulating these tiny arthropods), not surprisingly salivary glands and guts are infected in larvae and ovaries are infected in females (90). Interestingly, larvae that fail to transmit may retain the agent to the adult stage (85) and pass it to their progeny, suggesting the existence of minimum required doses for infectivity by bite.

CONCLUSION

It seems likely that routine use of molecular methods will uncover heretofore unrecognized species of rickettsiae from fleas and mites, which have been poorly studied by rickettsiologists but are the most diverse species of the vector arthropod groups. The life cycles of the insect-transmitted rickettsioses differ slightly from those of the tick-transmitted ones, in that reactivation probably does not occur because the time between blood meals is relatively short. Furthermore, their transmission is not dependent on delivery by salivary secretions but occurs through contamination with feces containing infectious bacteria. The mite-transmitted rickettsioses would be expected through phylogenetic arguments to have life cycles most similar to those transmitted by ticks, but for both rickettsialpox and scrub typhus the presence or absence of reactivation remains undescribed. Because mites feed relatively quickly it may be that reactivation does not occur. For all rickettsioses, however, perpetuation appears to rely upon inheritance, with the apparent exception of epidemic typhus, although the natural cycle for enzootic (flying squirrel) typhus should be examined carefully for a TOT component.

REFERENCES

1. Ricketts HT. The transmission of Rocky Mountain spotted fever by the bite of the wood tick (*Dermacentor occidentalis*). J Am Med Assoc 1906; 47:358.
2. Cowdry EV. The distribution of rickettsia in the tissues of insects and arachnids. J Exp Med 1923; 37:431–458.
3. Goodacre SL, Martin O, Thomas CFG, Hewitt GM. Wolbachia and other endosymbiont infections in spiders. Mol Ecol 2003; 15:517–527.
4. Kikuchi Y, Sameshima S, Kitade O, Kojima J, Fukatsu T. Novel clade of *Rickettsia* spp. from leeches. Appl Environ Microbiol 2002; 68:999–1004.
5. Burgdorfer W, Friedhoff KT, Lancaster JL. Natural history of tick-borne spotted fever in the USA. Bull WHO 1966; 35:149–153.
6. Wolbach SB, Todd JL, Palfrey FW. The Etiology and Pathology of Typhus. Cambridge, Massachusetts: Harvard University Press, 1922.

7. Spencer RR, Parker RR. Rocky Mountain spotted fever: infectivity of fasting and recently fed ticks. Pub Health Rep 1923; 38:333.
8. Parola P, Paddock C, Raoult D. Tick-borne rickettsioses around the world: emerging diseases challenging old concepts. Clin Microbiol Rev 2005; 18(4):719–756.
9. Paddock CD, Sumner JW, Comer JA, et al. *Rickettsia parkeri*: a newly recognized cause of spotted fever rickettsiosis in the United States. Clin Infect Dis 2004; 38:805–811.
10. Woodward TE. Murine and epidemic typhus: how close is their relationship? Yale J Biol Med 1982; 55:335.
11. Ricketts HT. A microorganism which apparently has a specific relationship to Rocky Mountain spotted fever. J Am Med Assoc 1909; 52:379.
12. Wolbach SB. Studies on Rocky Mountain spotted fever. J Med Res 1919; 41:1–197.
13. Davis GE. Experimental transmission of the spotted fevers of the United States, Colombia, and Brazil by the argasid tick *Ornithodoros parkeri*. Public Health Rep 1943; 58:1201–1208.
14. Parker RR, Philip CB, Jellison WL. Rocky Mountain spotted fever: potentialities of tick transmission in relation to geographical occurrence in the United States. Am J Trop Med Hyg 1933; 8:341–379.
15. Parker RR, Bell JF, Chalgren WS, Thrailkill FB, McKee MT. The recovery of starians of Rocky Mountain spotted fever and tularemia from ticks of the eastern United States. J Infect Dis 1952; 91:231–237.
16. Parker RR, Kohls GM, Steinhaus EA. Rocky Mountain spotted fever: spontaneous infection in the tick *Amblyomma americanum*. Pub Health Rep 1943; 58:721–729.
17. McDade JE, Newhouse VF. Natural history of *Rickettsia rickettsii*. Ann Rev Microbiol 1986; 40:287–309.
18. Childs JE, Paddock CD. The ascendancy of *Amblyomma americanum* as a vector of pathogens affecting humans in the United States. Ann Rev Entomol 2003; 48:307–337.
19. Sexton DJ. Rocky Mountain spotted fever. In: Service MW, ed. The Encyclopedia of Arthropod-transmitted Infections. New York: CABI Publishing, 2001:437–442.
20. Bozeman FM, Shirai A, Humphries JW, Fuller HS. Ecology of Rocky Mountain spotted fever. II. Natural infection of wild mammals and birds in Virginia and Maryland. Am J Trop Med Hyg 1967; 16:48.
21. Lundgren DL, Nichols PS, Thorpe BD. Experimental infection of lagomorphs with *Rickettsia rickettsii*. Am J Trop Med Hyg 1968; 17:213.
22. Norment BR, Burgdorfer W. Susceptibility and reservoir potential of the dog to spotted fever-group rickettsiae. Am J Vet Res 1984; 45(1706):1710.
23. Parola P, Raoult D. Ticks and tickborne bacterial diseases in humans: an emerging infectious threat. Clin Infect Dis 2001; 32(6):897–928. Erratum: Clin. Inf. Dis. 33:749.
24. Rehacek J. *Rickettsia slovaca*, the organism and its ecology. Acta Sci Nat Brno 1984; 18:1–50.
25. Hayes SF, Burgdorfer W, Aeschlimann A. Sexual transmission of spotted fever group rickettsiae by infected male ticks: detection of rickettsiae in immature spermatozoa of *Ixodes ricinus*. Infect Immun 1980; 27:638–642.
26. Philip CB. Some epidemiological considerations in Rocky Mountain spotted fever. Pub Health Rep 1959; 74:595–600.
27. Rudakov N, Samoilenko I, Yakimemko VV, et al. The re-emergence of Siberian tick typhus: field and experimental observations. In: Raoult D, Brouqui P, eds. Rickettsiae and Rickettsial Diseases at the Turn of the Third Millennium. Paris: Elsevier, 1999: 269–273.
28. Kelly PJ, Mason P. Transmission of a spotted fever group rickettsia by *Amblyomma hebraeum* (Acari: Ixodidae). J Med Entomol 1991; 28:596–600.
29. Burgdorfer W, Aeschlimann A, Peter O, Hayes SF, Philip RN. *Ixodes ricinus* vector of a hitherto undescribed spotted fever group agent in Switzerland. Acta Trop 1979; 36:357–367.
30. Goddard J. Experimental infection of lone star ticks, *Amblyomma americanum* (L.), with *Rickettsia parkeri* and exposure of guinea pigs to the agent. J Med Entomol 2003; 40(5):686–689.
31. Matsumoto K, Brouqui P, Raoult D, Parola P. Transmission of *Rickettsia massiliae* in the tick, *Rhipicephalus turanicus*. Med Vet Entomol 2005; 19(3):263–270.
32. Macaluso KR, Sonenshine DE, Ceraul SM, Azad AF. Rickettsial infection in *Dermacentor variabilis* (Acari: Ixodidae) inhibits transovarial transmission of a second Rickettsia. J Med Entomol 2002; 39(6):809–813.
33. Burgdorfer W, Brinton LP. Mechanisms of transovarial infection of spotted fever Rickettsiae in ticks. Ann NY Acad Sci 1975; 266:61–72.
34. Burgdorfer W. Investigation of transovarial transmission of *Rickettsia rickettsii* in the wood tick *Dermacentor andersoni*. Exp Parasitol 1963; 14:152.
35. Niebylski ML, Peacock MG, Schwan TG. Lethal effect of *Rickettsia rickettsii* on its tick vector (*Dermacentor andersoni*). Appl Environ Microbiol 1999; 65(2):773–778.
36. Blanc G, Caminopetros J. Epidemiological and experimental studies on Boutonneuse fever done at the Pasteur Institute in Athens. Arch Inst Pasteur Tunis 1932; XX(343):394.
37. Matsumoto K, Brouqui P, Raoult D, Parola P. Experimental infection models of ticks of the *Rhipicephalus sanguineus* group with *Rickettsia conorii*. Vector Borne Zoonotic Dis 2005; 5(4): 363–372.

38. Santos AS, Bacellar F, Santos-Silva M, Formosinho P, Gracio AJ, Franca S. Ultrastructural study of the infection process of *Rickettsia conorii* in the salivary glands of the vector tick *Rhipicephalus sanguineus*. Vector Borne Zoonotic Dis 2002; 2(3):165–177.
39. Socalovski, unpublished.
40. Kelly PJ, Matthewman LA, Mason PR, Courtney S, Katsande C, Rukwava J. Experimental infection of dogs with a Zimbabwean strain of *Rickettsia conorii*. J Trop Med Hyg 1992; 95(5):322–326.
41. Weyer F. Rickettsiae and lice. In: Kazar J, Ormsbee RA, Tarasevich IN, eds. Rickettsiae and Rickettsial Diseases. Bratislava: Veda, 1978:515–521.
42. Houhamdi L, Raoult D. Experimentally infected human body lice (*Pediculus humanus humanus*) as vectors of *Rickettsia rickettsii* and *Rickettsia conorii* in a rabbit model. Am J Trop Med Hyg 2006; 74(4): 521–525.
43. Demma LJ, Traeger MS, Nicholson WL, et al. Rocky Mountain spotted fever in Arizona associated with an unexpected tick vector. N Engl J Med 2005; 353:587–594.
44. Raoult D, Roux V. Rickettsioses as paradigms of new or emerging infectious diseases. Clin Microbiol Rev 1997; 10(4):694–719.
45. Parola P, Beati L, Cambon M, Raoult D. First isolation of *Rickettsia helvetica* from *Ixodes ricinus* ticks in France. Eur J Clin Microbiol Infect Dis 1998; 17(2):95–100.
46. Burgdorfer W, Ormsbee RA, Schmidt ML, Hoogstraal H. A search for the epidemic typhus agent in Ethiopian ticks. Bull World Health Organ 1973; 48:563–569.
47. Medina-Sanchez A, Bouyer DH, Alcantara-Rodriguez V, et al. Detection of a typhus group rickettsia in amblyomma ticks in the state of Nuevo Leon, Mexico. Ann NY Acad Sci 2005; 1063:327–332.
48. Burgdorfer W, Hayes SF, Mavros AJ. Nonpathogenic rickettsiae in *Dermacentor andersoni*: a limiting factor for the distribution of *Rickettsia rickettsii*. In: Burgdorfer W, Anacker RL, eds. Rickettsiae and Rickettsial Diseases. New York: Academic Press, 1981:585–594.
49. Spencer RR, Parker RR. Rocky Mountain spotted fever: infectivity of fasting and recently fed ticks. Pub Health Rep 1923; 38(333):339.
50. Katavolos P, Armstrong PM, Dawson JE, Telford SR III. Duration of tick attachment required for transmission of human granulocytic ehrlichiosis. J Infect Dis 1998; 177:1422–1425.
51. Wike DA, Burgdorfer W. Plaque formation in tissue cultures by *Rickettsia rickettsi* isolated directly from whole blood and tick hemolymph. Infect Immun 1972; 6(5):736–738.
52. Wike DA, Ormsbee RA, Tallent G, Peacock MG. Effects of various suspending media on plaque formation by rickettsiae in tissue culture. Infect Immun 1972; 6(4):550–556.
53. Hayes SF, Burgdorfer W. Reactivation of *Rickettsia rickettsii* in *Dermacentor andersoni* ticks: an ultrastructural analysis. Infect Immun 1982; 37:779–785.
54. Gilford JH, Price WH. Virulent–avirulent conversions of *Rickettsia rickettsii* in vitro. Proc Natl Acad Sci USA 1955; 41:870–873.
55. Rovery C, Renesto P, Crapoulet N, et al. Transcriptional response of *Rickettsia conorii* exposed to temperature variation and stress starvation. Res Microbiol 2005; 156(2):211–218.
56. Mulenga A, Macaluso KR, Simser JA, Azad AF. Dynamics of Rickettsia–tick interactions: identification and characterization of differentially expressed mRNAs in uninfected and infected *Dermacentor variabilis*. Insect Mol Biol 2003; 12(2):185–193.
57. Gaon JA, Murray ES. The natural history of recrudescent typhus (Brill Zinsser disease) in Bosnia. Bull WHO 1966; 35:133.
58. Bozeman FM, Williams NS, Stocks NI, et al. Ecologic studies on epidemic typhus infection in the eastern flying squirrel. In: Kazar J, Ormsbee RA, Tarasevich IN, eds. Rickettsiae and Rickettsial Diseases. Bratislava: Veda, 1978:493–504.
59. Ito S, Vinson JW, Whitecarver J. Ultrastructural observations of *Rickettsia typhi* in the human body louse. In: Kazar J, Ormsbee RA, Tarasevich IN, eds. Rickettsiae and Rickettsial Diseases. Bratislava: Veda, 1978:53–64.
60. Strong RP, Swift HF, Opie EL, et al. Trench Fever. Report of Commission, Medical Research Committee, American Red Cross. London: Oxford University Press, 1918.
61. Krampitz HE, Kleinschmidt A. Grahamella Brumpt 1911 biologische und morphologische Untersuchungen. Z Tropenmed Parasitol 1960; 11:336–352.
62. Kosoy MY, Saito EK, Green D, Marston EL, Jones DC, Childs JE. Experimental evidence of host specificity of Bartonella infection in rodents. Comp Immunol Microbiol Infect Dis 2000; 23:221–238.
63. Farhangazad A, Traub R, Wisseman CL. *Rickettsia mooseri* infection in the flea *Leptopsylla segnis* and *Xenopsylla cheopis*. Am J Trop Med Hyg 1983; 32:1392.
64. Farhangazad A, Traub R. Transmission of murine typhus rickettsiae by *Xenopsylla cheopis*, with notes on experimental infection and effects of temperature. Am J Trop Med Hyg 1985; 34:555.
65. Snyder JC, Wheeler CM. The experimental infection of the human body louse, *Pediculus humanus corporis*, with murine and epidemic louse borne typhus strains. J Exp Med 1945; 82:1–20.
66. Sikora H. Beitrage zur Kenntnis der Rickettsien. Arch Schiffs Tropenhygien Leipzig 1918; xxii:442–446.
67. Adams JR, Schmidtmann ET, Azad AF. Infection of colonized cat fleas, *Ctenocephalides felis* (Bouché), with a rickettsia-like microorganism. Am J Trop Med Hyg 1990; 43:400–409.
68. Schriefer ME, Sacci JB Jr, Dumler JS, Bullen MG, Azad AF. Identification of a novel rickettsial infection in a patient diagnosed with murine typhus. J Clin Microbiol 1994; 32:949–954.

69. Higgins JA, Radulovic S, Schriefer ME, Azad AF. *Rickettsia felis*: a new species of pathogenic rickettsia isolated from cat fleas. J Clin Microbiol 1996; 34:671–674.
70. Wedincamp J, Foil LD. Vertical transmission of *Rickettsia felis* in the cat flea (Ctenocephalides felis Bouche). J Vector Ecol 2002; 27:96–101.
71. Parola P, Miller RS, McDaniel P, et al. Emerging rickettsioses of the Thai–Myanmar border. Emerg Infect Dis 2003; 9:592–595.
72. Rolain JM, Bourry O, Davoust B, Raoult D. *Bartonella quintana* and *Rickettsia felis* in Gabon. Emerg Infect Dis 2005; 11(11):1742–1743.
73. Bitam I, Parola P, Dittmar de la Cruz K, et al. First molecular detection of *Rickettsia felis* in fleas from Algeria. Am J Trop Med Hyg 2006; 74:532–535.
74. Stevenson HL, Labruna MB, Montenieri JA, Kosoy MY, Gage KL, Walker DH. Detection of *Rickettsia felis* in a New World flea species, *Anomiopsyllus nudata* (Siphonaptera: Ctenophthalmidae). J Med Entomol 2005; 42(2):163–167.
75. Gross L. How Charles Nicolle of the Pasteur Institute discovered that epidemic typhus is transmitted by lice: reminiscences from my years at the Pasteur Institute in Paris. Proc Natl Acad Sci USA 1996; 93:10539–10540.
76. Fuller HS, Murray ES, Snyder JC. Studies of human body lice, *Pediculus humanus corporis*. I. A method for feeding lice through a membrane and experimental infection with *Rickettsia prowazekii*, *R. mooseri*, and *Borrelia novyi*. Publ Health Rep 1949; 64:1287.
77. Silverman DJ, Boese JL, Wisseman CL Jr. Ultrastructural studies of *Rickettsia prowazeki* from louse midgut cells to feces: search for "dormant" forms. Infect Immun 1974; 10:257–263.
78. Houhamdi L, Fournier PE, Fang R, Lepidi H, Raoult D. An experimental model of human body louse infection with *Rickettsia prowazekii*. J Infect Dis 2002; 186:1639–1646.
79. Sergent E, Foley H, Vialette C. Sur des formes microbiennes abondantes dans les corps des poux infectes par le typhus exanthematique, et toujours absentes dans les poux temoins, non typhiques. Mem Soc Biol 1914; lxxvii(2):101.
80. Turell MJ, Rossignol PA, Spielman A, Rossi CA, Bailey CL. Enhanced arboviral transmission by mosquitoes that concurrently ingested microfilariae. Science 1984; 225:1039–1041.
81. Sonenshine DE, Bozeman FM, Williams MS, et al. Epizootiology of epidemic typhus (*Rickettsia prowazekii*) in flying squirrels. Am J Trop Med Hyg 1980; 29:277.
82. Huebner RJ, Stamps P, Armstrong C. Rickettsialpox—a newly recognized rickettsial disease. I. Isolation of the etiological agent. Publ Health Rep 1946; 61:1605–1614.
83. Fuller HS. Studies of rickettsialpox. III. Life cycle of the mite vector, *Allodermanyssus sanguineus*. Am J Hyg 1954; 59:236–239.
84. Philip CB, Hughes LE. The tropical rat mite, *Liponyssus bacoti*, as an experimental vector of rickettsialpox. Am J Trop Med Hyg 1948; 28:697–705.
85. Rapmond G, Upham RW, Kundin WD, Manikumaran C, Chan TC. Transovarian development of scrub typhus rickettsiae in a colony of vector mites. Trans Roy Soc Trop Med Hyg 1969; 63:251–258.
86. Lerdthusnee K, Khlaimanee N, Monkanna T, et al. Efficiency of Leptotrombidium chiggers (Acari: Trombiculidae) at transmitting *Orientia tsutsugamushi* to laboratory mice. J Med Entomol 2002; 39:521–525.
87. Traub R, Wisseman CL, Jones MR, OKeefe JJ. The acquisition of *Rickettsia tsutsugamushi* by chiggers (trombiculid mites) during feeding process. Ann NY Acad Sci 1975; 266:91–114.
88. Walker JS, Chan CT, Manikumaran C, Elisberg BL. Attempts to infect and demonstrate transovarial transmission of *Rickettsia tsutsugamushi* in three species of Leptotrombidium mites. Ann NY Acad Sci 1975; 266:80–90.
89. Frances SP, Watcharapichat P, Phulsuksombati D, Tanksul P. Transmission of *Orientia tsutsugamushi*, the aetiological agent of scrub typhus, to cofeeding mites. Parasitology 2000; 120:601–607.
90. Roberts LW, Robinson DM, Rapmund G, Walker JS, Gan E, Ram S. Distribution of *Rickettsia tsutsugamushi* in organs of *Leptotrombidium fletcheri* (Prostigmata: Trombiculidae). J Med Entomol 1975; 12:345–348.

4 | Murine Typhus

Yanis Tselentis and Achilleas Gikas
Laboratory of Clinical Bacteriology, Parasitology, Zoonoses, and Geographical Medicine, University of Crete, Crete, Greece

INTRODUCTION

Murine typhus, also known as endemic typhus, is a flea-borne infectious disease caused by *Rickettsia typhi*. The disease occurs sporadically in environments where rats and humans live in close proximity and typically in temperate and subtropical seaboard regions during warm months of the year. The illness is less commonly diagnosed in developed countries than in the developing part of the world due to improved hygiene and rat control efforts. It is difficult to establish the true incidence because of the difficulty in distinguishing murine typhus from other causes of rash and fever.

R. typhi is a member of the typhus group of rickettsiae that also includes the agent responsible for epidemic typhus, *R. prowazekii*. These organisms are obligate intracellular, gram-negative bacteria that can only be grown in tissue culture, cells of experimental animals, or chick embryos. *R. typhi* (or *R. mooseri*), the causal agent of endemic typhus, is carried by the rat flea *Xenopsylla cheopis*, and typically infects humans in markets, grain stores, breweries, and garbage depots. It usually causes a mild form of illness, but severe forms of the disease can also occur.

HISTORY

The identification of the clinical entity known widely today as the endemic or murine typhus, the distinction from the classical—known from archaic periods—epidemic (or louse-borne) typhus and the isolation of its causal agent, as well as the full comprehension of this microorganism's life cycle were not accomplished until the first decades of the twentieth century.

Paullin probably made the first clinical description of a "milder form of typhus" in 1913 in Atlanta (1). In 1917, Neill used blood from cases of typhus fevers in Texas and injected it in the peritoneum of male guinea pigs, which led to scrotal swelling and inflammation, along with hemorrhage beneath the tunica, a few days later (2–4). This was later known as the Neill–Mooser's reaction, due to the extension of Neill's experiments by Mooser in 1928, who used blood obtained from cases with typhus fever in Mexico. Mooser adopted the local word *tabardillo*, which means red cloak to refer to this disease that had been known in Mexico since the Spanish occupation during the sixteenth century. These studies contributed in distinguishing the endemic from the classic or louse-borne typhus where this reaction was not observed (4–6).

In 1923, in the Annual Reports of the Department of Health of Palestine, there was a reference to a mild course of typhus fever, similar to Brill's disease and different from the classic form of typhus (5). Stuart in 1924 made the first comprehensive study on typhus in Palestine, and in 1926 the possibility of a vector other than the louse was implied, in the Annual Reports of the Department of Health of Palestine (5). Fletcher and Lesslar (7) also made observations on the endemic type of typhus fever in Malaya in 1925.

In 1926, Maxcy (8), an epidemiologist who had studied typhus in the southern United States, suggested the transmission of the disease from fleas (*X. cheopis*) to humans. Maxcy's theory was validated by two different groups in 1931. The first group, Dyer et al. (9,10), were the first to isolate the suggested new "virus" from fleas in a drugstore in Baltimore during an outbreak of three cases of typhus. The owner of the drugstore (Dr. J. Lipsky) and two of his clerks were involved. It is of interest that the initial diagnosis was typhoid fever, but the negative results of the blood culture and the Widal reaction, combined with a titer of 1:320 of the Proteus OX-19 reaction, led to the final diagnosis of endemic typhus fever. The second group, Mooser et al. (11), recovered the responsible microorganism from the brains of rats in a prison in Mexico City, where several inmates had presented typhus fever. The work of these two groups helped elucidate the epidemiological cycle of the disease by revealing the reservoir (rat) and the vector (flea).

The latter group of scientists also made a series of observations on various characteristics of Mexican typhus and other entities, such as Brill's disease.

In 1932, Lépine was the first to describe the disease in Greece when he revealed the microorganism in similar studies on the brains of rats during investigations on cases of endemic typhus (12–14). In 1932, Stuart and Krikorian from Palestine announced the possibility of transmitting the disease from humans to rabbits and guinea pigs (5,15). During 1933, Marcandier and Pirot conducted similar studies on sporadic cases of the disease on a Mediterranean man-of-war (2). Studies of Lépine, Lorandos, Lemiere (1934), Combiesco et al. (1935) led to isolation of the "virus" from cats and dogs (5,12–14). Moreover, Le Chuiton et al. in 1935 proved that the transmission of the disease by mouth was effective in animal experiments (5).

In 1935–1936, Chilean researchers Suarez, Palacios, Chavez, and Sesnic and Giroud in Tunisia identified and asymptomatic cases of murine typhus (confirmed by a positive Weil–Felix reaction or animal cultures) (5,6). In 1936, Krigler and Comaroff confirmed the existence of the endemic type of typhus in Palestine (2,5).

In 1938, Wolbach attempted to explain the difference in mortality rates of typhus fever on rich and poor classes, suggesting that poorer classes gain immunity to the disease due to mild attacks during childhood. Moreover, it was marked that patients who recovered from endemic typhus fever were also immune, or suffered from a milder form of disease when infected by epidemic typhus and vice versa (5,16).

Late reports established the worldwide distribution of endemic typhus, involving Kuwait, Thailand, North Africa, Egypt, Australia, Russia, France, and South America (5,17). The incidence of *R. typhi* infections declined in the second half of the twentieth century (18–20), enhanced by rat control programs in the United States in the 1940s (17). However, murine typhus has began to reappear during the last decades [confirmed by seroepidemiological studies by Al-Awadi et al. (1982) in Kuwait, Botros et al. (1989) in Egypt, Brown et al. (1989) in Thailand, Duffy et al. (1990) in Thailand, and Dumler et al. (1991) in the United States, especially in developing countries, leading us to the conclusion that it is a reemerging disease (14,18).

Tselentis et al. reported the reappearance of the disease in Europe after almost half a century in 1986 on the Greek island of Euboea. This was followed by other reports in Greece, mainly on the island of Crete (14,21).

Finally, it should be noted that the name initially given to the microorganism responsible for the endemic form of typhus was *R. mooseri* (today also known as *R. typhi*), in honor of Herman Mooser, as his detailed studies and the revelations he made on various aspects of the disease enlightened the modern medical society and led the way for his contemporaries into further investigations regarding several parameters of medical research and methodology.

EPIDEMIOLOGY—LIFE CYCLE

The rat flea *X. cheopis* mainly transmits *R. typhi* (22,23). Occasionally, other flea species or arthropod vectors have been reported to transmit *R. typhi*, including the cat flea *Ctenocephalides felis*, the mouse flea *Leptopsyllia segnis*, and lice, mites, and ticks (22,24,25). The flea remains infected for life, but neither its lifespan nor its reproductive activities are affected (22,24–26). The primary reservoirs are the rats belonging to the subgenus *Rattus*, mainly *Rattus norvegicus* and *R. rattus* (22), but various rodents and other wild and domestic animals, such as house mice, cats, opossums, shrews, and skunks, have also been seen to act occasionally as hosts (22). Rats serve not only as simple hosts, but also as amplifying hosts by making rickettsiae in their blood available for the bloodsucking vectors (22), although they remain rickettsemic for a limited period, approximately 7 to 12 days after inoculation (25).

After a rickettsemic blood meal from an infected rat, the flea becomes infected. Rickettsia in turn enters the midgut epithelial cells of the flea, where it multiplies and can persist for life without causing any damage. The bacterium is then released in the gut lumen and excreted with the feces. Rickettsia is then transmitted back to a susceptible vertebrate host upon subsequent feeding (22). Besides horizontal transmission—from flea to vertebrate host to uninfected flea—it is supported that the bacterium is additionally maintained in fleas by transovarial and transstadial transmission, but to a lesser extent (22,25).

Humans are infected through fleas. While feeding on a human host, the flea defecates, and the irritation caused by the bite causes the host to scratch and thus inoculate the rickettsiae, which is excreted in the flea feces, into the flea-bite site or skin abrasions. Rickettsiae can persist into the flea feces for several years (22,25) and they are also thought to infect humans via inhalation or contamination of the conjunctiva (22,25). The role of humans in the natural cycle of *R. typhi* is secondary, as they are only accidental hosts.

Murine typhus is found throughout the world, in environments ranging from hot and humid to cold and montane or semiarid (22), but is most prevalent in warmer countries (25). The fact that the patients usually mark a rather mild course and present with nonspecific symptoms makes it difficult to establish the true incidence of the disease, and so the number of reported cases does not reflect the true prevalence (24,25). Many reports illustrate that murine typhus is an emerging disease with worldwide distribution since it is found in areas not previously known to be endemic for this disease (27,28). In the United States, most cases occur in south Texas and southern California (18), whereas outbreaks have been reported worldwide (22,26,29–33). The seasonal and geographical distribution of the disease is strongly associated with the distribution of its hosts and vectors. Most cases occur in late summer or early autumn, as in Texas where cases are reported on April to June (18). This seasonal variation directly correlates with the abundance of the vector fleas (22), whereas human outbreaks and endemic foci are mainly described in areas with large rat populations (22,24). The distribution of murine typhus in many coastal areas is attributed to the introduction of infected rats and their fleas from ships, such as on the island of Euboea, where the installation of an endemic focus is attributed to the rats being transferred to this region via ships carrying wood (22,34).

In a study performed in Greece, the increase in human cases is noticed simultaneously with an increase in rat population of this area (14). In addition, there is a direct association between the incidence decline of murine typhus and the induction of rat and flea control programs by the public health services (22,24,35). Murine typhus can also occur in travelers returning from endemic regions (24,26).

PATHOPHYSIOLOGY

The clinical manifestations, laboratory abnormalities, and complications of the disease correlate with the underlying histopathology. Still, only few autopsy studies that give an accurate description of the pathologic effect of rickettsia on the various tissues exist.

The main finding is a systemic endothelial injury, a lymphohistiocytic vasculitis affecting almost any organ, with consequent interstitial pneumonitis, interstitial myocarditis, interstitial nephritis, portal triaditis, gastrointestinal tract vasculitis, and meningitis (26,36).

The frequent finding of transaminase elevation is attributed to the infiltrates found in the portal endothelium and the hepatic sinusoidal with occasional pseudogranuloma formation. Although swelling and necrosis of the hepatocytes were present, there was also evidence of rapid hepatocellular regeneration (36,37).

In some cases of severe murine typhus, with renal involvement and renal failure, renal biopsy revealed multifocal perivascular interstitial nephritis (38). Prerenal azotemia and hypoperfusion of the kidneys, secondary to loss of intravascular volume, due to increased vascular permeability caused by rickettsia, is another cause for renal failure (26). Hematuria, when present, is attributed to the infection of the glomerular endothelial cells and the hemorrhages of the urinary mucosa (36).

Thrombocytopenia, as well as leukopenia, is consistent with the consumption of platelets and leukocytes at the site of vascular inflammation (26). Hypoalbuminemia, electrolyte disturbances, and hypovolemia are attributed to the increased microcirculation permeability, causing leakage of serum, albumin, electrolytes, and intravascular volume from damaged capillaries (36). This increased vascular permeability may also lead, in most severe cases, to vasogenic cerebral edema and noncardiogenic pulmonary edema (39).

In one case with spleen involvement, computed tomography demonstrated intrasplenic pseudoaneurysms, infarcts, and hemorrhages, nonspecific findings consistent with vasculitis (40).

PATHOGENESIS

The recent complete genome analysis of *R. typhi* revealed 42 genes, suggested to be involved in pathogenesis (41). Those genes have to do with the escape of the bacterium from the defensive mechanisms of the host cell, mainly from the phagolysosome, and its intracellular survival, as well as with the production of hemolysins (41).

After adherence of the rickettsia to a protein-dependent receptor on the host-cell membrane, the cytoskeletal rearrangements at the attachment site result in rickettsial entry into the host cell by induced phagocytosis (42). The bacterium in turn escapes from the early phagosomes prior to phagolysosomal fusion, into the cytosol where it multiplies, avoiding the intracytoplasmic host-defensive mechanisms and acquiring the essential nutrients (e.g., glutamate, amino acids, adenosine diphosphate/adenosine triphosphate transporter) for its growth (42). The consequent membrane lysis allows the exit and hematogenous spread of rickettsiae toward vascular endothelial cells of almost every organ, causing disseminated vasculitis.

A phospholipase A2–like mechanism has been suggested as being responsible for the entry of rickettsia into the host cell, as well as for the exit from the phagosome and the cell (41,43,44), but its pathogenic role has still not been proven (42). The *pldA* gene, encoding a protein with phospholipase D activity, is found in *R. conorii* but is also present in the *R. typhi* genome; its functional role is yet to be determined (41). Host cell injury is also attributed to the generation of reactive oxygen species (ROS) produced by endothelial cells, whereas the simultaneous down-regulation of enzymes that protect the cells from oxidative injury leads to damage of the cellular membranes through lipid peroxidation (39). It is believed that the host-cell damage is attributed to both ROS and phospholipase A2–like activity, acting synergistically. Although lacking in knowledge about the endothelial cell alterations that account for increased vascular permeability, it is suggested that the pathogenic sequence includes hematogenous dissemination of rickettsiae throughout the vascular endothelial cells (mostly in brain and lungs), increased vascular permeability and edema, immunity mediated by NK cells and cytotoxic T-lymphocytes, as well as the release of inflammatory cytokines and antibodies. The activity of nitric oxide on the interendothelial tight junctions contributes to the above pathogenic mechanisms, while the activation of coagulation factors is believed to have a preventive role in vascular damage (45).

The activation of the endothelium after rickettsial infection leads to the production of cytokines and subsequent activation of the innate immune response (46). Interferon (IFN)-γ and tumornecrosis factor (TNF)-α are the two cytokines considered essential for the immune clearance of rickettsiae (42,46,47), which indicates the importance of cellular immunity as both these cytokines are produced by T lymphocytes and natural killer (NK) cells (46). Indeed, CD8 T lymphocytes play a crucial role in effective clearance of the rickettsiae, whereas NK cells contribute to the early immune response by secreting IFN-γ (42,47,48). Although CD8 T-lymphocytes are suggested to target and eliminate rickettsia-infected endothelial cells and macrophages by inducing apoptosis, cell necrosis is still believed to be the commonest mechanism of rickettsia-infected cells removal (42,49).

LABORATORY DIAGNOSIS

The early diagnosis of murine typhus is based chiefly on clinical suspicion since no reliable diagnostic test is available on the early phase of the illness. Thus, the presence of the typical clinical findings, in combination with a compatible epidemiological background, should raise the suspicion of the disease, while awaiting laboratory confirmation.

When choosing a diagnostic method, one must take into account its specificity, sensitivity, cost, the amount of antigen required, and its commercial availability.

Collection and Storage of Specimens

Specimens must be collected before antimicrobial therapy begins. Serological diagnosis requires sera from a blood sample of 10 mL. Samples can be preserved at −20°C for months without risk of degradation of the antibodies (50). Culture requires a blood sample of at least 5 mL, collected in heparin- or citrate-containing tubes. The leukocyte cell buffy coat is then collected and stored at −70°C, or in liquid nitrogen if culture is delayed for more than 24 hours. Ethylene diamine tetraacetic acid (EDTA) should not be used because it is harmful to the cell monolayers (50). For molecular diagnosis polymerase chain reaction (PCR), the blood sample is collected in an EDTA tube and stored at −20°C when the test has been delayed for more than 24 hours (50).

Pathological Examination

Because murine typhus has a low fatality rate, only very few autopsy studies have been performed (24). In one fatal case of an 81-year-old woman in Texas, the necropsy revealed the pathologic effect of rickettsia infection in various tissues (36). The most prominent finding was vascular injury, with consequent inflammatory vasculitis, in the visceral organs. The lung biopsy revealed injury of the pulmonary microcirculation with consequent diffuse alveolar damage, alveolar hemorrhages, and increased vascular permeability. Bronchi examination showed diffuse mucosal hyperemia and copious luminal mucus. Petechiae and vasculitis were present in the central nervous system.

Heart examination demonstrated interstitial mononuclear myocarditis in the absence of myocardial fiber necrosis. In the urinary tract, glomerular endothelial infection and urinary mucosal hemorrhages were observed. As in other organs, the gastrointestinal tract involvement consisted of vasculitis, whereas infection of the hepatic sinusoids was the main finding from the liver. Similar findings have been reported in other pathological examination (37). Splenic pathological examination performed in one case with splenic involvement, which required splenectomy, showed splenomegaly with multiple infarctions, focal capsular rupture, and intraparenchymal acute hemorrhage (40). Skin lesions are characterized by obliterative thrombovasculitis and perivascular nodules resembling epidemic typhus autopsy findings (17).

Isolation—Culture

In the past, embryonated chicken egg-yolk sacs and guinea pigs were widely used for the isolation of rickettsia. Today, these methods are being replaced by cell culture systems (51). The microorganism can be isolated by inoculation of specimens onto conventional cell cultures (Vero cells). The most recent technique is the centrifugation shell vial method (51), in which specimens are inoculated onto Vero or L929 cells on a coverslip within the shell vial and the ensuing centrifugation enhances the attachment and penetration of rickettsiae into cells (50). The technique allows the identification of new rickettsiae and ensures early diagnosis because it can give a positive result within three days from sampling, before the antibody titer rises (52). The delay between sampling and inoculation onto shell vials as well as the use of antibiotic therapy prior to sampling, are important factors that limit the possibility of a positive culture (50,51). However, the need for biosafety Level-3 laboratories does not allow its widespread use (50).

Molecular Methods

An adequately equipped laboratory is required in order to perform molecular methods. They are based on DNA amplification (PCR) targeting various rickettsial genes. The genes that are specific for the typhus group rickettsia are the *rrs*, *gltA*, *ompB*, and gene *D*. PCR is a rapid, sensitive, and specific method and is considered the technique of choice for early diagnosis of the disease because it can give a positive result before seroconversion (50,51). It is a significant tool in detecting rickettsiae in blood, skin biopsies, and ticks, and it is also used for differentiating the various species of rickettsia (51,53,54).

Serological Diagnosis

1. The Weil–Felix test (Weil and Felix, 1916): The test is based on the fact that *Proteus vulgaris* and rickettsia share some common antigens, as the lipopolysaccharide (LPS) from the typhus group rickettsiae and *P. vulgaris* OX-19 contain similar epitopes (55). During rickettsial infection, patients produce antibodies that react strongly with the Proteus strains OX-19 and OX-2. Antibodies are detectable 5 to 10 days after the onset of illness (51) and are mainly of the IgM subclass (56), thus being useful for the diagnosis of acute disease only. Due to the poor sensitivity and specificity of the method, it is no longer in use (51,57).
2. Indirect immunofluorescence assay (IFA): This is the reference method for the serodiagnosis of rickettsia in most laboratories (50,51). It is both sensitive and specific and allows the detection of IgG and IgM antibodies simultaneously. Antibodies are usually detected 7 to 15 days after disease onset (50). It can be used for both diagnosis and seroepidemiological studies (51). Individual laboratories determine their cut-off titers by taking into account the endemicity and seroprevalence of the disease in each area. Indicative cut-off titers from the Unité des Rickettsies (Marseille, France) have established IgG titers ≥1/64 and/or IgM ≥1/32 as suggestive of rickettsia infection (50). Serological diagnosis requires an IFA titer greater than or equal to the cut-off titer or a fourfold rise in antibody titer to *R. typhi* antigen, as measured by IFA, in acute- and convalescent-phase specimens, ideally taken after two and four weeks from disease onset, respectively (50,51).
3. Immunoperoxidase assay: This is an alternative technique to IFA used in laboratories lacking a UV microscope, in which peroxidase is used instead of fluorescein. It is both sensitive and specific (51,58). Its advantages, compared to IFA, are that it provides permanent preparations for re-examination and that it does not require a fluorescence microscope (59).
4. Complement fixation (CF): Although highly specific, the CF test lacks sensitivity, especially in the early stages of the disease, as it detects antibodies after the second week of the disease or even at the end of the fourth week (60). It is thus useful only for seroepidemiologic studies (51).
5. Enzyme-linked immunosorbent assay: Equally sensitive and specific to IFA (61,62), this test can be used for both acute cases and seroepidemiologic studies (51), because it can detect antibodies at a single dilution of serum up to a year from illness (62). The main disadvantage of this method is that it is time-consuming (51).
6. Western blotting: This is the most specific and sensitive test, detecting the early antibodies of the disease at an earlier stage compared to IFA (51,63). It helps in differentiating true-positive from false-positive results attributed to cross-reactions between biogroups and between species, by detecting group-specific antigens (51,63). As other serological methods detect the LPS and O antigens, which are common not only between rickettsial groups but also between other bacterial species (*Proteus* spp. and *Legionella* spp.), Western blotting can be used for the confirmation of diagnosis made by other methods in doubtful cases (51,63). It is also a very important tool for seroepidemiologic studies (64). The limitations of this technique are that it is time-consuming and is only available in reference laboratories.
7. Line blot assay: This test is based on the application of an antigen to nitrocellulose in a linear pattern with an ink pen point (65). More than 45 antigens are detected simultaneously with a single antibody (65). The test detects primarily group-reactive antigens rather than species-specific antigens (66). The line blot assay shows similar sensitivity and specificity to the microimmunofluorescence (MIF) assay (66).
8. Microagglutination: This test is less sensitive than the IFA and CF tests and shows the most cross reactions of all methods (67). Another major disadvantage to this test is the need for large amounts of purified antigen, as antibodies react with entire rickettsial cells (51).
9. Indirect hemagglutination test: Sheep or human erythrocytes, coated with erythrocyte-sensitizing substance (ESS), which is specific for rickettsiae, react with both IgM and IgG antibodies (68). It is both sensitive and specific with acute-phase sera, and so it is only used for the detection of acute disease (51). This simple method is less sensitive than IFA and does not require special technical training or advanced equipment in order to be performed (69).
10. Latex agglutination test: The latex test uses ESS adsorbed to latex particles as antigens (70). It is a simple and rapid method (results are obtained within 45 minutes), with sensitivity

comparable to that of mIFA (70). It mainly detects IgM antibodies in the first week after the appearance of symptoms, but no antibodies are detected after two months (51). Its major disadvantage is the cost of reagents needed (51). It is useful in small nonequipped laboratories (71).

11. Cross-adsorption: This technique is used to eliminate false-positive results through cross reactions between bacteria sharing common antigens. In case of *R. typhi* infection, IgM cross reactions with Legionella and Proteus OX-19 may lead to false diagnosis (72). The need for a large amount of antigen is an important drawback to this method (51).

CLINICAL MANIFESTATIONS

As the disease is currently found less frequently, its clinical presentation can be easily confused. A high index of suspicion is necessary for establishing diagnosis, depending mainly on epidemiological grounds, as the classic triad of fever, headache, and rash, which are considered the prominent manifestations of the disease, is of limited usefulness for an immediate or early diagnosis.

The illness usually presents with an abrupt onset of symptoms following an incubation period of 6 to 14 days (73). In our study of 83 consecutive cases of murine typhus in the island of Crete, Greece (14), the most common clinical manifestations were: fever (100%), headache (88%), chills (87%), and rash (80%). Forty-nine patients (59%) presented with rash, whereas 17 additional patients (20%) developed rash during hospitalization. Similar rates were found in another study at the island of Euboea, Greece (34).

Other investigators report the following most common presenting symptoms: fever (in 96% of cases), followed by headache (45%), chills (44%), and nausea (33%). Rash at presentation was observed in only 18% of patients, but over the course of illness, 54% to 63% developed rash (18,73).

Rash in these reports appears at various intervals after the onset of fever, with a median onset at six days and a range of up to 18 days. The appearance of the rash is described as macular (in 49%), maculopapular (29%), papular (14%), petechial (6%), and morbilliform (3%). It most frequently affects the trunk (72–88%), but it is also found on the extremities. Involvement of the palms (38–55%), soles, or face has been rarely noted. Spread of the rash from the trunk to the extremities and from the extremities to the trunk appears to be equally frequent (18,73).

In our series, four patients (5%) had both spleen and liver enlargement, whereas isolated liver or spleen enlargement was observed in 19 (23%) and in 18 (22%) patients, respectively (14). Lymphadenopathy was noted in three patients (4%) (14). Other symptoms such as malaise, anorexia, myalgia, cough, perspiration, conjunctivitis, nausea, joint pain, and so on. were less common (Table 1).

Central nervous system abnormalities were involved in a small part of our series (9.6%), which concurs with earlier studies where it was stated that endemic typhus rarely causes neuropsychiatric disorders (74).

Gastrointestinal symptoms, as a result of the vascular damage caused by *R. typhi*, were few (18%) and mild in our patient population, a difference from previous studies regarding gastrointestinal symptoms that can be owed to our high index of suspicion of the disease that led to earlier administration of treatment in our patients (14). However, one series of 97 pediatric patients presented with a different variety of symptoms, as the clinical triad of fever, headache, and rash was noted in only 49%, while GI symptoms were noted in a higher percentage (77 out of 97 children) (75).

Laboratory Abnormalities

The most prominent biochemical abnormality observed in our patients was the elevation of aminotransferases (in 85% of our patients), a finding that is in agreement with previous studies (18).

The most frequent laboratory abnormalities in patient populations with murine typhus are: mildly elevated serum aspartate aminotransferase levels (90%), elevated alanine aminotransferase levels (73%), elevated lactate dehydrogenase levels (87%), mild hyponatremia

TABLE 1 Murine Typhus in Crete: Clinical Manifestations, Main Clinical Signs and Complications in 83 Patients

	Number of patients	Percentage
Clinical manifestations		
Fever	83/83	100.0
Headache	73/83	88.0
Chills	72/83	86.7
Rash	66/83	79.5
Malaise	46/83	55.4
Anorexia	44/83	53.0
Myalgia	37/83	44.6
Nonproductive cough	23/83	27.7
Perspiration	21/83	25.3
Conjuctivitis	21/83	25.6
Nausea-vomiting	15/83	18.1
Arthralgia	10/83	12.0
Abdominal pain	9/83	10.8
Diarrhea	9/83	10.8
CNS involvement	8/83	9.6
Confusion	8/83	9.6
Iritis	2/83	2.4
Clinical signs and complications		
Splenomegaly	19/83	22.8
Hepatomegaly	18/83	21.6
Lymphadenopathy	3/83	3.6
Pulmonary infiltrates	4/83	4.8
Pleural effusion	2/83	2.4
Acute renal failure	4/83	4.8
DIC	1/83	1.2

Abbreviations: CNS, central nervous system; DIC, disseminated intravascular coagulation.
Source: From Ref. 14.

(60%), and hypocalcemia (79%) (14). Fifteen percent of our patients had elevated levels of alkaline phosphatase during the first week of hospitalization (Table 2). Both normal and high values have been reported in the literature, but no convincing explanation for this disagreement has been given (18,76).

Hypoalbuminemia was found in all published series, including ours (14), which may be interpreted by vascular damage resulting in albumin leakage. The presence of this abnormality in 60% of patients one month later indicates that this damage takes a long time to be repaired (18,73,76,77).

The white blood cell count showed that in a small number of cases (6 of 83 in our series) leukopenia occurs early, as others had previously indicated. In advanced stages, the white blood cell count is normal or even elevated (18). The earliest and the most prominent hematological abnormality, found in 51% of our patients, was thrombocytopenia, suggesting consumption of platelets at the sites of rickettsial-mediated vascular injury (14).

TABLE 2 Main Laboratory Abnormalities in 83 Greek Patients with Murine Typhus

Laboratory abnormalities	Mean value	Percentage of patients	Normal range of values
AST	74 U/L	86%	12–32 U/L
LDH	320 U/L	82%	89–221 U/L
ALT	64 U/L	64%	4–36 U/L
CPK	329 U/L	42%	26–174 U/L
Sodium	136 mEq/L	37%	136–142 mEq/L

Abbreviations: ALT, alanine aminotransferase; AST, aspartate aminotransferase; CPK, creatine kinase; LDH, lactate dehydrogenase.
Source: Adapted from Ref. 14.

Complications

The clinical course of murine typhus is usually uncomplicated, and fatalities are uncommon (<5%) (18). Although most patients experience mild illness, mental confusion and other neuropsychiatric disorders (seizures, stupor, prostration, lethargy) as well as signs and symptoms indicating renal (vide infra), hepatic (jaundice), pulmonary (pleural effusion, respiratory failure), and cardiac dysfunction may occur in severe cases. Any organ may be affected, and, if left untreated, multiple organ dysfunction syndrome may occur.

When complications do occur, the most frequent is mild renal insufficiency (presenting with azotemia/proteinuria), which occurs in a minority of patients (22%) as a result of various mechanisms, including decreased renal perfusion (prerenal) and acute interstitial nephritis (78).

Cardiac abnormalities include minimal electrocardiographic abnormalities, peripheral cyanosis, and cold sweating, but clinical evidence of cardiac failure is unusual. A possible life-threatening situation is the infection of a patient with G6PD insufficiency, where severe hemolysis may lead to serious anemia and acute renal failure. The first description of a case involving G6PD insufficiency and murine typhus was in Vietnam, where an American soldier developed acute renal failure and severe hemolysis (19).

Although this association was also found in fulminant Rocky Mountain spotted fever (*R. rickettsii*) and severe infection with the agent of boutonneuse fever (*R. conorii*), it has never been conclusively established and it has been proposed that G6PD-associated hemolysis may somehow aggravate or potentiate vasculitis (79).

In our studies, the clinical course was complicated by acute renal failure (14,34). In the latter series, where 83 cases were involved, acute renal failure was observed in four patients (5%), pulmonary infiltrates in four patients (5%), and pleural effusion was present in two of them (2%). The fact that the complication rates were so low can be interpreted by the earlier administration of treatment in our patients because of the high index of suspicion of the disease.

Differential Diagnosis

The differential diagnosis of murine typhus, which is similar to but has a milder clinical course than that of epidemic typhus, includes Rocky Mountain spotted fever, ehrlichiosis, meningococcemia, measles, typhoid fever, bacterial and viral meningitis, viral hemorrhagic fever, secondary syphilis, leptospirosis, toxic shock syndrome, Kawasaki disease, and fevers acquired in the tropics and malaria, which should always be excluded by the examination of blood films.

TREATMENT

Endemic typhus is a disease with a good prognosis. Complete clinical recovery is observed over a period of 15 days from initiation of symptoms, even if not treated at all (77), which confers long-lasting immunity to reinfection (26).

The mortality rate is minimal. For example, in one large series, only two of 80 patients died (80), whereas in our series (involving 83 patients), these were no fatalities (14). The antibiotics that have been proved sufficient for therapy of patients with endemic typhus are tetracycline and chloramphenicol.

The drug of choice not only for nonpregnant adults, but also for children of all ages is doxycycline. The recommended dosage for adults is 100 mg orally every 12 hours (81) and for children 5 mg/kg/day in two doses up to a maximum dose of 100 mg per dose. Intravenous administration has been mentioned in severe cases (82). It has been stated that although the manufacturer of doxycycline does not publish dosage recommendations for children younger than the age of eight years (83), the danger of teeth discoloration has been proved to be minimal, when short-term therapy of 7 to 10 days for rickettsioses is applied (84). It is also proposed that children weighing less than 45 kg should receive 0.9 mg/kg/day in two divided doses. Children weighing more than 45 kg should receive the adult dose (24).

The optimal duration of therapy has not been assessed in clinical studies. Duration of 7 to 15 days is recommended (81), or for at least 48 hours after the patient has become afebrile. Therapeutic regimens with a single dose of 200 mg of doxycycline have been tested with adequate results (85). The use of tetracycline is contra-indicated during pregnancy, as it may cause liver damage to the mother and teeth abnormalities to the fetus.

In vitro studies using cell cultures for the evaluation of *R. typhi* susceptibility to antibiotics, by the methods of immunofluorescence and quantitative PCR DNA, have exhibited doxycycline as the most potent antibiotic, presenting the smaller minimum inhibitory concentration (MIC) (20,86).

Clinical trials have shown that response to doxycycline is rapid, as defervescence occurs in two to three days with a mean of 35 hours, ranging from 4 to 66 hours in one study (85). In our clinical study regarding the effectiveness of different antibiotic regimens in terms of duration of the fever, we found a mean of 2.9 days for defervescence after the administration of doxycycline. Additionally, the response observed after treatment with chloramphenicol or ciprofloxacin was 4.0 and 4.2 days for defervescence, respectively (87).

Chloramphenicol is considered to be effective as an alternative antibiotic (85,87) when tetracycline is contra-indicated, although it has a 1:25,000 to 1:40,000 risk of fatal aplastic anemia, which has limited its use. Chloramphenilol is the drug of choice for pregnant patients, except for the parturient, due to the danger of gray syndrome for the infant (24). However, relapse of the disease has been reported in patients who were treated with chloramphenicol (88).

There are no in vitro studies in the literature regarding *R. typhi* susceptibility to chloramphenicol. Earlier studies using embryonated eggs demonstrated minimal efficacy of this antibiotic (89). Chloramphenicol is administered in four divided doses of 50 mg/kg/day, orally or intravenously, up to a maximum dose of 2 g/day, until four to five days after the patient becomes afebrile (24).

Fluoroquinolones (ciprofloxacin, ofloxacin, pefloxacin, and levofloxacin) have been proved effective on *R. typhi* in vitro in cell cultures, although their exact potency has not been tested clinically. Ciprofloxacin is the only fluoroquinolone used on a clinical level, on a small number of patients, presenting controversial results (87,90,91).

Other antibiotics, indicated from in vitro studies to be effective on *R. typhi*, but with no clinical application, include rifampicin, thiamphenicol, macrolides, erythromycin, clarithromycin, josamycin (20,86), as well as telithromycin (20,92), while amoxicillin, gentamycin, and trimethoprime—sulfamethoxazole were shown to be ineffective.

PREVENTION

Prevention of murine typhus is directed primarily at controlling the flea vector and the mammalian reservoirs of infection. The incidence of endemic typhus has decreased as a result of the reduction of rat and rat-flea populations. This has been accomplished by the motivation of several rat-control activities, such as eliminating rodents from food depots, granaries, and residences; rat trapping and application of rodenticides; and dusting harborages with carbaryl or permethrin for flea control (26). All suspected cases of murine typhus should be reported to local health authorities due to the danger of epidemic spread. No effective vaccine is available for murine typhus.

REFERENCES

1. Zarafonetis CJD. The typhus fevers. In: Internal Medicine in World War II. Vol. II, Chapter VII. Medical Department, United States Army, 1963:221–223.
2. Kligler IJ, Comaroff R. An epidemic outbreak of murine typhus in a labour group in an inland village in Palestine. Trans R Soc Trop Med Hyg 1936; 30:363–368.
3. Neill MH. Experimental typhus in Guinea pigs. In: A Description of a Scrotal Lesion in Guinea pigs Infected with Mexican Typhus. Vol. 33. Washington: Pub. Health Rep, 1917:1105.
4. Mooser H. An American type of typhus. Trans R Soc Trop Med Hyg 1928; 22:175–176.
5. Reitler R, Btesh S, Marberg K. Endemic typhus in Palestine. Trans R Soc Trop Med Hyg 1939; 33:197–212.
6. Mooser H. Experiments relating to pathology and etiology of Mexican typhus (Tabardillo): clinical course and pathologic anatomy of Tabardillo in guinea pigs. J Infect Dis 1928; 43:241–260.
7. Fletcher W, Lesslar JE. Tropical typhus in the Federated Malay States. Bull Inst Med Res 1925; 2:1–58.
8. Maxcy KF. An epidemiological study of endemic typhus (Brill's disease) in the southeastern United States. Pub Health Rep 1926; 41:2967–2995.
9. Dyer RE, Rumreich A, Badger LF. Typhus fever: a virus of the typhus type derived from fleas collected from wild rats. Pub Health Rep 1931; 46:334–338.

10. Quintal D. Historical aspects of the rickettsioses. Clin Dermatol 1996; 14:237–242.
11. Mooser H, Castaneda MR, Zinsser H. Mexican typhus from rat to rat by polyplax spinulosus. J Exp Med 1931; 54:567–575.
12. Lépine P. Sur la présence dans l'encéphale des rat captures à Athenes d'un virus revêtant les caractères expérimentaux du typhus exanthématique (virus mexicain). C R Acad Sci 1932; 194:401–403.
13. Lorandos N. Cases of endemic typhus (Brill's disease) in Athens. Med Athens 1934; 42:639–641.
14. Gikas A, Doukakis S, Pediaditis IJ, et al. Murine typhus in Greece: epidemiological, clinical, and therapeutic data from 83 cases. Trans R Soc Trop Med Hyg 2002; 96:250–253.
15. Stuart G, Krikorian K. Typhus v. rabies. Trans R Soc Trop Med Hyg 1932; 25:353–366.
16. Wolbach SB. Typhus. In: Musser Internal Medicine. Philadelphia: Lea & Febiger, 1938.
17. Baxter J. The typhus group. Clin Dermatol 1996; 14:271–275.
18. Dumler JS, Taylor JP, Walker DH. Clinical and laboratory features of murine typhus in Texas, 1980 through 1987. J Am Med Assoc 1991; 266:1365–1370.
19. Whelton A, Donadio JV Jr, Elisberg BL. Acute renal failure complicating rickettsial infections in glucose-6-phosphate dehydrogenase-deficient individuals. Ann Intern Med 1968; 69:323.
20. Rolain JM, Stuhl L, Maurin M, et al. Evaluation of antibiotic susceptibilities of three rickettsial species including *Rickettsia felis* by a quantitative PCR DNA assay. Antimicrob Agents Chemother 2002; 46(9):2747–2751.
21. Tselentis Y, Edlinger E, Alexious G, et al. An endemic focus of murine typhus in Europe. J Infect 1986; 13:91–92.
22. Azad AF. Epidemiology of murine typhus. Annu Rev Entomol 1990; 35:553–569.
23. Chaniotis B, Psarulaki A, Chaliotis G, et al. Transmission cycle of murine typhus in Greece. Ann Trop Med Parasitol 1994; 88(6):645–647.
24. Sexton DJ. Murine Typhus. In: Rose BD, ed. MA, USA: Waltham, 2005.
25. Raoult D, Roux V. Rickettsioses as paradigms of new or emerging infectious diseases. Clin Microbiol Rev 1997; 10(4):694–719.
26. Dumler JS, Walker DH. *Rickettsia typhi* (murine typhus). In: Mandell, Douglas and Bennett's Principles and Practice of Infectious Diseases. 5th ed. Philadelphia: Churchill-Livingstone, 2000:2053–2055.
27. Roberts S, Hill P, Croxson M, et al. The evidence for rickettsial disease arising in New Zealand. NZ Med J 2001; 114:370.
28. Letaief AO, Kaabia N, Chakroun M, et al. Clinical and laboratory features of murine typhus in central Tunisia: a report of seven cases. Int J Infect Dis 2005; 9(6):331–334.
29. Al-Awadi AR, Al-Kazemi N, Ezzat G, et al. Murine typhus in Kuwait in 1978. Bull WHO 1982; 60:283–289.
30. Duffy PE, Le Buillouzic H, Gass RF, et al. Murine typhus identified as a major cause of febrile illness in a camp for displaced Khmers in Thailand. Am J Trop Med Hyg 1990; 43:520–526.
31. Fan MY, Walker DH, Yu SR, et al. Epidemiology and ecology of rickettsial diseases in the People's Republic of China. Rev Infect Dis 1987; 9:823–840.
32. Woodruff PW, Morrill JC, Burans JP, et al. A study of viral and rickettsial exposure and causes of fever in Juba, southern Sudan. Trans R Soc Trop Med Hyg 1988; 82:761–766.
33. Tissot-Dupont H, Brouqui P, Faugere B, et al. Prevalence of antibodies to *Coxiella burnetii*, *Rickettsia conorii*, and *Rickettsia typhi* in seven African countries. Clin Infect Dis 1995; 21:1126–1133.
34. Tselentis Y, Babalis U, Chrysanthis D, et al. Clinicoepidemiological study of murine typhus on the Greek island of Evia. Eur J Epidemiol 1992; 8(2):268–272.
35. Centers for Disease Control and Prevention. Outbreak of murine typhus—Texas. Morb Mortal Wkly Rep 1983; 32:131–132.
36. Walker DH, Parks FM, Betz TG, et al. Histopathology and immunohistologic demonstration of the distribution of *Rickettsia typhi* in fatal murine typhus. Am J Clin Pathol 1989; 91:720.
37. Binford CH, Ecker HD. Endemic (murine) typhus: report of autopsy findings in three cases. Am J Clin Pathol 1947; 17:797–806.
38. Silpapojakul K, Mitarnun W, Ovartlarnporn B, et al. Liver involvement in murine typhus. Q J Med 1996; 89(8):623–629.
39. Olano JP. Rickettsial infection. 4th International Conference on Rickettsiae and Rickettsial Diseases, Book of abstracts (L3), Spain, June 18–21, 2005.
40. Radin R, Hirbawi IA, Henderson RW. Splenic involvement in endemic (murine) typhus: CT findings. Abdom Imaging 2001; 26:298–299.
41. McLeod MP, Qin X, Karpathy SE, et al. Complete genome sequence of *Rickettsia typhi* and comparison with sequences of other rickettsiae. J Bacteriol 2004; 186(17):5842–5855.
42. Walker DH, Valbuena GA, Olano JP. Pathogenic mechanisms of diseases caused by Rickettsia. Ann NY Acad Sci 2003; 990:1–11.
43. Schmiela DH, Millera VL. Bacterial phospholipases and pathogenesis. Microbes Infect 1999; 1:1103–1112.
44. Walker DH, Feng HM, Popov VL. Rickettsial phospholipase A2 as a pathogenic mechanism in a model of cell injury by typhus and spotted fever group rickettsiae. Am J Trop Med Hyg 2001; 65(6):936–942.

45. Woods ME, Koo P, Wen G, et al. Nitric oxide (NO) as a mediator of increased microvascular permeability during rickettsial infection. 4th International Conference on Rickettsiae and Rickettsial Diseases, Book of Abstracts (0–59), Spain, June 18–21, 2005.
46. Valbuena G, Feng HM, Walker DH. Mechanisms of immunity against rickettsiae: new perspectives and opportunities offered by unusual intracellular parasites. Microbes Infect 2002; 4:625–633.
47. Walker DH, Popov VL, Feng HM. Establishment of a novel endothelial target mouse model of a typhus group rickettsiosis: evidence for critical roles for gamma interferon and CD8 T lymphocytes. Lab Invest 2000; 80(9):1361–1372.
48. Billings AN, Feng HM, Olano JP, et al. Rickettsial infection in murine models activates an early anti-rickettsial effect mediated by NK cells and associated with production of gamma interferon. Am J Trop Med Hyg 2001; 65(1):52–56.
49. Walker DH, Olano JP, Feng HM. Critical role of cytotoxic T lymphocytes in immune clearance of rickettsial infection. Infect Immun 2001; 69(3):1841–1846.
50. Brouqui P, Bacellar F, Baranton G, et al. ESCMID Study Group on Coxiella, Anaplasma, Rickettsia and Bartonella; European Network for Surveillance of Tick-Borne Diseases. Guidelines for the diagnosis of tick-borne bacterial diseases in Europe. Clin Microbiol Infect 2004; 12:1108–1132.
51. La Scola B, Raoult D. Laboratory diagnosis of rickettsiosis: current approaches to diagnosis of old and new rickettsial diseases. J Clin Microbiol 1997; 35(11):2715–2727.
52. Marrero M, Raoult D. Centrifugation–shell vial technique for rapid detection of Mediterranean spotted fever rickettsia in blood culture. Am J Trop Med Hyg 1989; 40:197–199.
53. Azad AF, Webb L, Carl M, et al. Detection of rickettsiae in arthropod vectors by DNA amplification using the polymerase chain reaction. Ann NY Acad Sci 1990; 590:557–563.
54. Tzianabos T, Anderson BE, McDade JE. Detection of *Rickettsia rickettsii* DNA in clinical specimens by using polymerase chain reaction technology. J Clin Microbiol 1989; 27(12):2866–2868.
55. Amano KI, Kyohno K, Aoki S, et al. Serological studies of the antigenic similarity between typhus group rickettsiae and Weil–Felix test antigens. Microbiol Immunol 1995; 39:63–65.
56. Amano KI, Hatakeyama H, Okutta M, et al. Serological studies of antigenic similarity between Japanese spotted fever rickettsiae and Weil–Felix test antigens. J Clin Microbiol 1992; 30:2441–2444.
57. Kaplan JE, Schonberger LB. The sensitivity of various serologic tests in the diagnosis of Rocky Mountain spotted fever. Am J Trop Med Hyg 1986; 35(4):840–844.
58. Kelly DJ, Wong PW, Gan E, et al. Comparative evaluation of the indirect immunoperoxidase test for the serodiagnosis of rickettsial disease. Am J Trop Med Hyg 1988; 38:400–406.
59. Yamamoto S, Minamishima Y. Serodiagnosis of Tsutsugamushi Fever (Scrub Typhus) by the indirect immunoperoxidase technique. J Clin Microbiol 1982; 15(6):1128–1132.
60. Shepard CC, Redus MA, Tzianabos T, et al. Recent experience with the complement fixation test in the laboratory diagnosis of rickettsial diseases in the United States. J Clin Microbiol 1976; 4:277–283.
61. Dobson ME, Azad AF, Dasch GA, et al. Detection of murine typhus infected fleas with an enzyme-linked immunosorbent assay. Am J Med Hyg 1989; 40(5):521–528.
62. Clements ML, Dumler JS, Fiset P, et al. Serodiagnosis of Rocky Mountain spotted fever: comparison of IgM and IgG enzyme-linked immunosorbent assays and indirect fluorescent antibody test. J Infect Dis 1983; 148(5):876–880.
63. Teysseire N, Raoult D. Comparison of Western immunoblotting and microimmunofluorescence for diagnosis of Mediterranean Spotted fever. J Clin Microbiol 1992; 30(2):455–460.
64. Babalis T, Dupont HT, Tselentis Y, et al. *Rickettsia conorii* in Greece: comparison of a microimmunofluorescence assay and Western blotting for seroepidemiology. Am J Trop Med Hyg 1993; 48(6):784–792.
65. Raoult D, Dasch GA. The line blot: an immunoassay for monoclonal and other antibodies: its application to the serotyping of gram-negative bacteria. J Immunol Methods 1989; 125(1–2):57–65.
66. Raoult D, Dasch GA. Line blot and Western blot immunoassays for diagnosis of Mediterranean spotted fever. J Clin Microbiol 1989; 27:2073–2079.
67. Newhouse VF, Shepard CC, Redus MD, et al. A comparison of the complement fixation, indirect fluorescent antibody, and microagglutination tests for the serological diagnosis of rickettsial diseases. Am J Trop Med Hyg 1979; 28(2):387–395.
68. Anacker RL, Philip RN, Thomas LA, et al. Indirect hemagglutination test for detection of antibody to *Rickettsia rickettsii* in sera from humans and common laboratory animals. J Clin Microbiol 1979; 10:677–684.
69. Shirai A, Dietel JW, Osterman JV. Indirect hemagglutination test for human antibody to typhus and Spotted Fever group rickettsiae. J Clin Microbiol 1975; 10:677–684.
70. Rawlings JA, Elliott LB, Little LM. Comparison of a latex agglutination procedure with the microimmunofluorescence test for *Rickettsia typhi*. J Clin Microbiol 1985; 21(3):470–471.
71. Hechemy KE, Osterman JV, Eisemann CS, et al. Detection of typhus antibodies by latex agglutination. J Clin Microbiol 1981; 13:214–216.
72. Raoult D, Dasch GA. Immunoblot cross-reactions among *Rickettsia*, *Proteus* spp. and *Legionella* spp. in patients with Mediterranean spotted fever. FEMS Immunol Med Microbiol 1995; 11:13–18.
73. Betz TG, Rawlings JA, Taylor JP, et al. Endemic typhus in Texas. Tex Med 1983; 79:48–53.

74. Samra Y, Shaked Y, Maier MK. Delayed neurologic display in murine typhus: report of two cases. Arch Intern Med 1989; 149:949–951.
75. Whiteford SF, Taylor JP, Dumler JS. Clinical, laboratory, and epidemiologic features of murine typhus in 97 Texas children. Arch Pediatr Adolesc Med 2001; 155:396.
76. Woodward TE. Murine typhus fever: clinical signs, symptoms, and pathophysiology. In: Walker DH, ed. Biology of Rickettsial Diseases. Boca Raton, FL: CRC Press, 1988:79–92.
77. Stuart BM, Pullen RL. Endemic (murine) typhus fever: clinical observations of 180 cases. Ann Intern Med 1945; 23:520–536.
78. Shaked Y, Shpilberg O, Samra Y. Involvement of the kidneys in Mediterranean spotted fever and murine typhus. Q J Med 1994; 87(2):103–107.
79. Walker DH. Rocky Mountain spotted fever: a seasonal alert. Clin Infect Dis 1995; 20:1111.
80. Fergie JE, Purcell K, Wanat D. Murine typhus in south Texas children. Pediatr Infect Dis J 2000; 19:535.
81. Raoult D, Drancourt M. Antimicrobial therapy of rickettsial diseases. Antimicrob Agents Chemother 1991; 35:2457–2462.
82. Masahla R, Merkin-Zaborsky H, Matar M, et al. Murine typhus presenting as subacute meningoencephalitis. J Neurol 1998; 245(10):665–668.
83. Abramson JS, Givner LB. Should tetracycline be contraindicated for therapy of presumed Rocky Mountain spotted fever? Pediatrics 1990; 86:123.
84. Committee on Infectious Diseases of the American Academy of Pediatrics. Report of the committee on Infectious Diseases. 22nd ed. Elk Grove Village, IL: American Academy of Pediatrics, 1991:407.
85. Silpapojakul K, Chayakul P, Krisanapan S. Murine typhus in Thailand: clinical features, diagnosis and treatment. Q J Med 1993; 86(1):43–47.
86. Rolain JM, Maurin M, Vestris G, et al. In vitro susceptibilities of 27 rickettsiae to 13 antimicrobials. Antimicrob Agents Chemother 1998; 42(7):1537–1541.
87. Gikas A, Doukakis S, Pediaditis J, et al. Comparison of the effectiveness of five different antibiotic regimens on infection with *Rickettsia typhi*: therapeutic data from 87 cases. Am J Trop Med Hyg 2004; 70(5):576–579.
88. Shaked Y, Samra Y, Maier MK, et al. Relapse of rickettsial Mediterranean spotted fever and murine typhus after treatment with chloramphenicol. J Infect 1989; 18(1):35–37.
89. Jackson EB. Comparative efficacy of several antibiotics on experimental rickettsial infections in embryonated eggs. Antibiot Chemother 1951; 1:231–241.
90. Laferl H, Fournier PE, Seiberl G, et al. Murine typhus poorly responsive to ciprofloxacin: a case report. J Travel Med 2002; 9(2):103–104.
91. Strand O, Stromberg A. Ciprofloxacin treatment of murine typhus. Scand J Infect Dis 1990; 22(4):503–504.
92. Rolain JM, Maurin M, Bryskier A, et al. In vitro activities of telithromycin (HMR 3647) against *Rickettsia rickettsii*, *Rickettsia conorii*, *Rickettsia africae*, *Rickettsia typhi*, *Rickettsia prowazekii*, *Coxiella burnetii*, *Bartonella henselae*, *Bartonella quintana*, *Bartonella bacilliformis*, and *Ehrlichia chaffeensis*. Antimicrob Agents Chemother 2000; 44(5):1391–1393.

5 | Louse-Borne Epidemic Typhus

Linda Houhamdi
Faculté de Médecine, Unité des Rickettsies, Institut Fédératif de Recherche 48, Centre National de Recherche Scientifique, Université de la Méditerranée, Marseille, France

Didier Raoult
Faculté de Médecine, Unité des Rickettsies, Université de la Méditerranée, Marseille, France

HISTORY AND EPIDEMIOLOGY OF EPIDEMIC TYPHUS

The life-threatening louse-borne epidemic typhus, also named "jail fever," caused by a rickettsia of typhus group, *Rickettsia prowazekii*, and vectorized by the human body louse, is one of the most dangerous arthropod-borne diseases. Zinsser (1) stated that epidemic typhus has probably caused more deaths than all of the wars in history. The origin of typhus is controversial. Some authors consider it to be an old European disease that caused the Athens plague. Others believe that the reservoir is extra-human and is of American origin, as shown by its presence in isolates from flying squirrels, *Glaucomys volans volans* (2), and their fleas and lice.

It is difficult to confirm that past diseases classically considered to be typhus were in fact epidemic typhus, before the description of its clinical and epidemiological entities (3,4) during the sixteenth century (when the presence of an exanthema allowed its distinction from typhoid fever). However, the Napoleonic Wars were an example of the terrible consequences of a combination of war and cold. The Grand Army marched to Moscow with 550,000 men and only 3000 came back. It is likely that 20% of the troops died of typhus (1,5). Typhus reemerged during World War I, but the Russians experienced the most terrible outbreak during the revolution between 1917 and 1925, when 25 million people were infected and three million died (6). During World War II, typhus was prevalent in Northern Africa and in Central and Eastern Europe, where terrible outbreaks occurred in concentration camps (7). Typhus has slowly declined since the end of the World War II, and the last reports of outbreaks were in Africa (2,8–12). Only a few reports have mentioned its presence in the Americas, such as in Guatemala (13), in U.S.A. (2,8–10,14), and in China (15). Until the last decades, typhus was considered a disease of the past, and in 1995 it was suspected to be prevalent only in Ethiopia (16). No cases had been recorded in Eastern Europe (including Russia, since the 1980s), nor in Africa (Rwanda, Burundi, Uganda, and Nigeria), which were regular foci (17). Few data were obtained from other mountainous tropical countries (such as Tibet, Nepal, or Peru), which were still louse-infested. However, since 1995, typhus has dramatically reemerged (Fig. 1). A large outbreak was reported in Burundi in 1997 during the civil war (18–20), in which 100,000 people were estimated to be infected. Small outbreaks were observed in Russia in 1997 (21) and in Peru in 1998 (22). Sporadic cases were reported in Northern Africa (23,24) and in France in a homeless (25).

As it has the most serious epidemic potential of all rickettsiae, louse-borne epidemic typhus should be considered a serious threat, even in developed countries (26–32), when body lice are prevalent. Epidemic typhus is currently considered as a potential bioterrorism agent (category B, Centers for Disease Control and Prevention).

THE CAUSATIVE AGENT: *RICKETTSIA PROWAZEKII*
Bacteriology of *R. prowazekii*

R. prowazekii (Fig. 2) belongs to the Rickettsiales order of which the members are short (0.8–2-μm long and 0.3–0.5-μm diameter), Gram-negative bacillary microorganisms that retain basic fuchsin when stained by the Gimenez method (33). Rickettsiae live only intracellularly, but not enclosed in a vacuole (34,35). The genome of 1.1 Mb of *R. prowazekii*, consisted of a single circular chromosome, has been completely sequenced (36).

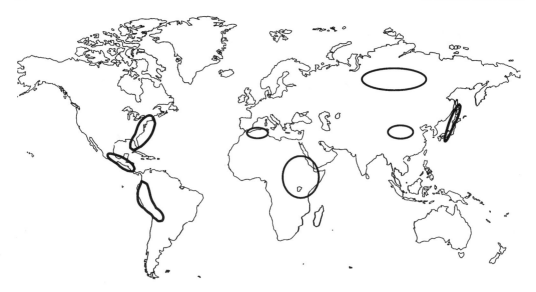

FIGURE 1 Geographical distribution of louse-borne epidemic typhus according to detection and/or isolation of R. prowazekii from patients or human body lice.

Traditional identification methods used in bacteriology cannot be applied to rickettsiae because of their strictly intracellular nature. For a long time, serological typing by microimmunofluorescence with mouse antisera has remained the reference method for the identification of rickettsiae (37). The usefulness of restriction fragment length polymorphism analysis of polymerase chain reaction (PCR)-amplified fragments of the citrate synthase (38) and the outer membrane protein B (39) was described. The advent of molecular taxonomic methods has enabled the determination of phylogenetic relationships between bacterial species (40) and placed *Rickettsia* species within the α subgroup of Proteobacteria (41). Phylogenetic analysis of the rickettsiae is based on comparisons of 16S rRNA and citrate synthase (42–44) gene sequences, and more recently the multispacer typing method (45).

Origin of *Rickettsia prowazekii*

Because the human body louse itself is probably 5000 to 10,000 years old, the pathogens strictly associated with it represent a recent evolution, as indicated by the fact that they appear to be strictly confined to humans (46). The fact that *R. prowazekii* is so aggressive to the louse is also in favor of its recent apparition as a louse/human pathogen.

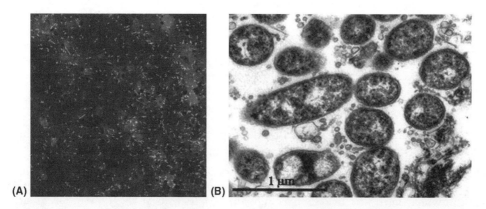

FIGURE 2 **(A)** *R. prowazekii* in the digestive cells of experimentally infected human body louse [immunofluorescence staining, confocal microscopy; original magnification: ×600] and in their feces **(B)** [transmission electron microscopy].

There are conflicting theories regarding the origin of *R. prowazekii*, but one of the most consistent is that it is a recent pathogen that first appeared in America, where the only nonhuman reservoir was found to be flying squirrels (2). The fact that *R. prowazekii* could use the louse as a vector meant that the Spanish imported the body louse, which led to epidemic typhus sometime in sixteenth century (46). It could be speculated that after infection of a louse-infested human, contaminated by the flying squirrel reservoir, the disease spread from Mexico, where it was described by the Aztec (46). This theory may be challenged by the report of the presence of *R. prowazekii* in *Amblyomma* ticks in Ethiopia and in Mexico.

Reservoir of *R. prowazekii*

The human body louse is the only established vector for *R. prowazekii*. Lice die of their infection with *R. prowazekii* and do not transmit their infection to their progeny, the main reservoir (except in the United States, where the flying squirrels are implicated) appears to be in humans. To contaminate lice and allow transmission, bacteremia may occur and be prolonged. *R. prowazekii* is not eradicated at the apparent end of the disease. Nicolle (47) reported that chronic asymptomatic bacteremia could be observed. Humans who contact typhus retain some rickettsiae for the rest of their lives. However, the bacterium remains present, leading immune-depressed patients to relapse, known as "Brill-Zinsser disease," a milder but bacteremic form of typhus (48). The bacteremia may then allow feeding lice to become infected and to start a new epidemic. Consequently, until all humans who have had typhus are dead, typhus can constitute a threat. This fact has been highlighted in Burundi in 1997, where after 20 years without any reported cases, a huge outbreak of typhus followed an outbreak of lice in refugee camps (18). Several cases of Brill-Zinsser disease have been recently reported in Europe (49–51).

THE VECTOR: HUMAN BODY LOUSE
Introduction

The threat posed by lice is not only associated to the louse infestation considered as a disease in itself known as "pediculosis." Indeed, the human body lice, *Pediculus humanus humanus*, or *P. h. corporis* (Fig. 3), are recognized as vectors of three human infections that are reemerging: epidemic typhus, relapsing fever (caused by *Borrelia recurrentis*) and trench fever (caused by *Bartonella quintana*). Only the human body lice can transmit human pathogens. They live in clothes and multiply when conditions such as cold weather, lack of hygiene, or war are present. Its prevalence reflects the socioeconomic level of the society (52). Currently, the infestation by the human body louse is reemerging, and it is increasingly described in the poorest populations of developed and industrialized countries (26–29).

Origin and Future of Lice

Lice have been recognized for thousands of years as human parasites. Ancient lice and eggs have been recognized on 5000-year-old mummified Egyptians (53), on Pompeii's conserved bodies (53), pre-Columbian Incas (1), and in soldiers of Napoleon's Grand Army in Vilnius (5). Lice have recently served as a paradigm for host–parasite coevolution (54). Thus, speciation of the louse

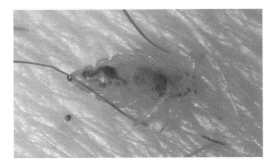

FIGURE 3 The human body louse, *Pediculus humanus humanus* (or *P. h. corporis*), while feeding on the skin.

predates the human colonization of America, which makes it one of the first ever human pathogens. It was thought in the past that the two *Pediculus* species (the human head and body lice) are homogenous and that the human body louse diverged from the head louse, its ancestor, when humans started wearing clothes, as the new subspecies specifically adapted to life in clothing (55). However, it has been recently found that the modern human lice were divided into two lineages (Fig. 4): the first contained only head lice of the New World (U.S. and Honduras), which had a very ancient origin (ca. 1.18 million years ago), and the other has a worldwide distribution (57). The worldwide lineage comprised two phyla: the first contained the human lice of the sub-Saharan Africa and the second contained those of the other geographical regions of the world (Americas, Europe, North Africa, and Asia) (56). Each phylum was secondarily divided into two subgroups: one made of head lice and the other comprising body lice (56) (Fig. 4).

It was expected, as with many infectious diseases, that lice would slowly disappear as civilization progressed and standards of hygiene improved (58). However, this has not been the case (59), and the body louse is reemerging. In fact, wars and social changes are rapidly promoting an increase in the numbers of body lice (58). The number of refugees and displaced people, which are associated with a recrudescence in body louse infestation, is rapidly increasing (60), even more surprisingly in developed countries (25–32).

Anatomy, Life Cycle, and Physiology of the Human Body Louse

The body louse head is short and constricted, with two antennae. The thorax is compact, and the seven-segment abdomen is long and membranous (Fig. 3). The cuticle (the extern revetment) may be colored, and the degree of coloration may reflect the skin color of their host (61). Body lice are defenseless, and their only natural enemy is their host (61).

The louse's life cycle begins as an egg, laid in the folds of clothing (but nowhere else). As the body louse is highly susceptible to cold, the eggs are usually attached to inner clothing, close to the skin, by an adhesive produced by the mother's accessory gland (53). Females lay about eight eggs a day, and because they do not have a sperm storage organ, they must mate before laying eggs. When held at a constant temperature (i.e., when clothes are not removed), the eggs will hatch six to nine days after being laid. The emerging louse immediately moves onto the skin to feed before returning to the clothing, where it remains until feeding again. The growing louse molts three times, usually at days 3, 5, and 10 after hatching. After the final molt, the mature louse will typically live for another 20 days.

Local louse populations vary in size, dynamics, and sex ratio (the ratio of males to females is about 1/6) (62). Population density is variable; usually only a few lice are observed on the same host, although anecdotal reports have mentioned people infected with "thousands of lice." Theoretically, a pair of mating lice can generate 200 lice during their one-month lifespan. Moreover, Evans and Smith (63) calculated that a population can increase by as much as 11% per day, but this rate is rarely observed. Although merely theoretical, this calculation shows how rapidly an outbreak of louse infestation could develop (55).

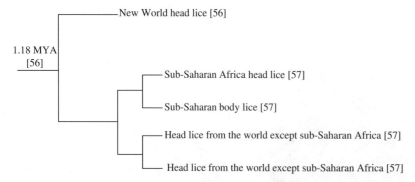

FIGURE 4 Representative cladogram of the reported phylogenetic relationships between human head and body lice according to the comparison of "18S rRNA" (56) and "COI and *Cyt*b" (57) sequences.

The body lice are a strictly hematophagous ectoparasites in all the stages. The louse's only method of rehydration is to feed on blood. The small diameter of the proboscis (the alimentary canal) prevents the rapid uptake of blood; thus, frequent, small meals are necessary (53). A louse typically feeds five times a day. Digestion of the blood meal is rapid and remain liquefied (64). Louse feces are extremely dry and powdery, with water content on only 2% (53). Feces contain a large amount of ammonium, which acts as an attractant for other lice. Sensory glands in the antennae of lice identify this stimulant (55).

Humidity is a critical factor for lice, which are susceptible to rapid dehydration (53). The optimal humidity for survival is in the range 70% to 90% (61); they cannot survive when this value falls below 40%. Conversely, under conditions of extremely high humidity, louse feces become sticky and can fatally adhere lice to clothing. Temperature is also highly influenced on the louse's physiology. Lice prefer a temperature of between 29°C and 32°C (61). Lice are able to maintain this temperature range by nestling in clothing. However, if a host becomes too hot because of fever or heavy exercise, infesting lice will leave him. Body lice die at 50°C, and this temperature is critical when washing clothes, as water or soap alone will not kill lice. Although eggs can survive at lower temperatures, their durability is limited to about 16 days.

In conclusion, several points are pertinent as bases for the control of the infestation with the body lice, to understand the epidemiology of the louse-borne infectious diseases and to use the adapted tools to control and to eradicate the body lice and the infectious diseases they transmit.

Epidemiology of Human Body Louse

Because lice live in clothing, their prevalence is determined by the weather, humidity, poverty, and lack of hygiene. Consequently, they are more prevalent during the colder months, and louse-transmitted diseases, especially epidemic typhus, are more frequently reported during winter and early spring (6).

Infestation with body lice and louse-transmitted diseases are also being increasingly reported among homeless and deprived populations in inner cities of developed countries (26–32). Interestingly, in western Europe, a large proportion of homeless migrants come from Eastern Europe, the historical source of many louse-transmitted outbreaks (30). It seems that social and hygienic decline provoked by the civil wars, and the economical instability and the natural catastrophes underlie all body louse infestations.

R. PROWAZEKII AND HUMAN BODY LOUSE
Infection of Human Body Louse with *R. prowazekii*

Transmission of epidemic typhus by the human body louse was demonstrated by Charles Nicolle, who obtained the Nobel Prize for this discovery (65,66).

The louse acquires *R. prowazekii* after feeding on a bacteremic-infected human, but does not become infective until five to seven days later (55). In the louse, when the obligate intracellular *R. prowazekii* are ingested with the infected blood meal, they only infect the epithelial cells of the first part of the louse's digestive tract (67,68) where they multiply. As a result of its excessive growth, infected epithelial cells enlarge and eventually burst five days postinfection, releasing the rickettsiae (Fig. 2A) into the gut lumen (67). Massive quantities of rickettsiae (Fig. 2B) are discharged in the feces starting from the fifth day postinfection (67), where it can remain viable, and then, infective for up to 100 days (55). The rupture of digestive epithelium allows the ingested blood to diffuse through the intestine to the hemolymph (the blood of the body louse) and the louse becomes red (53). Typhus has also been named "red louse disease" (Fig. 5). As ruptured epithelial cells are not replaced, infection with *R. prowazekii* leads to the death of the louse shortly thereafter (67). The fact that *R. prowazekii* is not motile could explain why it does not spread in its vector and is the only *Rickettsia* species unable to be transmitted transovarially to its progeny in its vector.

Detection of *R. prowazekii* in Human Body Louse

The human body louse is sterile, unless infected following feeding on a bacteremic host (55). The detection of *R. prowazekii* in the infected louse and/or in their feces is possible by

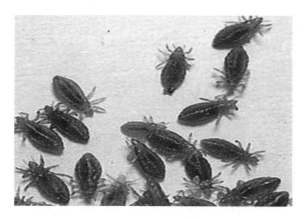

FIGURE 5 Human body lice infected with *R. prowazekii*. The dead infected lice presented a red color: "the red louse disease."

immunodetection (67,69), cell culture (67), and transmission electron microscopy (67,70). More recently, the association of amplification of specific fragments and analysis of the PCR products has been shown to be effective to obtain rapid and specific identification (71–73).

In countries where no medical and biological facilities are available, lice are a convenient tool in epidemiological studies of body-lice-transmitted diseases instead of blood. When outbreaks are suspected, or during a routine survey, lice collected in plastic tubes can be easily transported or shipped to laboratories equipped for analysis; the bacterial DNA is preserved even after the death of the insect. We have been able to show the usefulness of the detection of bacterial DNA in lice by PCR in several cases over the last years (74). Sporadic cases of typhus had been reported in Africa (17), but in 1995, *R. prowazekii* was characterized by sequencing the PCR product amplified from lice collected from patients in a jail in Burundi (18). This observation predated a massive outbreak of epidemic typhus in 1997 in refugee camps after the civil war (18).

PATHOPHYSIOLOGY OF EPIDEMIC TYPHUS

Transmission of *R. prowazekii* from the louse to the human occurs by contamination of the bite site with feces containing rickettsiae or by contamination of conjunctivae or mucous membranes with the crushed bodies or feces of infected lice (55). Infection through aerosols of feces-infected dust has been reported and provides the main risk of contraction of typhus for the physicians who are in contact with the patients infested with the infected lice (6). The threat of typhus as a biological weapon lies in its stability in the dried louse feces and in its infection by inhalation of an aerosol.

After inoculation to humans, rickettsiae spread throughout the body via the bloodstream, and enter endothelial cells, that is, their target cells, where they proliferate intracellularly until the cell bursts and releases rickettsiae into the extracellular space, the blood. *R. prowazekii* has the ability to injure cells directly in the absence of immune and inflammatory responses. Cellular injury results in the pathological hallmarks of all rickettsial infections: widespread vasculitis with increased vascular permeability, edema, and activation of humoral inflammatory and coagulation mechanisms. As illness advances, progressive endothelial damage leads to widespread vascular dysfunction. In severe infection, endothelial damage results in permeability changes and the passage of plasma and plasma proteins from the intravascular compartments to the interstitium. In addition, endothelial injury leads to disruption of vessel integrity, manifesting as microscopic and macroscopic foci of hemorrhage (75).

Thrombopenia often occurs in patients with advanced and severe illness. Vasculitis may be accompanied by mural and intimal thrombi in small vessels surrounded by inflammatory infiltrates consisting of macrophages, lymphocytes, and plasma cells. These lesions may occur focally throughout the central nervous system (CNS), where they are called "typhus nodules." These lesions may be associated with secondary changes induced by minute foci of hemorrhage. As the vasculitis of *R. prowazekii* infection is generalized, virtually any organ may be involved (76,77).

CLINICAL MANIFESTATIONS OF EPIDEMIC TYPHUS

After an incubation period of 10 to 14 days, epidemic typhus begins abruptly. The majority of patients with epidemic typhus develop a malaise and nonspecific constitutional symptoms (anorexia, chills, headache, myalgias, arthralgias, and fever) (17). In a recent study in Burundi, a crouching attitude due to myalgia, named "sutama," was reported (18). A cough is frequent, as well as confusion and stupor. There is no eschar of inoculation at the site of the lice biting. Most patients develop a skin rash that classically begins on the trunk and spreads to the periphery. A macular, maculopapular, or petechial rash may appear in 20% to 60% of cases, which may be difficult to detect on dark-skinned persons. The face, the hands palm, and the foot plants are saved. Rarely, patients with severe cases may develop gangrene of the distal extremities, necessitating amputation. The majority of patients with epidemic typhus manifest one or more abnormalities of function of the CNS, such as signs of meningeal irritation or signs of focal or generalized cortical dysfunction ranging from seizures to confusion, drowsiness, and coma as well as hearing loss (78). Myocarditis, pulmonary involvement (interstitial pneumonitis, bronchitis, or bonchiolitis) (79), thrombocytopenia, jaundice, and abnormal liver function tests may occur in severe cases. Without treatment, the disease is fatal in 10% to 30% of patients.

Recrudescent typhus or Brill-Zinsser disease is comparable to the primo-infection. It is less severe, however, with a natural fatality of 1.5%. It can appear in patients who had totally recovered from epidemic typhus, years after the onset of the first infection (48–51).

BIOLOGICAL DIAGNOSIS OF EPIDEMIC TYPHUS

The diagnosis of epidemic typhus is usually suggested by the presence of typical clinical findings such as fever, headaches, and skin rash in patients infested with body lice or in persons who are living in crowded, cold, and unhygienic circumstances. Thrombocytopenia and an increase of the hepatic enzymes may be observed particularly in severe cases. Typhus often occurs in clusters, but it may also occur as isolated illness.

The diagnosis of epidemic typhus is based on serology with indirect immunofluorescence being the reference method (80,81). Serological testing may also be performed on blood collected as drops on filter paper on a large scale for field samples (82). Cross-reactions occur within the typhus group (18), between typhus and spotted fever agents (83), and between *Rickettsia*, *Legionella*, and *Proteus* species (84). A diagnosis of recent epidemic or endemic (due to *R. typhi* and transmitted by the flea) typhus rickettsial infection can be established by demonstrating a fourfold or greater rise in titer of antibody in properly collected acute and convalescent serum samples. Epidemic and endemic typhus cannot be differentiated by serology unless, in specialized laboratories, Western blot associated to cross-adsorption techniques of sera are done (18,19,85). The immunofluorescent antibody test can distinguish between IgM and IgG antibody responses. Differentiation between increases in IgG and IgM antibody titers may not help to distinguish between a primary infection and Brill-Zinsser disease (86).

Biopsy of a skin rash can lead to a definitive diagnosis by demonstrating the characteristic changes of rickettsial vasculitis and the presence of rickettsiae in tissue by use of fluorescent antibody conjugates. As with other rickettsial diseases, a diagnosis of epidemic typhus can be confirmed by culture (87) and PCR technology (18,19,88) from blood (82,87) and/or lice (18,73,74) at a few large medical or research centers.

TREATMENT OF EPIDEMIC TYPHUS

In vitro susceptibility has been tested in lice (89,90) and in cells (91,92). Tetracycline and chloramphenicol are the effective treatments for epidemic typhus (93,94). Most patients treated with either antibiotic improve markedly within 48 hours after initiation of therapy. The prompt reaction to this treatment could be diagnostic for the infection. In fact, failure to show a response within 48 to 72 hours of starting empirical treatment is often considered to be clinical evidence that a rickettsial disease is not present. In areas of the world where diagnostic facilities are unavailable or inaccessible, chloramphenicol is widely used as an empirical treatment, as its broad spectrum includes other serious illness (meningococcemia and typhoid fevers) that can initially mimic epidemic typhus. However, many physicians prefer to use tetracycline for all typhus diseases, as it is cheaper and safer (55). A single dose of 200 mg of doxycycline, the reference treatment, is extremely efficient (18,95). Few or no relapses are observed (94–96) with this treatment, which should be prescribed for any suspected case, including those in children, as the risk of tooth staining with such a regimen is not demonstrated.

Ciprofloxacin should be avoided, following evidence from a case report of a patient misdiagnosed as having typhoid who died from typhus after treatment with this compound, despite in vitro efficiency (49).

VACCINATION

The first vaccine was developed by Weigl in Poland from infected lice from 1920 to 1930. Lice were inoculated intrarectally with viable R. prowazekii. Then, Weigl allowed the lice to feed on himself and his coworkers twice a day, permitting the rickettsiae to multiply in the intestinal cells of the arthropods (97). Many lice were necessary to produce vaccine (100 infected lice for a single dose of vaccine). The Madrid E nonpathogenic strain (98), the Cox vaccine egg (on egg embryonated), and the Durand vaccine (developed in the rat) were also used successfully (97). However, because antibiotic treatment is so efficient, vaccine was not considered a priority. The huge outbreak in Africa in 1997 has resulted in a different opinion as to the potential use of a vaccine.

CONTROL AND PREVENTION OF EPIDEMIC TYPHUS

Louse eradication is the most important preventive measure and is essential in the control of epidemic typhus outbreaks. As body lice live only in clothing, where they also lay their eggs, the simplest method of delousing is to remove and destroy all clothing. Thoroughly washing and boiling clothes can also effectively destroy lice. Dusting of all clothing with 10% dichlorodiphenyltrichloroethane, 1% malathion, or 1% permethrine (as in the protocol of the World Health Organisation) is also a rapid and effective method of killing body lice and reduces the risk of reinfestation (55). Although protective vaccines have been developed, they have not been widely used because effective antibiotic treatments are readily available.

REFERENCES

1. Zinsser H. Rats, Lice, and History. Londres: Broadway House, 1935:1–301.
2. Bozeman FM, Masiello SA, Williams MS, Elisberg BL. Epidemic typhus rickettsiae isolated from flying squirrels. Nature 1975; 255(5509):545–547.
3. Hardy A. Urban famine or urban crisis? Typhus in the Victorian city. Med Hist 1988; 32(4):401–425.
4. Gelston AL, Jones TC. Typhus fever: report of an epidemic in New York City in 1847. J Infect Dis 1977; 136(6):813–821.
5. Raoult D, Dutour O, Houhamdi L, et al. Evidence for louse-transmitted diseases in soldiers of Napoleon's grand army in Vilnius. J Infect Dis 2006; 193(1):112–120.
6. Patterson KD. Typhus and its control in Russia, 1870–1940. Med Hist 1993; 37(4):361–381.
7. Weiss K. The role of rickettsioses in history. In: Walker DH, ed. Biology of Rickettsial Diseases. 1st ed. Boca Raton, FL: CRC Press, 1988:1–14.
8. McDade JE, Shepard CC, Redus MA, Newhouse VF, Smith JD. Evidence of Rickettsia prowazekii infections in the United States. Am J Trop Med Hyg 1980; 29(2):277–284.
9. Ackley AM, Peter WJ. Indigenous acquisition of epidemic typhus in the eastern United States. South Med J 1981; 74(2):245–247.
10. Russo PK, Mendelson DC, Etkind PH, Garber M, Berardi VP, Gilfillan RF. Epidemic typhus (Rickettsia prowazekii) in Massachusetts: evidence of infection. N Engl J Med 1981; 304(19):1166–1168.
11. Sonenshine DE, Bozeman FM, Williams MS, et al. Epizootiology of epidemic typhus (Rickettsia prowazekii) in flying squirrels. Am J Trop Med Hyg 1978; 27(2, pt 1):339–349.
12. Bozeman FM, Sonenshine DE, Williams MS, Chadwick DP, Lauer DM, Elisberg BL. Experimental infection of ectoparasitic arthropods with Rickettsia prowazekii (GvF-16 strain) and transmission to flying squirrels. Am J Trop Med Hyg 1981; 30(1):253–263.
13. Romero A, Zeissig O, Espana D, Rizzo L. Tifus exantematico en Guatemala. Bol Sanit Panam 1977; 83(3):223–236.
14. Agger WA, Songsiridej V. Epidemic typhus acquired in Wisconsin. Wis Med J 1985; 84(1):27–30.

15. Fan MY, Walker DH, Yu SR, Liu QH. Epidemiology and ecology of rickettsial diseases in the People's Republic of China. Rev Infect Dis 1987; 9:823–840.
16. WHO Working Group on Rickettsial Diseases. Rickettsioses: a continuing disease problem. Bull WHO 1982; 60:157–164.
17. Perine PL, Chandler BP, Krause DK, et al. A clinico-epidemiological study of epidemic typhus in Africa. Clin Infect Dis 1992; 14(5):1149–1158.
18. Raoult D, Ndihokubwayo JB, Tissot-Dupont H, et al. Outbreak of epidemic typhus associated with trench fever in Burundi. Lancet 1998; 352(9125):353–358.
19. Raoult D, Roux V, Ndihokubwaho JB, et al. Jail fever (epidemic typhus) outbreak in Burundi. Emerg Infect Dis 1997; 3(3):357–360.
20. Bise G, Coninx R. Epidemic typhus in a prison in Burundi. Trans R Soc Trop Med Hyg 1997; 91(2):133–134.
21. Tarasevich I, Rydkina E, Raoult D. Outbreak of epidemic typhus in Russia. Lancet 1998; 352(9134):1151.
22. Raoult D, Birtles RJ, Montoya M, et al. Survey of three bacterial louse-associated diseases among rural Andean communities in Peru: prevalence of epidemic typhus, trench fever, and relapsing fever. Clin Infect Dis 1999; 29(2):434–436.
23. Mokrani K, Fournier PE, Dalichaouche M, Tebbal S, Aouati A, Raoult D. Reemerging threat of epidemic typhus in Algeria. J Clin Microbiol 2004; 42(8):3898–3900.
24. Niang M, Brouqui P, Raoult D. Epidemic typhus imported from Algeria. Emerg Infect Dis 1999; 5(5):716–718.
25. Brouqui P, Stein A, Dupont HT, et al. Ectoparasitism and vector-borne diseases in 930 homeless people from Marseilles. Medicine (Baltimore) 2005; 84(1):61–68.
26. Rydkina EB, Roux V, Gagua EM, Predtechenski AB, Tarasevich IV, Raoult D. *Bartonella quintana* in body lice collected from homeless persons in Russia. Emerg Infect Dis 1999; 5(1):176–178.
27. Van Der Laan JR, Smit RB. Back again: the clothes louse (*Pediculus humanus* var. *corporis*). Ned Tijdschr Geneeskd 1996; 140(38):1912–1915.
28. Jackson LA, Spach DH. Emergence of *Bartonella quintana* infection among homeless persons. Emerg Infect Dis 1996; 2(2):141–144.
29. Koehler JE, Quinn FD, Berger TG, Leboit PE, Tappero JW. Isolation of *Rochalimaea* species from cutaneous and osseous lesions of bacillary angiomatosis. N Engl J Med 1992; 327(23):1625–1631.
30. Brouqui P, Houpikian P, Tissot-Dupont H, et al. Survey of the seroprevalence of *Bartonella quintana* in homeless people. Clin Infect Dis 1996; 23(4):756–759.
31. Drancourt M, Mainardi JL, Brouqui P, et al. *Bartonella* (*Rochalimaea*) *quintana* endocarditis in three homeless men. N Engl J Med 1995; 332(7):419–423.
32. Brouqui P, La Scola B, Roux V, Raoult D. Chronic *Bartonella quintana* bacteremia in homeless patients. New Engl J Med 1999; 340(3):184–189.
33. Weiss E, Moulder JW. Order I, *Rickettsiales*, Gieszczkiewicz 1939. In: Krieg NR, Holt JG, eds. Bergey's Manual of Systematic Bacteriology. 1st ed. Baltimore, MD: Williams and Wilkins, 1984:687–703.
34. Teysseire N, Chiche-Portiche C, Raoult D. Intracellular movements of *Rickettsia conorii* and *R. typhi* based on actin polymerization. Res Microbiol 1992; 143:821–829.
35. Teysseire N, Boudier JA, Raoult D. *Rickettsia conorii* entry into Vero cells. Infect Immun 1995; 63(1):366–374.
36. Andersson SG, Zomorodipour A, Andersson JO, et al. The genome sequence of *Rickettsia prowazekii* and the origin of mitochondria. Nature 1998; 396(6707):133–140.
37. Philip RN, Casper EA, Burgdorfer W, Gerloff RK, Hughes LE, Bell EJ. Serologic typing of rickettsiae of the spotted fever group by microimmunofluorescence. J Immunol 1978; 121(5):1961–1968.
38. Regnery RL, Spruill CL, Plikaytis BD. Genotypic identification of rickettsiae and estimation of intraspecies sequence divergence for portions of two rickettsial genes. J Bacteriol 1991; 173(5):1576–1589.
39. Beati L, Finidori JP, Gilot B, Raoult D. Comparison of serologic typing, sodium dodecyl sulfate–polyacrylamide gel electrophoresis protein analysis, and genetic restriction fragment length polymorphism analysis for identification of rickettsiae: characterization of two new rickettsial strains. J Clin Microbiol 1992; 30(8):1922–1930.
40. Woese CR. Bacterial evolution. Microbiol Rev 1987; 51(2):221–271.
41. Relman DA, Lepp PW, Sadler KN, Schmidt TM. Phylogenetic relationships among the agent of bacillary angiomatis, *Bartonella bacilliformis*, and other alpha-proteobacteria. Mol Microbiol 1992; 6(13):1801–1807.
42. Stothard DR, Fuerst PA. Evolutionary analysis of the spotted fever and typhus groups of *Rickettsia* using 16S rRNA gene sequences. Syst Appl Microbiol 1995; 18:52–61.
43. Roux V, Raoult D. Phylogenetic analysis of the genus *Rickettsia* by 16S rDNA sequencing. Res Microbiol 1995; 146(5):385–396.
44. Roux V, Rydkina E, Eremeeva M, Raoult D. Citrate synthase gene comparison, a new tool for phylogenetic analysis, and its application for the rickettsiae. Int J Syst Bacteriol 1997; 47(2):252–261.
45. Zhu Y, Fournier PE, Ogata H, Raoult D. Multispacer typing of *Rickettsia prowazekii* enabling epidemiological studies of epidemic typhus. J Clin Microbiol 2005; 43(9):4708–4712.

46. Marchette NJ, Stiller D. Ecological Relationships and Evolution of the Rickettsiae. 1st ed. Boca Raton, FL: CRC Press, 1982:1–165.
47. Nicolle C. Destin des Maladies Infectieuses. Paris: France Lafayette, 1934:1–215.
48. Green CR, Fishbein D, Gleiberman I. Brill-Zinsser: still with us. J Am Med Assoc 1990; 264(14):1811–1812.
49. Zanetti G, Francioli P, Tagan D, Paddock CD, Zaki SR. Imported epidemic typhus. Lancet 1998; 352(9141):1709.
50. Stein A, Purgus R, Olmer M, Raoult D. Brill-Zinsser disease in France. Lancet 1999; 353(9168):1936.
51. Turcinov D, Kuzman I, Herendic B. Failure of azithromycin in treatment of Brill-Zinsser disease. Antimicrob Agents Chemother 2000; 44(6):1737–1738.
52. Meinking TL, Taplin D. Infestations: pediculosis. In: Eischmann EP, ed. Sexually Transmitted Diseases: Advances in Diagnosis and Treatment. Vol. 24. Basel: Curr. Probl. Dermatol., 1996:157–163.
53. Burgess IF. Human lice and their management. In: Baker JR, Muller R, Rollinson D, eds. Advances in Parasitology. Vol. 36. London: Academic Press, 1995:271–342.
54. Hafner MS, Nadler SA. Phylogenetic trees support the coevolution of parasites and their hosts. Nature 1988; 332(6161):258–259.
55. Raoult D, Roux V. The body louse as a vector of reemerging human diseases. Clin Infect Dis 1999; 29(4):888–911.
56. Yong Z, Fournier PE, Rydkina E, Raoult D. The geographical segregation of human lice preceded that of *Pediculus humanus capitis* and *Pediculus humanus humanus*. C R Biol 2003; 326(6):565–574.
57. Reed DL, Smith VS, Hammond SL, Rogers AR, Clayton DH. Genetic analysis of lice supports direct contact between modern and archaic humans. PLoS Biol 2004; 2(11):1972–1983.
58. Wilson ME. Infectious diseases: an ecological perspective. Br Med J 1995; 311(7021):1681–1684.
59. Raoult D. Infectious disease: return of the plagues. Lancet 1998; 352(suppl 4):SIV18.
60. Toole MJ, Ronald DTM, Waldman RJ. Refugees and displace persons: war, hunger, and public health. J Am Med Assoc 1993; 270(5):600–605.
61. Maunder JW. The appreciation of lice. Proc R Inst Great Brit 1983; 55:1–31.
62. Marshall AG. The sex ratio in ectoparasitic insects. Ecol Entomol 1981; 6:155–174.
63. Evans FC, Smith FE. The intrinsic rate of natural increase for the human louse *Pediculus humanus* L. Am Nat 1952; (86):299–310.
64. Vaughan JA, Azad AF. Patterns of erythrocyte digestion by bloodsucking insects: constraints on vector competence. J Med Entomol 1993; 30(1):214–216.
65. Gross L. How Charles Nicolle of the Pasteur Institute discovered that epidemic typhus is transmitted by lice: reminiscences from my years at the Pasteur Institute in Paris. Proc Natl Acad Sci USA 1996; 93(20):10539–10540.
66. Nicolle C, Comte C, Conseil E. Transmission expérimentale du typhus exanthématique par le pou du corps. C R Acad Sci Paris 1909; 146:486–489.
67. Houhamdi L, Fournier PE, Fang R, Lepidi H, Raoult D. An experimental model of human body louse infection with *Rickettsia prowazekii*. J Infect Dis 2002; 186(11):1639–1646.
68. Weigl R. Further studies on *Rickettsia rochalimae*. J Trop Med Hyg 1924; 27:14–15.
69. Fang R, Houhamdi L, Raoult D. Detection of *Rickettsia prowazekii* in body lice and their feces by using monoclonal antibodies. J Clin Microbiol 2002; 40(9):3358–3363.
70. Silverman DJ, Boese JL, Wisseman CL Jr. Ultrastructural studies of *Rickettsia prowazekii* from louse midgut cells to feces: search for "dormant" forms. Infect Immun 1974; 10(1):257–263.
71. Azad AF, Webb L, Carl M, Dasch GA. Detection of rickettsiae in arthropod vectors by DNA amplification using the polymerase chain reaction. Ann NY Acad Sci 1990; 590:557–563.
72. Higgins JA, Azad AF. Use of polymerase chain reaction to detect bacteria in arthropods: a review. J Med Entomol 1995; 32(3):213–222.
73. Roux V, Raoult D. Body lice as tools for diagnosis and surveillance of reemerging diseases. J Clin Microbiol 1999; 37(3):596–599.
74. Fournier PE, Ndihokubwayo JB, Guidran J, Kelly PJ, Raoult D. Human pathogens in body and head lice. Emerg Infect Dis 2002; 8(12):1515–1518.
75. Walker DH. Pathology and pathogenesis of the vasculotropic rickettsioses. In: Walker DH, ed. Biology of Rickettsial Disease. 1st ed. Boca Raton, FL: CRC Press, 1988:115–138.
76. Wolbach SB, Todd JL, Palfrey FW. The Etiology and Pathology of Typhus. Cambridge: Harvard University Press, 1922:3–222.
77. Walker DH. The role of the host factors in severity of spotted fever and typhus rickettsioses. Ann Rev Microbiol 1991; 540:10–19.
78. Friedmann I, Frohlich A, Wright A. Epidemic typhus fever and hearing loss: a histological study (Hallpike collection of temporal bone sections). J Laryngol Otol 1993; 107(4):275–283.
79. Diab SM, Araj GF, Fenech FF. Cardiovascular and pulmonary complications of epidemic typhus. Trop Geog Med 1989; 41(1):76–79.
80. La Scola B, Raoult D. Laboratory diagnosis of rickettsioses: current approaches to diagnosis of old and new rickettsial diseases. J Clin Microbiol 1997; 35(11):2715–2727.

81. Ormsbee RA, Peacock MG, Philip R, et al. Serologic diagnosis of epidemic typhus fever. Am J Epidemiol 1977; 105(3):261–271.
82. Fenollar F, Raoult D. Diagnosis of rickettsial diseases using samples dried on blotting paper. Clin Diagn Lab Immunol 1999; 6(4):483–488.
83. Ormsbee RA, Peacock MG, Philip R, et al. Antigenic relationships between the typhus and spotted fever groups of rickettsiae. Am J Epidemiol 1978; 108(1):53–59.
84. Raoult D, Dasch GA. Immunoblot cross-reactions among *Rickettsia*, *Proteus* spp. and *Legionella* spp. in patients with Mediterranean spotted fever. FEMS Immunol Med Microbiol 1995; 11(1):13–18.
85. La Scola B, Rydkina L, Ndihokubwayo JB, Vene S, Raoult D. Serological differentiation of murine typhus and epidemic typhus using cross-adsorption and Western blotting. Clin Diagn Lab Immunol 2000; 7(4):612–616.
86. Eremeeva ME, Balayeva NM, Raoult D. Serological response of patients suffering from primary and recrudescent typhus: comparison of complement fixation reaction, Weil-Felix test, microimmunofluorescence, and immunoblotting. Clin Diagn Lab Immunol 1994; 1(3):318–324.
87. Birg ML, La Scola B, Roux V, Brouqui P, Raoult D. Isolation of *Rickettsia prowazekii* from blood by shell vial cell culture. J Clin Microbiol 1999; 37(11):3722–3724.
88. Carl M, Tibbs CW, Dobson ME, Paparello S, Dasch GA. Diagnosis of acute typhus infection using the polymerase chain reaction. J Infect Dis 1990; 161(4):791–793.
89. Klimchuk ND. Comparative study of the action of different antibiotics and combined preparations on *Rickettsia prowazekii*. In: Kazar J, Ormsbee RA, Tarasevich IV, eds. Rickettsiae and Rickettsial Diseases. Bratislava: VEDA Publishing House of the Slovak Academy of Sciences, 1978:529–536.
90. Boese JL, Wisseman CL Jr, Walsh WT, Fiset P. Antibody and antibiotic action on *Rickettsia prowazekii* in body lice across the host–vector interface, with observations on strain virulence and retrieval mechanisms. Am J Epidemiol 1973; 98(4):262–282.
91. Rolain JM, Maurin M, Vestris G, Raoult D. In vitro susceptibilities of 27 rickettsiae to 13 antimicrobials. Antimicrob Agents Chemother 1998; 42(7):1537–1541.
92. Ives TJ, Manzewitsch P, Regnery RL, Butts JD, Kebede M. In vitro susceptibilities of *Bartonella henselae*, *B. quintana*, *B. elizabethae*, *Rickettsia rickettsii*, *R. conorii*, *R. akari*, and *R. prowazekii* to macrolide antibiotics as determined by immunofluorescent-antibody analysis of infected Vero cell monolayers. Antimicrob Agents Chemother 1997; 41(3):578–582.
93. Woodward WE. Typhus, typhoid and T.E.W. Md Med J 1989; 38(10):813–816.
94. Krause DW, Perine PL, McDade JE, Awoke S. Treatment of louse-borne typhus fever with chloramphenicol, tetracycline or doxycycline. East Afr Med J 1975; 52(8):421–427.
95. Perine PL, Krause DW, Awoke S, McDade JE. Single-dose doxycycline treatment of louse-borne relapsing fever and epidemic typhus. Lancet 1974; 2(7883):742–744.
96. Huys J, Kayhigi J, Freyens P, Berghe GV. Single-dose treatment of epidemic typhus with doxycycline. Chemotherapy 1973; 18(5):314–317.
97. Woodward TE. Rickettsial vaccines with emphasis on epidemic typhus: initial report of an old vaccine trial. S Afr Med J 1986; (suppl):73–76.
98. Clavero G, Perez-Gallardo F. Estudio experimental da una cepa apatogenica immunizante de *Rickettsia prowazekii*. Rev Sanidad Hlg Pub 1943; 17:1–27.

6 | Rickettsialpox

Christopher D. Paddock
Infectious Disease Pathology Activity, Division of Viral and Rickettsial Diseases, Centers for Disease Control and Prevention, Atlanta, Georgia, U.S.A.

Marina E. Eremeeva
Rickettsial Zoonoses Branch, Division of Viral and Rickettsial Diseases, Centers for Disease Control and Prevention, Atlanta, Georgia, U.S.A.

HISTORY

New York City holds many distinctions, but among the more unusual was its role in the discovery of the first and only known mite-borne spotted fever rickettsiosis. In February 1946, Benjamin Shankman, a New York City physician, evaluated an 11-year-old boy named Edmund Lohr Jr. from the Regency Park housing development in the Kew Gardens section of the borough of Queens. The child had a high fever, a papulovesicular lesion on his back, and axillary lymphadenopathy. Within the next several days, he developed a diffuse rash and his temperature rose to 40.5°C. Despite therapy with penicillin, the child remained ill for approximately one week. His recovery was complete, but during the next three months, Shankman saw approximately 20 additional patients from Regency Park with the same mysterious illness (1,2). By early summer, Shankman and several other clinicians, including Leo Sussman, Harry Zeller, and Joan Daly, had identified approximately 100 cases of the disease, referred as "Kew Gardens Mystery Fever" by local newspapers (1,3,4).

The New York City Department of Health initiated an investigation and within five months, the combined efforts of clinicians, epidemiologists, entomologists, and microbiologists culminated in the isolation and description of the causative agent, named *Rickettsia akari* from the Greek word for *mite* (5). Charles Pomerantz, a New York City exterminator and self-taught entomologist, is credited for first recognizing the role of rodents and mites in the transmission cycle of *R. akari* (1,6). The disease, named rickettsialpox by Huebner and colleagues for its rickettsial etiology and a clinical resemblance to chickenpox, was quickly characterized as a zoonosis that cycled among house mice (*Mus musculus*) from the bite of the house mouse mite, *Liponyssoides* (formerly *Allodermanyssus*) *sanguineus* (5,7). Ironically, Shankman was dissatisfied with the name assigned to this disease: "The name 'rickettsialpox' is proposed in the Public Health Reports . . . This is an unfortunate choice of terms. In the majority of cases there is no resemblance to chickenpox, for the lesions are more papular than vesicular" (8). A retrospective evaluation by the New York City Department of Health recognized a cluster of 10 probable cases from one large apartment house that had been identified several years earlier by a physician in the Riverdale section of the Bronx as "atypical chickenpox" (3).

During 1947 to 1951, 538 additional cases were identified in New York City (9). In 1949, Soviet investigators in the Ukraine identified a large outbreak of a disease they described as "vesicular rickettsiosis," and subsequently recognized as rickettsialpox (10,11). Rickettsialpox received considerable attention during the late 1940s and early 1950s; however, clinical and epidemiologic interests in this zoonosis dwindled during the subsequent five decades, and reporting of the disease diminished markedly. From 1969 to 1977, serum samples from only 12 patients were tested for evidence of this infection by the New York City Health Department Bureau of Laboratories, and only 45 cases of this disease were reported by the New York City Department of Health during 1980 to 1999 (12,13).

In 2001, intense public and clinician scrutiny regarding eschar-associated illnesses following the intentional release of *Bacillus anthracis* in the United States resulted in a noticeable increase in the number cases of rickettsialpox diagnosed at the Centers for Disease Control and Prevention (CDC). Approximately 20 confirmed cases of rickettsialpox from New York City, as well as several cases from cities in Maryland and New Jersey, were diagnosed at CDC during the six-month interval that followed this episode of bioterrorism (13, CDC, unpublished data). New York City remains the epicenter, historically and epidemiologically, for rickettsialpox. However, renewed interest in the natural history of R. akari, coupled with an increasing appreciation of the various rickettsial pathogens that cause eschar-associated illnesses in the United States and around the world (14), will likely prompt investigations that expand our knowledge of the distribution and magnitude of this unusual rickettsiosis.

MICROBIOLOGY
Cell Morphology and Staining Characteristics

The cellular structure of R. akari is similar to that of other Rickettsia species. Electron microscopy reveals rod-shaped bacteria 0.5 to 1.0 μm in length and 0.25 to 0.35 μm in width (15) (Fig. 1A and B). R. akari has an asymmetrical cell wall consisting of three layers: a 25- to 28-Å outer membrane and 25- to 40-Å inner membrane separated by a 30-Å periplasmic space. Intracellular R. akari may be surrounded by a capsule-like layer of 70 to 120 nm (16) similar to the S-layer described for R. rickettsii and R. prowazekii (17). Negative-contrast staining shows

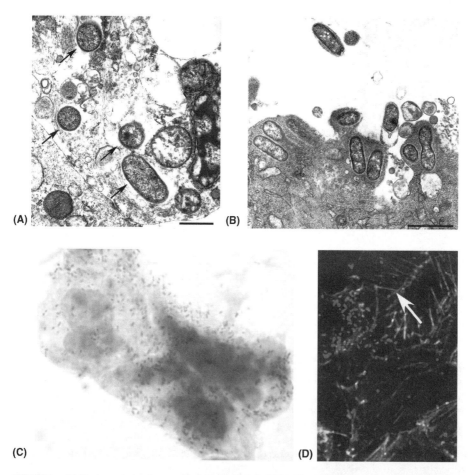

FIGURE 1 (**A**) Electron photomicrograph of R. akari (strain MK) in the cytosol of a Vero cell during a late-stage infection. Bar = 0.5 μm. (**B**) Release of R. akari (strain Croatian) through the filapodia of infected Vero cells. Rickettsiae outside the cell are surrounded by residual host cell cytoplasm and membrane. A rickettsia is exiting from this envelope near a deep invagination of the cell. Bar = 1 μm. (**C**) Giménez-stained R. akari in mouse peritoneal macrophages. (**D**) Microimmunofluorescence staining of actin tail polymerization by R. akari (strain MK) (arrow) in Vero cells exposed to R. akari for 96 hours and fixed with paraformaldehyde. Rickettsiae (dark gray) are stained using polyclonal mouse anti-R. akari serum and a Texas Red-labeled goat antimouse IgG antibody. Actin filaments (light gray) are stained with fluorescein-labeled phalloidin.

a net-like structure of the outer membrane comprised 7-nm subunits arranged in tetragons similar to other bacteria with protein S-layers (18).

R. akari does not stain well with conventional Gram's or eosin-azure-based techniques, but does stain with Giménez, Macchiavello's, and other related staining procedures that use carbol basic fuchsin (19). By this method (Fig. 1C), or by fluorescence microscopy using acridine orange stain, *R. akari* appear as small coccobacilli, diplococci, or diplobacilli in cell culture or smears made of infected yolk sacs or tissues of infected animals (10,20,21). *R. akari* may also be identified in host tissues using immunohistochemical stains or fluorescein-conjugated polyclonal antibodies (13,20,22–25).

R. akari resides predominantly in the cytoplasm of its host cell, but some bacteria may also situate within the host cell nucleus. Similar to other spotted fever group rickettsiae, *R. akari* induces the polymerization of actin in the host cell, allowing rickettsiae to move through the cytoplasm and invade the host cell nucleus (26,27) (Fig. 1D). In *R. akari*, this characteristic is likely regulated by a homologue of the *RickA* gene found in *R. conorii* and *R. rickettsii* (28,29).

Growth in Cell Culture and Plaque Formation

R. akari will grow in various cell lines of mammal, reptile, and arthropod origin (15,16,26,30,31). *R. akari* are phagocytosed by the host cell after inducing pseudopodia as observed in rabbit spleen fibroblast cells (32). Even when a high inoculation dose is used to achieve a 100% infection rate, only single rickettsiae are seen in the cytoplasm of infected cells during the first 48 hours following inoculation, after which the numbers of bacteria increase exponentially (32). Similar growth patterns have been described for *R. akari* in mouse macrophage-like P388D1 cells and mouse peritoneal macrophages (26). Following inoculation with *R. akari* at a multiplicity of infection of 50 plaque-forming units/cell, the percentage of infected cells increased from 25% to 92% at 24 and 96 hours after inoculation, respectively, in P388D1 cells, and from 18% to 78% during this same interval in peritoneal macrophages. The rate of infection in *R. akari*-infected cells was faster than that observed with *R. typhi*. In a similar manner, *R. akari* grown in mouse L929 fibroblasts appeared to accumulate faster and in higher numbers compared to *R. typhi* grown in the same cells (30).

R. akari produces lytic plaques in cultures of several cell lines (33–35). In primary chick embryo fibroblasts, *R. akari* forms plaques that are similar to those formed by *R. rickettsii* and *R. conorii* (33,34). In contrast, lytic plaques formed by *R. akari* in Vero cells or L929 mouse fibroblast cells take longer to appear and are 1.5 to 2.5 mm smaller than those plaques formed by *R. conorii* or *R. rickettsii* in the same cell lines (35).

Genetics and Phylogenetic Position

The genome of *R. akari* (strain Hartford) consists of a single 1,231,204-bp chromosome (GenBank AAFE01000001) with an estimated 1285 open reading frames (ORFs) and predicted coding capacity of 75.2%. The G + C% content (32.3%) is similar to those of other spotted fever group rickettsiae. The genome of *R. akari* is similar to other known rickettsial genomes, and encodes 33 tRNA genes, three ribosomal RNA genes (5S, 16S, and 23S), and three other RNA molecules [*ssrA* (tmRNA), *rnpB* (RNA component of ribonuclease P), and *srp* (signal recognition particle 4.5S RNA)]. Comparison of the genome sequence of *R. akari* to the genomes of other *Rickettsia* species reveals strong conservation of DNA sequences and specific gene orders at local operon and genome-wide levels (Fig. 2). As with other closely related bacteria, a cluster of multiple breaks and inversions has occurred opposite the origin of replication. Other regions of these genomes have experienced less frequent inversions. *R. akari* apparently shares more small conserved DNA elements with *R. felis* than with most other spotted fever group or typhus group rickettsiae. Compared with other rickettsial species for which full genome sequences are available, 63.8% of the putative ORFs encoded by the *R. akari* genome have the highest basic local alignment research tool (BLAST) similarity scores to proteins predicted for *R. felis*, followed by various other spotted fever group and typhus group rickettsiae (M. Eremeeva, unpublished data). In one investigation, genomic DNA of *R. akari* was evaluated using polymerase chain reaction (PCR) primers designed to amplify ORFs conserved between *R. prowazekii* and *R. conorii* (37). Amplicons were obtained with only 50 of 60 primer pairs, indicating nucleotide sequence variation around 5'- and 3'-ends of individual genes rather than the

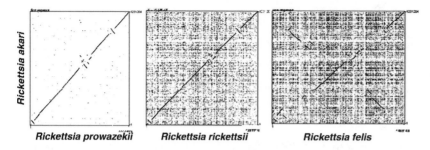

FIGURE 2 PipMaker plot comparison (36) of the genome sequences of *R. akari* with the genome sequences of *R. prowazekii*, *R. rickettsii*, and *R. felis*. The diagonal lines found in these three plots reveal strong conservation of DNA sequences and specific gene orders at both a local operon and genome-wide level among *Rickettsia*. A cluster of multiple breaks and inversions (*upper left–bottom right diagonals*) has occurred opposite the origin of replication (*middle* of PipPlots), but other parts of these genomes also have experienced inversions less frequently. Break sites often occur close to tRNA genes. The presence of a significant level of off-diagonal signal is seen in PipPlot pairwise comparisons of *R. rickettsii* and *R. felis* with *R. akari*. This signal appears to be due to the presence of numerous small conserved DNA elements scattered throughout rickettsial genomes.

absence of specific ORFs. The failure of primers to amplify conserved ORFs occurs more commonly as genetic relatedness between species decreases (37).

Because PCR studies failed to detect the 5' end of the rompA gene from *R. akari*, its absence was commonly accepted for this species (38). A 2502-bp sequence of tandem repeat region of *romp*A for *R. akari* (strain MK) has been described (39). However, *romp*A is present as a split gene in the complete genome sequence determined for *R. akari* (strain Hartford) and this strain lacks a tandem repeat region (40,41). This difference could be caused by passage history, strain variability, or variations of clone selected for the genomic project. The genome of *R. akari* (strain Hartford) encodes for nine other surface protein antigens (40,42). Five of these proteins, sca1 (1902 amino acids), sca2 (1795 amino acids), sca4 (1026 amino acids), sca5 (or rompB, 1655 amino acids), and sca6 (1483 amino acids), are encoded by complete ORFs. The other four proteins (sca3, sca7, sca8, and sca10) are encoded as split genes. The kinetics of expression of these proteins in vivo and their antigenic characteristics are largely unknown (40,41).

A comparison of rickettsial 16S rRNA gene sequences places *R. akari* in a cluster with *R. australis* and *R. felis* (43,44). A similar placement of *R. akari* is also obtained by analysis of individual protein coding genes *glt*A, *romp*B, *sca*4, *rpo*B (45,46), concatenated derived amino acid sequences of proteins encoding the type 4 secretion system, and by a genome-based comparison (47). *R. akari* is also grouped with *R. australis* and separated from other spotted fever group rickettsiae using monoclonal antibodies against cross-reacting epitopes of *R. conorii* lipopolysaccharide (LPS) and the 120-kDa protein antigen of *R. akari* (48); however, an extensive panel of monoclonal anti-*R. felis* antibodies identifies only a few cross-reacting protein epitopes between *R. akari* and *R. felis* (49). These data and previous evaluations using monoclonal anti-*R. akari* antibodies (50), further characterize the antigenic uniqueness of *R. akari*, suggested previously by microimmunofluorescence serotyping using polyclonal mouse antisera (51,52).

The one-dimensional sodium dodecyl sulfate–polyacrylamide gel electrophoresis profile of the proteins of *R. akari* differs from those of other *Rickettsia* species in the migration of at least six proteins (20,53–57). At least one high-molecular-weight protein contains epitopes that are recognized by mouse hyperimmune serum and exhibits an electrophoretic mobility shift following heat denaturation (58).

Several pieces of data suggest that a single ancestral strain of *R. akari* has been widely distributed around the globe. The protein profiles of isolates of *R. akari* obtained from the United States, the Ukraine, and Croatia are indistinguishable (58), and profiles of several U.S. isolates *R. akari* from the late 1940s and 1950s are identical to those of five U.S. strains isolated during 2001–2003 (20). Isolates of *R. akari* do not express significant intraspecies antigenic variation by cross-protection (11,59), complement fixation (60), microimmunofluorescence serotyping or Western blot assays (58). PCR multi-loci comparison of DNA of 14 strains of *R. akari*, isolated from rodents, mites, and humans from different continental origins between 1946 and 2003, reveals remarkable conservation in the genome of *R. akari* (41,61), and pulsed field gel electrophoresis of *R. akari* isolates demonstrates a similarly high degree of genetic homogeneity (60).

ECOLOGY AND NATURAL HISTORY
Arthropod Transmission
Liponyssoides sanguineus

R. akari is transmitted to several species of rodents by *L. sanguineus*, a hematophagous mesostigmatid mite in the family Dermanyssidae. Humans are not a regular component in the natural circulation of *R. akari*, and zoonotic transmission of this pathogen occurs only when a mite infected with rickettsiae is unable to locate its natural host and is forced to obtain a blood meal from a human host. *R. akari* has been isolated from various commensal and wild rodent species; however, transovarial and transstadial transmission of rickettsiae occurs in *L. sanguineus*, implicating the mite as an important or possibly the primary reservoir host of *R. akari*.

The house mouse mite was initially described in 1914 from specimens collected from rodents in Egypt during plague investigations by the Lister Institute (62). *L. sanguineus* was first identified in New York City in 1940 when a specimen was removed from candy in a hotel pastry department (63). The following year, an operator of a city exterminating company sent a specimen to the U.S. Department of Agriculture for identification, with a letter stating, "Aside from a purely academic interest in the animal, I have a problem to decide: namely, to whom do they belong, the landlord or tenant. The tenant originally complained of bed bugs . . . The tenant also claims that the 'bed bug' caused a rash (63)." The house mouse mite has been collected from at least 10 states in the United States, and from several countries in Eurasia and the Mediterranean basin (Table 1). Acarologists synonymized the genera *Allodermanyssus* and *Liponyssoides* in 1962 (75).

TABLE 1 Reported Collection Locations and Host Associations of the House Mouse Mite (*L. sanguineus*)

Location	Host	Year(s) of report(s)	Reference(s)
United States			
Washington, DC	NS	1909	(63)
Champaign, IL	*M. musculus*	1934	(64)
Tucson, AZ	*M. musculus*	1938	(63)
New York, NY[a]	*M. musculus*	1940, 1941, 1946	(63,65)
Philadelphia, PA	NS	1941	(63)
Salt Lake City, UT	*Rattus norvegicus*	1948	(64)
Indianapolis, IN	NS	1949	(64)
Boston, MA	*M. musculus*	1951	(66)
West Hartford, CT[a]	NS	1952	(67)
Brookline, MA	NS	1953	(68)
Ohio	*M. musculus*	1960	(69)
Columbia, SC	*M. musculus*	2002	(70)
Other Countries			
Egypt	*R. rattus*	1914, 1997, 1998	(62,71)
	Arvicanthis niloticus		
	Acomys dimidiatus		
	A. russatus		
	Dipodillus dasyurus		
	Sekeetamys calurus		
	Eliomys melanurus		
Ukraine[a]	*M. musculus*	1953	(72)
	R. norvegicus	1954	(11)
Armenia	*Cricetulus migratorius*	1953	(72)
	R. norvegicus		
Turkmenistan	NS	1968	(73)
Sicily	NS	1977	(74)

[a]*R. akari* isolated from mites collected at this location.
Abbreviation: NS, specimens not associated with a specific host or no host specified.

L. sanguineus is a nidocolous ectoparasite, most often found in proximity to rodent haborages that include nests and burrows, and in cracks and crevices close to nesting sites (72,76). The house mouse mite attaches to its host only long enough to obtain a blood meal, which it completes in as few as 15 minutes or as long as 36 hours (65). The life cycle involves five stages: egg, larva, protonymph, deutonymph, and adult. The rate of maturation may be influenced by the ambient temperature, but at 24°C, the interval from egg to adult is approximately 17 to 23 days (68). The larval stage does not feed and is relatively immobile. The protonymph and deutonymph are small (approximately 400–700 μm in length), active stages and each of these feed only once before molting to the next life stage.

Nonengorged adult female mites are approximately 650 to 750 μm in length and have two dorsal shields: a larger, tapered anterior plate, and a smaller, ovoid, posterior plate (Fig. 3A and B). The legs are long and slender, and the chelicerae are elongate and whip-like. Fully engorged females are 1.0 to 1.6 mm and appear bright red (65,72); as the mite digests its blood meal, it appears black, then colorless after the blood is fully digested (77). The adult male is approximately 700 μm in length and has a single dorsal shield (62). Adult male and female mites each obtain multiple blood meals, and the female mite oviposits 1 to 26 eggs within one to five days after each blood meal (62,68,72). In experimental settings, female *L. sanguineus* mites can complete up to five gonotrophic cycles. Parthenogenic development in the absence of male mites has been described (78).

Nymphal stage and adult mites are each capable of transmitting *R. akari* to susceptible hosts. Because mites do not defecate while feeding, introduction of rickettsiae to the vertebrate host presumably occurs during inoculation of infective salivary secretions at the bite site. The ability of rickettsiae to effectively pass among all life stages of *L. sanguineus* and the requirement by the house mouse mite to obtain multiple blood meals to complete its life cycle provide multiple opportunities for *L. sanguineus* to transmit *R. akari* to susceptible vertebrate hosts (68,79). *R. akari* has been isolated from *L. sanguineus* collected in the domiciles of patients with rickettsialpox (1,11,65,67,76,80). The observations made at the sentinel cluster in Kew Gardens, New York in 1946 and in an apartment house in West Hartford, Connecticut, where eight persons developed rickettsialpox during January 1952, are the most noteworthy. In these settings, flat and fully engorged mites were observed crawling on the external walls of incinerators used to burn household garbage in the basements of the dwellings. Huebner et al. described seeing as many as 100 mites on one incinerator (65) and recovered more than 100 mites from a mouse nest situated in a couch in the basement of a Kew Gardens apartment (76).

L. sanguineus is best known as an ectoparasite of *M. musculus*, but the house mouse mite has also been collected from various other rodents in the U.S.A., Eurasia, and Africa, including the brown rat, roof rat, gray dwarf hamster, African arvicanthus, eastern spiny mouse, golden spiny mouse, Wagner's dipodil, large-eared dormouse, and bushy-tailed jird (Table 1). House mouse mites have also been collected from a house mouse sold in a pet store (70) and from various laboratory rodents, including Mongolian gerbils (*Meriones unguiculatus*) and Egyptian gerbils (*M. libycus*) (81). However, surveys conducted by the U.S. Public Health Service during the 1940s suggest that *L. sanguineus* is not a common ectoparasite of peridomestic rats in

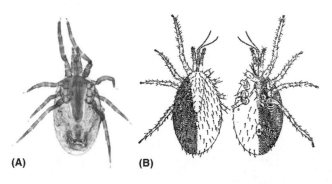

FIGURE 3 (**A**) Ventral aspect of an adult female *Liponyssoides* (=*Allodermanyssus*) *sanguineus* Hirst (Acari: Dermanyssidae) collected from a brown rat (*R. norvegicus*) in Salt Lake City, Utah, by Harmston on June 11, 1948 (64). Cleared specimen stained with acid fuchsin. (**B**) Dorsal (*left*) and ventral (*right*) aspects of an adult female *L. sanguineus*. *Source*: From Ref. 77.

the eastern United States. Investigators identified house mouse mites on 92 (10%) of 963 *M. musculus* trapped in New York City, but on none of 121 *Rattus* spp. trapped from the same areas, and no specimens of *L. sanguineus* were recovered from 4070 *R. rattus* and *R. norvegicus* collected in nine southeastern states during 1945–1948 (64). The proclivity of *L. sanguineus* to take blood meals from larger vertebrate hosts is also suggested by serologic surveys identifying antibodies reactive with *R. akari* in dogs in New York City and in feral and pet cats in California (82,83). Collectively, these data suggest that the house mouse mite is an opportunistic feeder, whose hosts may include various native or commensal rodents, dogs, cats, and humans, when its preferred host, the house mouse, is not available.

Other Potential Vectors

Liponyssus bacoti, the tropical rat mite, becomes infected with *R. akari* when it obtains a blood meal from a rickettsemic mouse, and may transmit *R. akari* transovarially to its progeny; however, the tropical rat mite does not appear to be an efficient vector of *R. akari* (84). The human body louse (*Pediculus humanus humanus*) can acquire *R. akari* by feeding on infected mice, and rickettsiae will generally proliferate in the louse midgut epithelial cells without apparent harm to the insect (85,86). Lice infected with *R. akari* do not transmit the agent when allowed to feed on human volunteers; however, the feces of infected lice cause disease when inoculated into mice, suggesting that lice or other ectoparasites of rodents could be involved in the transmission of *R. akari* to susceptible hosts (85).

Vertebrate Hosts
Mus musculus

M. musculus is a commensal rodent that is ubiquitously distributed throughout the world. In the original 1946 outbreak in New York, investigators quickly recognized an association between abundance of house mice and human cases of rickettsialpox. Large populations of *M. musculus* were found infesting each of two housing developments where cases of rickettsialpox were identified (76). At Kew Gardens, approximately 60 mice were trapped in apartment basements where rodent harborage existed in store rooms and incinerator ashpits, and *R. akari* was subsequently isolated from a mouse trapped at this location (7). Individual mice may be infested by 1 to 20 *L. sanguineus* mites that are most often localized to the rump of the mouse (64,76).

Although dose-dependent morbidity and mortality is observed in house mice infected with *R. akari*, wild *M. musculus* can recover from infection and develop immunity to subsequent infection with *R. akari*. Wild house mice, trapped at a focus of infection in New York City, had complement fixing antibodies reactive with *R. akari* and survived intraperitoneal challenge with concentrations of *R. akari* that were uniformly lethal to naive inbred laboratory mice and to wild house mice trapped at a nonendemic focus from northern Virginia. Serum samples of the two later groups of mice had no demonstrable anti-*R. akari* antibodies (7). In a similar manner, complement fixing antibodies were present in the sera of several mice trapped at a millinery in downtown Boston where human cases of rickettsialpox had occurred; however, rickettsial isolates were obtained only from mice without detectable antibodies reactive with *R. akari* (66). These data suggest that *M. musculus* may function more as an amplifying host than as a true natural reservoir of *R. akari*. Nonetheless, house mice undoubtedly play an important role in the ecology of rickettsialpox by supporting the proliferation of mite populations and providing a means by which mites are situated in proximity to humans (9).

Despite broad geographic distributions of the vector mite and the house mouse (Table 1), confirmed reports of rickettsialpox are relatively sparse and sporadic, suggesting that the occurrence of this disease in human populations may not simply reflect the convergent endemicities of *L. sanguineus*, *R. akari*, and *M. musculus*. In this context, conditions that favor the parasitism of humans by *L. sanguineus* may have the greatest impact on the epidemiologic activity of rickettsialpox (9). In 1983, Krinsky (87) suggested that lymphocytic choriomeningitis virus (LCMV) infection in house mouse populations could force the emergence of rickettsialpox in humans. In some settings, mice that are acutely infected with LCMV, a broadly distributed, rodent-borne, Old World arenavirus may die or develop acute disease, making these potentially undesirable hosts for infective mites. In these settings, *L. sanguineus* might be more likely seek a human host (87). As circumstantial evidence, Krinsky cited remarks made by Huebner and colleagues that early attempts to isolate *R. akari* from *M. musculus* trapped at Kew Gardens were complicated by frequent LCMV infections in mice at this location (7).

Other Potential Hosts

R. akari has been isolated from tissues of naturally infected *R. norvegicus* rats in the Ukraine (10) and from a reed vole (*Microtus fortis pelliceus*) trapped on the Korean peninsula (88). In the case of *M. fortis pelliceus*, infection with *R. akari* appears to be relatively uncommon: only one of 11 trapped voles was infected, and none of 174 other Korean rodents trapped in the general vicinity of the infected vole showed evidence of infection with *R. akari* by serologic or isolation procedures (88). Other species of wild rodents, including the cotton rat (*Sigmodon hispidus*) and the yellow-necked mouse (*Apodemus flavicollis*), are susceptible to infection with *R. akari*, and those animals that survive the infection develop robust anti-*R. akari* antibody titers (66,89). Antibodies reactive with *R. akari* have also been detected in several species of wild rodents in Orange County, California, including 45 (23%) of 197 *Peromyscus maniculatus*, one of one *P. eremecus*, and one of two *Neotoma fuscipes* (90). Collectively, these findings suggest that in some regions of the world, sylvatic cycles that involve native rodents may exist in addition to the classic urban cycle that involves house mice.

A serosurvey of New York City dogs identified antibodies reactive with spotted fever group rickettsiae in 24 (7.7%) of 311 canine serum samples (82). Twenty (83%) of the positive animals resided in Manhattan or the Bronx, the boroughs presently associated with the greatest number of reported cases of rickettsialpox (13). A serologic cross-adsorption method identified *R. akari* as the probable infecting agent in six (86%) of seven seropositive canine serum specimens that were evaluated by this technique, suggesting that *R. akari* may cycle among some companion animals in addition to commensal rodents (82).

EPIDEMIOLOGY
Geographic Distribution

Rickettsialpox is a notifiable disease in New York City, and during 1989–2000, a median of one (range 0–10) confirmed case was reported each year by the city health department (13). Populations of the vector mites and rodent hosts are documented throughout the U.S.A. (Table 1), and various studies suggest that substantial rates of infection occur among inhabitants of other urban areas (90,91); however, every U.S. case series of rickettsialpox published during the last 50 years describes a patient cohort that resided within the geographical boundaries of New York City (13,22,24,92,93). This observation suggests that most contemporary clinicians beyond the borders of New York City are relatively unfamiliar with rickettsialpox despite the documented or inferred occurrence of *R. akari* in several other U.S. cities (66,80, 90,91,94–97) (Table 2). From 1960 to 1971, cases of rickettsialpox were optionally reported by certain states to the U.S. Public Health Service. During this interval, cases were documented from Arkansas, Delaware, New Mexico, New York, Pennsylvania, and Utah; however, no corresponding clinical or laboratory data accompanied these reports (110–115). A broader use of confirmatory methods, particularly cell culture isolation and PCR evaluation of eschar biopsy specimens, will undoubtedly expand the recognized distribution of rickettsialpox in the United States (20).

Soviet investigators identified rickettsialpox in the Ukraine in 1949 and extensively studied the disease and its epidemiology during the early 1950s (10,11,72,79,116,117). However, in a manner similar to U.S. endeavors, interest in this relatively benign rickettsiosis waned during subsequent decades. Curiously, relatively few cases of rickettsialpox have been confirmed from Europe. Serologic surveys or occasional case reports from Albania, France, Germany, and Italy have identified low titers of antibodies reactive to *R. akari* in some persons (107,109, 118); however, no confirmed cases have been identified in any of these countries. *R. akari* was isolated from the blood of a patient from Zadar, Croatia, in 1991 (58), and rickettsialpox was diagnosed

TABLE 2 Reported Locations of Confirmed and Suspected Cases of Rickettsialpox, and of Persons with Serologic Reactivity to *R. akari*

Location	Year(s) reported	Laboratory evidence	Reference(s)
United States			
New York, NY	1946–2003	Serology, culture, IHC, PCR	(5,12,13,20,22,24,92,93,98,99)
Boston, MA	1950, 1951	Serology	(94,96)
Hartford, CT	1952	Serology	(67,80)
Philadelphia, PA	1952	Serology	(97)
Brookline, MA	1953	Serology	(68)
Cleveland, OH	1956	Serology	(95)
Newark, NJ	1991	Serology, IHC	(CDC, unpublished data)
Baltimore, MD	1999, 2001	Serology, IHC	(91; CDC, unpublished data)
Trenton, NJ	2002	IHC	(CDC, unpublished data)
Concord, NC	2002	Serology	(100)
Los Angeles, CA	2006	Serology	(90)
Other countries			
Ukraine	1950	Serology, culture	(10,11)
Central African Republic	1952	Serology	(101,102)
South Africa	1954	Serology	(103)
Bosnia-Herzegovina	1956	Serology	(104)
Albania	1961	Serology	(105)
Costa Rica	1971	Serology	(106)
Germany	1981	Serology	(107)
Croatia	1996	Serology, culture	(58)
Turkey	2003	Serology	(108)
France	2005	Serology	(109)

Abbreviations: CDC, Centers for Disease Control; IHC, immunohistochemistry; PCR, polymerase chain reaction.

in a child from Nevpehir in central Turkey using a serologic cross-adsorption assay (108). Rickettsiologists continue to identify various novel pathogens as causes of febrile, eschar-associated illnesses (14), and it is likely that continued emphasis on laboratory methods that provide a species-level diagnosis, including molecular and culture-based techniques, will uncover cases of rickettsialpox in new regions of this subcontinent.

Cases of rickettsialpox, identified by serologic assays, have been reported from South Africa (103,119), and from the Central African Republic (101,102); however, several clinically similar, eschar-associated spotted fever group rickettsioses, including infections caused by *R. africae*, *R. conorii*, and *R. aeschlemannii*, also exist in Africa (14), that may result in antibodies that cross-react with antigens of *R. akari*. By example, 91 (63%) of 144 serum specimens collected from the Central African Republic demonstrated antibodies reactive with *R. rickettsii* when tested using an indirect immunofluorescence antibody (IFA) assay, and 20% of these demonstrated titers ≥640. When these specimens were analyzed further by microagglutination assays for *R. rickettsii*, *R. conorii*, and *R. akari*, approximately half reacted with *R. conorii*, but none reacted with either *R. rickettsii* or *R. akari*, suggesting that a spotted fever group rickettsia other than *R. akari* was responsible for the serologic reactivity in this region (120).

Little is known about the distribution of *R. akari* in Southeast Asia other than its isolation from a reed vole on the Korean peninsula (88) and one unconfirmed report that described the detection of DNA of *R. akari* in a human serum specimen from a Korean patient (121). From a serosurvey of commensal rodents on Samar Island in the Philippines, none of 47 *M. musculus* and none of 49 *R. rattus* had evidence of antibodies reactive with *R. akari* (122).

Patient Demographics, Seasonality, and Risk Factors

Rickettsialpox has been described in patients of all ages, from infants as young as six months, to adults as old as 92 years (4,13). In most patient series, the disease occurs equally among males and females (6,10,11,24,116). Cases are documented from all months of the year. Epidemics of rickettsialpox in New York City and the Ukraine during the late 1940s were

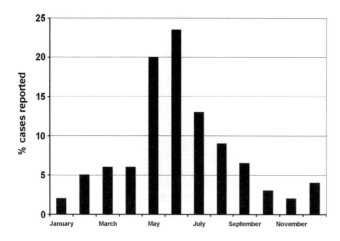

FIGURE 4 Reported cases of rickettsialpox in the Ukraine, by month, during 1949–1950. *Source*: From Refs. 10, 116.

notable for a predominance of cases during May to August (6,10) (Fig. 4); however, recent reports suggest a more sporadic and continuous distribution of cases in New York City throughout the year (13,22,24).

Serologic surveys from the last several years have identified antibodies reactive with spotted fever group rickettsiae in approximately 8% to 16% of several indigent inner city cohorts in New York City, Baltimore, and Los Angeles. The use of cross-adsorption techniques on the serum specimens from these three cohorts revealed that the majority of these infections were most likely attributable to *R. akari*. These results suggest that the activities of some urban inhabitants, particularly the homeless, the poor, and injection drug users, may place them at increased risk for rickettsialpox (90,91,98). Only one report describes specifically rickettsialpox in an immunocompromised individual (23). The patient was an HIV-seropositive woman with a CD4 + T-lymphocyte count of 482 cells/µL. Her clinical course was typical of the disease; however, the impact of immune suppression of the severity of rickettsialpox remains largely unknown.

Laboratory- and field-acquired cases of rickettsialpox are described by several early investigators who worked with the pathogen, including rickettsiologist Jellison (65). A technician working with the MK strain of *R. akari* at the Harvard School of Public Health developed a vesicular exanthem and enanthem accompanied by fever, photophobia, nausea, and severe headache, that responded to chloramphenicol; no eschar was identified, and the presumed route of exposure was through the respiratory or conjunctival mucous membranes during the manipulation of chicken yolk sacs infected with *R. akari* (123). Rose (99) briefly described a case of laboratory-acquired rickettsialpox that began as an eschar just inside the nostril of a patient, seven days after he had worked with the agent. This patient developed fever on the tenth day and a papulovesicular rash on the 12th day, following exposure to *R. akari*.

Temporal and Spatial Characteristics

In a manner similar to other spotted fever rickettsioses, cases of rickettsialpox often cluster in time and space, and simultaneous or consecutive illnesses (in some reports as many as eight) have been identified among family members or other residents from a single common location (2,4,6,9,11,92,124). Except for the 1946 epidemic in Queens, most cases in New York City have been reported from northern Manhattan and in the adjacent borough of the Bronx (24,92,124,125). A recent study that documented the geographical distribution of cases in New York City during 2001–2002 identified a pattern that closely resembled area case distributions reported during 1946–1952 and reflected persistent foci of this urban zoonosis (13). Approximately two-thirds of the New York City cases observed during 2001 and 2002 originated from the Upper West End of Manhattan Island and in the Bronx, with few or no cases from the southern tip of Manhattan, Staten Island, Brooklyn, and Queens, similar to the recognized distribution of cases during the late 1940s (124,126). Persistent urban foci have also been described in the Ukraine (11,116).

Epidemics of rickettsialpox are well described (6,9,10). Because this disease is an arthropod-borne zoonosis, ecological factors that govern populations of rodent reservoirs or their ectoparasites undoubtedly influence the emergence of this disease in human populations. During the epidemiologic investigation of the sentinel New York City outbreak in 1946, tenants of Kew Gardens housing development reported sightings of mice in courtyards and some apartments; however, mice were particularly abundant in the basements of these buildings, which also housed incinerators that were connected by a chute to the upper floors and functioned to burn household garbage for the six to nine families that resided in each building. The proper functioning of the incinerators required a laborer to regularly ignite the trash and routinely clean the incinerator to ensure that garbage did not accumulate in the upper compartment. Because of a workforce shortage during World War II, incinerators were not regularly fired, basements became cluttered, and garbage accumulated in many of the incinerators long enough to provide ample food that allowed house mice to proliferate (6). In one Ukrainian city, an outbreak of rickettsialpox was attributed to the local geography of the downtown district that facilitated the accumulation of large numbers of commensal rodents: the central business and residential districts were surrounded by a river and by several ponds that limited the egress of populations of mice and rats that had concentrated in this area of the city (117).

Prevention

Only one study has assessed the impact of rodent and mite control to diminish the spread of rickettsialpox. In this investigation, workers described the impact of commensal rodent elimination in a Ukrainian city where an epidemic of rickettsialpox had recently occurred (117). Various interventions to eliminate harborages, including street and yard cleaning and closing large holes and burrows with cement, were followed by application of a rodenticide and dichlorodiphenyltrichloroethane (DDT) to the most extensively infested apartment and office buildings and groceries. Two interventions in March and June 1952 sealed approximately 17,000 rodent nests and sprayed 1,700,000 m^2 of businesses and residences with DDT. These efforts resulted in an estimated 90% to 95% decrease in mouse and rat infestations, and an approximately 60% to 80% reduction in the numbers of rickettsialpox cases in this city during 1952, compared with the two preceding years (117). It is evident from this work that reduction of commensal rodent and house mouse mite populations is effective in controlling epidemics of rickettsialpox; nonetheless, house mice are ubiquitous residents of most urban areas, and it is unlikely that the risk of acquiring rickettsialpox can be eliminated entirely.

CLINICAL DISEASE
Incubation Period

Because nonengorged *L. sanguineus* mites are minute (e.g., <1 mm), attach for only short periods to obtain blood (e.g., minutes to hours), and inflict a painless bite, patients almost never identify the actual infective exposure (127). In rare cases where an initial exposure is known with certainty, a primary lesion develops at the bite site within seven days, and systemic manifestations occur within 10 days, following the mite bite (4,99). Estimated limits of the incubation period range from 6 to 15 days (126).

In a study from the Ukraine during the early 1950s, 1 mL of blood from a patient with rickettsialpox, collected on the fifth day of illness, was inoculated subcutaneously into a healthy volunteer (116). A 2-cm, indurated, erythematous lesion was observed at the site of inoculation on day 2 and was followed by headache, meningeal signs, and generalized weakness in the volunteer eight days later. Eleven days after the inoculation, the volunteer developed myalgias, and fever as high as 39.3°C. A papulovesicular rash appeared three days following the onset of systemic manifestations and persisted until day 17; the rash was distributed on the trunk, upper and lower extremities, face, and scalp. The volunteer's fever persisted for seven days, and his myalgias and headache lasted an additional four and five days, respectively, following lysis of the fever. Inflammation at the inoculation site increased during the febrile period but resolved when his temperature decreased and completely disappeared after two months (116).

Cutaneous and Mucosal Manifestations
The Primary Lesion
The primary lesion of rickettsialpox represents the site of inoculation of rickettsiae from the bite of an infected *L. sanguineus* mite and is described for 83% to 100% of patients in several large series (10,13,22,24,99,127,128). In its early stages, this lesion is a firm, nonpruritic, erythematous papule that soon enlarges and develops a central vesicle containing clear or opaque fluid. The lesion is generally painless and is often described by patients as a pimple, boil, or insect bite. Eventually, the vesicle ruptures and a dark brown or black crust develops over the lesion, forming the characteristic eschar (Fig. 5A). The eschar often is surrounded by a larger zone of erythema. Primary lesions range in size from 0.5 to 2.5 cm and are located, in order of decreasing frequency, on the upper extremities, lower extremities, back and shoulders, neck, face, chest, and abdomen. Eschars have also been reported uncommonly in the nostril and on the scalp, axillae, vulva, penis, buttocks, and perineum (8,22,99,127). Two eschars are occasionally identified on separate anatomic sites (12,99,127). Regional lymph nodes are often enlarged and tender. Lymphangitis has not been described in any U.S. cases series, but has been described on rare occasion in the Ukraine (10). The eschar generally persists for three to four weeks and heals to form a small depressed scar (22,127).

The Exanthem
A cutaneous eruption develops in most patients within one to four days following the onset of fever. This eruption is characterized by small (2–10 mm), discrete, erythematous maculopapules distributed on the extremities, abdomen, back, chest and face, and only rarely on the palms and soles (99,128). After two to three days, some lesions become indurated and develop a small vesicle containing cloudy fluid at the apex, described by initial investigators as "a window framed in the top of the papule" (127) (Fig. 5B). Many lesions never develop further than papules, and some vesicles never exceed the size of a pinhead and dry rapidly. The number of papules varies from 5 to >100, although most patients develop approximately 20 to 30 of these lesions. The rash is neither painful nor pruritic and generally resolves within four to seven days to leave small hyperpigmented spots (24,99,127). The severity of the rash does not reflect the severity of the systemic manifestations (2).

The Enanthem
Vesicular lesions involving the mucous membranes of the oral cavity have been reported in approximately 17% to 26% of patients in various series. The enanthem is characterized by small (2–4 mm) vesicles, maculopapules, or erosions that may occur on the tongue, soft palate, uvula, tonsils, pharynx, or buccal mucosae (22,99,123,127–129). The mucosal lesions, noticeable for as few as 48 hours, are typically more ephemeral than the cutaneous lesions and are easily missed without careful examination (99).

Systemic Manifestations
Patients with rickettsialpox generally experience sudden onset of fever, diaphoresis, lassitude, myalgias, and headache two to seven days following the appearance of the primary lesion (128). In patients who do not receive specific antibiotic therapy, these symptoms persist for approximately 7 to 10 days (116,127,128). Remittant fever and malaise are invariably reported. The usual peak temperature is 38°C to 40°C, although it may rise to 41°C (92,127). A headache, usually frontal and occasionally severe, is described in approximately 90% to 100% of patients (3,127). Myalgias are frequently reported and are most commonly described as backache (128,130). Other less frequently described findings include conjunctivitis (Fig. 5C), splenomegaly, pharyngitis, nausea, and vomiting (24,99,127).

Rickettsialpox is generally described as a relatively benign, self-limited illness; however, central nervous system signs severe enough to warrant lumbar puncture have been documented, including photophobia, vertigo, pain on movement of the eyes, and nuchal rigidity. The cerebrospinal fluid specimens of the few patients for whom this specimen has been examined showed no abnormalities (99). Most patients show a mild-to-moderate leukopenia ($2.4–4.0 \times 10^9$ leukocytes/L) that returns to normal levels approximately two to three weeks

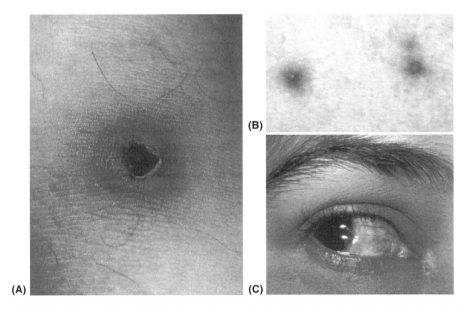

FIGURE 5 (*See color insert.*) (**A**) Eschar on the arm of a New York City patient with rickettsialpox. *R. akari* was subsequently isolated in cell culture from this lesion (20). (**B**) Papulovesicular rash on the upper back of a New York City patient with rickettsialpox. The patient had approximately 20 to 30 similar lesions on her back and face, and first noted the rash three days after the appearance of an eschar. (**C**) Conjunctival injection in a patient with rickettsialpox.

after the acute illness (10,92,116,126). Serial blood cell measurements of an HIV-infected patient acutely infected with *R. akari* revealed transient mild decreases in the absolute numbers of leukocytes and platelets during the acute stage of the infection, suggesting that rickettsialpox may cause a more generalized myelosuppression (23). Large atypical mononuclear cells, with vacuolated cytoplasm that resemble the cells associated with infectious mononucleosis, may appear transiently in the peripheral blood smears of some patients during the early stages of the illness (99). In contemporary case series, patients with rickettsialpox are hospitalized infrequently. No deaths have been attributed to infection with *R. akari* (13,22,24,92).

Differential Diagnosis

The differential diagnosis of a patient with an eschar encompasses various infectious and noninfectious syndromes, including trauma, spider bite, erythema gangrenosum, factitial dermatitis, herpes simplex, herpes zoster, aspergillosis, and several diseases caused by agents associated with bioterrorism (e.g., *Francisella tularensis*, *Yersinia pestis*, *Burkholderia pseudomallei*, and *B. anthracis*) (13,20,22,93). Occasionally, rickettsialpox may even mimic some sexually transmitted diseases. Shankman described a patient with an ulcerated lesion on his penis and bilateral inguinal adenopathy for whom his initial differential diagnosis included chancroid, granuloma inguinale, syphilis, and herpes simplex; however, a papular rash appeared three days later and allowed Shankman to establish the diagnosis of rickettsialpox (8). The eschar of rickettsialpox is indistinguishable from the primary lesions associated with many other rickettsioses, including African tick bite fever, boutonneuse fever, Siberian tick typhus, Queensland tick typhus, scrub typhus, and a recently described rickettsiosis in the Americas caused by *R. parkeri* (20,131,132). In this context, a careful clinical history that includes questions about recent travel and potential exposures to rodents or arthropods can provide important clues for distinguishing among these diseases. It is also important for physicians to obtain, whenever possible, appropriate clinical specimens (i.e., eschar biopsy samples) which allow a pathogen-specific diagnosis (20).

PATHOGENESIS
Entry, Intracellular Growth, and Host Cell Responses

Entry of *R. akari* into the host cell is accomplished by induced phagocytosis (32). Intracellular *R. akari* undergoes binary fission, and accumulates to large numbers within 96 hours, without causing apparent structural damage to their host cells (15,16,32). In the host cell cytoplasm, *R. akari* is capable of active movement, first documented using stop action cinemicrography (32) and later characterized as the ability *R. akari* to induce polymerization of unipolar actin tails (27). In the initial cinemicrographic studies, the speed of movement of *R. akari* was higher than those observed for *R. conorii* or *R. sibirica*. Actin-based motility is also the propulsive force that allows *R. akari* to penetrate the nucleus of its host cell (27,32); however, differences in nuclear cytoskeletal proteins may influence the number of host cell nuclei that are penetrated by *R. akari* (32). *R. akari* exits its host cell through filopodia that detach and rupture immediately after release from the cell membrane. Extracellular rickettsiae are often seen surrounded by cellular membrane and fragments of the host cytoplasm (Fig. 1B). *R. akari* loses directed movement soon after leaving the cell, and only Brownian movement is observed in cell-free rickettsiae (32).

Vero cells infected with *R. akari* do not show obvious cytopathologic changes until late in the course of the infection. L929 cells infected with *R. akari* demonstrate cytotoxic effects earlier in the infection and these morphologic changes correlate with decreased thymidine incorporation by the cells (30). In contrast, mouse peritoneal macrophages appear to be relatively resistant to infection with *R. akari* perhaps because of activation of the transcriptional factor NF kappa B in these cells (26). It is unknown if this activation also modulates apoptotic responses of human macrophages infected with *R. akari* in vivo, or if *R. akari* triggers an antiapoptotic mechanism similar to the mechanism described for *R. rickettsii* in human endothelial cells (133).

Infection of primary mouse macrophages with *R. akari* induces in vitro secretion of IL-1β and IL-6, and the kinetics of cytokine production are different from those measured when the cells are infected with *R. typhi*. The secretion of TNF-α was also slightly increased but no measurable changes were reported for several other cytokines including interferon gamma, IL-10, IL-12, and TGF-β (26).

Immune Responses to *R. akari*

The host immune responses to infection with *R. akari* have been characterized partially in various studies. Athymic and thymus-intact BALB/c mice treated with antibiotics survive intraperitoneal infection with 2.5×10^8 rickettsiae, and develop robust titers of antirickettsial antibodies (134). However, only euthymic mice develop postinfection immunity to subsequent challenge with *R. akari*. The passive transfer of anti-*R. akari* antibodies, or the transplantation of splenic cells from mice that had recovered from infection, will protect susceptible immunocompetent mice from fatal infection with *R. akari*. Macrophages from athymic or euthymic mice will destroy opsonized *R. akari* in vitro, even though infection in the presence of antibody does not occur in vivo. These results suggest a crucial role for T-cell-mediated activation of macrophages in recovery from infection with *R. akari* (134). Murine antibody responses to *R. akari* and other spotted fever group rickettsiae appear as early as three to five days following infection. Athymic mice produce predominantly IgM antibody, and both IgM and IgG antibodies were produced by thymus-intact mice (135).

Several studies demonstrate variability of different inbred mouse strains and outbred stocks in resistance to lethal infection with *R. akari*. The susceptibility of mouse strains depend primarily on macrophage competence (136–141). Of many mouse strains tested, C3H/HeJ and other mouse lineages with defective macrophage function are particularly susceptible to lethal infection with *R. akari* (136,138). Peritoneal macrophages from mouse strains resistant to lethal effects of *R. akari* infection show high levels of tumoricidal and rickettsiacidal activities within two to four days after intraperitoneal inoculation of *R. akari*, and most of these mice clear the infection by day 4 (139). In contrast, macrophages from susceptible mouse strains do not exhibit nonspecific tumor cytotoxicity and these mice die within 8 to 10 days after inoculation with *R. akari*. Activation of macrophages from susceptible animals can be achieved by lymphokine treatment (prior to or after infection with *R. akari*) or nonspecifically by infection with BCG strain of *Mycobacterium bovis* (139).

C3H/HeJ mice have a dominant negative mutation in the cytoplasmic domain of the TLR4 receptor (142). TLR4 may represent the primary LPS-signaling receptor that control diverse functions contributing to host resistance to Gram-negative bacteria, including stimulation of early cytokine expression, recruitment and activation of phagocytic cells, and eventual establishment of cell-mediated adaptive immunity (143,144). *R. akari* is tropic for macrophages in human tissues (25) and in Swiss Webster mice following intravenous inoculation with *R. akari* (58); however, the specific cell-signaling events following entry of *R. akari* into host macrophages and the specific rickettsial targets of protective immunity are unknown.

Animal Models of Infection

Most animal models of rickettsialpox have used the yolk sacs of embryonated chicken eggs infected with *R. akari*, or tissue suspensions from infected rodents as the infective inoculum. In these investigations, animals have been infected by intraperitoneal, intracerebral, intravenous, or intranasal routes of exposure (10,21,58,59,145). In this context, the disease manifestations observed from these models may not necessarily represent the pathology of natural infections in animals that follow from percutaneous inoculation of salivary secretions of an infecting mite.

Domestic mice and outbred white Swiss Webster mice inoculated intraperitoneally, intranasally, intracerebrally, or intravenously with *R. akari* develop ruffled fur, closed eyelids, rapid breathing, and anorexia, followed by death 5 to 14 days after exposure (7,21,58,59,145). Intraperitoneal inoculation causes massive accumulation of rickettsiae in the liver, spleen, and peritoneal fluid, with necrosis in the liver and spleen, and occasionally in the kidneys, brain, and lung (21,59,145). White mice inoculated intraperitoneally with a concentrated suspension of *R. akari* (strain Toger) exhibit weight-dependent mortality. All mice weighing 6 to 8 g die within 10 days of infection, 50% of mice weighing 10 to 12 g die within five days, and mice weighing 16 to 18 g show no clinical signs of illness (60). Intranasal inoculation of *R. akari* in mice causes a rickettsial pneumonia and death of the animal within three to five days (59). Intracerebral inoculation results in a massive accumulation of rickettsiae in the leptomeninges and death within four days following inoculation (145). Rickettsiae can be detected in the brain, liver, lungs, and kidneys of mice 4 to 11 days following subcutaneous inoculation with *R. akari*, and persist in the spleen for as long as 18 to 24 days following inoculation (21).

Histological changes in mice infected by intraperitoneal inoculation are most prominent in regional lymph nodes, liver, and spleen (145). Infection of lymph nodes is associated with swelling of blood vessels and progressive proliferation of endothelium and reticular cells in sinuses and follicles. Proliferation is detected two to three days following inoculation, and necrotic changes appear on day 4. Rickettsiae accumulate in reticular cells and endothelial sinuses. Liver changes include hyperplasia of Kupffer cells and infiltration of the infected area by polymorphonuclear leukocytes. By day 5 after inoculation, dystrophic and necrotic changes are detected which often coincide with the appearance of inflammatory and thrombotic foci; numerous rickettsiae are detected in liver cells on days 4 to 7 following inoculation. Rickettsial infection of the spleen causes hyperplasia and swelling of reticular sinuses, dystrophic and necrotic changes occur on day 4 following inoculation, and massive accumulation of rickettsiae is often accompanied by vasculitis, proliferation of endothelium, and foci of inflammation. Similar changes are rare in mice infected subcutaneously. Intravenous infection causes severe hepatic injury and disseminated vascular lesions. In these animals, rickettsiae are detected in macrophages of the splenic red pulp, in detached endothelial cells, and in circulating monocytes (58).

The brown rat (*R. norvegicus*) does not demonstrate clinical symptoms following intraperitoneal inoculation with *R. akari* but may develop a low-level persistent infection that can be detected by passage of rat tissue suspensions into naïve guinea pigs (59). White laboratory rats infected by intraperitoneal inoculation develop fever and mild periorchitis (59,145). Histopathologic changes in the peritoneum include proliferation of connective tissue, infiltration with polymorphonuclear leukocytes, and hypervascularization of viscera. Similar changes occur in the tunica vaginalis, and myocarditis and nephritis are occasionally observed (145). Cotton rats (*S. hispidus*) are highly susceptible to intraperitoneal infection with *R. akari*. After an eight-day incubation period, the animals appear motionless, with markedly ruffled fur and partially closed eyelids. The spleen and liver become enlarged, and numerous intracellular rickettsiae and hemorrhagic exudates can be seen in the peritoneal cavity (59).

Intraperitoneal inoculation of *R. akari* in guinea pigs (*Cavia porcelus*) causes fever, peritonitis, and periorchitis, but the animals typically recover (59,60,145). All strains from endemic foci in the Ukraine are pathogenic for guinea pigs and most cause fever to 40°C for three to eight days; however, infection with the Askalunin strain of *R. akari* results in a milder febrile response (60). Histologic examination of the peritoneum during the first days after inoculation reveals endothelial swelling and lymphocytic infiltrates. Periorchitis is characterized by adherence of the testes to the inflamed and thickened tunica vaginalis, and by altered spermatogenesis (145). Regional lymph nodes and the spleen become enlarged five to six days following inoculation and are accompanied by hyperplasia of reticular and endothelial cells. Swelling and hyperplasia of Kupffer cells and single-cell hepatocyte necrosis are seen in livers of infected guinea pigs. Subcutaneous infection of guinea pigs causes cutaneous erythema within three days, followed by infiltration and necrosis of the infected area, and subsequent formation of an eschar (59).

ANTIBIOTIC SUSCEPTIBILITY AND THERAPY

The in vivo efficacy of tetracyclines and chloramphenicol antibiotics against *R. akari* was recognized soon after the initial clinical recognition of rickettsialpox (146,147). Chloramphenicol and chlortetracycline (aureomycin) were utilized as effective therapies for patients with rickettsialpox as early as 1949 (148), and oxytetracycline (terramycin) was used therapeutically beginning in 1950 (149). Most patients defervesce and show improvement of constitutional symptoms (e.g., headache and myalgias) within one day after starting therapy with these drugs. Tetracyclines, particularly doxycycline, remain the drugs of choice for the treatment of rickettsialpox. In two contemporary case series documenting antibiotic responses in 28 patients who received tetracycline or doxycycline treatment for rickettsialpox, fever and other systemic symptoms resolved in most patients within 24 hours, and all patients became asymptomatic within 48 hours (22,24). Interestingly, two young children in these same studies were treated using erythromycin and became afebrile within the same interval, despite in vitro data to suggest that *R. akari* is relatively resistant to erythromycin (35). Experimental studies and some anecdotal clinical data indicate that several other antibiotics, including penicillins, sulfa-containing antimicrobials, streptomycin, and cephalosporins, are ineffective therapies for infection with *R. akari* (2,20,150,151).

Detailed in vitro evaluation of the susceptibility of *R. akari* to various antibiotics using dye uptake and plaque assays indicate that *R. akari* is highly susceptible to doxycycline with a minimal inhibitory concentration (MIC) of 0.06 to 0.125 μg/mL. These assays also show that thiamphenicol, a derivative of chloramphenicol, and rifampin are effective at 0.5 to 2.0 and 0.006 to 1.0 μg/mL, respectively (35). Tetracyclines and chloramphenicol exert bacteriostatic activity in Swiss Webster mice infected with *R. akari*; although these antibiotics prevent the development of disease and death, viable rickettsiae can be detected in the mice for as long as 40 days after antibiotic treatment (152).

R. akari is also susceptible to various fluoroquinolones in vitro, including ciprofloxacin, oflaxacin, and pefloxacin, with MICs that range between 0.5 and 2.0 μg/mL (35). Josamycin has the lowest MIC (0.5–1.0 μg/mL) of the macrolide antibiotics, including pristinamycin (1–8 μg/mL) and clarithromycin (0.5–4.0 μg/mL). MICs of 0.25 and 2 μg/mL have been determined for azithromycin and clarythromycin, respectively, using IFA analysis of infected Vero cell monolayers (153). Erythromycin has bacteriostatic effects against *R. akari*, but only at high MICs (e.g., 2–8 μg/mL), as determined by a dye uptake assay (35), and 16 μg/mL using an IFA assay (153). In a similar manner, some beta-lactam and aminoglycoside antibiotics have in vitro bacteriostatic activity against *R. akari* at very high concentrations. *R. akari* grown in mouse fibroblast cell culture will form spheroblasts when treated with 50 to 100 μg/mL of penicillin or 250 to 1500 μg/mL of vancomycin; however, even high concentrations of penicillin do not inhibit bacterial replication (154).

LABORATORY DIAGNOSIS
Serology

The diagnosis of rickettsialpox is confirmed most often by serologic testing. Complement fixation assays were the first tests developed to detect antibodies reactive with *R. akari*. Most patients show negligible or low titers (≤16) during the first 10 days of illness; however, by three weeks patients generally demonstrate titers ≥64 (99).

Patients with rickettsialpox typically do not develop agglutinating antibodies against the OX-19, OX-2, and OX-K antigens of *Proteus vulgaris* (i.e., negative Weil–Felix reactions). Although low titers against one or more of these antigens are occasionally observed in some patients, a negative Weil–Felix test is considered a relatively characteristic serologic feature of rickettsialpox (3,10,99,155).

The microimmunofluorescence or IFA assay is the test of choice for the serologic diagnosis of rickettsioses (13,22,24,58,91,98,100,108). Diagnostic antibody titers (i.e., ≥64) are frequently lacking during the acute phase of the illness. For example, a recent study of 22 rickettsialpox patients tested by IFA showed that only 11 (50%) of these patients had diagnostic IFA titers against *R. akari* in the first serum specimen, collected a median of seven days (range 3–29) after the onset of symptoms. All 11 patients for whom a second sample was obtained, collected a median of 41 days (range 16–72) after onset, showed diagnostic antibody, with a geometric mean titer for the group of 798 (range 256–4096) (13).

A major caveat in the interpretation of almost all commonly used serologic techniques is the high cross-reactivity among antigens of rickettsiae in the spotted fever group. This cross-reactivity is caused by group-specific LPS and species-specific protein antigens (55,156). The method of antigen preparation, including purification, heating, and inactivation, can affect the results of rickettsial agglutination and complement fixation assays (157). The interpretation of serologic results should be done in the context of the epidemiologic situation and, when possible, more specific assays should be used to corroborate the diagnosis. Cross-adsorption tests have been used to confirm some cases of rickettsialpox (91,98,100,108). Only one high-molecular-weight protein of *R. akari* is detected by Western blotting when reacted with mouse polyclonal antiserum (58) or convalescent-phase human serum (158). Western blot analysis has been used effectively to exclude the diagnosis of rickettsialpox in some circumstances when IFA testing indicated high titers of antibody cross-reactive with *R. akari* (159).

Cell Culture Isolation

During the decade that followed the discovery of *R. akari*, several isolates were obtained from humans, rodents, and house mouse mites. Recovery of the pathogen was typically accomplished by inoculating whole blood from febrile patients, or triturates of infected rodent or mite tissues into the peritoneal cavity of mice. These isolates were often then passed in guinea pigs and chicken yolk sacs to obtain a noncontaminated, robust strain. The MK (Kaplan) strain of *R. akari* was isolated from blood obtained from a 20-year-old patient of Shankman's named Marjory Kaplan (1,5). Additional isolates were soon recovered from patients in New York City (5,99,127) and the Ukraine (10). *R. akari* was also isolated from *L. sanguineus* and *M. musculus* in New York and other northeastern U.S. cities (7,65–67), from *R. norvegicus*, *M. musculus*, and *L. sanguineus* in the Ukraine (10,11,59), and from *M. fortis pelliceus* in Korea (88). More recently, isolates of *R. akari* have been obtained in Vero cells inoculated with patient blood (58) or triturates of eschar biopsy specimens (20).

Histopathology and Immunohistochemistry

The cutaneous histopathology of the primary lesion demonstrates extensive necrosis of the epidermis and dermis, with subjacent perivascular and periadnexal inflammatory cell infiltrates and occasional panniculitis (Fig. 6A). The histopathology of rash is typically more variable and age-dependent, but papules generally reveal edema of the papillary dermis, spongiosis, mononuclear infiltrates of the epidermis, vacuolar degeneration of the basal cell layer, and perivascular and periadnexal inflammation. Fully developed papulovesicles show subepidermal vesicle formation that is a relatively characteristic histopathologic feature of rickettsialpox (24,92) (Fig. 6B). Inflamed blood vessels demonstrate varying degrees of endothelial swelling, blurring or obliteration of the vessel wall by inflammatory cell infiltrates, mural necrosis, extravasation of red cells, or fibrin thrombi. Lymphocytes and macrophages comprise the predominant inflammatory cell types (Fig. 6C), although neutrophils are occasionally present in and around necrotic foci (24). These infiltrates may involve hair follicles, sebaceous and eccrine sweat glands, erector pili muscles, or nerve twigs (24,160,161).

Several immunohistochemistry studies have identified the cellular targets of infection and distribution of *R. akari* in the cutaneous lesions of rickettsialpox using a polyclonal rabbit anti-*R. rickettsii* antibody (13,20,22,24) or a monoclonal antibody directed against the LPS of *R. conorii* (25), that cross-react with other spotted fever group rickettsiae, including *R. akari* (Fig. 6D). *R. akari* is found predominantly in macrophages in the perivascular and periadnexal inflammatory cell infiltrates of eschars and papulovesicles, and only rarely in vascular endothelial cells of these lesions (20,25) (Fig. 6E). Rickettsiae and rickettsial antigens are characteristically distributed in greater abundance in eschars than in the papulovesicles. In this context, biopsy specimens of eschars provide the best sample for diagnostic evaluation (20,22).

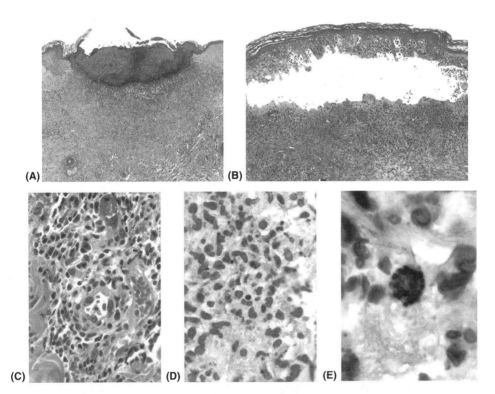

FIGURE 6 (*See color insert.*) Cutaneous histopathology of rickettsialpox and immunohistochemical localization of *R. akari*. (**A**) A primary lesion (eschar), demonstrating extensive epidermal and dermal necrosis, with perivascular and periadnexal inflammation (original magnification: ×12.5, hematoxylin and eosin stain). (**B**) Papulovesicular lesion showing prominent subepidermal vesicle (original magnification: ×25, hematoxylin and eosin stain). (**C**) Perivascular inflammatory cell infiltrate, comprised predominantly of lymphocytes and macrophages, with swelling of vascular endothelium of involved vessel (original magnification: ×100, hematoxylin and eosin stain). (**D**) *R. akari* distributed in a perivascular inflammatory cell focus in an eschar (original magnification: ×100, immunoalkaline phosphatase with rabbit anti-*R. rickettsii* antibody and naphthol fast-red, with hematoxylin counterstain). (**E**) Coccoid intracellular *R. akari* in a macrophage in the perivascular infiltrate of an eschar (original magnification: ×158, immunoalkaline phosphatase with rabbit anti-*R. rickettsii* antibody and naphthol fast-red, with hematoxylin counterstain).

Molecular Methods

The complete and recently available nucleotide sequence of the *R. akari* genome and other species of *Rickettsia* provides many targets to design specific diagnostic tools for accurate and reliable identification of *R. akari*. However, relatively few data are available that describe the utility of PCR for the diagnosis of rickettsialpox. Nested PCR has been used to amplify a fragment of the *Rickettsia* genus-specific 17-kDa outer membrane protein gene from eschar biopsy samples from rickettsialpox patients (20). Of seven samples that were positive for spotted fever rickettsiae by immunohistochemical stain, six gave positive PCR signals whose specificity could be confirmed by DNA sequencing. At least two studies report detection of *R. akari* DNA in serum samples of patients with an acute febrile illness using nested PCR of the 120-kDa protein (rompB) gene (121,162); however, these results have been questioned because of technical inconsistencies (163).

CONCLUSION

Sixty years has passed since rickettsialpox emerged in one of the largest metropolitan centers in the world. Rickettsialpox remains one of the most peculiar of the spotted fever rickettsioses, in terms of its global but predominantly urban occurrence, its mite vector, and its relatively benign clinical course. The cosmopolitan distributions of *R. akari*, *L. sanguineus*, and *M. musculus* suggest that many previously unrecognized cases of rickettsialpox remain to be identified in several continents. An intensified clinical focus on eschar-associated diseases, and an emphasis on coupling traditional diagnostic methods (e.g., cell culture isolation) with contemporary molecular techniques (e.g., PCR and nucleotide sequencing), will undoubtedly expand the magnitude of this fascinating and unusual rickettsial disease.

ACKNOWLEDGMENTS

We gratefully acknowledge the following individuals for their assistance: Vsevolod L. Popov, University of Texas Medical Branch, Galveston, for Figure 1A and B; Suzanna Radulovic, School of Medicine, University of Maryland, Baltimore, for Figure 1C; Barry M. OConnor, University of Michigan, for providing the specimen of *L. sanguineus* in Figure 2A; The National Pest Management Association, Fairfax, VA, for permission to reproduce Figure 2B; Tamara Koss, Columbia University College of Physicians and Surgeons, New York, NY, for Figure 5A and B; Oleg Mediannikov, The Gamaleya Research Institute, Moscow, for assistance with obtaining many of the original Russian articles; Gregory A. Dasch, CDC, Atlanta, for useful suggestions and review of the manuscript, and Mitesh Patel and Cynthia Goldsmith, CDC, Atlanta, GA, for assistance in preparing the figures.

REFERENCES

1. Rouéche B. The alerting of Mr. Pomerantz. The New Yorker 1947; 23:28–37.
2. Shankman B. Report of an outbreak of endemic febrile illness, not yet identified, occurring in New York City. NY State J Med 1946; 46:2156–2159.
3. Greenberg M, Pellitteri O. Rickettsialpox. Bull NY Acad Med 1947; 23:338–351.
4. Sussman LN. Kew Gardens' spotted fever. NY Med 1946; 2:27–28.
5. Huebner RJ, Stamps P, Armstrong C. Rickettsialpox—a newly discovered rickettsial disease. I. Isolation of the etiological agent. Public Health Rep 1946; 45:1605–1614.
6. Greenberg M, Pellitteri OJ, Jellison WL. Rickettsialpox—a newly discovered rickettsial disease. III. Epidemiology. Am J Pub Health 1947; 37:860–868.
7. Huebner RJ, Jellison WL, Armstrong C. Rickettsialpox—a newly recognized rickettsial disease. V. Recovery of *Rickettsia akari* from a house mouse (*Mus musculus*). Public Health Rep 1947; 62:777–780.
8. Shankman B. A new rickettsial illness occurring in New York City: supplementary report. NY State J Med 1947; 47:711.
9. Nichols E, Rindge ME, Russell GG. The relationship of the habits of the house mouse and the mouse mite (*Allodermanyssus sanguineus*) to the spread of rickettsialpox. Ann Intern Med 1953; 39:92–102.
10. Kulagin SM. Characteristics of endemic rickettsioses. Zh Mikrobiol Epidemiol Immunobiol 1952; 12:3–10 (in Russian).

11. Levi MI, Kiselev RI, Tchueva GI, Kislyakova LN. Epidemiology of vesicular rickettsiosis. Ann Kharkov Mechnikov Res Inst 1954; 20:285–291 (in Russian).
12. Wong B, Singer C, Armstrong D, Millian SJ. Rickettsialpox: case report and epidemiologic review. J Am Med Assoc 1979; 242:1998–1999.
13. Paddock CD, Zaki SR, Koss T, et al. Rickettsialpox in New York City: a persistent urban zoonosis. Ann NY Acad Sci 2003; 990:36–44.
14. Parola P, Paddock CD, Raoult D. Tick-borne rickettsioses around the world: emerging diseases challenging old concepts. Clin Microbiol Rev 2005; 18:719–756.
15. Gudima OS, Alimov ZA. Ultrastructure and some peculiarities of an interaction with the cell of the causative agent of vesicular rickettsiosis—*Dermacentroxenus murinus* Kulagin (1951). Zh Mikrobiol Epidemiol Immunobiol 1974; 7:8–10 (in Russian).
16. Popov VL, Barkhatova OI. Interaction of *Rickettsia akari* with the host cell in vitro: multiplication, development of spheroplast-like forms and destruction in phagosomes. Zh Mikrobiol Epidemiol Immunobiol 1984; 2:23–27 (in Russian).
17. Silverman DJ, Wisseman CL Jr. Comparative ultrastructural study on the cell envelopes of *Rickettsia prowazekii*, *Rickettsia rickettsii*, and *Rickettsia tsutsugamushi*. Infect Immun 1978; 21:1020–1023.
18. Palmer EL, Martin ML, Mallavia L. Ultrastructure of the surface of *Rickettsia prowazeki* and *Rickettsia akari*. Appl Microbiol 1974; 28:713–716.
19. Giménez DF. Staining rickettsiae in yolk-sac cultures. Stain Technol 1964; 39:135–140.
20. Paddock CD, Koss T, Eremeeva ME, et al. Isolation of *Rickettsia akari* from eschars of patients with rickettsialpox. Am J Trop Med Hyg 2006; 75:732–738.
21. Kiselev RI. Experimental studies of the pathogenesis of vesicular rickettsiosis in domestic mice. Ann Kharkov Mechnikov Res Inst 1954; 20:279–284 (in Russian).
22. Koss T, Carter EL, Grossman ME, et al. Increased detection of rickettsialpox in a New York City hospital following the anthrax outbreak of 2001: use of immunohistochemistry for the rapid confirmation of cases in an era of bioterrorism. Arch Dermatol 2003; 139:1545–1552.
23. Sanders S, Di Costanzo D, Leach J, et al. Rickettsialpox in a patient with HIV infection. J Am Acad Dermatol 2003; 48:286–289.
24. Kass EM, Szaniawski WK, Levy H, et al. Rickettsialpox in a New York City hospital, 1980 to 1989. N Engl J Med 1994; 331:1612–1617.
25. Walker DH, Hudnall SD, Szaniawski WK, Feng HM. Monoclonal antibody-based immunohistochemical diagnosis of rickettsialpox: the macrophage is the principal target. Mod Pathol 1999; 12:529–533.
26. Radulovic S, Price PW, Beier MS, et al. *Rickettsia*–macrophage interactions: host cell responses to *Rickettsia akari* and *Rickettsia typhi*. Infect Immun 2002; 70:2576–2582.
27. Radulovic S, Troyer JM, Beier MS, Azad AF. *Rickettsia*-induced actin assembly requires expression of an actA gene homolog. 98th General Meeting of the American Society for Microbiology. Atlanta, Georgia: 1998.
28. Gouin E, Egile C, Dehoux P, et al. The RickA protein of *Rickettsia conorii* activates the Arp2/3 complex. Nature 2004; 427:457–461.
29. Jeng RL, Goley ED, D'Alessio JA, et al. A *Rickettsia* WASP-like protein activates the Arp2/3 complex and mediates actin-based motility. Cell Microbiol 2004; 6:761–769.
30. Weiss E, Newman LW, Grays R, Green AE. Metabolism of *Rickettsia typhi* and *Rickettsia akari* in irradiated L cells. Infect Immun 1972; 6:50–57.
31. Řeháček J, Brezina R, Majerská M. Multiplication of rickettsiae in tick cells in vitro. Acta Virol 1968; 12:41–43.
32. Kokorin IN, Kiet CD. Vital observations and cinematography of intracellular development of *D. muris* and its interaction with cells. Zh Mikrobiol Epidemiol Immunobiol 1976; 5:50–52 (in Russian).
33. Wike DA, Tallent G, Peacock MG, Ormsbee RA. Studies of the rickettsial plaque assay technique. Infect Immun 1972; 5:715–722.
34. McDade JE, Stakebake JR, Gerone PJ. Plaque assay system for several species of *Rickettsia*. J Bacteriol 1969; 99:910–912.
35. Rolain JM, Maurin M, Vestris G, Raoult D. In vitro susceptibilities of 27 rickettsiae to 13 antimicrobials. Antimicrob Agents Chemother 1998; 42:1537–1541.
36. Schwartz S, Zhang Z, Frazer KA, et al. PipMaker—a web server for aligning two genomic DNA sequences. Genome Res 2000; 10:577–586.
37. Dasch GA, Yu Q, Eremeeva ME. Consensus primer PCR analysis of genomes of *Rickettsia* spp. International Conference on Rickettsiae and Rickettsial Diseases. Slovenia: Ljubljana, 2002. [abstract O-63].
38. Eremeeva M, Yu X, Raoult D. Differentiation among spotted fever group rickettsiae species by analysis of restriction fragment length polymorphism of PCR-amplified DNA. J Clin Microbiol 1994; 32:803–810.
39. Gilmore RD. Comparison of the *rompA* gene repeat regions of *Rickettsiae* reveals species-specific arrangements of individual repeating units. Gene 1993; 125:97–102.
40. Blanc G, Ngwamidiba M, Ogata H, et al. Molecular evolution of rickettsia surface antigens: evidence of positive selection. Mol Biol Evol 2005; 22:2073–2083.

41. Eremeeva ME, Hassel TC, Lemon-Steiner H, et al. A genome-based comparison of fourteen strains of *Rickettsia akari*. 18th Sesquiannual Meeting of the American Society for Rickettsiology [abstract 7]. MD: Rocky Gap, 2003.
42. Eremeeva ME, Madan A, Malek J, Dasch GA. Analysis of the genome sequence of *Rickettsia akari*, *R. sibirica*, and *R. rickettsii*: implications for their pathology. American Society for Microbiology and the Institute for Genomic Research Conference on Microbial Genomes [abstract 79]. LA: New Orleans, 2003.
43. Stothard DR, Fuerst PA. Evolutionary analysis of the spotted fever and typhus groups of *Rickettsia* using 16S rRNA sequences. Syst Appl Microbiol 1995; 18:52–61.
44. Roux V, Raoult D. Phylogenetic analysis of the genus *Rickettsia* by 16S rDNA sequencing. Res Microbiol 1995; 146:385–396.
45. Roux V, Rydkina E, Eremeeva M, Raoult D. Citrate synthase gene comparison, a new tool for phylogenetic analysis, and its application for the rickettsiae. Int J Syst Bacteriol 1997; 47:252–261.
46. Sekeyova Z, Roux V, Raoult D. Phylogeny of *Rickettsia* spp. inferred by comparing sequences of 'gene D', which encodes an intracytoplasmic protein. Int J Syst Evol Microbiol 2001; 51:1353–1360.
47. Eremeeva ME, Madan A, Shaw CD, Tang K, Dasch GA. New perspectives on rickettsial evolution from new genome sequences of *Rickettsia*, particularly *R. canadensis*, and *Orientia tsutsugamushi*. Ann NY Acad Sci 2005; 1063:47–63.
48. Xu W, Raoult D. Taxonomic relationships among spotted fever group rickettsiae as revealed by antigenic analysis with monoclonal antibodies. J Clin Microbiol 1998; 36:887–896.
49. Fang R, Raoult D. Antigenic classification of *Rickettsia felis* by using monoclonal and polyclonal antibodies. Clin Diagn Lab Immunol 2003; 10:221–228.
50. McDade JE, Black CM, Roumillat LF, Redus MA, Spruill CL. Addition of monoclonal antibodies specific for *Rickettsia akari* to the rickettsial diagnostic panel. J Clin Microbiol 1988; 26:2221–2223.
51. Pickens EG, Bell EJ, Lackman DB, Burgdorfer W. Use of mouse serum in identification and serologic classification of *Rickettsia akari* and *Rickettsia australis*. J Immunol 1965; 94:883–889.
52. Philip RN, Casper EA, Burgdorfer W, et al. Serologic typing of rickettsiae of the spotted fever group by microimmunofluorescence. J Immunol 1978; 121:1961–1968.
53. Obiejski MK, Palmer EL, Tzianabos T. Proteins of purified rickettsiae. Microbios 1974; 11:61–76.
54. Pedersen CE, Walters VD. Comparative electrophoresis of spotted fever group rickettsial proteins. Life Sci 1978; 22:583–587.
55. Anacker RL, Mann RE, Gonzales C. Reactivity of monoclonal antibodies to *Rickettsia rickettsii* with spotted fever and typhus group rickettsiae. J Clin Microbiol 1987; 25:167–171.
56. Cwikel BJ, Ighbarieh J, Sarov I. Antigenic polypeptides of Israeli spotted fever isolates compared with other spotted fever group rickettsiae. Ann NY Acad Sci 1990; 590:381–388.
57. Xu W, Raoult D. Distribution of immunogenic epitopes on the two major immunodominant proteins (rOmpA and rOmpB) of *Rickettsia conorii* among the other rickettsiae of the spotted fever group. Clin Diagn Lab Immunol 1997; 4:753–763.
58. Radulovic S, Feng HM, Morovic M, et al. Isolation of *Rickettsia akari* from a patient in a region where Mediterranean spotted fever is endemic. Clin Infect Dis 1996; 22:216–220.
59. Lavrushina TT, Korenblit RS, Kiselev RI. Study of biological properties of rickettsial strains "Zh" and "Z-M". Ann Kharkov Mechnikov Res Inst 1954; 20:259–264 (in Russian).
60. Eremeeva M, Balayeva N, Ignatovich V, Raoult D. Genomic study of *Rickettsia akari* by pulsed-field gel electrophoresis. J Clin Microbiol 1995; 33:3022–3024.
61. Eremeeva ME, Balayeva NM, Ignatovich VF, Raoult D. Proteinic and genomic identification of spotted fever group rickettsiae isolated in the former USSR. J Clin Microbiol 1993; 31:2625–2633.
62. Hirst S. On the parasitic acari found on the species of rodents frequenting human habitations in Egypt. Bull Entomol Res 1914; 5:215–229.
63. Ewing SA. A second introduced rat mite becomes annoying to man. Proc Helminth Soc Wash 1942; 9:74–75.
64. Pratt HD, Lane JE, Harmston FC. New locality records for *Allodermanyssus sanguineus*, vector of rickettsialpox. J Econ Entomol 1949; 42:414–415.
65. Huebner RJ, Jellison WL, Pomerantz C. Rickettsialpox—a newly recognized rickettsial disease. IV. Isolation of a rickettsia apparently identical with the causative agent of rickettsialpox from *Allodermanyssus sanguineus*, a rodent mite. Public Health Rep 1946; 61:1677–1682.
66. Fuller HS, Murray ES, Ayres JC, Snyder JC, Potash L. Studies of rickettsialpox. II. Recovery of the causative agent from house mice in Boston, Massachusetts. Am J Hyg 1951; 54:82–100.
67. Eustis EB, Fuller HS. Rickettsialpox. II. Recovery of *Rickettsia akari* from mites, *Allodermanyssus sanguineus*, from West Hartford, Conn. Proc Soc Exp Biol Med 1952; 80:546–549.
68. Fuller HS. Studies of rickettsialpox. III. Life cycle of the mite vector, Allodermanyssus sanguineus. Am J Hyg 1954; 59:236–239.
69. Masters CO. Arthropods of medical importance in Ohio. Ohio J Sci 1960; 60:332–334.
70. Reeves WK, Cobb KD. Ectoparasites of house mice (*Mus musculus*) from pet stores in South Carolina, U.S.A. Comp Parasitol 2005; 72:193–195.
71. El-Kady GA, Makled KM, Morsy TA, Morsy ZS. Rodents, their seasonal activity, ecto- and blood-parasites in Saint Catherine area, South Sinai Governorate, Egypt. J Egypt Soc Parasitol 1998; 28:815–826.

72. Kulagin SM, Zemskaya AA. The mite *Allodermanyssus sanguineus* Hirst as a vector of vesicular rickettsiosis. In: Questions of Regional Experimental Parasitology and Medical Zoology. Moscow: Medgiz, 1953:34–40 (in Russian).
73. Zemskaya AA, Pchelkina AA. On the infection of various species of gamasidae mites with *Rickettsia burneti* in natural foci of Q fever. Zh Mikrobiol Epidemiol Immunobiol 1968; 45:130–132 (in Russian).
74. Dardanoni L, Lavagnino A. Spunti di entomologia regionale in riferimento alle rickettsiosi. Minerva Med 1977; 68:2385–2386.
75. Sheals JG. The status of the genera *Dermanyssus, Allodermanyssus* and *Liponyssoides* (Acari, Mesostigmata). Verhandlungen der XI Internationaler Kongress fur Entomologie, Wien, Vienna, 1960, Vol. 2, 1962:473–476.
76. Huebner RJ. Rickettsialpox—general considerations of a newly recognized rickettsial disease. In: Moulton FR, ed. Rickettsial Diseases of Man. Washington, DC: American Association for the Advancement of Science, 1948:113–117.
77. Baker EW, Evans TM, Gould DJ, Hull WB, Keegan HL. A manual of parasitic mites of medical or economic importance. New York: National Pest Control Association, 1956:18–21.
78. Osipova NZ. Multiplication of ticks *Allodermanyssus sanguineus* Hirst. Meditsinsk Parazitol Parazit Bolezni 1967; 36:36–40 (in Russian).
79. Kiselev RI, Voltchanetskaya GI. Role of the mite *Allodermanyssus sanguineus* in the epidemiology of vesicular rickettsiosis. In: Pavlovskyi EN, Petrishcheva PA, Sayeuchina DN, Olsuf'eva MG, eds. Natural Focality of Diseases of Humans and Regional Epidemiology. Leningrad: Medgiz, 1955:248–252 (in Russian).
80. Rindge ME. Connecticut has first rickettsialpox outbreak. Conn Health Bull 1952; 66:73–75.
81. Levine JF, Lage AL. House mouse mites infesting laboratory rodents. Lab Animal Sci 1984; 34:393–394.
82. Comer JA, Vargas MC, Poshni I, Childs JE. Serologic evidence of *Rickettsia akari* infection among dogs in a metropolitan city. J Am Vet Med Assoc 2001; 218:1780–1782.
83. Case JB, Chomel B, Nicholson W, Foley JE. Serological survey of vector-borne zoonotic pathogens in pet cats and cats from animal shelters and feral colonies. J Feline Med Surg 2006; 8:111–117.
84. Philip CB, Hughes LE. The tropical rat mite, *Liponyssus bacoti*, as an experimental vector of rickettsialpox. Am J Trop Med 1948; 28:697–705.
85. Weyer F. The behavior of *Rickettsia akari* in the body louse after artificial infection. Am J Trop Med 1952; 1:809–820.
86. Weyer F. Weitere Beobachtungen und Versuche über das Verhalten von Rickettsien in Kleiderläusen. Z Tropenmed Parasitol 1961; 12:97–117.
87. Krinsky WL. Does epizootic lymphocytic choriomeningitis prime the pump for epidemic rickettsialpox? Rev Infect Dis 1983; 5:1118–1119.
88. Jackson EB, Danauskas JX, Coale MC, Smadel JE. Recovery of *Rickettsia akari* from the Korean reed vole *Microtus fortis pelliceus*. Am J Hyg 1957; 66:301–308.
89. Řeháček J, Úrvölgyi J, Kocianová E, Jedlička L. Susceptibility of some species of rodents to rickettsiae. Folia Parasitol 1992; 39:265–284.
90. Bennett SG, Comer JA, Smith H, Webb JP. Serologic evidence of *Rickettsia akari* infection in wild rodents in Orange County and humans in Los Angeles County, California. In press.
91. Comer JA, Tzianabos T, Flynn C, Vlahov D, Childs JE. Serologic evidence of rickettsialpox (*Rickettsia akari*) infection among intravenous drug users in inner-city Baltimore, Maryland. Am J Trop Med Hyg 1999; 60:894–898.
92. Brettman LR, Lewin S, Holzman RS, et al. Rickettsialpox: report of an outbreak and a contemporary review. Medicine (Baltimore) 1981; 60:363–372.
93. Saini R, Pui JC, Burgin, S. Rickettsialpox: report of three cases and a review. J Am Acad Dermatol 2004; 51:S65–S70.
94. Franklin J, Wasserman E, Fuller HS. Rickettsialpox in Boston: report of a case. N Engl J Med 1951; 244:509–511.
95. Hoeprich PD, Kent GT, Dingle JH. Rickettsialpox: report of a serologically proved case in Cleveland. N Engl J Med 1956; 254:25–27.
96. Pike G, Cohen S, Murray ES. Rickettsialpox: report of a serologically proved case occurring in a resident of Boston. N Engl J Med 1950; 243:913–915.
97. LaBoccetta AC, Israel HL, Perri AM, Sigel MM. Rickettsialpox: report of four apparent cases in Pennsylvania. Am J Med 1952; 13:413–422.
98. Comer JA, Diaz T, Vlahov D, Monterroso E, Childs JE. Evidence of rodent-associated *Bartonella* and *Rickettsia* infections among intravenous drug users from Central and East Harlem, New York City. Am J Trop Med Hyg 2001; 65:855–860.
99. Rose HM. The clinical manifestations and laboratory diagnosis of rickettsialpox. Ann Intern Med 1949; 31:871–883.
100. Krusell A, Comer JA, Sexton DJ. Rickettsialpox in North Carolina: a case report. Emerg Infect Dis 2002; 8:727–728.

101. Le Gac P, Giroud P, Le Henaff A, Baup G. Épidémie familiale de rickettsiose varicelliforme dans un village de l'Oubangui-Chari (A.E.F.). Bull Soc Pathol Exot 1952; 45:19–23.
102. Le Gac P, Giroud P. Rickettsiose vésiculeuse en Oubangui-Chari (A.E.F.). Bull Soc Pathol Exot 1951; 44:413–415.
103. Gear J. The rickettsial diseases of southern Africa: a review of recent studies. S Afr J Clin Sci 1954; 5:158–175.
104. Gaon J, Terzin AL. Some viral and rickettsial infections in Bosnia and Herzegovina: a sero-epidemiological study. Bull World Health Org 1956; 15:299–316.
105. Brezina R, Urvölgyi J, Rosický B, et al. Rickettsioses and infections caused by viruses of the psittacosis–ornithosis–mammalian pneumonia group, in Albania. J Hyg Epidemiol Microbiol Immunol 1961; 85:85–88.
106. Peacock MG, Ormsbee RA, Johnson KM. Rickettsioses of Central America. Am J Trop Med Hyg 1971; 20:941–949.
107. Weber K. Serological study with rickettsial antigens in erythema chronicum migrans. Dermatologica 1981; 163:460–467.
108. Ozturk MK, Gunes T, Coker C, Radulovic S. Rickettsialpox in Turkey. Emerg Infect Dis 2003; 9:1498–1499.
109. Brouqui P, Stein A, Dupont HT, et al. Ectoparasitism and vector-borne diseases in 930 homeless people from Marseilles. Medicine (Baltimore) 2005; 84:61–68.
110. Centers for Disease Control. Annual supplement: reported incidence of notifiable diseases in the United States, 1960. Morb Mortal Wkly Rep 1961; 9:1–24.
111. Centers for Disease Control. Annual supplement: reported incidence of notifiable diseases in the United States, 1961. Morb Mortal Wkly Rep 1962; 10:1–28.
112. Centers for Disease Control. Annual supplement: reported incidence of notifiable diseases in the United States, 1962. Morb Mortal Wkly Rep 1963; 11:1–28.
113. Centers for Disease Control. Annual supplement: reported incidence of notifiable diseases in the United States, 1964. Morb Mortal Wkly Rep 1965; 13:1–56.
114. Centers for Disease Control. Annual supplement: reported incidence of notifiable diseases in the United States, 1970. Morb Mortal Wkly Rep 1971; 19:1–60.
115. Centers for Disease Control. Annual supplement: reported incidence of notifiable diseases in the United States, 1971. Morb Mortal Wkly Rep 1972; 20:1–68.
116. Kiselev RI, Zhdanov VM, Alexandrova NN. Clinico-epidemiological characteristics of vesicular rickettsiosis. Ann Kharkov Mechnikov Res Inst 1954; 20:253–257 (in Russian).
117. Kiselev RI, Voltchanetskaya GI. Complete elimination of rats and mites as the means of prevention of vesicular rickettsiosis. Zh Mikrobiol Epidemiol Immunobiol 1955; 12:28–33 (in Russian).
118. Badiali C. Ricerche sull'eventuale presenza di anticorpi anti-*R. akari*. Nuovi Ann Ig Microbiol 1957; 8:422–425.
119. Garavelli PL. Rickettsialpox: descrizione di due casi clinici importati dal Sud Africa. Recent Prog Med 2005; 96:609–610.
120. Gonzalez JP, Fiset P, Georges AJ, Saluzzo JF, Wisseman CL. Approche sérologique sur l'incidence des rickettsioses en République Centrafricaine. Bull Soc Pathol Exot 1985; 78:153–156.
121. Choi YJ, Lee SH, Park KH, et al. Evaluation of PCR-based assay for diagnosis of spotted fever group rickettsiosis in human serum samples. Clin Diagn Lab Immunol 2005; 12:759–763.
122. Camer A, Masangkay J, Satoh H, et al. Prevalence of spotted fever rickettsial antibodies in dogs and rodents in the Philippines. Jpn J Infect Dis 2000; 53:162–163.
123. Sleisenger MH, Murray ES, Cohen S. Rickettsialpox case due to laboratory infection. Pub Health Rep 1951; 66:311–316.
124. Greenberg M. Endemic features of rickettsialpox. NY State J Med 1948; 48:502–506.
125. Paterson PY, Taylor W. Rickettsialpox. Bull NY Acad Med 1966; 42:579–587.
126. Greenberg M. Rickettsialpox in New York City. Am J Med 1948; 4:866–874.
127. Greenberg M, Pellitteri O, Klein IF, Huebner RJ. Rickettsialpox—a newly recognized rickettsial disease. II. Clinical observations. J Am Med Assoc 1947; 133:901–906.
128. Barker LP. Rickettsialpox. J Am Med Assoc 1947; 141:1119–1123.
129. Colman RS. Rickettsialpox—a new rickettsial disease with oral manifestations. Oral Surg Oral Med Oral Pathol 1950; 3:1257–1259.
130. Rose HM. Rickettsialpox. NY State J Med 1948; 48:2266–2271.
131. Paddock CD. *Rickettsia parkeri* as a paradigm for multiple causes of tick-borne spotted fever in the Western Hemisphere. Ann NY Acad Sci 2005; 1063:315–326.
132. Paddock CD, Sumner JW, Comer JA, et al. *Rickettsia parkeri*: a newly recognized cause of spotted fever rickettsiosis in the United States. Clin Infect Dis 2004; 38:805–811.
133. Clifton DR, Goss RA, Sahni SK, et al. NF-kappa B-dependent inhibition of apoptosis is essential for host cell survival during *Rickettsia rickettsii* infection. Proc Natl Acad Sci USA 1998; 95:4646–4651.
134. Kenyon RH, Pedersen CE. Immune responses to *Rickettsia akari* infection in congenitally athymic nude mice. Infect Immun 1980; 28:310–313.

135. Jerrells TR, Eisemann CS. Role of T-lymphocytes in production of antibody to antigens of *Rickettsia tsutsugamushi* and other *Rickettsia* species. Infect Immun 1983; 41:666–674.
136. Anderson GW Jr, Osterman JV. Host defenses in experimental rickettsialpox: genetics of natural resistance to infection. Infect Immun 1980; 28:132–136.
137. Anderson GW Jr, Osterman JV. Host defenses in experimental rickettsialpox: resistance of C3H mouse sublines. Acta Virol 1980; 24:294–296.
138. Meltzer MS, Nacy CA. Macrophages in resistance to rickettsial infection: susceptibility to lethal effects of *Rickettsia akari* infection in mouse strains with defective macrophage function. Cell Immunol 1980; 54:487–490.
139. Nacy CA, Meltzer MS. Macrophages in resistance to rickettsial infection: strains of mice susceptible to the lethal effects of *Rickettsia akari* show defective macrophage rickettsicidal activity in vitro. Infect Immun 1982; 36:1096–1101.
140. Kyet CD. Differences in the interlinear sensitivity of mice to the causative agents of rickettsialpox. Zh Mikrobiol Epidemiol Immunobiol 1977; 3:78–81 (in Russian).
141. Kokorin IN, Kyet CD, Miskarova ED, Abrosimova GE. Differences in the susceptibility of mouse lines to the rickettsialpox agent. Acta Virol 1978; 22:497–501.
142. Poltorak A, He X, Smirnova I, et al. Defective LPS signaling in C3H/HeJ and C57BL/10ScCr mice: mutations in Tlr4 gene. Science 1998; 282:2085–2088.
143. Medzhitov R. Toll-like receptors and innate immunity. Nat Rev Immunol 2001; 1:135–145.
144. Pasare C, Medzhitov R. Toll-like receptors: linking innate and adaptive immunity. Adv Exp Med Biol 2005; 560:11–18.
145. Kokorin IN. Histopathology of vesicular rickettsiosis in guinea pigs, white rats, and mice. Archiv Patologii 1957; 11:3–9 (in Russian).
146. Wong SC, Cox HR. Action of aureomycin against experimental rickettsial and viral infections. Ann NY Acad Sci 1948; 51:290–305.
147. Smadel JE, Jackson EB, Cruise AB. Chloromycetin in experimental rickettsial infections. J Immunol 1949; 62:49–65.
148. Rose HM, Kneeland Y, Gibson CD. Treatment of rickettsialpox with aureomycin. Am J Med 1950; 9:300–307.
149. Rose HM. The experimental and clinical evaluation of terramycin against *Rickettsia akari* (rickettsialpox). Ann NY Acad Sci 1950; 53:385–394.
150. Smadel JE, Jackson EB, Gauld RL. Factors influencing the growth of rickettsiae. I. Rickettsiostatic effect of streptomycin in experimental infections. J Immunol 1947; 57:273–284.
151. Rose HR. The treatment of rickettsialpox with antibiotics. Ann NY Acad Sci 1955; 55:1019–1026.
152. Kekcheeva NK. Effect of chemotherapy on the course of experimental infection and immunity in vesicular rickettsiosis in mice. Zh Mikrobiol Epidemiol Immunobiol 1955; 6:64–67 (in Russian).
153. Ives TJ, Manzewitsch P, Regnery RL, Butts JD, Kebede M. In vitro susceptibilities of *Bartonella henselae*, *B. quintana*, *B. elizabethae*, *Rickettsia rickettsii*, *R. conorii*, *R. akari*, and *R. prowazekii* to macrolide antibiotics as determined by immunofluorescent-antibody analysis of infected Vero cell monolayers. Antimicrob Agents Chemother 1997; 41:578–582.
154. Barkhatova OI, Popov VL, Kekcheeva NK, Prozorovskii SV. Electron microscopic characteristics of penicillin and vancomycin effect on *Rickettsia conorii* and *Rickettsia akari* in vitro. Antibiotiki 1984; 29:580–585 (in Russian).
155. Jacobson JM, Desmond EP, Kornblee LV, Hirschman SZ. Positive Weil–Felix reactions in a case of rickettsialpox. Int J Dermatol 1989; 28:271–272.
156. Vishwanath S. Antigenic relationships among the rickettsiae of the spotted fever and typhus groups. FEMS Microbiol Lett 1991; 65:341–344.
157. Dasch GA, Weiss E. Characterization of the Madrid E strain of *Rickettsia prowazekii* purified by renografin density gradient centrifugation. Infect Immun 1977; 15:280–286.
158. Raoult D, Paddock CD. *Rickettsia parkeri* infection and other spotted fevers in the United States. N Engl J Med 2005; 353:626–627.
159. Zavala-Velazquez JE, Ruiz-Sosa J, Vado-Solis I, Billings AN, Walker DH. Serologic study of the prevalence of rickettsiosis in Yucatan: evidence for a prevalent spotted fever group rickettsiosis. Am J Trop Med Hyg 1999; 61:405–408.
160. Dolgopol VB. Histologic changes in rickettsialpox. Am J Pathol 1948; 48:119–133.
161. Hershberger LR, Huebner RJ. A report on the histopathology of the cutaneous lesions of a case of rickettsialpox. Public Health Rep 1947; 62:1740–1742.
162. Choi YJ, Jang WJ, Ryu JS, et al. Spotted fever group and typhus group rickettsioses in humans, South Korea. Emerg Infect Dis 2005; 11:237–244.
163. Fournier PE, Rolain JM, Raoult D. Rickettsioses in South Korea, materials and methods. Emerg Infect Dis 2006; 12:531.

7 | Flea-Borne Spotted Fever

Abir Znazen
Laboratoire de Microbiologie, Centre Hospitalo-Universitaire, Habib Bourguiba Sfax, Tunisie

Didier Raoult
Faculté de Médecine, Unité des Rickettsies, Université de la Méditerranée,
Marseille, France

INTRODUCTION AND HISTORY

Flea-borne spotted fever (also called cat flea typhus) is an emerging rickettsiosis due to *Rickettsia felis*, which belongs to the spotted fever group (SFG) of *Rickettsia*. *R. felis* is hosted by fleas, as are *R. typhi*, *Bartonella henselae*, *Wolbachia pipientis*, and *Yersinia pestis* (1). This *Rickettsia* was probably first detected in cat fleas *Ctenocephalides felis* in 1918 (2). It was rediscovered in 1990, when cat fleas (*C. felis*) were examined as possible vectors of *R. typhi*. In Orange County California, where infected rats are difficult to document, cases of murine typhus were reported. Epidemiologic studies were performed and demonstrated that cases were associated with seropositive domestic cats and opossums. The latter were heavily infested with *C. felis*. When fleas were investigated for *R. typhi*, a newly identified *Rickettsia*-like organism was observed by electron microscopy in midgut epithelial cells of *C. felis* (3). The agent was characterized by molecular biology techniques and named the Elb agent for the EL Laboratory in Soquel, California. The bacterium was detected in 1994 by polymerase chain reaction (PCR) in a blood sample obtained from a patient in Texas (4). *R. felis* has been considered as a member of the typhus group (TG) *Rickettsiae* based on its reactivity with anti-*R. typhi* antibodies. However, genetic analysis of the common 17-kDa antigen gene (*htrA*) and the 16S rRNA placed *R. felis* as a member of the SFG (5,6). In 1997, *R. felis* was detected in two other flea species in the United States, *C. felis* and *Pulex irritans* (1). In 1994 and 1995, isolation of the Elb agent was reported and the name *R. felis* was proposed on the basis of its origin in the cat flea (4,7). These early works were not pursued or confirmed and may have resulted from a contamination of cell culture *R. typhi*. Moreover, in the described conditions of isolation, suspected isolates of *R. felis* were not able to grow. Finally, the authors reported that their tests for antibiotic susceptibility were hampered by *R. typhi* contamination (8). In retrospect, it appears that the results described *R. typhi*. The definitive characterization of *R. felis* was achieved in 2001 when culture conditions were established. Indeed, *R. felis* was cultivated using *Xenopus laevis* tissue culture (XTC) cells and in mosquito cells (labuna AEM) at relatively low temperatures (optimally at 28°C) and did not grow at 37°C (9). The Elb agent was characterized as a unique SFG *Rickettsia*, and the name *R. felis* was validated (10,11).

Subsequent cases of "flea-borne spotted fever" were reported from Europe and South and Central America (9,12,13) that had been diagnosed by PCR and/or serologic tests. The whole genome of this bacterium has been recently sequenced and revealed more phenotypic and genotypic properties that were surprisingly different from other bacteria of the same genus (14).

PHYLOGENY AND TAXONOMIC POSITION

At present, *Rickettsiae* are divided into three groups, namely the SFG, the TG, and *R. bellii* (14–16). Attempts to define the classification of *R. felis* have proved problematic since first isolations were contaminated by *R. typhi* (11). Molecular data classified *R. felis* into the SFG *Rickettsiae*. In fact, on the bases of 16S rDNA, a 17-kDa protein antigen, a citrate synthase encoding gene, *rompB* gene, and the *metK*, *ftsY*, *polA*, and *dnaE* genes, *R. felis* appeared to be more closely related to *R. akari* and *R. australis*, a distinct clade of the SFG (5,6,10,17–20). In addition, *OmpA* gene has been described in almost all the members of the SFG and has been reported to be an excellent tool in characterizing *Rickettsia* species (21). *R. felis* has been reported to carry the *OmpA* gene, which placed it closer to the SFG rather than to the TG *Rickettsiae*. Recently, *sca2* gene (surface-cell antigen), which belongs to a family of genes coding for proteins that play a role in adhesion to host cells (15,22), was identified and demonstrated to be a good tool for *Rickettsia* phylogeny. *R. felis* appeared to be more closely related to *R. akari* and *R. autralis* (23).

When *R. felis* could be obtained in culture, monoclonal and polyclonal antibodies were generated permitting further phenotypic characterization. In fact, sodium dodecyl sulfate–polyacrylamide gel electrophoresis and immunoblotting showed that it was closely related to the SFG *Rickettsiae*. Serotyping by the micro immuno fluorescence (MIF) assay demonstrated its intensive antigenic relations with the SFG *Rickettsiae* rather than the TG *Rickettsiae* (24). Antigenic analysis of murine antisera to *R. felis* and monoclonal antibodies against *R. felis* and other *Rickettsia* species showed that it phenotypically clustered with *R. australis*, *R. akari*, and *R. montanensis*.

EPIDEMIOLOGY, FLEAS, AND *RICKETTSIA FELIS* RELATIONSHIPS

Rickettsioses are zoonoses vectorized by arthropods. *R. felis* is the only species of SFG that is transmitted by fleas. Humans can be infected after flea bites (1). Since its discovery, *R. felis* has been associated with fleas throughout the world, and published data has demonstrated its wide geographic distribution. It has been detected in fleas in Brazil (25), in Africa including Ethiopia (9), Gabon, and Algeria (26), in Europe including Spain (25), France (27), the United Kingdom (28,29), and Cyprus (30), in Asia including Thailand (31) and Afghanistan (32), and in New Zealand (33). The involvement of cat fleas and domesticated mammals including rodents, hedgehogs, cats, dogs, and recently monkeys (34) in the transmission cycle must be further investigated, as they may act as reservoir of *R. felis*.

The Vector

Fleas are found worldwide on mammals and are vectors of several zoonoses of public health importance. *Y. pestis*, the causative agent of plague (35), and *R. typhi*, the etiologic agent of murine typhus, are maintained in a zoonotic cycle involving rats (*Rattus rattus* and *R. norvegicus*) and the rat flea, *Xensopsylla cheopis*. For *R. felis* and also *R. typhi*, the zoonotic cycle has been shown to involve opossums and cat flea that are more related to humans (36). In addition to *Rickettsia*, cat fleas have been found to carry *Bartonella* species, especially *B. quintana*, the agent of bacillary angiomatosis (27,34). The rapid spread of these pathogens to human populations is due to the frequent feeding behavior and extraordinary mobility of fleas.

To date, five species of fleas have been associated with *R. felis*: *C. felis* (1), *C. canis* (37), *P. irritans* (1), *Anomiopsyllus nudata*, and recently *Archaeopsylla erinacei* (26). From all these species, the cat flea, *C. felis*, is one of the most frequent external parasites of companion animals worldwide (38). *C. felis* is generally regarded as the predominant species to find on dogs, cats, and opossums (38). In the United States opossums were found to be the most heavily infested with the cat flea, *Ctencephalides felis* (1). *C. felis* was found to be infected with *R. felis* by PCR, with infection rates at 3.8% in the United States (1) and up to 12% in the United Kingdom (28). In the United States, *R. felis* was also detected in opossum tissue (36,39). Recently, *R. felis* has been detected in *C. felis* fleas parasitizing rats in Cyprus (30). As *C. felis* has a worldwide distribution and infestation with these fleas is very common, flea-borne spotted fever may occur worldwide (Fig. 1).

Rickettsia felis and Fleas Relationships

The rickettsial relationship with their arthropod hosts is considered stable. Acquisition, propagation, dissemination, and transmission of *R. typhi* in fleas have been well studied through experimental infections (40). The dynamics of *R. felis* infection have not yet been studied in detail experimentally, but the microorganism has been observed by electron microscopy in gut epithelial linings, tracheal matrix, muscle, ovaries, and epithelial sheath of the testes (3). The high rates of infection in laboratory colonies of fleas and the presence of *R. felis* in their eggs and newly emerged nonblood-fed specimens indicate that the maintenance of this rickettsiosis occurs by transovarial transmission. However, fleas may acquire *R. felis* from rickettsemic hosts

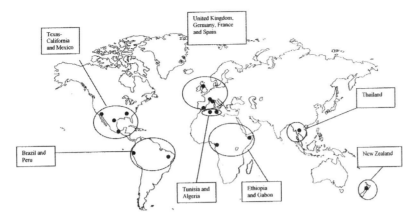

FIGURE 1 Distribution of *R. felis* worldwide: *R. felis* detected in fleas and reported cases of flea-borne spotted fever.

and then pass on the infection to their progeny by transovarial transmission. *R. felis* infection is not lethal to fleas. There is no evidence that massive infection of flea midgut affects the feeding behavior and survival of the infected fleas (1).

DESCRIPTION OF THE AGENT
The Bacteriology

R. felis belongs to the order *Rickettsiales*. It is a small (0.8–2 μm in length and 0.3–0.5 μm in diameter), rod-shaped, Gram-negative bacilli that retains basic fuchsin when stained by the Gimenez method (15,41). *R. felis* is an obligate intracellular bacterium. The culture of this *Rickettsia* was a great challenge. First, it was reported in 1995 to grow in cell culture at 37°C and to have phenotypic characteristics of TG *Rickettsia* (1,42,43). However, genotyping studies showed that it clustered in the SFG *Rickettsiae*. Lately, the same group reported that their cultures were contaminated (8). Later, *R. felis* could be obtained in culture from fleas, with isolations from 19 of 20 macerated flea samples positive by PCR for the organism (9). XTC-2 cells were used to grow the bacterium by shell vial centrifugation technique (9,44). These cells, derived from *X. laevis*, grow at 28°C and are used for *Bunyaviridae*, including *Bunyaviruses*, α-viruses, *flaviviruses*, and *rhabdoviruses* cultures (45). Besides, many arthropod-borne pathogenic microorganisms grow more rapidly in the laboratory at lower temperatures than that in the human body (46). In fact, optimal temperature growth of the TG of *Rickettsiae* is 35°C and of the SFG is 32°C (47). Other SFG rickettsia or arthropod-borne bacteria, such as the *Wolbachia* species (48), may also be cultivated more effectively at lower temperatures using this cell line. The culture allowed researchers to identify and more specifically characterize *R. felis* (11).

When grown on XTC-2 cells, *R. felis* induces cytopathic foci and plaques formation at nine days. First, the bacterium was detected only in the cytoplasm of infected cells (11), and then it was shown that it is also present in the nucleus (Fig. 2) (49). This culture system allowed purification of the bacterium. Thus, mouse polyclonal anti-*R. felis* antibodies were generated to detect the bacterium by immunofluorescence. The culture of *R. felis* permitted production of antigens for serologic diagnosis to test its susceptibility to antibiotics, and also to sequence its genome (14).

Molecular Characterization

Genome sequencing is a strategy used to characterize fastidious microorganisms. Indeed, it allows phenotypic property identification, culture condition definition, development of molecular diagnostic tools, detection of gene coding for antibiotic resistance, and epidemiologic studies of the bacterium. To date, 11 *Rickettsia* species genomes have been sequenced: *R. prowazekii*, *R. typhi*, *R. conorii*, *R. sibirica*, *R. rickettsi*, *R. africae*, *R. slovaca*, *R. massiliae*,

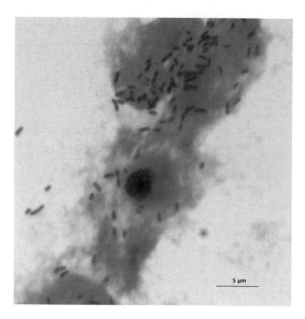

FIGURE 2 *R. felis* growing in XTC-2 cells with multiplication within the nucleus. Gimenez staining magnification: ×1000 (49).

R. canadensis, R. belli, and *R. akari* (50–54). The genome of *R. felis* showed many surprising characteristics. The chromosome is circular and longer (1485 Mb) than other previously sequenced *Rickettsiae*. It shows colinearity to other *Rickettsia* genomes, but it is more frequently interrupted by inversions/translocations. What is surprising is the presence of two plasmids. One of them apparently contains the equipment to allow conjugative plasmid transfer. This is the first *Rickettsia* genome harboring a plasmid. In addition, compared to *R. conorii, R. sibirica, R. prowazekii*, and *R. typhi, R. felis* had 530 specific open reading frames (ORFs). Consistently, the *R. felis* genome exhibits more paralogs in several identified gene families and unidentified gene families than other *Rickettsiae*. These families included a high number of transposases (82), *tnp*. The genome *R. felis* was demonstrated to carry more *sca* genes than other *Rickettsia* species sequenced genomes, that is, nine versus five, respectively (14). Also a high number (22) of ankyrin repeats *ank*, more than any bacteria sequenced so far, were identified. These are genes containing protein–protein interaction motifs involved in many steps of cell-cycle regulation. For adaptation to its eukaryotic host, *R. felis* exhibits 11 TPR-containing genes that play a role in protein–protein interaction. For adaptation to its environment, *R. felis* was found to carry the highest number (14) of *spoT* genes. These genes encode for enzymes controlling alarmone (55). Also, 11 tetratricopeptide repeat containing protein gene, *tpr*, and five families of chromosomal toxin–antitoxin (TAT) system genes (16 toxin and 14 antitoxin genes) are found. These specific genes of *R. felis* are also associated with protein interactions. TAT cassettes were demonstrated to increase cell survival during nutritional stress. In fact, during starvation, they control alarmone secretion that downregulates RNA synthesis.

Pathogenicity Factors

Sequencing the genome of *R. felis* allowed postgenomic analysis and characterization of many host-invasion and pathogenicity factors (49). In addition to the higher number of *sca* genes, which are involved in the adhesion to the host cell (56), pili-associated genes were found. The presence of pili on the surface of a *Rickettsia* was first observed by electron microscopy when *R. felis* showed small hair-like projections projecting from its surface. These pili are probably involved in the attachment of the bacteria to other cells (Fig. 3). A second type of long pili was observed, known as sex pili. These pili may be specialized in conjugation. As spreading factors, the *R. felis* plasmids were shown to carry genes coding to a hyaluronidase and patatin-like protein. Furthermore, based on the presence of a *RickA* homologue gene in the genome, immunofluorescence assays were performed and showed that *R. felis* can use the actin

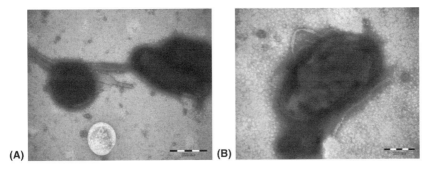

FIGURE 3 Visualization of *R. felis* pili by transmission electron microscopy. (**A**) Sexual pilus observed between two bacteria. (**B**) *R. felis* also possesses small appendages likely to be fimbriae pili (14).

cytoskeleton to disseminate through eukaryotic cells, as demonstrated for other SFG *Rickettsiae* (57). Another *R. felis* pathogenicity factor that was suggested from genomic analyses and experimentally confirmed was its hemolytic property. In fact, *R. felis* genome was found to carry three ORFs encoding for patatin-like proteins and one for phospholipase D (14).

PHYSIOPATHOLOGY

Inoculation to humans occurs through contact between wounds or abraded skin with feces from infected flea or through flea bites (1). Infection begins in the site of inoculation and then disseminates through the bloodstream. *Rickettsiae* infect the endothelial cells lining the blood vessels. *R. felis* was demonstrated to carry *sca* genes coding for proteins, permitting its attachment to target cells. After phagocytosis, *Rickettsiae* escape from the phagosome and then multiplicate in the cytoplasm. *R. felis*, as all SFG *Rickettsia*, can disseminate in the nucleus as its genome showed the presence of a *RickA* homologue gene. An eschar will develop in the site of inoculation due to the ischemia with the perivascular lymphoplasmocytes reaction responsible for the necrosis. From this initial site, *Rickettsia* will disseminate through the bloodstream. The generalized vascularitis due to infection of endothelial cells is responsible for the cutaneous rash (58).

PATHOGENICITY AND CLINICAL FEATURES

The pathogenic role of *R. felis* in humans was demonstrated by PCR and/or serologic tests in many patients throughout the world (7,9,12,13). In 2000 in Mexico, three patients with fever, exanthem, headache, and central nervous system involvement were diagnosed as infected by *R. felis* by specific PCR on blood or skin and seroconversion to rickettsial antigens (12). Since then, high antibody titers to *R. felis* were found in two French patients with clinical rickettsial disease and 2 of 16 Brazilian patients with febrile rash (9). Serum of one of the Brazilian patients had specific sequences of *R. felis* (9). In 2002, two cases of typical spotted fevers were reported in an adult couple in Germany (13). Clinical features included fever, marked fatigue, headache, generalized maculopapular rash, and a single black, crusted, cutaneous lesion surrounded by a halo (on the woman's right thigh and the man's abdomen). The man had enlarged, painful lymph nodes in the inguinal region. Serologic techniques discriminated *R. felis* infection among several *Rickettsiae* for the woman and this was confirmed by detection of *R. felis* DNA in the woman's sera. Although no laboratory evidence of *R. felis* infection was obtained for the man, the simultaneous occurrence of symptoms similar to those observed in his wife strongly suggested infection with the same microorganism (13). Recently, the first case of *R. felis* infection documented by serology in Asia was reported (59). Finally, serological evidence of *R. felis* infection in eight cases in Sfax, Tunisia, North Africa) has been reported (60) and in the Canary Islands (61). Clinical characteristics of all reported cases are presented in Table 1.

TABLE 1 Clinical Data of Patients Reported with Flea-Borne Spotted Fever

No.	Country	Fever	Eschar	Cutaneous rash	Central nervous system involvement	Other signs
1	U.S.A.	Yes	Yes	Yes	Yes	
2	Mexico	Yes	No	Yes	Yes	Conjunctivitis + diarrhea
3	Mexico	Yes	No	Yes	Yes	
4	Mexico	Yes	No	Yes	Yes	Vomiting + diarrhea
5	Brazil	Yes	—	Yes	No	
6	Brazil	Yes	—	Yes	Yes	
7	France	Yes	No	Yes	No	
8	France	Yes	No	Yes	No	
9	Germany	Yes	Yes	Yes	No	Lymph nodes + splenomegaly
10	Germany	Yes	Yes	Yes	No	Splenomegaly
11	Thailand	Yes	No	No	No	Vomiting
12	Tunisia	Yes	No	Yes	No	
13	Tunisia	—	—	—	No	
14	Tunisia	Yes	No	No	No	
15	Tunisia	Yes	No	Yes	No	Interstitial pneumopathy
16	Tunisia	Yes	No	Yes	No	Lymph nodes
17	Tunisia	Yes	No	Yes	No	Lymph nodes
18	Tunisia	Yes	No	Yes	No	
19	Tunisia	Yes	No	Yes	No	

DIAGNOSIS PROCEDURES

Common nonspecific laboratory abnormalities in flea-borne spotted fever may be the same in all rickettsioses. They include mild leucopenia, anemia, and thrombocytopenia. Hyponatremia, hypoalbuminemia, and hepatic and renal abnormalities may also occur (15).

Specific diagnosis of rickettsioses is based mainly on serological tests (62). Microimmunofluorescence is currently considered as the reference method. One limitation of serology is the cross-reactivity that might occur between the antigens of organisms within the same genus and, occasionally, in different genera (63). Antisera to *R. felis* have been demonstrated to have cross-reactivities with *R. rickettsii*, *R. conorii*, and *R. typhi*, which are the only commercially available antigens (24). It seems unlikely that *R. felis* infection could be detected by use of these antigens, and therefore, it is suggested that for the diagnosis of *R. felis* infections, it may be necessary to include a specific antigen for serologic assays. However, when the whole genome of *R. felis* has been sequenced, this demonstrated genetic similarity between *R. felis* and *R. typhi* but with some genes missing from the *R. conorii* genome, possibly explaining the differential cross-reactivity (14). Interestingly, *R. felis* may be the major cause of cross reactions between *R. typhi* and *R. conorii* or other tick-borne spotted fever agents. Cross reactions between these two groups of *Rickettsia* in patients have been puzzling, as this is not reported in experimentally infected guinea pigs and mice (64). Recently, cross-reacting sera with both *R. typhi* and *R. conorii* were demonstrated to be in fact caused by *R. felis* infection (60).When antigens to *R. felis* are not available, this is a good screening method for this infection.

At the "unite des rickettsies," referral center of *Rickettsia* in France, a rickettsial antigen is considered to represent the agent of infection when titers of IgG or IgM antibody against this antigen are at least two serial dilutions higher than titers of IgG or IgM antibody against other rickettsial antigens. When differences in titers between several antigens are lower than two dilutions, Western blot assays and, if needed, cross absorption studies are performed (59). Thus, serology should only be considered the first step toward diagnosing or recognizing a rickettsial disease. In order to differentiate infections within rickettsial antigens, cross absorption of sera followed by Western blotting can be done (62,65). However, this technique is time- and antigen-consuming.

Even though all reported cases of flea-borne spotted fever have been diagnosed by serology or PCR, isolation in cell cultures, particularly using the shell vial technique, remains the ultimate diagnostic method for rickettsial infection (44). Moreover, culture is only available in biosafety Level 3 laboratories (62). *R. felis* can be cultivated only on XTC-2 cells at low temperature (27) or on mosquito cell line (636 REF AEM 2006 R. FELIS) (9). So, diagnosis of flea-borne spotted fever must be suspected prior to the use of appropriate cells and adequate culture conditions. Isolation of *R. felis* can be performed routinely using buffy coat preparations of heparinized or EDTA-anticoagulated whole blood, skin biopsy specimens, or fleas if available.

PCR and sequencing methods are now used as sensitive and rapid tools to detect and identify *Rickettsiae* in blood and skin biopsies. Primers amplifying sequences of several genes have been used including *OmpA*, *OmpB*, *gltA*, and gene D (27,31). Fleas may also be subject to PCR. They are essentially used as epidemiological tools to detect the presence of a pathogen in a specific area (32).

TREATMENT

Susceptibility of *R. felis* to a wide range of antibiotics was studied by quantitative PCR assay (66). Like SFG *Rickettsia*, *R. felis* was susceptible to doxycycline, fluoroquinolones, telithromycin, and rifampin and resistant to trimethoprim sulfamethoxazole, β-lactams, and erythromycin. In fact, genome of *R. felis* was shown to carry a gene coding to β-lactamases of class C and D, streptomycin-resistant protein, and multidrug transport-system protein (14). Doxycycline, rifampin, and fluoroquinolones have already been demonstrated as the most effective antibiotics in vitro against all strains of *Rickettsiae* (67,68,72,73). For *R. felis*, MICs (μg/mL) ranged from 0.06 to 0.125 for doxycyline, from 0.06 to 0.25 for rifampin, and from 0.5 to 1 for ciprofloxacin. Thus, doxycycline (200 mg/day) remains the treatment of choice for all spotted fever rickettsioses, including those found in children (15,69). All reported cases of flea-borne spotted fever have been treated with doxycyline. Similar to other spotted fever rickettsioses, treatment during pregnancy and childhood was studied. Macrolides have been demonstrated to represent a safe alternative to doxycycline. In theses compounds, only josamycin efficacy has been tested for the treatment of Mediterranean spotted fever (70). For *R. felis*, telithromycin, with MIC at 1 μg/mL, may be the most adapted antibiotherapy.

The exact treatment duration is not fully determined. Usually, the exact duration of appropriate antibiotic therapy for SFG rickettsioses is generally related more to clinical response than to a precise number of days. However, for most rickettsial infections, therapy should be prescribed for up to two or three days after the patient's fever has abated.

PREVENTION

As no vaccine is available, prevention is essentially based on rodent control. Sanitary measures with rodenticides must be undertaken especially in agglomerations. Prevention includes action on fleas by regularly spraying insecticides in the environment. For this purpose, chemistry has been developed that has shown marked cat-flea control (71).

REFERENCES

1. Azad AF, Radulovic S, Higgins JA, Noden BH, Troyer JM. Flea-borne rickettsioses: ecologic considerations. Emerg Infect Dis 1997; 3(3):319–327.
2. Sikora H. Beitrage Zur Kenntni Der Rickettsien. Arch Inst Cardiol Mex 1918; 43:400–409.
3. Adams JR, Schmidtmann ET, Azad AF. Infection of colonized cat fleas, *Ctenocephalides felis* (Bouché), with a rickettsia-like microorganism. Am J Trop Med Hyg 1990; 43(4):400–409.
4. Higgins JA, Radulovic S, Schriefer ME, Azad AF. *Rickettsia felis*: a new species of pathogenic rickettsia isolated from cat fleas. J Clin Microbiol 1996; 34(3):671–674.
5. Azad AF, Sacci JB, Nelson WM, Dasch GA, Schmidtmann ET, Carl M. Genetic characterization and transovarial transmission of a typhus-like rickettsia found in cat fleas. Proc Natl Acad Sci USA 1992; 89:43–46.
6. Stothard DR, Fuerst PA. Evolutionary analysis of the spotted fever and typhus groups of *Rickettsia* using 16s rRNA gene sequences. Syst Appl Microbiol 1995; 18:52–61.
7. Schriefer ME, Sacci JBJR, Dumler JS, Bullen MG, Azad AF. Identification of a novel rickettsial infection in a patient diagnosed with murine typhus. J Clin Microbiol 1994; 32(4):949–954.
8. Radulovic S, Higgins JA, Jaworski DC, Azad AF. In vitro and in vivo antibiotic susceptibilities of Elb rickettsiae. Antimicrob Agents Chemother 1996; 40(12):2912.

9. Raoult D, La Scola B, Enea M, et al. A flea-associated rickettsia pathogenic for humans. Emerg Infect Dis 2001; 7(1):73–81.
10. Bouyer DH, Stenos J, Crocquet-Valdes P, et al. *Rickettsia felis*: molecular characterization of a new member of the spotted fever group. Int J Syst Evol Microbiol 2001; 51:339–347.
11. La Scola B, Meconi S, Fenollar F, Roux V, Rolain JM, Raoult D. Emended description of *Rickettsia felis* (Bouyer et al., 2001), a temperature-dependant cultured bacterium. Int J Syst Evol Microbiol 2002; 52(part 6):2035–2041.
12. Zavala-Velasquez JE, Sosa-Ruiz JA, Zavala-Castro J, et al. *Rickettsia felis*—the etiologic agent of three cases of rickettsiosis in Yucatan. Lancet 2000; 356:1079–1080.
13. Richter J, Fournier PE, Petridou J, Häussinger D, Raoult D. *Rickettsia felis* infection acquired in Europe and documented by polymerase chain reaction. Emerg Infect Dis 2002; 8(2):207–208.
14. Ogata H, Renesto P, Audic S, et al. The genome sequence of *Rickettsia felis* identifies the first putative conjugative plasmid in an obligate intracellular parasite. PLoS Biol 2005; 3(8):1391–1402.
15. Raoult D, Roux V. Rickettsioses as paradigms of new or emerging infectious diseases. Clin Microbiol Rev 1997; 10(4):694–719.
16. Stothard DR, Clark JB, Fuerst PA. Ancestral divergence of *Rickettsia bellii* from the spotted fever and typhus groups of *Rickettsia* and antiquity of the genus *Rickettsia*. Int J Syst Bacteriol 1994; 44(4):798–804.
17. Andersson SGE, Stothard DR, Fuerst P, Kurland CG. Molecular phylogeny and rearrangement of rRNA genes in *Rickettsia* species. Mol Biol Evol 1999; 16(7):987–995.
18. Roux V, Raoult D. Phylogenetic analysis of the genus *Rickettsia* by 16s rDNA sequencing. Res Microbiol 1995; 146:385–396.
19. Roux V, Rydkina E, Eremeeva M, Raoult D. Citrate synthase gene comparison, a new tool for phylogenetic analysis, and its application for the rickettsiae. Int J Syst Bacteriol 1997; 47:252–261.
20. Moron CG, Bouyer DH, Yu X-J, Foil LD, Croquet-Valdes P, Walker DH. Phylogenetic analysis of the *Rompb* genes of *Rickettsia felis* and *Rickettsia prowazekii* European-human and North American flying-squirrel strains. Am J Trop Med Hyg 2000; 62(5):598–603.
21. Fournier PE, Roux V, Raoult D. Phylogenetic analysis of spotted fever group rickettsiae by study of the outer surface protein Rompa. Int J Syst Bacteriol 1998; 48:839–849.
22. Uchiyama T, Uchida T, Walker DH. Species-specific monoclonal antibodies to *Rickettsia japonica*, a newly identified spotted fever group rickettsia. J Clin Microbiol 1990; 28:1177–1180.
23. Ngwamidiba M, Blanc G, Ogata H, Raoult D, Fournier PE. Phylogenetic study of *Rickettsia* species using sequences of the autotransporter protein-encoding gene *Sca*2. Ann NY Acad Sci 2005; 1063:94–99.
24. Fang R, Raoult D. Antigenic classification of *Rickettsia felis* by using monoclonal and polyclonal antibodies. Clin Diagn Lab Immunol 2003; 10(2):221–228.
25. Oliveira RP, Galvao MAM, Mafra CL, et al. *Rickettsia felis* in *Ctenocephalides* spp. fleas, Brazil. Emerg Infect Dis. In Press.
26. Bitam I, Parola P, De La Cruz KD, et al. First molecular detection of *Rickettsia felis* in fleas from Algeria. Am J Trop Med Hyg 2006; 74(4):532–535.
27. Rolain JM, Franc M, Davoust B, Raoult D. Molecular detection of *Bartonella quintana*, *B. koehlerae*, *B. henselae*, *B. clarridgeiae*, *Rickettsia felis*, and *Wolbachia pipientis* in cat fleas, France. Emerg Infect Dis 2003; 9(3):338–342.
28. Kenny MJ, Birtles RJ, Day MJ, Shaw SE. *Rickettsia felis* in the United Kingdom. Emerg Infect Dis 2003; 9(8):1023–1024.
29. Shaw SE, Kenny MJ, Tasker S, Birtles RJ. Pathogen carriage by the cat flea *Ctenocephalides felis* (Bouche) in the United Kingdom. Vet Microbiol 2004; 102(3–4):183–188.
30. Psaroulaki A, Antoniou M, Papaeustathiou A, Toumazos P, Loukaides F, Tselentis Y. First detection of *Rickettsia felis* in *Ctenocephalides felis* fleas parasitizing rats in Cyprus. Am J Trop Med Hyg 2006; 74(1):120–122.
31. Parola P, Sanogo OY, Lerdthusnee K, et al. Identification of *Rickettsia* spp. and *Bartonella* spp. from the Thai–Myanmar border. Ann NY Acad Sci 2003; 990:173–181.
32. Marie JL, Fournier PE, Rolain JM, Briolant S, Davoust B, Raoult D. Molecular detection of *Bartonella quintana*, *B. elizabethae*, *B. koehlerae*, *B. doshiae*, *B. taylorii*, and *Rickettsia felis* in rodent fleas collected in Kabul, Afghanistan. Am J Trop Med Hyg 2006; 74(3):436–439.
33. Kelly PJ, Meads N, Theobald A, Fournier PE, Raoult D. *Rickettsia felis*, *Bartonella henselae*, and *B. clarridgiae*, New Zealand. Emerg Infect Dis 2004; 10(5):967–968.
34. Rolain JM, Bourry O, Davoust B, Raoult D. *Bartonella quintana* and *Rickettsia felis* in Gabon. Emerg Infect Dis 2005; 11(11):1742–1744.
35. Perry RD, Fetherston JD. *Yersinia pestis*—etiologic agent of plague. Clin Microbiol Rev 1997; 10(1):35–66.
36. Williams SG, Sacci JBJR, Schriefer ME, et al. Typhus and typhus-like rickettsiae associated with opossums and their fleas in Los Angeles County, California. J Clin Microbiol 1992; 30(7):1758–1762.
37. Parola P, Cornet JP, Sanogo YO, et al. Detection of *Ehrlichia* spp., *Anaplasma* spp., *Rickettsia* spp., and other *Eubacteria* in ticks from the Thai–Myanmar border and Vietnam. J Clin Microbiol 2003; 41(4):1600–1608.

38. Rust MK, Dryden MW. The biology, ecology, and management of the cat flea. Annu Rev Entomol 1997; 42:451–473.
39. Schriefer ME, Sacci JBJR, Taylor JP, Higgins JA, Azad AF. Murine typhus: updated roles of multiple urban components and a second typhus-like rickettsia. J Med Entomol 1994; 31(5):681–685.
40. Farhang-Azad A, Traub R, Sofi M, Wisseman CL Jr. Experimental murine typhus infection in the cat flea, *Ctenocephalides felis* (Siphonaptera: Pulicidae). J Med Entomol 1984; 21(6):675–680.
41. Weiss E, Moulder JW. Order I *Rickettsiales*, Gieszczkiewicz 1939. In: Krieg NR, Holt JG, eds. Bergey's Manual of Systematic Bacteriology. 1st ed. Baltimore, MD: Williams and Wilkins, 1984:687–703.
42. Radulovic S, Higgins JA, Jaworski DC, Dasch GA, Azad AF. Isolation, cultivation, and partial characterization of the Elb agent associated with cat fleas. Infect Immun 1995; 63(12):4826–4829.
43. Radulovic S, Higgins JA, Jaworski DC, Azad AF. In vitro and in vivo antibiotic susceptibilities of Elb rickettsiae. Antimicrob Agents Chemother 1995; 39(11):2564–2566.
44. Vestris G, Rolain JM, Fournier PE, et al. Seven years' experience of isolation of *Rickettsia* spp. from clinical specimens using the shell vial cell culture assay. Ann NY Acad Sci 2003; 990:371–374.
45. Watret GE, Pringle CR, Elliott RM. Synthesis of bunyavirus-specific proteins in a continuous cell line (Xtc-2) derived from *Xenopus laevis*. J Gen Virol 1985; 66:473–482.
46. Maurin M, Birtles RJ, Raoult D. Current knowledge of *Bartonella* species. Eur J Clin Microbiol Infect Dis 1997; 16:487–506.
47. Weiss E, Moulder JW. The rickettsias and chlamydias. In: Kreig NR, Holt JG, eds. Bergey's Manual of Systematic Bacteriology. Baltimore, MD: Williams and Wilkins, 1984:687–739.
48. O'Neill SL, Pettigrew MM, Sinkins SP, Braig HR, Andreadis TG, Tesh RB. In vitro cultivation of *Wolbachia pipientis* in an *Aedes albopictus* cell line. Insect Mol Biol 1997; 6(1):33–39.
49. Ogata H, Robert C, Audic S, et al. *Rickettsia felis*, from culture to genome sequencing. Ann NY Acad Sci 2005; 1063:26–34.
50. Andersson SGE, Zomorodipour A, Andersson JO, et al. The genome sequence of *Rickettsia prowazekii* and the origin of mitochondria. Nature 1998; 396(6707):133–140.
51. Mcleod MP, Qin X, Karpathy SE, et al. Complete genome sequence of *Rickettsia typhi* and comparison with sequences of other rickettsiae. J Bacteriol 2004; 186(17):5842–5855.
52. Ogata H, Audic S, Renesto-Audiffren P, et al. Mechanisms of evolution in *Rickettsia conorii* and *R. prowazekii*. Science 2001; 293(5537):2093–2098.
53. Malek JA, Wierzbowski JM, Tao W, et al. Protein interaction mapping on a functional shotgun sequence of *Rickettsia sibirica*. Nucleic Acids Res 2004; 32(3):1059–1064.
54. Ogata H, La SB, Audic S, et al. Genome sequence of *Rickettsia bellii* illuminates the role of amoebae in gene exchanges between intracellular pathogens. PLoS Genet 2006; 2(5):E76.
55. Rovery C, Renesto P, Crapoulet N, et al. Transcriptional response of *Rickettsia conorii* exposed to temperature variation and stress starvation. Res Microbiol 2005; 156(2):211–218.
56. Uchiyama T. Adherence to and invasion of Vero cells by recombinant *Escherichia coli* expressing the outer membrane protein Rompb of *Rickettsia japonica*. Ann NY Acad Sci 2003; 990:585–590.
57. Gouin E, Welch MD, Cossart P. Actin-based motility of intracellular pathogens. Curr Opin Microbiol 2005; 8(1):35–45.
58. Fenollar F, Raoult D. *Rickettsia*. In: Libbey J, ed. Bactéries, Champignons et Parasites Transmissibles de la Mère à L'enfant. Paris: Eurotext Ed., 2002:262–274.
59. Parola P, Miller RS, Mcdaniel P, et al. Emerging rickettsioses of the Thai–Myanmar border. Emerg Infect Dis 2003; 9(5):592–595.
60. Znazen A, Rolain JM, Hammami A, Jemaa MB, Raoult D. *Rickettsia felis* infection, Tunisia. Emerg Infect Dis 2006; 12(1):138–140.
61. Perez-Arellano JL, Fenollar F, Angel-Moreno A, et al. Human *Rickettsia felis* infection, Canary Islands, Spain. Emerg Infect Dis 2005; 11(12):1961–1964.
62. La Scola B, Raoult D. Laboratory diagnosis of rickettsioses: current approaches to the diagnosis of old and new rickettsial diseases. J Clin Microbiol 1997; 35(11):2715–2727.
63. Parola P, Raoult D. Ticks and tickborne bacterial diseases in humans: an emerging infectious threat. Clin Infect Dis 2001; 32(6):897–928.
64. Hechemy KE, Raoult D, Eisemann C, Han Y, Fox JA. Detection of antibodies to *Rickettsia conorii* with a latex agglutination test in patients with Mediterranean spotted fever. J Infect Dis 1986; 153(1):132–135.
65. La Scola B, Rydkina L, Ndihokubwayo JB, Vene S, Raoult D. Serological differentiation of murine typhus and epidemic typhus using cross-adsorption and Western blotting. Clin Diagn Lab Immunol 2000; 7(4):612–616.
66. Rolain JM, Sthul L, Maurin M, Raoult D. Evaluation of antibiotic susceptibilities of three rickettsial species including *Rickettsia felis* by a quantitative PCR DNA assay. Antimicrob Agents Chemother 2002; 46(9):2747–2751.
67. Rolain JM, Maurin M, Vestris G, Raoult D. In vitro susceptibilities of 27 rickettsiae to 13 antimicrobials. Antimicrob Agents Chemother 1998; 42(7):1537–1541.
68. Ives TJ, Marston EL, Regnery RL, Butts JD. In vitro susceptibilities of *Bartonella* and *Rickettsia* spp. to fluoroquinolone antibiotics as determined by immunofluorescent antibody analysis of infected Vero cell monolayers. Int J Antimicrob Agents 2001; 18:217–222.

69. Purvis JJ, Edwards MS. Doxycycline use for rickettsial disease in pediatric patients. Pediatr Infect Dis J 2001; 19(9):871–874.
70. Bella F, Font B, Uriz S, et al. Randomized trial of doxycycline versus josamycin for Mediterranean spotted fever. Antimicrob Agents Chemother 1990; 34:937–938.
71. Rust MK. Advances in the control of *Ctenocephalides felis* (cat flea) on cats and dogs. Trends Parasitol 2005; 21(5):232–236.
72. Raoult D, Gallais H, De Micco P, Casanova P. Ciprofloxacin therapy for Mediterranean spotted fever. Antimicrob Agents Chemother 1986; 30:606–607.
73. Gudiol F, Pallares R, Carratala J, et al. Randomized double-blind evaluation of ciprofloxacin and doxycycline for Mediterranean spotted fever. Antimicrob Agents Chemother 1989; 33:987–988.

Section II: TICK-BORNE RICKETTSIOSES

8 | Rocky Mountain Spotted Fever

James E. Childs
Department of Epidemiology and Public Health, Yale University School of Medicine,
New Haven, Connecticut, U.S.A.

Christopher D. Paddock
Infectious Disease Pathology Activity, Division of Viral and Rickettsial Diseases, Centers for Disease Control and Prevention, Atlanta, Georgia, U.S.A.

HISTORY

> The name spotted fever I consider a good one, for this reason: To the laity it bodes grave responsibility. We well know that certain diseases afflicting a patient to a profound degree are inconsistent with life. Many of these cases terminating fatally with the best skill and untiring energy an intelligent physician can give them, we then feel the burden is somewhat lightened, and the responsibility of life is shared by family and friends if they are prepared for the inevitable.
>
> McCullough (1)

To the inhabitants of western Montana at the beginning of the twentieth century, the term "spotted fever" invoked a level of fear atleast as intense as the words "Ebola" or "bird flu" now elicit among contemporary residents of the United States. Mortality statistics from Montana during the early 1900s convey spotted fever's devastating consequences: from 1904 to 1913, 96 (63%) of 153 patients diagnosed with spotted fever died from this disease (2). Rocky Mountain spotted fever (RMSF), the prototypic and most severe of all the spotted fever rickettsioses, is also a disease steeped in the history of scientific exploration of arthropod-borne infections. The first investigators to study this tick-transmitted zoonosis were a remarkable amalgam of clinicians, pathologists, epidemiologists, entomologists, and microbiologists who provided the foundation for the science of rickettsiology.

The earliest records of RMSF date to 1873 (3). Early western inhabitants and physicians grimly referred to this life-threatening illness as "spotted fever" or "black measles" for the dark and extensive petechial rash (Fig. 1A and B), and "blue disease" or "black fever" to describe the dusky appearance of moribund patients (1). References to the disease as a unique clinical entity appeared during the late 1890s (4,5). Pioneering investigations into the etiology of RMSF were initiated in 1902 by pathologists Wilson and Chowning (6). Their investigation included careful questioning of older residents of the Bitterroot Valley, including trappers, American Indians, and Roman Catholic priests, none of whom could recall the occurrence of the disease prior to 1873. They examined several patients during the acute illness, conducted autopsies, and mapped the locations of over 100 RMSF cases, in addition to summarizing existing clinical information. They correctly concluded that "spotted fever" was a disease of the capillary circulation, caused by a noncultivable infectious agent with a wild animal reservoir. Unfortunately, these valid conclusions were overshadowed and subsequently questioned, because Wilson and Chowning misconstrued the etiologic agent by identifying an artefactual intraerythrocytic parasite (*Pyroplasma hominis*) in the hypochromic and sludged red cells of an afflicted patient (2,6,7).

In 1906, Howard Taylor Ricketts, a pathologist from the University of Chicago, arrived in the Bitterroot Valley to pursue studies on spotted fever. During the next three years, Ricketts conducted a series of elegant, insightful, and ultimately legendary experiments that: provided definitive evidence that spotted fever was transmissible from the blood of ill patients to naïve hosts; demonstrated that ticks could acquire the pathogen from an infected animal and transmit it to a

---

The findings and conclusions in this chapter are those of the authors and do not necessarily reflect the views of the U.S. Department of Health and Human Services.

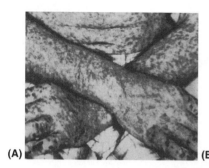 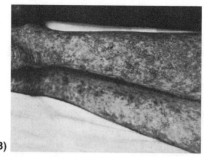

FIGURE 1 (**A** and **B**) The classical petechial or "spotted" rash of late-stage RMSF on moribund patients from western Montana during the early twentieth century. *Abbreviation*: RMSF, Rocky Mountain spotted fever. *Source*: Courtesy of Rocky Mountain Laboratories, National Institutes of Allergy and Infectious Diseases.

naïve animal; documented robust immunity to reinfection among experimentally infected animals; identified the agent in peripheral blood of patients and in tissues of the Rocky Mountain wood tick, *Dermacentor andersoni*; and experimentally demonstrated vertical transmission of the infectious agent from infected female ticks to their progeny (8). Intensive study of RMSF continued in western Montana for several decades following Ricketts' discoveries by a impressive collection of scientists assembled at the Rocky Mountain Laboratories in Hamilton that included Parker, Spencer, Davis, Philip, Jellison, and Cox (9).

The American West provided the background for the initial clinical recognition and descriptions of RMSF; however, physicians soon identified cases of tick-borne spotted fever from the eastern and southeastern United States and Central and South America. Clinically and epidemiologically compatible cases of RMSF were described from New York State as early as 1912; however, the first clinically recognized, laboratory confirmed case east of the Rocky Moutains was documented in an Indiana child in 1925 (10,11). In 1931, Badger et al. (12,13) from the National Institutes of Health described cases of RMSF in Delaware, Maryland, North Carolina, Pennsylvania, Virginia, and Washington, DC, firmly establishing the widespread distribution of RMSF in the United States. Contemporary diagnostic methods have permitted the retrospective confirmation of a fatal case of spotted fever in a Maryland patient that occurred in 1901 (14). Interestingly, this patient had been diagnosed with typhus by the renowned physician, William Osler. In this context, RMSF existed in the eastern United States long before its formal clinical recognition, and that prior to this time, other cases of spotted fever were also probably diagnosed as louse-borne typhus.

During the early 1930s, South American and United States investigators recognized that variously named febrile exanthems in Brazil—"São Paulo exanthematic typhus," "Minas Gerais exanthematic typhus," and "Brazilian spotted fever"—were most likely infections with *Rickettsia rickettsii* (15,16). During the next several decades, RMSF was confirmed in Columbia, Mexico, Canada, Panama, Costa Rica, and Argentina. One century after the pioneering studies of Wilson, Chowning, and Ricketts, investigators in the Western Hemisphere continue to discover new aspects of this dreaded and fascinating disease.

AGENT
Microbiology

R. rickettsii is an obligatory intracellular pathogen in the order Rickettsiales of the alpha subgroup of proteobacteria. It is phylogenetically related to various intracellular endosymbionts, such as *Wolbachia*, and intracellular organelles, such as mitochondria (17). These small ($1.0–2.0 \times 0.3–0.7$ μm), Gram-negative, coccobacillary bacteria have the capacity to infect and replicate in the cytosol and occasionally in the nucleus of vertebrate cells (e.g., endothelium, vascular smooth muscle, and macrophages) and invertebrate cells (e.g., hemocytes and salivary gland epithelium). *R. rickettsii* stains poorly with conventional Gram techniques, but stains well with Wolbach's Giemsa, Gimenez, Macchiavello, and Castañeda stains. In ticks, rickettsiae appear more pleomorphic and stain more deeply than in vertebrate tissues.

Genome

The complete genome sequence of *R. rickettsii* has not been fully characterized, but contains 1,257,710 bp with an estimated 1365 to 2849 open reading frames (ORFs) (18); the computational annotation status can be found at the PathoSystems Resource Integration Center Website. The genome of *R. rickettsii* presumably contains considerable inactivated genetic material in the process of spontaneous degeneration, in common with other *Rickettsia* species that have evolved for a highly specialized obligatory intracellular niche (19,20).

Natural History

The reservoir hosts for *R. rickettsii* include several species of ticks from several genera, including *Dermacentor*, *Rhipicephalus*, and *Amblyomma* (Fig. 2) (21–23). In its acarine host, rickettsiae infect and replicate in several cell types, including ovaries, salivary gland and midgut epithelium, and hemocytes (24). Transstadial and transovarial transmission of rickettsiae in tick hosts is central to the maintenance of *R. rickettsii* in nature (25,26), and presumably contributes to persistent high-risk foci for human infection (see "Case Clustering and Factors Influencing the Persistence of Rocky Mountain Spotted Fever Foci"). However, fitness costs associated with vertical transmission of *R. rickettsii*, as demonstrated for infected *D. andersoni* (27), may necessitate episodes of horizontal transmission of rickettsiae among ticks feeding on an infected vertebrate intermediary host. In this context, vertebrates are the source of blood for species of reservoir-host ticks, and may also provide a route by which *R. rickettsii* is transmitted to noninfected ticks during blood meal acquisition (28).

Vertebrates from which *R. rickettsii* has been isolated, and some of which have proven capable of sustaining a rickettsemia sufficient to infect various stages of *Dermacentor* spp. ticks, include domestic dogs, field voles (*Microtus pennsylvanicus*) (29,30), pine voles (*M. pinetorum*), white-footed mice (*Peromyscus leucopus*), cotton rats (*Sigmodon hispidus*), cottontail rabbits (*Sylvilagus floridanus*), Rocky Mountain cottontail rabbits (*S. nuttallii*), snowshoe hares (*Lepus americanus*), opossums (*Didelphis virginiana*), chipmunks (*Tamias amoenus*), and golden-mantled ground squirrels (*Spermophilus lateralis*) (21,31,32). The significance of birds as reservoir hosts for *R. rickettsii* remains unproven (28).

Cell Tropisms and Intracellular Pathophysiology

Harvard pathologist Simeon Burt Wolbach was the first to demonstrate *R. rickettsia* in human tissues using a modified Giemsa stain. His meticulous and detailed descriptions of rickettsiae in the tissues of patients with fatal RMSF established the foundation for the current understanding of the pathogenesis of this disease:

> The organisms are found in apparently uninjured endothelium of normal vessels, in areas of proliferated endothelium of the intima of vessels, in hyaline necrosed intima of more advanced lesions, in apparently normal and necrosed smooth muscle fibers of vessels with lesions and in endothelial cells in the perivascular zones of proliferation. They occasionally occur within endothelial cells in

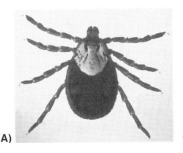 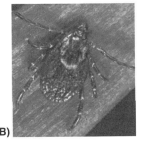 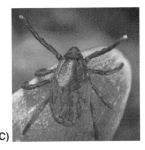

FIGURE 2 Adult, nonengorged, female stages of various tick species definitively implicated in the transmission of *R. rickettsii* in the United States. (**A**) *D. andersoni* (the Rocky Mountain wood tick). (**B**) *D. variabilis* (the American dog tick). (**C**) *Rhipicephalus sanguineus* (the brown dog tick). *Source*: (**B**) and (**C**) are courtesy of James Gathany, CDC.

dilated lymphatics ... The largest masses are seen in smooth muscle cells of affected arteries and veins and occasionally they occur in enormous numbers in such cells (33).

R. rickettsii primarily infects vascular endothelial cells, and permissible mammalian cell lines for the bacterium's isolation, culture, and experimental manipulation include immortalized human microvascular endothelial cells and primary embryonic human endothelial cells (34,35). Other permissive cell lines include Vero E6 cells (36–38), and some derived from primary blood monocytes, macrophages, and bone marrow (39). On several occasions, Vero cell culture has proven to be an effective means of isolating R. rickettsii from North and South American locations (22,40).

Genes are differentially expressed in the target organs of reservoir-host ticks infected by Rickettsia spp. as compared to uninfected controls. Of 54 gene transcripts which are differentially expressed in female D. andersoni ticks infected with R. montanensis, nine have significant homology to genes coding for proteins primarily involved with cell structure, movement, and cell-to-cell interactions (41). The putatively identified overexpressed proteins include a vasodilator-stimulated phosphoprotein-like molecule and a V-ATPase associated with actin assembly, and potentially linked to actin-based motility of spotted fever rickettsiae within the tick host (see "Clinical Disease"). The V-ATPase is associated with clathrin-coated vesicles involved with receptor-mediated endocytosis—a process by which rickettsiae enter cells—in addition to cell-to-cell interactions (41).

Once introduced into a mammalian host, R. rickettsii preferentially attaches to vascular endothelium via the outer membrane protein A (rOmpA) (42). Adherence and penetration of Vero cells has been achieved by recombinant Escherichia coli expressing the rOmpB protein (43), indicating a potential role for both major outer surface proteins in cell adhesion and uptake. Internalization of R. rickettsii within the mammalian cell may be mediated by phospholipase of rickettsial origin as demonstrated with a Vero cell system (44).

Experimental manipulations using human endothelial cells have permitted elucidation of pathophysiological effects coincident with the intracellular entry of R. rickettsii. Infection by R. rickettsii causes a significant reduction in key enzymes involved in the protection of endothelial cells from oxidative injury (45) resulting in increased levels of intracellular peroxides accompanied by ultrastructural indications of cell injury (46). Highly cytopathic strains of R. rickettsii rapidly damage cells and release large amounts of cytoplasmic lactate dehydrogenase, indicative of oxidative injury (47). Infection by R. rickettsii induces heme oxygenase (HO-1) expression in host endothelial cells (48), which may serve a protective function against oxidative injury.

Endothelial cell infection by R. rickettsii activates the nuclear transcription factor-κβ (NF-κβ) which exerts an antiapoptotic effect (49) by inhibiting proteins in the caspase family which mediate apoptosis (50); inhibition of apoptosis is essential for host cell survival and site persistence of active infection (51). Activation of catalytic I kinases by R. rickettsii, is an important upstream signaling event for activation of NF-κβ (52). Inhibition of NF-kB in infected cells rapidly results in apoptosis, suggesting that selective inhibition of catalytic kinases may be a target for reducing intracellular survival of R. rickettsii and the intracellular inflammatory changes associated with infection (52).

Cell-to-cell transmission or transfer of R. rickettsii is achieved by active propulsion of rickettsiae by means of directionally polymerized actin (Fig. 3) (53). Expression of the rickettsial surface protein RickA (54) activates the Arp2/3 complex initiating polymerization of new actin fibers and organizing the fibers into Y-branched arrays. The polymerization process initiated by R. conorii varies from that of Listeria and Shigella (55), although the process in R. rickettsii appears qualitatively similar (54). Variation in actin polymerization by different intracellular bacteria has been recently reviewed (56).

The RickA gene of R. rickettsii (ORFB4) (19) and a related gene in R. conorii (RC0909) (20,57) are only found in spotted fever group rickettsiae (54). Of note is the potential for interaction between rOmpA and RickA for accelerating cell-to-cell spread of rickettsiae. The ompA gene of R. peacockii, an endosymbiont of ticks which can competitively exclude R. rickettsii from infecting tick cells (58), contains three premature stop codons (59). The nonfunctional ompA gene of R. peacockii renders this bacterium incapable of polymerizing actin and presumably underlies this organism's slow growth rate and weak infectivity.

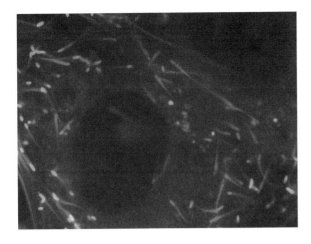

FIGURE 3 Actin-based motility as demonstrated by *R. rickettsii* in infected Vero cells. Actin is stained with rhodamine phalloidin (*gray*). Bacteria are stained with a fluorescein-conjugated rabbit anti-*R. rickettsii* antibody (*white*). *Source*: Courtesy of Matthew Welch, University of California, Berkeley.

CLINICAL DISEASE

RMSF is a systemic illness that can involve endothelial cells of capillaries and small-to-medium-sized vessels of all tissues and organs; however, the signs and symptoms of early disease resemble many other infectious syndromes, and even in areas where the awareness of the disease is reasonably high, as many as 60% to 75% of patients with RMSF receive an incorrect diagnosis on their first visit for medical care (60–62). Approximately one week (range 3–12 days) following the bite of an infected tick, the disease begins with abrupt onset of fever and is often accompanied by headache, nausea, vomiting, anorexia, and generalized myalgia, especially in the muscles of the lumbar region, thigh, and calf. The fever is typically high (39–41°C) and is accompanied by a severe frontal headache (60,63,64). Other findings recorded consistently but with varying frequency include irritability, altered mental status, abdominal pain, splenomegaly, conjunctival injection, and periorbital edema (65,66).

Rash, considered the hallmark feature of RMSF, is generally absent until the second to fourth day of fever. Although the evolution and character of the rash can help distinguish this disease from other acute febrile exanthems, clinicians must not rely on the presence of a distinctly petechial rash before establishing an early diagnosis. The rash begins as small (1–5 mm), pink, blanching macules, typically on the wrists, ankles, and forearms that evolve to maculopapules (Fig. 4). Within 24 hours, it spreads centrally to involve the legs, buttocks, arms, axillae, trunk, neck, and face. The entire body may be involved, including the mucous membranes of the palate and pharynx (64–66). Characteristics of the rash considered "classic" for RMSF, that is, petechial lesions and a distribution that includes the palms and soles, occur in as many as 60% and 80% of patients, respectively; however, these features are frequently not observed until the fifth day or later of the illness (60,63,65–67). Patients with a petechial rash

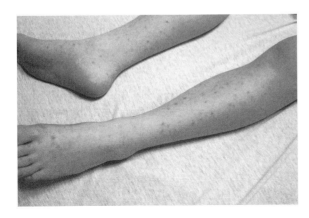

FIGURE 4 Maculopapular rash on the lower extremities of a child with RMSF. *Abbreviation*: RMSF, Rocky Mountain spotted fever. *Source*: Courtesy of Gary Marshall, University of Louisville School of Medicine.

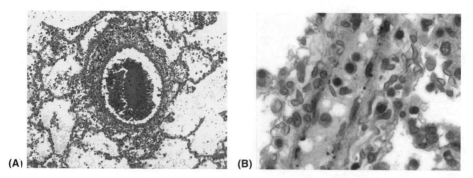

FIGURE 5 (*See color insert.*) Histopathology and immunohistochemical localization of *R. rickettsii* in the tissues of a Brazilian patient with fatal RMSF. (**A**) Arteriole in the lung showing transmural lymphohistiocytic inflammatory infiltrate (original magnification: ×50, hematoxylin and eosin stain). (**B**) Intracellular rickettsiae in endothelial cells and intravascular mononuclear cells in a pulmonary arteriole (original magnification: ×158, polyclonal rabbit anti-*R. rickettsii* antibody, immunoalkaline phosphatase with naphthol fast-red and hematoxylin counterstain). *Abbreviation*: RMSF, Rocky Mountain spotted fever.

are often severely ill. In some severe cases, petechiae may coalesce to form large ecchymoses. In approximately 10% of patients, the rash may be fleeting, evanescent, atypical in distribution, or entirely absent. These findings are most often described for black patients in whom some of the early and subtle features of the rash may be obscured (68,69). Children are less likely than adults to present without a rash (62).

The histopathologic lesion of RMSF involves a generalized and predominantly lymphohistiocytic vascultis (Fig. 5A), that occurs in response to rickettsial infection of the vascular endothelium (Fig. 5B). The life-threatening pathophysiologic consequence of infection and inflammation is microvascular damage and increased vascular permeability that results, sometimes catastrophically, in edema, localized hemorrhage, and hypoperfusion of one or more organ systems. Severe manifestations may include pulmonary edema and hemorrhage, cerebral edema, myocarditis, renal failure, disseminated intravascular coagulopathy, and gangrene (70,71). In untreated patients who survive their illness, the natural course of fever terminates after approximately two to three weeks (72).

Antibiotic Therapy

Before the introduction of effective antirickettsial therapies in the late 1940s, approximately 10% of children and 30% of adults with RMSF died of the infection (64,73,74). Despite the current availability of effective treatment and advances in medical care, approximately 2% to 6% of patients still die from RMSF. The majority of deaths are attributable to delayed diagnosis and failure to initiate specific antibiotic treatment within the first several days of the illness (75,76). Timely administration of effective antibiotic therapy is crucial, because at least half of all deaths occur within the first eight days of the disease (77). The recommended therapy for RMSF is doxycycline, administered in a dose of 100 mg twice daily (orally or intravenously) for adults or 2.2 mg/kg body weight per dose administered twice daily (orally or intravenously) for children weighing more than 45 kg (100 lbs) (65).

Host Factors, Immune Clearance, and Immunity

Cultured strains of *R. rickettsii* show variable degrees in virulence when evaluated in vitro in human endothelial cell cultures (47,78); however, particular host and pathogen factors responsible for disease severity remain poorly understood. Cases of subclinical or mild RMSF are considered rare, and usually are based solely on nonspecific serologic evidence of past infection. In this context, it is possible that cases of "atypical" or "mild" RMSF actually represent infections with spotted fever rickettsiae other than *R. rickettsii*. Various host factors have been associated epidemiologically with severe or fatal RMSF, including advanced age, male gender, and black race (69). The only genetically determined risk factor that has been clearly linked with severe RMSF is glucose-6-phosphate dehydrogenase (G6PD) deficiency, a sex-linked condition that occurs in approximately 12% of the U.S. black male population. G6PD was initially identified as a cause of massive intravascular hemolysis in black soldiers in Vietnam infected with *R. typhi* and *Orientia tsutsugamushi* (79), and later associated with fulminant RMSF (disease that terminates fatally within five days of onset) in black male patients (80). The exact pathogenic mechanism for hemolysis and increased severity of RMSF that occurs in patients with this phenotype remains to be determined.

Even after the discoveries of chloramphenicol and tetracycline in the mid-1940s, astute clinicians recognized that antibiotic therapy for RMSF, although remarkable in its impact, needed to work in tandem with the host immune response. In 1949, Harrell (66), a physician from North Carolina with considerable experience in caring for patients with RMSF, wrote, "In the long run, the patient must still cure himself. No supportive therapy will be helpful unless the patient's immune response can conquer the organism." Immune clearance of rickettsial infections in humans is largely dependent on cellular immune functions involving T-lymphocytes; the CD8+ T-lymphocytes are crucial to controlling infection and enhancing survivorship (81). In experiments primarily involving *R. conorii*, infected endothelial cells and macrophages were targeted by cytotoxic CD8+ lymphocytes (CTL), which provide MHC-I-restricted CTL activity, indicating this function was more important than IFN-γ production. Expression of CXCR3 ligands, the chemokines CXCL9/10 which target CD8+ T-lymphocytes, was significantly higher in *R. conorii*-infected cells, and upregulation of these transcripts occurred four days before tissue invasion by CD8+ T-lymphocytes (82).

Because RMSF is a relatively rare disease, knowledge of long-term immunity following naturally acquired infections is based primarily on relatively few anecdotal reports. Parker (83) commented that the degree and duration of immunity appeared to be related to the severity of the primary infection, and that authenticated second infections, including some that proved fatal, had been reported eight years or longer after the initial infection. Solid immunity against challenge with *R. rickettsii* was identified in six male volunteers for as long as 17 months following their recovery from experimentally induced RMSF. Although four of these men developed fourfold or greater rises in complement fixing antibodies or Weil–Felix agglutinins, none developed signs or symptoms of RMSF, suggesting that active infection offers significant immunity that is demonstrable for at least several years (84).

One report describes the isolation of *R. rickettsii* from an inguinal lymph node removed from an asymptomatic 50-year-old man approximately one year after he had recovered from a severe episode of RMSF (85). Interestingly, the second isolate, identified as the "Matthews strain," produced only a minimal febrile response in male guinea pigs, with little or no scrotal reaction. In contrast, the primary isolate of *R. rickettsii*, obtained from the patient's blood one year earlier, caused fever and scrotal changes characteristic of a highly virulent strain. These investigators suggested that the apparent attenuation in virulence may have been caused by prolonged contact with the host immune system and resulted in a persistent infection (85); however, unlike the well-established examples of persistent and recrudescent infections that occur with *R. prowazekii*, this phenomenon remains otherwise largely undescribed for *R. rickettsii*.

EPIDEMIOLOGY
Geographic Distribution

RMSF is endemic to regions of North, Central, and South America, and cases have been reported from Canada to Argentina, although some countries between these north–south extremes have yet to describe cases. The greatest numbers of RMSF fatalities have been reported from the United States and Brazil, although there is undoubtedly surveillance bias in the reporting of disease and mortality throughout the endemic region, including the United States (see "Transmission").

The distribution of RMSF in the United States reflects the distribution and abundance of the primary tick vector *D. variabilis* (the American dog tick) in central and eastern states and *D. andersoni* in western states (Fig. 6). The eastern and central states of North Carolina, Oklahoma, and Arkansas demarcate a belt of high-endemicity RMSF with incidence decreasing to the north and south. Montana and Wyoming report the highest incidence of RMSF in the West. The impact of *R. sanguineus* (the brown dog tick) on the distribution of RMSF in the

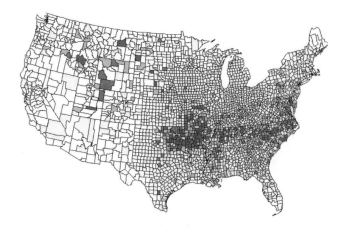

FIGURE 6 (*See color insert.*) Annual incidence of RMSF in the United States, 1997–2002, by county of occurrence (cases per million population: *tan* = 0.01–5; *pink* = 5–15; *brown* = 15–30; *red* = 30–511). The annual incidence was computed by case reports submitted to CDC through mandated reporting to the National Electronic Telecommunications Surveillance System and census data on residents per county. *Abbreviations*: RMSF, Rocky Mountain spotted fever; CDC, Centers for Disease Control and Prevention. *Source*: From Ref. 86.

United States is incompletely defined, although it is likely that cases of RMSF caused by this tick occur in other regions in United States, as well as in Mexico (where the vector status of the brown dog tick was first recognized in the 1940s) (87) and in other countries in the Western Hemisphere.

Transmission

RMSF almost always results from the transmission of rickettsiae to a human host by a tick as it obtains a blood meal from that host (88). Recognized tick vectors of *R. rickettsii* include at least four species of ixodid ticks—*D. andersoni*, *D. variabilis*, *R. sanguineus*, and *Amblyomma cajenennse* (the Cayenne tick) (11,22,28). Because *R. rickettsii* is passaged transovarially and transstadially, all hematophagous stages of these ticks are potentially capable of transmitting rickettsiae to a susceptible human host. The "grace period," or interval during which attached *D. andersoni* ticks may be removed from a vertebrate host before *R. rickettsii* can be transmitted, ranges from 2 to 20 hours (average 10 hours) (89,90).

Other recognized, albeit rare, routes of transmission of *R. rickettsii* to human hosts include blood transfusion (91), and inoculation of rickettsiae through mucous membranes following contact with fingers contaminated during the crushing of infected ticks removed manually from a human or animal, most notably the domestic dog (30,92,93).

Seasonality

Approximately 90% of reported cases of RMSF occur during the months of April through September in the temperate United States (76,93,94). This period coincides with the greatest host-seeking activity of the *Dermacentor* spp. ticks that serve as the principal vectors of *R. rickettsii* (95,96). However, sporadic cases of RMSF are reported during all months of the year including the winter months (97). In Brazil, tick surveys in the County of Pedreira documented peak numbers of larvae and nymphs of *A. cajennense* between June and October, the months coinciding with the most reports of RMSF in Brazil (98).

Incidence

The incidence of RMSF in the United States fluctuated markedly during the interval from 1920 to 2002 (99) (Fig. 5). The lowest incidence (approximately one case per million) occurred in 1950s following the death of Parker, the Director of the Rocky Mountain Laboratories in Hamilton, Montana. For nearly 30 years, Parker was the driving force behind RMSF surveillance activities in the United States, and his death in 1949 is believed by some to have created an artefactual decline in the number of recorded cases of this disease. Since the 1980s, and the active collection of passive data and voluntary CRFs at CDC, the incidence of RMSF has varied from approximately 1.5 to 5.0 cases per million (Fig. 7).

The reported incidence of RMSF in the United States is usually greatest among persons less than 20 years of age and those greater than 50 years of age (76,94). Surveillance data from

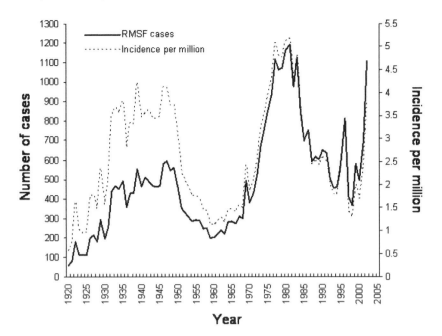

FIGURE 7 Annual incidence of RMSF from 1920 to 2002. *Abbreviation*: RMSF, Rocky Mountain spotted fever. *Source*: From Ref. 99.

1997 to 2002 found the lowest incidence among the age groups more than 5 and 10 to 19 years have resulted from changes in antibiotic treatment or simply the product of random variation in reporting (86). The lack of national surveillance for spotted fever in Brazil and other South and Central American countries precludes definitive statements about age-specific incidence over much of the extensive region where RMSF is endemic. However, as in the United States, the greatest number of reported RMSF deaths have occurred in children or young adults less than 20 years of age (100–102).

Most cases of severe rickettsial disease are confirmed by serologic testing and on this basis are attributed to RMSF caused by *R. rickettsii*. However, the recent description of *R. parkeri* as a cause of rash-associated febrile illness (103) in the United States highlights the fallibility of ascribing etiologic diagnoses for spotted fever rickettsioses based solely on the results of serologic tests.

Case Clustering

Outbreaks of RMSF in the United States and Brazil periodically occur within families or small communities (22,100,104), and among military personnel training at specific sites (105,106). These occurrences have also focused attention on one of the most striking features of the epidemiology of RMSF, the persistence of endemic foci over time. Spatially clustered outbreaks of RMSF have been documented in the United States and Mexico since 1904 [see Ref. (104) for a review]. Recent clusters of disease occurred in 2003 and 2004 in the United States (22,107) and in 1995 and 2000 in Brazil (100). The number of spotted fever cases per cluster has ranged from two to nine (Fig. 8), but these values are likely an underestimate as retrospective or prospective investigations have not been universally conducted to identify additional cases linked to a specific site or family. Endemic foci for RMSF have been documented to persist for decades within small regions or communities, as is the situation on Cape Cod and other offshore islands of Massachusetts (60,108), and endemic RMSF has been documented for over a century in the Bitterroot Valley of Montana.

Familial clusters of RMSF may only be detected when active investigations, initiated after the death of an index case, reveal a pattern of persistent *R. rickettsii* transmission at a site. As an example, prospective studies in Tennessee identified three confirmed cases of RMSF in one

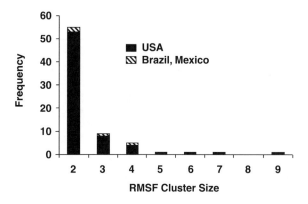

FIGURE 8 The frequency distribution of cluster size for familial or site-specific outbreaks of spotted fever in the United States and Central and South America. *Source*: From Refs. 22, 100, 104, 107.

family occurring within a month of the death of the index case. Retrospective investigation revealed that an additional family member had died of RMSF, as confirmed by immunostaining of tissues taken at autopsy, 27 months preceding the death of the index case (104).

In several instances, the onset of RMSF in humans has been preceded by the same disease occurring among pet dogs (109–111), and in several instances the death of a dog has alerted health providers to the nature of the pet owner's illness. In 2003, a resident of Mississippi became ill with RMSF two weeks after two pet dogs had died of suspected RMSF (112). Although appropriate antibiotic therapy was initiated immediately after disease onset, because of a high level of suspicion of RMSF, the patient died of the infection (112). In a more unusual setting where clinical suspicion of RMSF would be low, a patient residing in New York City was rapidly diagnosed and successfully treated for RMSF two weeks after a pet dog had died of confirmed RMSF; information on RMSF in the patient's dog had been provided to the patient's physician (113).

Factors Influencing the Persistence of Rocky Mountain Spotted Fever Foci

Although the exact mechanisms which favor persistence of RMSF at a focus are unknown, biologic interactions among the tick vector, the pathogen *R. rickettsii*, and the intracellular presence of other tick-associated rickettsial endosymbionts have been implicated as mediating factors. The majority of studies investigating the prevalence of *R. rickettsii* infection among *D. andersoni* and *D. variabilis* in the United States, and *A. cajennense* in Brazil, have found this agent in <1% of ticks examined (21,114–116) [Horta cited in Ref. (100)]. The low prevalence of *R. rickettsii* infections in natural tick populations may be largely regulated by the pathogenic effect that *R. rickettsii* exert on *Dermacentor* spp. ticks during the course of transovarial transmission (27) and the potential for competitive exclusion of *R. rickettsii* infection by other, nonpathogenic, endosymbiotic *Rickettsia* spp. that may be harbored by these ticks (117).

The clearest example of competitive exclusion involves *R. peacockii* which, in a manner similar to *R. rickettsii*, is transovarially transmitted in *D. andersoni* (58). The prevalence of *R. peacockii* infection within populations of *D. andersoni* ranges between 69% and 80% on the eastside of the Bitterroot valley in Montana (where RMSF is rarely reported) and where *R. rickettsii* is nearly absent (58,59,118). However, RMSF is endemic on the west side of the Bitterroot Valley, where approximately 1% of *D. andersoni* ticks are infected with *R. rickettsii* (116).

An observation of particular interest and potential importance for the understanding of virulence mechanisms involved in *R. rickettsii* infection has come from genetic studies of the nonpathogenic rickettsia *R. peacockii*. The slow growth and nonpathogenicity of *R. peacockii* in persistently infected *D. andersoni* cell lines mirrors the likely nonpathogenicity of this endosymbiont for humans (59). Genetic analyses of the *ompA* gene of *R. peacockii* obtained from Colorado and the east and westside of the Bitterroot Valley in Montana reveal three premature stop codons (59). Both rOmpA and RickA are localized to the surface of *R. rickettsii*, and the absence of rOmpA in *R. peacockii* coincides with an inability to polymerase actin (59). These data support the hypothesis that OmpA, in addition to, or possibly in conjunction with RickA, is required to initiate actin polymerization required for accelerated cell-to-cell spread of rickettsiae (54,57).

Mortality

RMSF is the most severe of all spotted fever rickettsioses and its fearsome reputation is closely linked with its capacity to rapidly kill otherwise healthy individuals; in this context, the case-fatality rate of RMSF in patients with untreated infection rivals some of the most deadly viral hemorrhagic fevers, including Ebola (119). Sporadic early reports of case-fatality rates of RMSF from the Bitterroot Valley and other endemic regions of the American West were as high as 70% (99). In Brazil, where RMSF is endemic to in at least five states, mortality was 40% in Minas Gerais State between 1981 and 1989 (100).

In the decade preceding the discovery of effective antimicriobial therapy for RMSF, aggregate U.S. mortality attributable to this disease was approximately 23% (120). Many RMSF patients receive an appropriate antibiotic during their course of infection and the number of RMSF deaths reported to CDC declined significantly during 1983–1998; nonetheless, the case fatality continues to range between 2% and 6% (Fig. 8) (76,93,120).

A review of 10 published reports outlining risk factors for fatal RMSF from 1970 to 1998 identified factors both consistently and variably associated with death over nearly three decades of study; factors which varied in significance over time were attributable to differences in methods and the advent of multiple logistic regression analyses which permit assessment of each factor's independent contribution to risk of death while controlling for the effects of other factors (99). The consistent features associated with increasing risk of death were increasing age of the patient, no known documentation of tick bite, a delay from disease onset to diagnosis, and lack of treatment with an effective antibiotic. In studies dating from 1981 to 1998 treatment with antibiotics other than tetracyclines, including chloramphenicol, increased risk of death (76,121,122). Risk factors of being male and nonwhite, which were identified as increasing the risk of fatal RMSF from 1970 to 1980, were not identified in any later studies using multivariate methods of analysis (99); it was hypothesized that the delay in diagnosis and treatment were more important factors than skin color or gender.

RMSF can mimic many other viral or bacterial diseases (101,123–125), and underestimates of mortality attributable to RMSF undoubtedly occur. Most RMSF deaths occur within seven to nine days following disease onset (8,75), and may precede the production of diagnostic levels of specific antibodies, often precluding a confirmatory diagnosis by most commonly used serologic tests (77).

Estimates of the mortality caused by RMSF in the United States have been determined by application of capture–recapture methods using two independent databases: case report forms (CRFs) voluntarily submitted to CDC from 1983 to 1998 and; the multiple cause-of-death (MCD) database compiled by the National Center for Health Statistics (120). Analyses indicated an estimated 612 deaths (95% confidence interval: 548–675) during the 16-year interval of study (RMSF deaths enumerated from CRFs and the MCD database totaled 224 and 304). These analyses suggested that 388 deaths, or 64% of all fatal cases of RMSF, were not reported to CDC during this period (120). The estimated total number of RMSF deaths dropped significantly from 1983 to 1997 (Fig. 9), and this decline was present in data obtained from both CRFs and MCD databases.

PREVENTION

The prevention or control of any tick-borne disease is most effectively achieved by personal protection measures to reduce the probability of a tick attaching and feeding on a human host. These measures include wearing appropriate clothing in tick-infested areas, such as light-colored long-sleeved clothes with pant cuffs tucked into socks, applying effective repellents directly on the skin, such as DEET (*N,N*-diethyl-*m*-toluamide) or spraying repellant on clothing, such as Permanone (containing the synthetic acaricide permethrin), followed by close inspection of the body to remove unattached and recently attached ticks. The directly applied repellents are often short-lived and are only partially effective when used on clothing (126). The synthetic pyrethroid compounds applied to clothing remain effective for weeks and after one or more washings (127).

Other measures of tick control include destruction of the vector tick, reduction of the density of host or reservoir species, habitat modification, public education, and professional

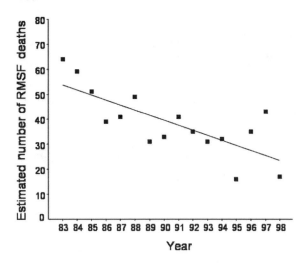

FIGURE 9 Estimated annual deaths caused by RMSF in the United States 1983–1997, obtained by capture–recapture methods comparing two independent databases. *Abbreviation*: RMSF, Rocky Mountain spotted fever. *Source*: From Ref. 120.

education (126). Public education about RMSF and the importance of applying repellents and acaricides to pet dogs was employed as a follow-up public health measure following the description of *R. sanguineus*-transmitted *R. rickettsii* in the southwestern United States (22). Professional education of physicians has been attempted in a few counties within Mississippi that reported an unusual number of fatal cases of RMSF (128), although the long-term effectiveness of such efforts remains to be evaluated.

One of the most effective means of preventing RMSF and other tick-borne infectious diseases is the prompt inspection for removal of crawling or attached ticks on skin or clothing after occupational or recreational activities that place individuals in areas inhabited by ticks (e.g., hunting, hiking, fishing, gardening, camping, or dog-walking). Because ticks must remain attached to their host for a minimum of several hours to transmit *R. rickettsii* (88,89), expeditious removal of ticks diminishes the likelihood of pathogen transmission. If a tick is found, it should be detached by using fine-tipped tweezers or forceps, grasping the body of the tick firmly and close to the skin as possible, and pulling with steady constant pressure. Removing ticks with bare hands should be avoided, and ticks should not be crushed between fingers after removal, as potentially infectious body fluids may contaminate the skin in this manner. No licensed vaccine exists for RMSF (65).

DIAGNOSTICS

There is no widely available, sensitive laboratory assay to confirm a diagnosis of acute RMSF. Decisions to treat are guided principally by epidemiologic clues garnered during a careful history, and by clinical findings (65,125,129). Most patients present for care within the first three days after onset of symptoms leaving a relatively narrow window of time during which antibiotic therapy dramatically reduces the risk of progression to severe illness or death. Because as few as 3% of patients possess the classic diagnostic triad of fever, rash, and a history of tick exposure during this interval (64), physician awareness of the seasonality and geographic distribution of the disease is critically important. A history of recent tick bite is helpful when present; however, the absence of this feature (as many as 40% of all cases) (62,75,93) should not dissuade the clinician from suspecting or treating for RMSF.

Abnormalities of routine laboratory tests include hyponatremia, hypoalbuminemia, anemia, and thrombocytopenia, reflecting vascular injury and increasing vascular permeability (71). Low serum sodium levels or diminished platelet counts occur in approximately 50% to 60% of all patients, and detecting these abnormalities may help to establish a presumptive diagnosis. The white blood cell count is generally normal when the patient first presents for care, although as many as 30% will eventually demonstrate a leukocytosis at some point in their illness (63).

A laboratory diagnosis may be made by serology, polymerase chain reaction assays, immunohistochemistry, or by isolation of rickettsiae in cell culture. Each of these assays are generally used to provide retrospective confirmation, and treatment and management decisions for acutely ill patients should never be delayed while waiting for the results of specialized confirmatory tests. The detection of antibodies reactive with *R. rickettsii* by use of the indirect immunofluorescence antibody assay is the most widely available and frequently used method to confirm RMSF. In approximately 50% of patients, diagnostic levels of antibody do not appear until the second week of disease. This test is best interpreted when paired serum samples, collected during the illness and approximately two to six weeks following the patient's recovery, are available for evaluation. Immunostaining of rash biopsy specimens has been used to diagnose patients in the acute stage of the illness; however, this assay is limited to specialized research laboratories (126). This assay may also be applied to tissues obtained at autopsy and has been used to confirm RMSF in patients for whom detectable levels of anti-*R. rickettsii* antibodies are absent or nondiagnostic (Fig. 5B) (77). Polymerase chain reaction assays can be used to detect rickettsial DNA in whole blood or tissue specimens; however, these methods demonstrate varying levels of sensitivity that may be affected by the type of the sample tested and by the timing of specimen collection during the course of the disease (130).

R. rickettsii can be isolated in the yolk sacs of embryonated hens' eggs and in several types of continuous cells lines, including monkey kidney (Vero) cells, chick embryo fibroblasts, and mouse L cells. However, these methods are primarily restricted to research laboratories and are seldom attempted. *R. rickettsii* is classified as a select agent (131) and should be handled in facilities using Biosafety Level 3 practices. Laboratories that perform culture isolation of *R. rickettsii* need to comply with federal regulations [42 C.F.R. (2004)] concerning registration and the use of select agents (www.cdc.gov/od/sap).

SPECIAL CONSIDERATIONS FOR LABORATORY PERSONNEL

Mucosal, transdermal, and aerosol exposures to *R. rickettsii* may result in RMSF and pose significant risks particularly for laboratory personnel who work with large volumes of rickettsiae (132–135). During the twentieth century, a surprisingly large number of investigators and laboratorians working with *R. rickettsii* developed RMSF, and several have died from the infection. In 1941, Parker reported that during several decades of experimental work with virulent strains of *R. rickettsii* at the Rocky Mountain Laboratories, 19 staff members had been infected, and that nine of these cases were fatal (Fig. 10) (135). In another laboratory, RMSF occurred among nine laboratory personnel from 1971 to 1976, presumably by inhalation of infectious aerosols containing *R. rickettsii* created during routine handling of cultured material; the affected persons had adhered to established protocols for handling hazardous agents (133). In February 1977, a glassware worker and a custodian employed by the Centers for Disease Control and Prevention in Atlanta, Georgia, died within five days following a laboratory exposure to *R. rickettsii*. Neither employee worked directly with the agent and despite a detailed investigation, the precise source of infection and mode of transmission were never confirmed; however, circumstantial evidence strongly suggested that both workers were exposed to *R. rickettsii* simultaneously, either in an autoclave area where contaminated laboratory materials were sterilized, or in a laboratory where the agent was cultured and processed (136).

CONCLUSION AND PROSPECTUS

> I arrived in Missoula, Montana, April 21, 1906, equipped for the bacteriologic and hematologic study of the so-called Rocky Mountain spotted fever and for the study of the infectious agent by means of animal inoculations.
>
> —Ricketts (8)

One hundred years have elapsed since Ricketts began his landmark investigations that would uncloak many of the mysteries that surrounded the dreaded "so-called Rocky Mountain spotted fever." Several remarkable scientific and medical achievements followed in subsequent decades

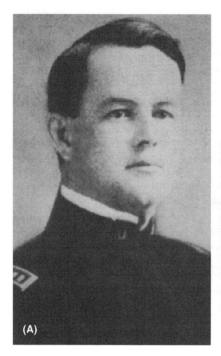 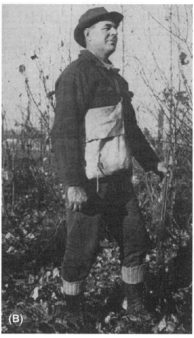

FIGURE 10 Two of several U.S. Public Health Service personnel who lost their lives to RMSF during laboratory investigations in Montana during the early twentieth century. (**A**) Thomas B. McClintic, Assistant Surgeon, U.S.P.H.S. (1912). (**B**) George H. Cowan, Field Assistant, U.S.P.H.S. (1924). *Source*: Courtesy of Rocky Mountain Laboratories, National Institutes of Allergy and Infectious Diseases.

that characterized the pathology, identified effective antibiotic therapy, and established various methods to confirm the diagnosis. Recently, the genome of *R. rickettsii* has been obtained and will eventually be dissected to reveal its molecular constituents; however, on a macroscopic scale, many fundamental aspects of the natural history of *R. rickettsii*, and the epidemiology of RMSF, remain unexplored. Consider the identification of *R. parkeri* as a cause of spotted fever in the Western Hemisphere in 2004 (103), and the confirmation of *R. sanguineus* as a vector of RMSF in the high desert of Arizona in 2005 (22). Each of these studies suggests a paradigm shift concerning the magnitude and ecology of RMSF in the United States, over a century after its formal description. In the case of *R. parkeri*, it is conceivable that the incidence of RMSF has been misrepresented by inclusion of other, less severe spotted fever rickettsioses (i.e., *R. parkeri* rickettsiosis) misdiagnosed as "RMSF" using nonspecific serologic assays (137,138). Hattwick et al. (69) recognized this possibility 30 years ago when they noted, "it is also possible that rickettsial diseases caused by agents other than *R. rickettsii* are being diagnosed as Rocky Mountain spotted fever."

Many confirmed and candidate pathogens of the spotted fever group, including *R. parkeri*, *R. massiliae*, *R. rhipicephali*, *R. amblyommii*, strains Tillamook and 364D, and *R. andeanae*, occur in human-biting ticks throughout the Americas (138–140). In this context, there exists a real need to better define the magnitude of RMSF and other spotted fever rickettsioses in the Western Hemisphere. This will require the development of more specific serologic and immunohistochemical assays, the resurrection of culture-based methods, and continued application of molecular techniques for the diagnosis of these varied infections (103,138–141). Renewed interest in spotted fever rickettsioses in Central and South America, reflected by the recent identification of spotted fever in Argentina and Peru (142,143) and by contemporary investigations of RMSF in Brazil, Columbia, and Mexico (100,102,144–146), suggests a period of rich scientific exploration of rickettsial diseases in this region of the world.

From a clinical perspective, further studies are needed to identify host factors that, in a manner similar to G6PD, predispose certain patients to fatal RMSF, and to use this information to educate specific high-risk cohorts, physicians, and public health professionals, that may benefit from intensified efforts at prevention, diagnosis, and treatment. Finally, there is a relentless need to educate physicians and other healthcare professionals about the early clinical recognition of RMSF, and the appropriateness of empirical therapy with doxycycline in adults and children (65,107,125,128,147).

In many respects, rickettsiology remains a scientific frontier, with ample room for new investigators (148). In 1973, Woodward (149), a clinician-investigator who had devoted approximately 30 years to the study of rickettsial diseases, commented on the need for new scientists to pursue the unanswered questions in rickettsiology: "There are opportunities for ... entomologists, epidemiologists, biologists, pathologists, and clinicians ... The small group of adventurers who thin out the weeds and wait for harvest would find a ready market for their produce." In 2006, many unsolved research questions exist for new investigators. One hundred years after Ricketts' discoveries, RMSF retains several of its mysteries, and continues to provide countless exciting opportunities for rickettsiologists and rickettsiology.

REFERENCES

1. McCullough GT. Spotted fever. Med Sentinel 1902; 10:225–228.
2. Ormsbee RA. A review: "Studies in *Pyroplasmosis hominis* ('spotted fever' or 'tick fever' of the Rocky Mountains)" by Louis B. Wison and William M. Chow. Rev Infect Dis 1979; 1:559–562.
3. Rucker WC. Rocky Mountain spotted fever. Public Health Rep 1912; 27:1465–1482.
4. Wood MW. Spotted fever as reported from Idaho. Rep Surgeon General US Army, 1896.
5. Maxey EE. Some observations on the so-called spotted fever of Idaho. Med Sentinel 1899; 7:433–438.
6. Wilson LB, Chowning WM. Studies in *Pyroplasmosis hominis* ("spotted fever" or "tick fever" of the Rocky Mountains). J Infect Dis 1904; 1:31–57.
7. Heyneman D. The blight of the Bitterroot, the mysterious Rocky Mountain spotted fever, and the significant role of Wilson and Chowning—a commentary. Wilderness Environ Med 2001; 12:118–120.
8. Ricketts HT. A summary of investigations of the nature and means of transmission of Rocky Mountain spotted fever. Contributions to Medical Science by Howard Taylor Ricketts, 1870–1910. Chicago: University of Chicago Press, 1911:278–372.
9. Philip RN. Rocky Mountain Spotted Fever in Western Montana. Hamilton, Montana: The Bitter Root Historical Society, 2000.
10. LaBier CR. Rocky Mountain spotted fever in Indiana. J Indiana Med Assoc 1925; 18:418–419.
11. Parker RR. Certain phases of the problem of Rocky Mountain spotted fever: a summary. Arch Pathol 1933; 15:398–429.
12. Badger LF, Dyer RE, Rumreich A. An infection of the Rocky Mountain type: identification in the eastern part of the United States. Public Health Rep 1931; 46:463–470.
13. Rumreich A, Dyer RE, Badger LF. The typhus–Rocky Mountain spotted fever group: an epidemiological and clinical study in the eastern and southeastern states. Public Health Rep 1931; 46:470–480.
14. Dumler JS. Fatal Rocky Mountain spotted fever in Maryland—1901. J Am Med Assoc 1991; 265:718.
15. Piza J, Salles-Gomes L, Meyer J, et al. Le typhus exanthematique a São Paulo. C R Seances Soc Biol Fil 1931; 106:1020–1022.
16. Parker RR, Davis GE. Protective value of convalescent sera of São Paulo exanthematic typhus against the virus of Rocky Mountain spotted fever. Public Health Rep 1933; 48:501–507.
17. Emelyanov VV. Evolutionary relationship of rickettsiae and mitochondria. FEBS Lett 2001; 501:11–18.
18. Eremeeva ME, Madan A, Shaw CD, et al. New perspectives on rickettsial evolution from new genome sequences of *Rickettsia*, particularly *R. canadensis*, and *Orientia tsutsugamushi*. Ann NY Acad Sci 2005; 1063:47–63.
19. Andersson JO, Andersson SG. Pseudogenes, junk DNA, and the dynamics of *Rickettsia* genomes. Mol Biol Evol 2001; 18:829–839.
20. Ogata H, Audic S, Renesto-Audiffren P, et al. Mechanisms of evolution in *Rickettsia conorii* and *R. prowazekii*. Science 2001; 293:2093–2098.
21. Burgdorfer W. Ecological and epidemiological considerations of Rocky Mountain spotted fever and scrub typhus. In: Walker DH, ed. Biology of Rickettsial Disease. Boca Raton, FL: CRC Press, 1988:34–50.
22. Demma LJ, Traeger MS, Nicholson WL, et al. Rocky Mountain spotted fever from an unexpected tick vector in Arizona. N Engl J Med 2005; 353:587–594.
23. Guedes E, Leite RC, Prata MC, et al. Detection of *Rickettsia rickettsii* in the tick *Amblyomma cajennense* in a new Brazilian spotted fever-endemic area in the state of Minas Gerais. Mem Inst Oswaldo Cruz 2005; 100:841–845.
24. Sonenshine DE. The Biology of Ticks. Oxford: Oxford University Press, 1993.
25. Burgdorfer W, Brinton LP. Mechanisms of transovarial infection of spotted fever rickettsiae in ticks. Ann NY Acad Sci 1975; 266:61–72.

26. Burgdorfer W. Vertical transmission of spotted fever group and scrub typhus rickettsiae. Curr Top Vector Res 1984; 2:77–92.
27. Niebylski ML, Peacock MG, Schwan TG. Lethal effect of *Rickettsia rickettsii* on its tick vector (*Dermacentor andersoni*). Appl Environ Microbiol 1999; 65:773–778.
28. Burgdorfer W. A review of Rocky Mountain spotted fever (tick-borne typhus), its agent, and its tick vectors in the United States. J Med Entomol 1975; 12:269–278.
29. Badger LF. Rocky Mountain spotted fever: susceptibility of the dog and sheep to the virus. Public Health Rep 1933; 48:795.
30. Price WH. The epidemiology of Rocky Mountain spotted fever. II. Studies on the biological survival mechanism of *Rickettsia rickettsii*. Am J Hyg 1954; 60:292–319.
31. McDade JE, Newhouse VF. Natural history of *Rickettsia rickettsii*. Annu Rev Microbiol 1986; 40:287–309.
32. Schriefer ME, Azad AF. Changing ecology of Rocky Mountain spotted fever. In: Sonenshine DE, Mather TN, eds. Ecological Dynamics of Tick-borne Zoonoses. New York: Oxford University Press, 1994:314–326.
33. Wolbach SB. The etiology of Rocky Mountain spotted fever: a preliminary report. J Med Res 1916; 34:121–128.
34. Dawson JE, Candal FJ, George VG, et al. Human endothelial cells as an alternative to DH82 cells for isolation of *Ehrlichia chaffeensis*, *E. canis*, and *Rickettsia rickettsii*. Pathobiology 1993; 61:293–296.
35. Silverman DJ, Bond SB. Infection of human vascular endothelial cells by *Rickettsia rickettsii*. J Infect Dis 1984; 149:201–206.
36. Heinzen RA. Rickettsial actin-based motility: behavior and involvement of cytoskeletal regulators. Ann NY Acad Sci 2003; 990:535–547.
37. Heinzen RA, Grieshaber SS, Van Kirk LS, et al. Dynamics of actin-based movement by *Rickettsia rickettsii* in Vero cells. Infect Immun 1999; 67:4201–4207.
38. Policastro PF, Hackstadt T. Differential activity of *Rickettsia rickettsii* opmA and ompB promoter regions in a heterologous reporter gene system. Microbiology 1994; 140:2941–2949.
39. Buhles WC, Huxsoll DL, Ruch G, et al. Evaluation of primary blood monocyte and bone marrow cell culture for the isolation of *Rickettsia rickettsii*. Infect Immun 1975; 12:1457–1463.
40. Melles HB, Colombo S, Lemos ER. Isolamento de *Rickettsia* em cultura de células vero. Rev Soc Bras Med Trop 1999; 32:469–473.
41. Macaluso KR, Mulenga A, Simser JA, et al. Differential expression of genes in uninfected and *Rickettsia*-infected *Dermacentor variabilis* ticks as assessed by differential-display PCR. Infect Immun 2003; 71:6165–6170.
42. Li H, Walker DH. rOmpA is a critical protein for the adhesion of *Rickettsia rickettsii* to host cells. Microb Pathog 1998; 24:289–298.
43. Uchiyama T. Adherence to and invasion of Vero cells by recombinant *Escherichia coli* expressing the outer membrane protein rOmpB of *Rickettsia japonica*. Ann NY Acad Sci 2003; 990:585–590.
44. Silverman DJ, Santucci LA, Meyers N, et al. Penetration of host cells by *Rickettsia rickettsii* appears to be mediated by a phospholipase of rickettsial origin. Infect Immun 1992; 60:2733–2740.
45. Devamanoharan PS, Santucci LA, Hong JE, et al. Infection of human endothelial cells by *Rickettsia rickettsii* causes a significant reduction in the levels of key enzymes involved in protection against oxidative injury. Infect Immun 1994; 62:2619–2621.
46. Hong JE, Santucci LA, Tian X, et al. Superoxide dismutase-dependent, catalase-sensitive peroxides in human endothelial cells infected by *Rickettsia rickettsii*. Infect Immun 1998; 66:1293–1298.
47. Eremeeva ME, Dasch GA, Silverman DJ. Quantitative analyses of variations in the injury of endothelial cells elicited by 11 isolates of *Rickettsia rickettsii*. Clin Diagn Lab Immunol 2001; 8:788–796.
48. Rydkina E, Sahni A, Silverman DJ, et al. *Rickettsia rickettsii* infection of cultured human endothelial cells induces heme oxygenase 1 expression. Infect Immun 2002; 70:4045–4052.
49. Joshi SG, Francis CW, Silverman DJ, et al. Nuclear factor kappa B protects against host cell apoptosis during *Rickettsia rickettsii* infection by inhibiting activation of apical and effector caspases and maintaining mitochondrial integrity. Infect Immun 2003; 71:4127–4136.
50. Joshi SG, Francis CW, Silverman DJ, et al. NF-kappaB activation suppresses host cell apoptosis during *Rickettsia rickettsii* infection via regulatory effects on intracellular localization or levels of apoptogenic and anti-apoptotic proteins. FEMS Microbiol Lett 2004; 234:333–341.
51. Clifton DR, Goss RA, Sahni S, et al. NF-kappa B-dependent inhibition of apoptosis is essential for host cell survival during *Rickettsia rickettsii* infection. Proc Natl Acad Sci USA 1998; 95:4646–4651.
52. Clifton DR, Rydkina E, Freeman RS, et al. NF-kappaB activation during *Rickettsia rickettsii* infection of endothelial cells involves the activation of catalytic IkappaB kinases IKKalpha and IKKbeta and phosphorylation-proteolysis of the inhibitor protein IkappaBalpha. Infect Immun 2005; 73:155–165.
53. Heinzen RA, Hayes SF, Peacock MG, et al. Directional actin polymerization associated with spotted fever group rickettsia infection of Vero cells. Infect Immun 1993; 61:1926–1935.
54. Jeng RL, Goley ED, D'Alessio JA, et al. A *Rickettsia* WASP-like protein activates the Arp2/3 complex and mediates actin-based motility. Cell Microbiol 2004; 6:761–769.
55. Gouin E, Gantelet H, Egile C, et al. A comparative study of the actin-based motilities of the pathogenic bacteria *Listeria monocytogenes*, *Shigella flexneri* and *Rickettsia conorii*. J Cell Sci 1999; 112:1697–1708.

56. Gouin E, Welch MD, Cossart P. Actin-based motility of intracellular pathogens. Curr Opin Microbiol 2005; 8:35–45.
57. Gouin E, Egile C, Dehoux P, et al. The RickA protein of *Rickettsia conorii* activates the Arp2/3 complex. Nature 2004; 427:457–461.
58. Niebylski ML, Schrumpf ME, Burgdorfer W, et al. *Rickettsia peacockii* sp. nov., a new species infecting wood ticks, *Dermacentor andersoni*, in western Montana. Int J Syst Bacteriol 1997; 47:446–452.
59. Baldridge GD, Burkhardt NY, Simser JA, et al. Sequence and expression analysis of the ompA gene of *Rickettsia peacockii*, an endosymbiont of the Rocky Mountain wood tick, *Dermacentor andersoni*. Appl Environ Microbiol 2004; 70:6628–6636.
60. Hazard GW, Ganz RN, Nevin RW, et al. Rocky Mountain spotted fever in the eastern United States: thirteen cases from the Cape Cod area of Massachusetts. N Engl J Med 1969; 280:57–62.
61. Linnemann CC Jr, Janson PJ. The clinical presentations of Rocky Mountain spotted fever: comments on recognition and management based on a study of 63 patients. Clin Pediatr 1978; 17:673–679.
62. Helmick CG, Bernard KW, D'Angelo LJ. Rocky Mountain spotted fever: clinical, laboratory, and epidemiological features of 262 cases. J Infect Dis 1984; 150:480–488.
63. Kaplowitz LG, Fischer JJ, Sparling PF. Rocky Mountain spotted fever: a clinical dilemma. In: Remington JS, Swartz MN, eds. Current Clinical Topics in Infectious Diseases. New York: McGraw-Hill, 1981:89–107.
64. Ong HA, Raffeto JF. Rocky Mountain spotted fever: an analysis of eighteen cases in children. J Pediatr 1940; 40:647–653.
65. Centers for Disease Control and Prevention. Diagnosis and management of tickborne rickettsial diseases: Rocky Mountain spotted fever, ehrlichiosis, and anaplasmosis—United States: a practical guide for physicians and other health-care and public health professionals. Morb Mortal Wkly Rep 2006; 55(RR-4):1–29.
66. Harrell GT. Rocky Mountain spotted fever. Medicine (Baltimore) 1949; 28:333–370.
67. Sexton DJ, Burgdorfer W. Clinical and epidemiologic features of Rocky Mountain spotted fever in Mississippi, 1933–1973. Southern Med J 1975; 68:1529–1535.
68. Sexton DJ, Corey GR. Rocky Mountain "spotless" and "almost spotless" fever: a wolf in sheep's clothing. Clin Infect Dis 1992; 15:439–448.
69. Hattwick MAW, O'Brien RJ, Hanson BF. Rocky Mountain spotted fever: epidemiology of an increasing problem. Ann Int Med 1976; 84:732–739.
70. Kirkland KB, Marcom PK, Sexton DJ, et al. Rocky Mountain spotted fever complicated by gangrene: report of six cases and review. Clin Infect Dis 1993; 16:629–634.
71. Elghetany MT, Walker DH. Hemostatic changes in Rocky Mountain spotted fever and Mediterranean spotted fever. Am J Clin Pathol 1999; 112:159–168.
72. Pincoffs MC, Guy EG, Lister LM, et al. The treatment of Rocky Mountain spotted fever with chloromycetin. Ann Intern Med 1948; 29:656–663.
73. Topping NH. Rocky Mountain spotted fever: a note on some aspects of its epidemiology. Public Health Rep 1941; 56:1699–1707.
74. Ross S, Schoenbach EB, Burke FG, et al. Aureomycin therapy of Rocky Mountain spotted fever. J Am Med Assoc 1948; 138:1213–1216.
75. Dalton MJ, Clarke MJ, Holman RC, et al. National surveillance for Rocky Mountain spotted fever, 1981–1992: epidemiologic summary and evaluation of risk factors for fatal outcome. Am J Trop Med Hyg 1995; 52:405–413.
76. Kirkland KB, Wilkinson WE, Sexton DJ. Therapeutic delay and mortality in cases of Rocky Mountain spotted fever. Clin Infect Dis 1995; 20:1118–1121.
77. Paddock CD, Greer PW, Ferebee TL, et al. Hidden mortality attributable to Rocky Mountain spotted fever: immunohistochemical detection of fatal, serologically unconfirmed disease. J Infect Dis 1999; 179:1469–1476.
78. Eremeeva ME, Klemt RM, Santucci-Domotor LA, et al. Genetic analysis of isolates of *Rickettsia rickettsii* that differ in virulence. Ann NY Acad Sci 2003; 990:717–722.
79. Whelton A, Donadio JV, Elisberg BL. Acute renal failure complicating rickettsial infections in glucose-6-phosphate dehydrogenase-deficient individuals. Ann Int Med 1968; 69:323–328.
80. Walker DH, Hawkins HK, Hudson P. Fulminant Rocky Mountain spotted fever: its pathologic characteristics associated with glucose-6-phosphate dehydrogenase deficiency. Arch Pathol Lab Med 1983; 107:121–125.
81. Walker DH, Olano JP, Feng HM. Critical role of cytotoxic T lymphocytes in immune clearance of rickettsial infection. Infect Immun 2001; 69:1841–1846.
82. Valbuena G, Bradford W, Walker DH. Expression analysis of the T-cell-targeting chemokines CXCL9 and CXCL10 in mice and humans with endothelial infections caused by rickettsiae of the spotted fever group. Am J Pathol 2003; 163:1357–1369.
83. Parker RR. Rocky Mountain spotted fever. J Am Med Assoc 1938; 110:1273–1278.
84. DuPont HL, Hornick RB, Dawkins AT, et al. Rocky Mountain spotted fever: a comparative study of the active immunity induced by inactivated and viable pathogenic *Rickettsia rickettsii*. J Infect Dis 1973; 128:340–344.

85. Parker RT, Menon PG, Merideth AM, et al. Persistence of *Rickettsia rickettsii* in a patient recovered from Rocky Mountain spotted fever. J Immunol 1954; 73:383–386.
86. Chapman AS, Murphy SM, Demma LJ, et al. Rocky Mountain spotted fever in the United States, 1997–2002. Vector Borne Zoonotic Dis. In press.
87. Bustamente ME, Varela G. Estudios de fiebre manchada en Mexico. Papel del *Rhipicephalus sanguineus* en la transmission de la fiebre manchada en la Republica Mexicana. Rev Inst Salub Enferm Trop 1947; 8:139–141.
88. McCalla LP. Direct transmission from man to man of the Rocky Mountain spotted (tick) fever. Med Sentinel 1908; 16:87–88.
89. Moore JJ. Time relationship of the wood-tick in the transmission of Rocky Mountain spotted fever. J Infect Dis 1911; 8:339–347.
90. Spencer RR, Parker RR. Rocky Mountain spotted fever: infectivity of fasting and recently fed ticks. Public Health Rep 1923; 38:333–339.
91. Wells GM, Woodward TE, Fiset P, et al. Rocky Mountain spotted fever caused by blood transfusion. J Am Med Assoc 1978; 239:2763–2765.
92. Spencer RR, Parker RR. Infection by means other than tick bites. Hyg Lab Bull 1930; 154:60–63.
93. Gordon JC, Gordon SW, Peterson E, et al. Epidemiology of Rocky Mountain spotted fever in Ohio, 1981: serologic evaluation of canines and rickettsial isolation from ticks associated with human case exposure sites. Am J Trop Med Hyg 1984; 33:1026–1031.
94. Treadwell TA, Holman RC, Clarke MJ, et al. Rocky Mountain spotted fever in the United States during 1993 through 1996. Am J Trop Med Hyg 2000; 63:21–26.
95. Clark KL, Oliver JH, McKechnie DB, et al. Distribution, abundance, and seasonal activities of ticks collected from rodents and vegetation in South Carolina. J Vector Ecol 1998; 23:89–105.
96. Eads RB, Smith GC. Seasonal activity and Colorado tick fever virus infection rates in Rocky Mountain wood ticks, *Dermacentor andersoni* (Acari: Ixodidae), in north-central Colorado, USA. J Med Entomol 1983; 20:49–55.
97. Lange JV, Walker DH, Wester TB. Documented Rocky Mountain spotted fever in wintertime. J Am Med Assoc 1982; 247:2403–2404.
98. de Lemos ER, Machado RD, Coura JR, et al. Epidemiological aspects of the Brazilian spotted fever: seasonal activity of ticks collected in an endemic area in Sao Paulo, Brazil. Rev Soc Bras Med Trop 1997; 30:181–185.
99. Childs JE, Paddock CD. Passive surveillance as an instrument to identify risk factors for fatal Rocky Mountain spotted fever: is there more to learn? Am J Trop Med Hyg 2002; 66:450–457.
100. Galvao MA, Dumler JS, Mafra CL, et al. Fatal spotted fever rickettsiosis, Minas Gerais, Brazil. Emerg Infect Dis 2003; 9:1402–1405.
101. Goncalves da Costa PS, Brigatte ME, Pereira DA, et al. Atypical fulminant *Rickettsia rickettsii* infection (Brazilian spotted fever) presenting as septic shock and adult respiratory distress syndrome. Braz J Infect Dis 2002; 6:91–96.
102. de Lemos ER, Rozental T, Villela CL. Brazilian spotted fever: description of a fatal clinical case in the State of Rio de Janeiro. Rev Soc Bras Med Trop 2002; 35:523–525.
103. Paddock CD, Sumner JW, Comer JA, et al. *Rickettsia parkeri*: a newly recognized cause of spotted fever rickettsiosis in the United States. Clin Infect Dis 2004; 38:805–811.
104. Jones TF, Craig AS, Paddock CD, et al. Family cluster of Rocky Mountain spotted fever. Clin Infect Dis 1999; 28:853–859.
105. Sanchez JL, Candler WH, Fishbein DB, et al. A cluster of tick-borne infections—association with military training and asymptomatic infections due to *Rickettsia rickettsii*. Trans R Soc Trop Med Hyg 1992; 86:321–325.
106. McCall CL, Curns AT, Singleton JS, et al. Fort Chaffee revisited: the epidemiology of tickborne diseases at a persistent focus. Vector Borne Zoonotic Dis 2001; 2:119–127.
107. Centers for Disease Control and Prevention. Fatal cases of Rocky Mountain spotted fever in family clusters—three states, 2003. Morb Mortal Wkly Rep 2004; 53:407–410.
108. Massachusetts Department of Health. On the alert for Rocky Mountain spotted fever. N Engl J Med 1975; 292:1127–1129.
109. Topping NH. The epidemiology of Rocky Mountain spotted fever. NY State J Med 1947; 47: 1585–1587.
110. Sexton DJ, Burgdorfer W, Thomas L, et al. Rocky Mountain spotted fever in Mississippi: survey for spotted fever antibodies in dogs and for spotted fever group rickettsiae in dog ticks. Am J Epidemiol 1976; 103:192–197.
111. Steinfeld HJ, Silverstein J, Weisburger W, et al. Deafness associated with Rocky Mountain spotted fever. Md Med J 1988; 37:287–288.
112. Elchos BN, Goddard J. Implications of presumptive fatal Rocky Mountain spotted fever in two dogs and their owner. J Am Vet Med Assoc 2003; 223:1450–1452.
113. Paddock CD, Brenner O, Vaid C, et al. Concurrent Rocky Mountain spotted fever in a dog and its owner. Am J Trop Med Hyg 2002; 66:197–199.
114. Pretzman C, Daugherty N, Poetter K, et al. The distribution and dynamics of *Rickettsia* in the tick population of Ohio. Ann NY Acad Sci 1990; 590:227–236.

115. Horta MC. Pesquisa de infecção por riquétsias do grupo da febre maculosa em humanos, caninos e em diferentes estádios de vida de Amblyomma cajennese, provenientes de uma área endêmica do estado de São Paulo, Brasil. Thesis Dissertation, Universidade de São Paulo, 2002.
116. Gage KL, Schrumpf ME, Karstens RH, et al. DNA typing of rickettsiae in naturally infected ticks using a polymerase chain reaction/restriction fragment length polymorphism system. Am J Trop Med Hyg 1994; 50:247–260.
117. Burgdorfer W, Hayes SF, Mavros AJ. Nonpathogenic rickettsiae in *Dermacentor andersoni*: a limiting factor for the distribution of *Rickettsia rickettsii*. In: Burgdorfer W, Anacker RL, eds. Rickettsiae and Rickettsial Diseases. New York: Academic Press, 1981:585–594.
118. Philip CB. Some epidemiological considerations in Rocky Mountain spotted fever. Public Health Rep 1959; 74:595–600.
119. Rollin PE, Ksiazek TG. Ebola haemorrhagic fever. Trans R Soc Trop Med Hyg 1998; 92:1–2.
120. Paddock CD, Holman RC, Krebs JW, et al. Assessing the magnitude of fatal Rocky Mountain spotted fever in the United States: comparison of two national data sources. Am J Trop Med Hyg 2002; 67:349–354.
121. Fishbein DB, Frontini MG, Giles R, et al. Fatal cases of Rocky Mountain spotted fever in the United States, 1981–1988. Ann NY Acad Sci 1990; 590:246–247.
122. Holman RC, Paddock CD, Curns AT, et al. Analysis of risk factors for fatal Rocky Mountain spotted fever: evidence for superiority of tetracyclines for therapy. J Infect Dis 2001; 184:1437–1444.
123. Zavala-Velazquez JE, Yu XJ, Walker DH. Unrecognized spotted fever group rickettsiosis masquerading as dengue fever in Mexico. Am J Trop Med Hyg 1996; 55:157–159.
124. Lowenstein R. Deadly viral syndrome mimics. Emerg Med Clin North Am 2004; 22:1051–1065.
125. Masters EJ, Olson GS, Weiner SJ, et al. Rocky Mountain spotted fever: a clinician's dilemma. Arch Intern Med 2003; 163:769–774.
126. Zaki MH. Selected tickborne infections—a review of Lyme disease, Rocky Mountain spotted fever, and babesiosis. NY State J Med 1989; 6:320–335.
127. Schreck CE, Snoddy EL, Spielman A. Pressurized sprays of permethrin or DEET on military clothing for personal protection against *Ixodes dammini* (Acari: Ixodidae). J Med Entomol 1988; 23:396–399.
128. O'Reilly M, Paddock C, Elchos B, et al. Physician knowledge of the diagnosis and management of Rocky Mountain spotted fever: Mississippi, 2002. Ann NY Acad Sci 2003; 990:295–301.
129. Woodward TE. Rocky Mountain spotted fever: epidemiological and early clinical signs are keys to treatment and reduced mortality. J Infect Dis 1984; 150:465–468.
130. Tzianabos T, Anderson BE, McDade JE. Detection of *Rickettsia rickettsii* DNA in clinical specimens by using polymerase chain reaction technology. J Clin Microbiol 1989; 27:2866–2868.
131. Centers for Disease Control and Prevention, National Institutes of Health. Biosafety in Microbiological and Biomedical Laboratories. Washington, DC: U.S. Government Printing Office, 1999.
132. Wolf GL, Cole CR, Carlisle HN, et al. The pathogenesis of Rocky Mountain spotted fever in monkeys, infected by inhalation. Arch Pathol 1967; 84:486–494.
133. Oster CN, Burke DS, Kenyon RH, et al. Laboratory-acquired Rocky Mountain spotted fever. N Engl J Med 1977; 297:859–863.
134. Johnson JE, Kadull PJ. Rocky Mountain spotted fever acquired in a laboratory. N Engl J Med 1967; 277:842–847.
135. Parker RR. Rocky Mountain spotted fever: results of fifteen years' prophylactic vaccination. Am J Trop Med 1941; 21:369–383.
136. Harden VA. Rocky Mountain Spotted Fever: History of a 20th Century Disease. Baltimore: The Johns Hopkins University Press, 1990, with Centers for Disease Control and Prevention. Fatal rocky mountain spotted fever–Georgia. Morb Mortal Wkly Rep 1977; 28:84.
137. Raoult D, Paddock CD. *Rickettsia parkeri* infection and other spotted fevers in the United States. N Engl J Med 2005; 353:626–627.
138. Paddock CD. *Rickettsia parkeri* as a paradigm for multiple cause of tickborne spotted fever in the Western Hemisphere. Ann NY Acad Sci 2005; 1063:315–326.
139. Parola P, Paddock CD, Raoult D. Tick-borne rickettsioses around the world: emerging diseases challenging old concepts. Clin Microbiol Rev 2005; 18:719–756.
140. Eremeeva ME, Bosserman EA, Demma LJ, Zambrand ML, Blau DM, Dasch GA. Isolation and identification of *Rickettsia massiliae* in *Rhipicephalus sanguineus* ticks from Arizona. Appl Environ Microbiol 2006; 72:5569–5577.
141. McDade JE. Diagnosis of rickettsial diseases: a perspective. Eur J Epidemiol 1991; 7:270–275.
142. Ripoll CM, Remondegui CE, Ordonez G, et al. Evidence of spotted fever and ehrlichial infections in a subtropical territory of Jujuy, Argentina. Am J Trop Med Hyg 1999; 61:350–354.
143. Schoeler GB, Moron C, Richards A, et al. Human spotted fever rickettsial infections. Emerg Infect Dis 2005; 11:622–624.
144. de Lemos ERS, Alvarenga FBF, Cintra ML, et al. Spotted fever in Brazil: a seroepidemiologic study and description of clinical cases in an endemic area in the state of São Paulo. Am J Trop Med Hyg 2001; 65:329–334.

145. Zavala-Castro JE, Zavala-Velázquez JE, Walker DH, et al. Fatal human infection with *Rickettsia rickettsii*, Yucatán, Mexico. Emerg Infect Dis 2006; 12:672–674.
146. Valbuena G, Olano J, Bouyer D, Walker D. Rocky mountain spotted fever in Colombia: a forgotten disease strikes again. Fourth international conference on Rickettsiae and Rickettsial Diseases [abstract P-168]. Spain: Logrono (La Rioja), 2005.
147. Centers for Disease Control and Prevention. Consequences of delayed diagnosis of Rocky Mountain spotted fever in children—West Virginia, Michigan, Tennessee, and Oklahoma, May–July 2000. Morb Mortal Wkly Rep 2000; 49:885–888.
148. Walker DH. *Rickettsia rickettsii*: as virulent as ever. Am J Trop Med Hyg 2002; 66:448–449.
149. Woodward TE. A historical account of the rickettsial diseases with a discussion of unsolved problems. J Infect Dis 1973; 127:583–594.

9 African Tick-Bite Fever

Mogens Jensenius
Department of Infectious Diseases, Ullevål University Hospital, Oslo, Norway

Lucy Ndip
Department of Biochemistry and Microbiology, University of Buea, Buea, Cameroon

Bjørn Myrvang
Department of Infectious Diseases and Center for Imported and Tropical Diseases, Ullevål University Hospital, Oslo, Norway

INTRODUCTION

The history of African tick-bite fever, probably an ancient disease in sub-Saharan Africa, contains several phases of scientific confusion. The first human cases were described almost 100 years ago in Mozambique and South Africa (1). At that time, however, the disease was confused with Mediterranean spotted fever caused by *Rickettsia conorii* and it was not until the mid-1930s that Pijper, a pathologist working in Pretoria, thoroughly described the distinct epidemiology and clinical picture of African tick–bite fever (2). More importantly, Pijper was also able to isolate the causative agent and demonstrated that it differed from *R. conorii* using cross-protection studies. Unfortunately, his isolate and data were later lost, and subsequent scientists were unable to reproduce Pijper's findings. As a result, African tick-bite fever was again erroneously recognized as a mere variant of Mediterranean spotted fever, and the observed difference in clinical presentation and epidemiology between the two entities were attributed to different host factors, such as age and risk behavior (3). The final breakthrough came several decades later, in 1992, when a spotted-fever group rickettsia was isolated in the blood of a 36-year-old Zimbabwean woman who presented with typical African tick-bite fever (4). This isolate was distinct from *R. conorii*, but indistinguishable from rickettsial strains isolated in *Amblyomma* ticks collected in Ethiopia and Zimbabwe some 20 years earlier (5,6); the species was later named *Rickettsia africae*. This newly identified species was later named *R. africae* (7).

Numerous studies published in the last 15 years have widened our concepts of African tick-bite fever, including its microbiology, entomology, epidemiology, clinical presentation, diagnosis, treatment, and possible prevention (3). Perhaps most importantly, we now know that the disease can be one of the most common causes of acute febrile disease in rural sub-Saharan Africa, particularly in visitors from abroad but also in indigenous populations. Moreover, recent case reports indicate that complications may be more common and potentially more severe than previously anticipated. In the following, we give an overview of the current status of African tick–bite fever.

CAUSATIVE ORGANISM

R. africae is a spotted-fever group rickettsia closely related to *R. parkeri* in North America and *R. sibirica* in Northeast Asia. Electron microscopy shows that the organism measures about $0.4 \times 1.0\,\mu m$, occurs free in the cytoplasm, and has an outer slime layer and a trilaminar cell wall (7). The latter contains immunogenic lipopolysaccharide antigens, which are responsible for extensive cross-reactivity with the other spotted fever group rickettsiae (8), whereas species-specific antigens are located in the rickettsial outer membrane proteins A and B (9,10).

TICK VECTORS

R. africae is transmitted by ixodid ticks of the genus *Amblyomma*, mainly *Amblyomma variegatum* (Fig. 1), in West, Central, and East Africa and in the eastern Caribbean, and *Amblyomma*.

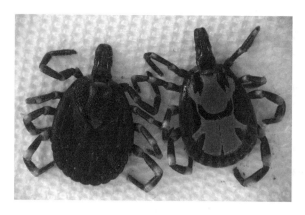

FIGURE 1 Male (*Right*) and female (*Left*) adult *A. variegatum*.

hebraeum in southern Africa (6,11,12). Both tick species prefer semihumid habitats with tall grass or bush and are not present in arid or urban areas. Cattle, wild game, and other ungulates constitute the principal hosts, although tick larvae and nymphs may also parasitize birds and rodents. In some areas, up to 90% of domestic cattle are infested with *Amblyomma* ticks (13). *A. hebraeum* and *A. variegatum* are active all year, but their number peaks during and after the rainy season, usually from January to May (14). Both species act not only as vectors of *R. africae*, but are also reservoirs in which the infection is maintained through transstadial transmissions (6). The rates of *R. africae* infection in *A. variegatum* and *A. hebraeum* ticks collected in endemic areas are typically high, and may exceed 50% (12,15). In contrast to most other ticks of human importance, *Amblyomma* ticks are hunter ticks and exhibit a notoriously aggressive behavior. Humans are usually attacked on the legs, but once on the skin the ticks may crawl around for hours before attaching, typically on moist skin behind the knee, in the groin, the perineum, or the axilla.

EPIDEMIOLOGY

R. africae has been isolated or detected in *Amblyomma* ticks or humans from 15 African countries (16). Seroepidemiological studies, however, indicate that its geographical distribution is far wider and probably covers most rural areas in more than 30 sub-Saharan African countries (Fig. 2) (17–19). *R. africae* was transferred with tick-infested cattle from West Africa to the New World some 200 years ago, and is today present on several West Indian islands, including Guadeloupe, Martinique, and St. Kitts (20–23).

Despite very high seropositivity rates in many areas, for example, >90% in southern Zimbabwe (19), reports on African tick-bite fever in indigenous populations are surprisingly

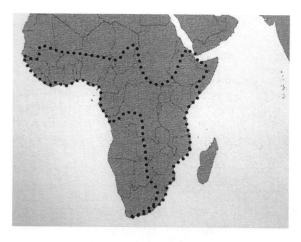

FIGURE 2 Estimated distribution of *R. africae* in Africa.

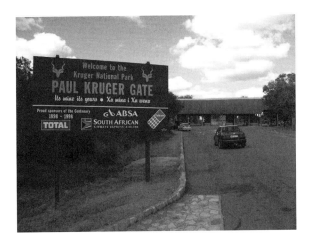

FIGURE 3 The Krüger National Park in the Mpumalanga Province, South Africa, a "hot spot" for travel-associated African tick-bite fever.

scarce. The reason for this is unknown but can partly be attributed to the frequently nonspecific clinical presentation and that skin eruptions, which are important diagnostic clues in rickettsioses, may easily be overlooked in pigmented skin. Also, the unavailability of specific laboratory tests, equipment, expertise, and the limited economic resources in most endemic countries may be responsible for the paucity of reports. Recent studies performed in Cameroon, however, indicate that African tick-bite fever may be common in indigenous populations. In a series of 234 febrile patients diagnosed as negative for malaria and typhoid fever, as many as 32% had IgM antibodies against spotted-fever group rickettsiae (24), and in another study, *R. africae* was confirmed by PCR as the cause of illness in 6% of 118 patients with fever of unknown etiology (25).

Nevertheless and despite these recent reports on indigenous populations, African tick-bite fever appears to primarily affect nonimmune visitors from abroad, in whom the disease may be second only to malaria as a cause of acute fever (25a). Since 1983, more than 350 cases among safari tourists, backpackers, hunters, sports competitors, students, foreign aid workers, and deployed soldiers have been published in the literature (3,26,27). Many international travelers are infected in South Africa, and notably in the national parks and game reserves situated in the northeastern parts of the country (Fig. 3) (28–31). The incidence of travel-associated African tick-bite fever may be surprisingly high, as was seen in a Norwegian cohort of 940 safari travelers in which the overall attack rate was 4%, ranging from 2% in leisure tourists to 25% in game hunters (32). In the same study, hunting, travel to southern Africa, and travel between November and April were identified as independent risk factors. Importantly and probably due to the aggressive nature of the Amblyomma ticks, most travel-associated cases of African tick-bite fever occur in clusters, which occasionally may present as spectacular outbreaks that may affect up to 100% of exposed subjects (33–37a).

PATHOGENESIS

The pathophysiological hallmark of African tick-bite fever, as well of other spotted-fever group rickettsioses, is the formation of focal or disseminated vasculitis (38). *R. africae* primarily invades the endothelial cells of smaller blood vessels, thereby triggering an increased secretion of von Willebrand factor, soluble E-selectin, and possibly other endothelium-associated mediators (39). Subsequent damage to the endothelium results in intramural and perivascular inflammation composed mainly of polymorphonuclear leukocytes and to a lesser extent of T-cells and macrophages (39a) (Fournier, personal communication). Recent studies indicate that inflammation and pro-coagulant processes are induced by *R. africae* in concert with platelet-derived soluble CD40 ligand, a transmembrane protein structurally related to tumor necrosis factor alpha (40). The clearance of *R. africae* from endothelial cells is characterized by increased circulating levels of cytokines, CC-chemokines, and CXC-chemokines (39). Secreted toxins appear not to be involved in the pathogenesis of African tick-bite fever.

CLINICAL FEATURES

R. africae infection is symptomatic in less than 50% of cases (41). The clinical course typically comprises an abrupt onset of fever, nausea, headache, and neck myalgia commencing 5 to 10 days after a tick bite (26,32). Most patients develop an inoculation eschar, a painless centimeter-large black crust surrounded by a red halo (Figs. 4 and 5), at the site of the tick bite. In 30% to 50% of the cases. Multiple eschars are seen. A painful regional lymphangitis (28), sometimes with a visible draining lymphangitis, is detected in half of the cases and may be found also in the absence of a frank eschar. Less frequent clinical signs of African tick-bite fever include a vesicular or maculopapular cutaneous rash (38), aphthous stomatitis (28), and arthralgia (3). Routine laboratory tests usually reveal lymphopenia and elevated serum C-reactive protein, whereas elevated serum liver enzymes and thrombocytopenia are seen in less than 40% of patients (42).

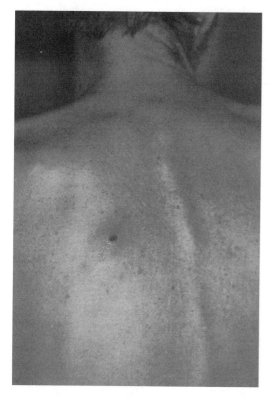

FIGURE 4 Inoculation eschar on the back of a 54-year-old Norwegian geologist infected with African tick-bite fever in Tanzania.

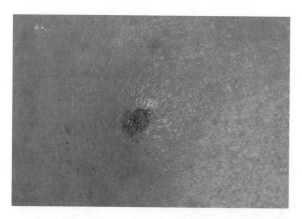

FIGURE 5 Close-up of eschar in Figure 4.

The majority of patients with African tick-bite fever develop a mild-to-moderately severe illness that either resolves spontaneously within 10 days or responds promptly to antirickettsial treatment (26,32,35,37). Complications are rarely seen but recent case reports have described patients presenting with long-lasting fever (43), reactive arthritis (32,44), subacute cranial or peripheral neuropathy (45), chronic fatigue (45), neuropsychiatric symptoms (36), and myocarditis (46). Interestingly, some of these complications may evolve despite preceding treatment with antirickettsial drugs and are likely to be caused by immunological mechanisms (45). No fatalities have ever been reported in African tick-bite fever.

MICROBIOLOGICAL DIAGNOSIS

For a detailed discussion on microbiological diagnosis of rickettsioses, readers are referred to Chapter 23. Briefly, the preferred microbiological test in African tick-bite fever is the immunofluorescence assay (47). Due to cross-reactions, commercial kits based on *R. conorii* or *R. rickettsii*, the agent of Rocky Mountain spotted fever in the Americas, are useful in this setting. It should be noted, though, that diagnostic antibody titers typically appear late or sometimes not at all in mild cases or in those treated with doxycycline (48). More sophisticated serological tests, for example, multiple-antigen immunofluorescence assay, where reactions to several ricketsial antigens including *R. africae* can be compared directly, Western blot, and cross-adsorption assays are only available at reference centers (49). Isolation of *R. africae* in cell cultures and antigen detection by immunohistochemistry or PCR are not widely available but should be attempted in unusual or complicated cases (39a,47,50).

TREATMENT

R. africae is in vitro susceptible to tetracyclines, chloramphenicol, rifampin, fluoroquinolones, newer macrolides, and ketolides (51,52). Most patients respond quickly to doxycycline when given 100 mg twice daily; treatment can usually be discontinued after three to seven days. From personal experience, we also consider fluoroquinolones, for example, ciprofloxacin 750 mg twice daily, as efficient, whereas the clinical role of other drugs is unknown (3). Patients with mild symptoms may not require any treatment at all (32).

PREVENTION

It is recommended that travelers to endemic areas should wear protective clothing, preferably impregnated or sprayed with permethrine or other acaricides, when walking in high grass and other typical tick habitats (16). Topical insect repellents may be used on exposed skin, but unfortunately most commercial repellents have only short-lasting efficacy against *Amblyomma* ticks (53,54). Daily inspection of the skin is advocated, and any attached tick should be removed swiftly. Removal of *Amblyomma* ticks, however, may be difficult because they have long mouthparts and can attach vigorously. Prophylactic treatment with antirickettsial drugs has not been studied and is currently not recommended. There is no vaccine against African tick-bite fever.

CONCLUSIONS

African tick-bite fever has recently emerged as one of the most common causes of flu-like illness in international travelers to sub-Saharan Africa, and should now be considered along with malaria and other tropical fevers when evaluating febrile returnees from this region. Its impact on indigenous populations is not as well known but may be significant as indicated by recent studies performed in central Africa. The clinical diagnosis is not always straightforward, but the presence of one or several inoculation eschars, neck myalgia, a vesicular cutaneous rash, and aphthous stomatitis are important clues. Complications are increasingly reported, and include subacute neuropathies and reactive arthritis. Treatment with doxycycline and ciprofloxacin appears to shorten the clinical course, and is recommended in cases with more pronounced symptoms. Travelers to endemic areas should be informed about the risk of contracting African tick-bite fever, and should be encouraged to protect themselves against tick bites.

REFERENCES

1. McNaught JG. A tick-borne fever in the Union of South Africa. J R Army Med Corps 1911; 16:505.
2. Pijper A, Crocker GC. Rickettsioses of South Africa. S Afr Med J 1938; 12:613–630.
3. Jensenius M, Fournier PE, Kelly P, Myrvang B, Raoult D. African tick bite fever. Lancet Infect Dis 2003; 3(9):557–564.
4. Kelly P, Matthewman L, Beati L, et al. African tick-bite fever: a new spotted fever group rickettsiosis under an old name. Lancet 1992; 340(8825):982–983.
5. Burgdorfer W, Ormsbee RA, Schmidt ML, Hoogstraal H. A search for the epidemic typhus agent in Ethiopian ticks. Bull World Health Organ 1973; 48:563–569.
6. Kelly PJ, Mason PR. Transmission of a spotted fever group rickettsia by *Amblyomma hebraeum* (Acari: Ixodidae). J Med Entomol 1991; 28(5):598–600.
7. Kelly PJ, Beati L, Mason PR, Matthewman LA, Roux V, Raoult D. *Rickettsia africae* sp. nov., the etiological agent of African tick bite fever. Int J Syst Bacteriol 1996; 46(2):611–614.
8. Hechemy KE, Raoult D, Fox J, Han Y, Elliott LB, Rawlings J. Cross-reaction of immune sera from patients with rickettsial diseases. J Med Microbiol 1989; 29(3):199–202.
9. Fournier PE, Roux V, Raoult D. Phylogenetic analysis of spotted fever group rickettsiae by study of the outer surface protein rOmpA. Int J Syst Bacteriol 1998; 48(pt 3):839–849.
10. Roux V, Raoult D. Phylogenetic analysis of members of the genus *Rickettsia* using the gene encoding the outer-membrane protein rOmpB (ompB). Int J Syst Evol Microbiol 2000; 50(pt 4):1449–1455.
11. Kelly PJ, Beati L, Matthewman LA, Mason PR, Dasch GA, Raoult D. A new pathogenic spotted fever group rickettsia from Africa. J Trop Med Hyg 1994; 97(3):129–137.
12. Parola P, Inokuma H, Camicas JL, Brouqui P, Raoult D. Detection and Identification of spotted fever group Rickettsiae and Ehrlichiae in African Ticks. Emerg Infect Dis 2001; 7(6):1014–1017.
13. Kelly PJ, Mason PR, Manning T, Slater S. Role of cattle in the epidemiology of tick-bite fever in Zimbabwe. J Clin Microbiol 1991; 29(2):256–259.
14. Norval RAI. Ticks of Zimbabwe. VII. The genus *Amblyomma*. Zimb Vet J 1983; 14:3–18.
15. Dupont HT, Cornet JP, Raoult D. Identification of rickettsiae from ticks collected in the Central African Republic using the polymerase chain reaction. Am J Trop Med Hyg 1994; 50(3):373–380.
16. Parola P, Raoult D. Ticks and tickborne bacterial diseases in humans: an emerging infectious threat. Clin Infect Dis 2001; 32(6):897–928.
17. Anstey NM, Tissot DH, Hahn CG, et al. Seroepidemiology of *Rickettsia typhi*, spotted fever group rickettsiae, and *Coxiella burnetti* infection in pregnant women from urban Tanzania. Am J Trop Med Hyg 1997; 57(2):187–189.
18. Dupont HT, Brouqui P, Faugere B, Raoult D. Prevalence of antibodies to *Coxiella burnetti*, *Rickettsia conorii*, and *Rickettsia typhi* in seven African countries. Clin Infect Dis 1995; 21(5):1126–1133.
19. Kelly PJ, Mason PR, Matthewman LA, Raoult D. Seroepidemiology of spotted fever group rickettsial infections in humans in Zimbabwe. J Trop Med Hyg 1991; 94(5):304–309.
20. Kelly PJ, Fournier PE, Parola P, Raoult D. A survey for spotted fever group Rickettsiae and Ehrlichiae in *Amblyomma variegatum* from St. Kitts and Nevis. Am J Trop Med Hyg 2003; 69(1):58–59.
21. Parola P, Vestris G, Martinez D, Brochier B, Roux V, Raoult D. Tick-borne rickettsiosis in Guadeloupe, the French West Indies: isolation of *Rickettsia africae* from *Amblyomma variegatum* ticks and serosurvey in humans, cattle, and goats. Am J Trop Med Hyg 1999; 60(6):888–893.
22. Parola P, Attali J, Raoult D. First detection of *Rickettsia africae* on Martinique, in the French West Indies. Ann Trop Med Parasitol 2003; 97(5):535–537.
23. Kelly PJ. *Rickettsia africae* in the West Indies. Emerg Infect Dis 2006; 12: 224–226.
24. Ndip LM, Bouyer DH, Travassos Da Rosa AP, Titanji VP, Tesh RB, Walker DH. Acute spotted fever rickettsiosis among febrile patients, Cameroon. Emerg Infect Dis 2004; 10(3):432–437.
25. Ndip LM, Fokam EB, Bouyer DH, et al. Detection of *Rickettsia africae* in patients and ticks along the coastal region of Cameroon. Am J Trop Med Hyg 2004; 71(3):363–366.
25a. Freedman DO, Weld LH, Kozarsky PE, et al. Spectrum of disease and relation to place of exposre among ill returned travellers. N Engl J Med 2006; 354(2):119–130.
26. Raoult D, Fournier PE, Fenollar F, et al. *Rickettsia africae*, a tick-borne pathogen in travelers to sub-Saharan Africa. N Engl J Med 2001; 344(20):1504–1510.
27. Jensenius M, Fournier PE, Raoult D. Rickettsioses and the international traveler. Clin Infect Dis 2004; 39(10):1493–1499.
28. Brouqui P, Harle JR, Delmont J, Frances C, Weiller PJ, Raoult D. African tick-bite fever: an imported spotless rickettsiosis. Arch Intern Med 1997; 157(1):119–124.
29. Fournier PE, Beytout J, Raoult D. Tick-transmitted infections in Transvaal: consider *Rickettsia africae*. Emerg Infect Dis 1999; 5(1):178–181.
30. Jensenius M, Hasle G, Henriksen AZ, et al. African tick-bite fever imported into Norway: presentation of 8 cases. Scand J Infect Dis 1999; 31(2):131–133.
31. McQuiston JH, Paddock CD, Singleton J Jr, Wheeling JT, Zaki SR, Childs JE. Imported spotted fever rickettsioses in United States travelers returning from Africa: a summary of cases confirmed by

laboratory testing at the Centers for Disease Control and Prevention, 1999–2002. Am J Trop Med Hyg 2004; 70(1):98–101.
32. Jensenius M, Fournier PE, Vene S, et al. African tick bite fever in travelers to rural sub-Equatorial Africa. Clin Infect Dis 2003; 36(11):1411–1417.
33. Caruso G, Zasio C, Guzzo F, et al. Outbreak of African tick-bite fever in six Italian tourists returning from South Africa. Eur J Clin Microbiol Infect Dis 2002; 21(2):133–136.
34. Consigny PH, Rolain JM, Mizzi D, Raoult D. African tick-bite fever in French travelers. Emerg Infect Dis 2005; 11:1804–1806.
35. Fournier PE, Roux V, Caumes E, Donzel M, Raoult D. Outbreak of *Rickettsia africae* infections in participants of an adventure race in South Africa. Clin Infect Dis 1998; 27(2):316–323.
36. Jackson Y, Chappuis F, Loutan L. African tick-bite fever: four cases among Swiss travelers returning from South Africa. J Travel Med 2004; 11(4):225–228.
37. Smoak BL, McClain JB, Brundage JF, et al. An outbreak of spotted fever rickettsiosis in U.S. Army troops deployed to Botswana. Emerg Infect Dis 1996; 2(3):217–221.
37a. Oostvogal PM, van Doornum GJ, Ferreira R, Vink J, Fenollar F, Raoult D. African tickbite fever in travellers. Swaziland Emerg Infect Dis 2007; 13(2):353–355.
38. Toutous-Trellu L, Peter O, Chavaz P, Saurat JH. African tick bite fever: not a spotless rickettsiosis! J Am Acad Dermatol 2003; 48(suppl 2):S18–S19.
39. Jensenius M, Ueland T, Fournier PE, et al. Systemic inflammatory responses in African tick-bite fever. J Infect Dis 2003; 187(8):1332–1336.
39a. Lepidi H, Fournier PE, Raoult D. Histologic features and immunodetection of African tick-bite fever eschar. Emerg Infect Dis 2006; 12(9):1332–1337.
40. Damås JK, Jensenius M, Ueland T, et al. Increased levels of soluble CD40L in African tick bite fever: possible involvement of TLRs in the pathogenetic interaction between *Rickettsia africae*, endothelial cells, and platelets. J Immunol 2006; 177:2699–2706.
41. Jensenius M, Hoel T, Raoult D, et al. Seroepidemiology of *Rickettsia africae* infection in Norwegian travellers to rural Africa. Scand J Infect Dis 2002; 34(2):93–96.
42. Jensenius M, Fournier PE, Hellum KB, et al. Sequential changes in hematologic and biochemical parameters in African tick bite fever. Clin Microbiol Infect 2003; 9(7):678–683.
43. Parola P, Jourdan J, Raoult D. Tick-borne infection caused by *Rickettsia africae* in the West Indies. N Engl J Med 1998; 338(19):1391.
44. Ding T, Lloyd G, Tolley H, Bradlow A. Tick bite fever and arthritis associated with travel to Africa. Ann Rheum Dis 2004; 63(12):1703–1704.
45. Jensenius M, Fournier P-E, Fladby T, et al. Subacute neuropathy in patients with African tick bite fever. Scand J Infect Dis 2006.
46. Bellini C, Monti M, Potin M, Dalle Ave A, Bille J, Greub G. Cardiac involvement in a patient with clinical and serological evidence of African tick-bite fever. BMC Infect Dis 2006; 38(2):114–118.
47. La Scola B, Raoult D. Laboratory diagnosis of rickettsioses: current approaches to diagnosis of old and new rickettsial diseases. J Clin Microbiol 1997; 35(11):2715–2727.
48. Fournier PE, Jensenius M, Laferl H, Vene S, Raoult D. Kinetics of antibody responses in *Rickettsia africae* and *Rickettsia conorii* infections. Clin Diagn Lab Immunol 2002; 9(2):324–328.
49. Jensenius M, Fournier PE, Vene S, Ringertz SH, Myrvang B, Raoult D. Comparison of immunofluorescence, Western blotting, and cross-adsorption assays for diagnosis of African tick bite fever. Clin Diagn Lab Immunol 2004; 11:786–788.
50. La Scola B, Raoult D. Diagnosis of Mediterranean spotted fever by cultivation of *Rickettsia conorii* from blood and skin samples using the centrifugation-shell vial technique and by detection of *R. conorii* in circulating endothelial cells: a 6-year follow-up. J Clin Microbiol 1996; 34(11):2722–2727.
51. Rolain JM, Maurin M, Vestris G, Raoult D. In vitro susceptibilities of 27 rickettsiae to 13 antimicrobials. Antimicrob Agents Chemother 1998; 42(7):1537–1541.
52. Rolain JM, Maurin M, Bryskier A, Raoult D. In vitro activities of telithromycin (HMR 3647) against *Rickettsia rickettsii, Rickettsia conorii, Rickettsia africae, Rickettsia typhi, Rickettsia prowazekii, Coxiella burnetii, Bartonella henselae, Bartonella quintana, Bartonella bacilliformis,* and *Ehrlichia chaffeensis.* Antimicrob Agents Chemother 2000; 44(5):1391–1393.
53. Jensenius M, Pretorius AM, Clarke F, Myrvang B. Repellent efficacy of four commercial DEET lotions against *Amblyomma hebraeum* (Acari: Ixodidae), the principal vector of *Rickettsia africae* in southern Africa. Trans R Soc Trop Med Hyg 2005; 99:708–711.
54. Pretorius AM, Jensenius M, Clarke F, Ringertz SH. Repellent efficacy of DEET and KBR 3023 against *Amblyomma hebraeum* (Acari: Ixodidae). J Med Entomol 2003; 40(2):245–248.

10 | Rickettsia conorii Infections (Mediterranean Spotted Fever, Israeli Spotted Fever, Indian Tick Typhus, Astrakhan Fever)

Clarisse Rovery and Didier Raoult
Faculté de Médecine, Unité des Rickettsies, Université de la Méditerranée, Marseille, France

BACKGROUND

Mediterranean spotted fever (MSF) was described by Conor and Bruch in Tunisia in 1910 (1) and was soon reported in other regions around the Mediterranean basin—the Black Sea littoral, India, the Middle East, and southern Africa. The disease was thereafter also known as "boutonneuse fever" because of a papular rather than macular rash. The typical inoculation eschar was described in 1925 in Marseille by Boinet and Pieri (2). In the early 1930s, the brown dog tick *Rhipicephalus sanguineus* was recognized as a vector in Europe (3), and a spotted-fever group rickettsia was shown to be the causative agent; this organism was named *Rickettsia conorii* in honor of the work of Conor.

R. conorii is an obligate intracellular Gram-negative, rod-shaped bacterium that measures 0.3 to 0.5 by 0.9 to 1.6 μm. It belongs to the genus *Rickettsia* order *Rickettsiales*. The advent of molecular taxonomic methods, especially 16S rDNA polymerase chain reaction (PCR) and DNA sequencing, has enabled the determination of phylogenetic relationships between bacterial species (4). The classification within *Rickettsiales* is continually modified as new data become available. Polyphasic taxonomy, which integrates phenotypic and phylogenetic data, seems to be particularly useful for rickettsial taxonomy (5,6). However, experts in the field of rickettsiology frequently disagree over species definitions. Until 2005, rickettsiae of the so-called *R. conorii* complex, including *R. conorii* strain Malish (the agent of MSF), Israeli spotted fever rickettsia (ISFR), *R. conorii* strain Indian [Indian Tick typhus rickettsia (ITTR)], and Astrakhan spotted fever rickettsia (AFR), were considered to be members of the same species. Phylogenetically, these rickettsiae constitute a homogeneous cluster supported by significant bootstrap values and are distinct from other *Rickettsia* species. Zhu et al. (7) estimated the degrees of genotypic variation among 31 isolates of *R. conorii*, one isolate of ITTR, two isolates and three tick amplicons of AFR, and two isolates of ISFR using multilocus sequence typing (MLST). Also, 16S rRNA and *gltA* genes, as well as three membrane-exposed protein-encoding genes, *ompA*, *ompB*, and *sca4* (formerly gene D), were incorporated in MLST. To further characterize the specifications of distinct MLST types, a prototype isolate was incorporated from each of these into a multispacer typing assay, which had previously been demonstrated to be more discriminant than MLST at the strain level for *R. conorii*. Furthermore, mouse serotypes were obtained for each of these MLST types. Using these results, Zhu et al. proposed to modify the nomenclature of the *R. conorii* species through the creation of the following subspecies: *R. conorii* subsp. *conorii* subsp. nov. (type strain Malish, ATCC VR-613), *R. conorii* subsp. *caspia* subsp. nov. (type strain A-167, formerly Astrakhan fever rickettsia), *R. conorii* subsp. *israelensis* subsp. nov. (type strain ISTT CDC1, formerly ISFR), and *R. conorii* subsp. *indica* subsp. nov. (type strain ATCC VR-597, formerly ITTR) (7).

Our knowledge about MSF has evolved over time. At first, it was thought that MSF was limited to certain regions of the world, that is, southern Europe, Africa, and India, but more and more countries, such as central Europe and Central and South Africa, have since reported MSF cases (Fig. 1). Serological techniques do not allow for differences between rickettsiae species of the spotted-fever group. Clinical descriptions based on serology surely include infections

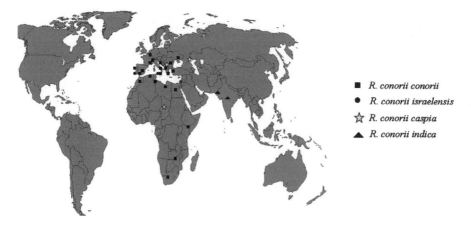

FIGURE 1 World map of the repartition of *R. conorii* species.

related to multiple species of rickettsiae and do not correspond to only one clinico-etiologic entity. In France, emerging rickettsioses, such as *R. sibirica mongolitimonae*, *R. slovaca*, *R. felis*, *R. helvetica* and *R. massilae*, have been recently described (8) and in Africa it is now known that *R. aeschlimannii*, *R. africae*, *R. conorii*, *R. sibirica mongolitimonae*, and *R. massiliae* are prevalent (8). The first series of patients describing MSF in these regions surely included those infected with these emerging rickettsioses. This confusion could explain atypical findings in the description of MSF such as winter cases, forms without rash in children, vesicular rash, and multiple eschars.

Another point that should be made is that *R. conorii* vector *Rh. sanguineus* is found throughout the world, but *R. conorii* is found only in some regions. Perhaps there is only an animal reservoir limited to some regions of the world and *Rh. sanguineus* may only be a vector of the disease. This was recently proposed in a study of *Rh. sanguineus* transmitting *R. rickettsii* infection in Arizona (9).

R. CONORII INFECTIONS
R. conorii conorii (Mediterranean Spotted Fever)

Three strains of *R. conorii conorii* include (*i*) Seven or Malish (the most common strain identified in our laboratory from France, Portugal, and North Africa), (*ii*) Kenyan, and (*iii*) Moroccan, which is apparently a unique isolate (D. Raoult, unpublished result). In 2001, the genome of *R. conorii* strain Seven was fully sequenced and revealed several unique characteristics among bacterial genomes (10,11), including long-palendromic-repeat fragments irregularly distributed throughout the genome. Further comparison of the *R. conorii* genome with that of *R. prowazekii* (the agent of the epidemic typhus and included in the typhus group genus of *Rickettsia*) provided additional data on the evolution of rickettsial genomes, the latter appearing to be a subset of the former (10). These data will provide insights into the mechanism of rickettsial pathogenicity (12) and new molecular diagnostic targets and new tools for phylogenetic and taxonomic studies.

Vector

R. conorii is transmitted by *Rh. sanguineus*, the brown dog tick. This bacterium does not normally infect humans during its natural cycle between its arthropod and vertebrate hosts, dogs. *Rh. sanguineus* probably has the most widespread distribution of all *Ixodid* ticks. Although it is widespread, its distribution is patchy in that it is confined to localities within urban, suburban, periurban, and rural areas in which there are both domestic dogs and human dwellings or man-made structures. It has traveled worldwide with domestic dogs and now is established in buildings as far north as Canada and Scandinavia and as far south as Australia. Although *Rh. sanguineus* has a worldwide distribution, *R. conorii* is confined to particular regions of the world, and has never been isolated in the United States (Fig. 1). *Rh. sanguineus* lives in peridomestic environments shared with dogs but has relatively low affinity for humans. Infection rates of *Rh. sanguineus* with rickettsiae are generally under 10% (13). Because of these circumstances, cases of MSF are sporadic and typically encountered in urban areas. The yellow dog tick, *Haemaphysalis leachi*, and *Rh. simus* have been suspected as vectors in southern Africa, but no isolate is currently available from these ticks.

Epidemiology

MSF is endemic in the Mediterranean area, including northern Africa and southern Europe. Cases continue to be identified in new locations within this region, as some cases were recently described in Malta (14), Turkey (15,16), Cyprus (17), Slovenia (18), Croatia (19), Greece (20), and Bulgaria (21). In Italy, the national incidence rate is 1.6 cases per 100,000 persons; however, considering the Sicily region, this incidence is much higher (10 cases per 100,000 persons) (22). In 2002, more than a half (498 of 890) of the cases of MSF identified in Italy and reported to the Ministry of Health came from Sicily. MSF is a reportable disease in Portugal (23), where the annual incidence rate of 9.8 cases per 100,000 persons was the highest of the rates of all Mediterranean countries in the 1990s (24). In some regions of Portugal, such as Bragança, the estimated incidence is as high as 56.5 cases per 100,000 persons (25). In Spain, estimated incidence was 23 to 45 cases per 100,000 persons in 1983–1985 (26,27). As with all rickettsioses, this rate likely underestimates the true incidence, and some authors suggest that there are seven times more cases than officially reported (24). Overall, in endemic countries, fluctuation in incidence has been noted, which peaked in 1982–1984 in Italy (28,29), and in South of France (30). In Spain, there was an almost constant increase in the number of cases between 1982 and 1988 (31). This may be due to variation in climatic conditions, such as an increase in temperature and the lack of rainfall (31–33). Some cases have also been sporadically reported in northern and central Europe, including Belgium (34), Switzerland (35), and northern France (36), where *Rh. sanguineus* is sometimes imported with dogs and survive in peridomestic environments providing acceptable microclimatic conditions, including kennels and houses (37). Sporadic cases in nonendemic countries are also frequently observed as a consequence of tourism (38,39), and in North America, MSF is one of the most frequently imported rickettsioses with African tick-bite fever (40,41). Notably, although *Rh. sanguineus* is prevalent in North America, no cases of MSF have been described until recently on that continent. MSF is also encountered infrequently in sub-Saharan Africa—in Kenya (42), Somalia (43), South Africa (44), Central African Republic (45), Somalia (46), and Togo (47)—and around the Black Sea (13). Although an MSF-like disease was described in Vladivostok in the eastern part of Russia in 1966 (48), no direct evidence of *R. conorii* infection has been reported there since that time. Figure 1 illustrates the distribution of *R. conorii* in the world. In Europe, cases are encountered in late summer. In France, most cases are diagnosed during July and August. This period is associated with the peak of activity of immature ticks that are smaller than adults and difficult to observe even when attached to the body (13). Similarly, most samples submitted for diagnostic evaluation in Portugal at the Center for Vectors and Infectious Disease Research, National Institute of Health, are received between July and September (23). In Croatia, more than 80% of cases occur between July and September, with a peak in August (49). To our knowledge, a recent report describing 22 *Rh. sanguineus* (one adult and 21 nymphs) attached to an alcoholic homeless man living with his dog near Marseille (50) was the first documentation of more than one *Rh. sanguineus* feeding on a human host. Because this infestation was associated with the highest summer temperatures noted in France during the past 50 years, it is possible that host-seeking and feeding behaviors of this tick were altered by unusual climatic circumstances (37).

Pathogenesis

When transmitted to a susceptible human host, *R. conorii* multiply in endothelial cells of small to medium vessels, causing a vasculitis that is responsible for the clinical and laboratory abnormalities occurring in MSF (37). After phagocytosis and internalization, the phagocytic vacuole is rapidly lysed, and rickettsiae escape the phagocytic digestion to multiply freely in the host cell cytoplasm and nucleus (13). Escape from vacuole is suspected to be mediated by an enzyme, with phospholipase A2 activity (51). However, the presence of a gene encoding a phospholipase D has been recently shown, and this gene may be a key factor for virulence (51). Rickettsiae can move from cell to cell by actin mobilization (52). *R. conorii* cells express a surface protein, RickA, which recruits Arp2/3, activates it, and induces actin polymerization (10,53). It is unknown how RickA is addressed to the bacterial surface and whether the type IV secretion system predicted by the genome sequence is involved in bacterial host cell interaction. The actin filaments present behind intracellular bacteria in the tails are long and unbranched. These filaments might form bundles, in particular, when bacteria spread from cell to cell, as shown previously (54).

Clinical Features

Males are more frequently ill than females [80% (55) and 59.7% (56), respectively], and this could be tied to occupation, tick contact, or specific susceptibility. After an asymptomatic incubation of six days (1–16 days) (56,57), the onset of MSF is abrupt and typical cases present with high fever (>39°C), flu-like symptoms (headache, chills, arthromyalgias), and a black eschar (tache noire) at the tick-bite site (13,55). Eschar is indolent and is usually localized on the trunk and the legs and arms (Fig. 2). Patients must be carefully examined as eschars can be localized on the scrotum in 2% of cases (56,58) or in an inguinal or axillar area. In children, we can find it frequently on the scalp, in retroauricular area (26,58–62). Eschars are rarely multiple. In Sicily, 7 of 645 children had multiple eschars (63). In four Spanish studies (26,57,64,65), multiple eschars were found, respectively, in 3%, 7.6%, 6.5%, and 11.5% of the patients, and involved more particularly children. However, the role of *R. aeschlimannii* circulating in *Hyalomma* sp. in Spain has to be considered in these cases of multiple eschars. Indeed, *Rh. sanguineus* has a low affinity to bite humans, and the infection rate by rickettsiae is low (less than 10%) (13). Thus, the probability of being bitten simultaneously by several infected *Rh. sanguineus* is quite low. Conversely, *Hyalomma marginatum* ticks readily bite humans, and persons may receive multiple simultaneous tick bites (8). In this context, it is possible that some cases of spotted fever acquired in southern Europe and presenting with several eschars are caused by *R. aeschlimannii*. In a few cases, the inoculation occurred through conjunctivae and patients presented with conjunctivitis (Fig. 3). Eschar is not retrieved in 14% to 28% of cases (56,64,65). In adults, regional adenopathy is not present as compared with lymphangitis-associated rickettsioses and this finding permits the discrimination between these two rickettsioses in endemic country (66). Regional adenopathy is more frequent in children, as it accounted for 33% to 74% of cases (26,59,61,67). Usually, rash follows fever within two to three days and is rarely delayed until the fifth day (57,58,62). The exanthema is initially macular and sparse, subsequently becoming maculopapular and generalized, often turning red-purple in color. The rash often involves the palms and soles, but spares the face (Fig. 4), and is present in all but 1% to 4% of cases. It can be purpuric in 1.4% to 16% of cases (Fig. 5) (56,64,65) and usually is associated with a severe form of MSF. Some authors (55,63,64) reported papulovesicular rash, but in these studies, rickettsialpox and *R. africae* cannot be excluded. In fact, as new species of Rickettsiae have been described to be coendemic with *R. conorii*, past clinical studies of MSF cases included the description of these emerging rickettsioses described as MSF. Gastrointestinal symptoms may be present in about 30% of patients (31,55,67) and are more likely to be present in children. The natural duration of illness is from 12 to 20 days (68). Defervescence and clinical improvement usually occurred within 48 hours of therapy (62). Generally, patients will recover within 10 days without any sequelae. Raoult and Roux (13) proposed in the last several years a diagnostic score to help clinicians for the diagnosis of MSF. It was recently presented as a helpful tool using clinical and epidemiological criteria only, when 62 consecutive charts of patients with suspected MSF were retrospectively reviewed in Tunisia (69).

Severe Forms of Mediterranean Spotted Fever

Severe forms, including major neurological manifestations and multiorgan involvement, may occur in 5% to 6% of MSF cases (70,71). Complications and death are very rare in infancy (24,26,61). The mortality rate is usually estimated around 2.5% among diagnosed cases (1.50% in the last decade in Portugal, including 2.58% in 1997) (23,70). In Portuguese series of cases, the fatality rates were 1.2% to 10% (24,72,73). Classic risk factors for severe forms include advanced age, immunocompromised situations, chronic alcoholism, glucose-6-phosphate-dehydrogenase deficiency, prior prescription of an inappropriate antibiotic, and delay in treatment (13). In 1997 in Beja, a southern Portuguese district, the case fatality rate in hospitalized patients with MSF was 32.3%, the highest obtained there since 1994. Interestingly, when risk factors for fatal outcome were studied in 105 patients hospitalized between 1994 and 1998, the

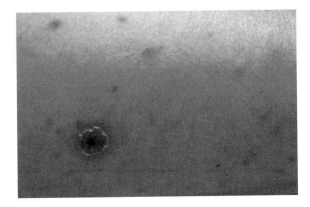

FIGURE 2 Eschar on the leg of a patient with Mediterranean spotted fever (MSF).

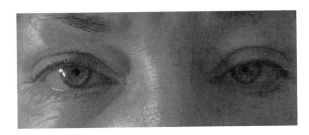

FIGURE 3 Conjunctivitis in a patient with Mediterranean spotted fever (MSF).

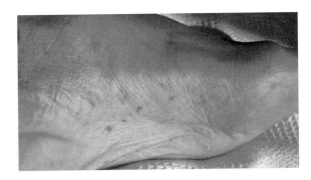

FIGURE 4 Plantar rash in a patient with Mediterranean spotted fever (MSF).

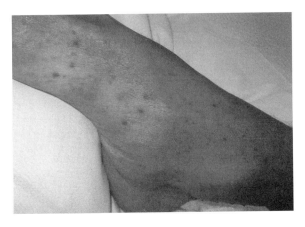

FIGURE 5 Purpuric rash in a patient with Mediterranean spotted fever (MSF).

risk of dying was significantly associated with diabetes, vomiting, dehydration, and uremia (24). Clinical presentation of these patients was unusual with only 20% with eschar (24). Some differences in the severity of MSF in different areas, even in the same country, such as Catalonia in northern Spain, have been noted. There, the disease seems to be milder than elsewhere in the country, as no fatalities were reported (65) in 227 MSF cases. In 78 admissions to the University Hospital in Barcelona (May 1986–October 1987), only five cases had complications (74). These differences suggest that severity is not only due to susceptibility of the host, but also to differences in virulence of strains.

R. conorii israelensis (Israeli Spotted Fever Rickettsia)

The first cases of rickettsial spotted fever in Israel, in the Haifa Bay area, were reported in 1946 (75) and the number of cases increased following the development of new settlements in the rural areas of this country (13). In 1971, the agent of Israeli spotted fever (ISF) was isolated from a patient (76). Two other antigenically identical agents were isolated from *Rh. sanguineus* ticks collected on the dogs of two patients with serologically documented ISF. These three isolates were rickettsiae closely related to, but slightly different from, *R. conorii* isolates obtained from patients with MSF (76). This observation has been confirmed by recent molecular studies (77–80), and Zhu et al. (7) proposed that the agent of Israeli spotted fever (ISF) constitutes a subspecies of *R. conorii* identified as *R. conorii* subsp. *israelensis* subsp. comb. nov.

One particularity of ISF is that the eschar at the inoculation site is absent in more than 90% of cases and resembles a small pinkish papule (81). The disease may be acquired even without direct contact with animals, through exposure to ticks in places where there are dogs, was reported (82). Several fatal cases and severe forms have been described, especially in children and in glucose-6-phosphate dehydrogenase deficiency (81,83,84).

In 1999, *R. conorii israelensis* was isolated from three patients living in semirural areas along the Tejo River in Portugal (85). None of these patients had traveled away from Portugal during the previous year, and none reported an eschar. All patients had severe disease and two patients died with septic shock and multiorgan failure. More recently, De Sousa et al. (86) reported the clinical data of 44 patients infected with *R. conorii israelensis* in Portugal between 1994 and 2004. Cases were confirmed by isolation of the rickettsia from blood or by PCR on skin biopsies. Absence of an eschar was noted in 54% of the patients. These findings call into question the concept that eschar is rare in ISF. A total of 10 out of 44 patients died. These clinical characteristics were not statistically different from those of 44 patients infected with *R. conorii conorii* in the same period (86).

R. conorii israelensis was also detected in Sicilian *Rh. sanguineus* ticks (87). A retrospective analysis, in western Sicily, from 1987 to 2001, identified, by molecular-sequence-based techniques, 5 out of 24 patients to be infected with *R. conorii israelensis* (22). In this series, the first reported case was in 1991. Among these five patients, three had severe disease and one died.

The occurrence of *R. conorii israelensis* in Portugal and Sicily indicates that the geographic distribution of ISF is wider than previously appreciated. These new cases also outline that *R. conorii israelensis* is a severe disease.

R. conorii caspia (Astrakhan Fever Rickettsia)

Since 1972, cases of a febrile exanthema have been described in patients living in rural areas in Astrakhan, a region of Russia located on the Caspian Sea. Prospective surveillance during 1983–1989 identified 321 cases of "Astrakhan fever." The number of cases increased each year, reaching 72 cases in 1988. Most patients were adults (94%), specifically males (61%), and occurred during summer months (85%, including 43% in August). The disease was similar to MSF; however, the presence of a tache noire was reported in only 23% of the patients. Conjunctivitis was frequent (32% of the cases). Headaches were noted in 92%, myalgias in 84%, hepatomegaly in 24%, and hearing loss in 14%. No fatal cases were reported (88). The Gamaleya Institute for Epidemiology and Microbiology in Moscow tested sera from patients with Astrakhan fever using the complement fixation test and observed the presence of antibodies reactive with *R. conorii* in 72% of patients (89). These results were also confirmed by microimmunofluorescence when tested at the Unité des Rickettsies in Marseille (90). Most of the patients had dogs and reported having contact with *Rh. sanguineus* dog ticks. The disease seemed to be transmitted by *Rh. sanguineus*, with 8% shown to be infected by the hemolymph test (89).

A rickettsial isolate was obtained from a patient with Astrakhan fever in 1991 (91). In 1992, it was shown by restriction-endonuclease digestion that DNA fragments of rickettsiae amplified from the blood of a patient were identical to those of rickettsial DNA amplified *Rh. sanguineus* ticks collected in Astrakhan, and related to those of *R. conorii* strain from Israel (92). Rickettsiae with identical genomic patterns were also found in *Rh. pumilio* ticks. This species usually feeds on domesticated and wild mammals, including rabbits and large rodents, but may occasionally bite humans (93).

By molecular methods, *R. conorii caspia* was detected in four *Rh. sanguineus*, including three collected on dogs and one taken from a soldier of the French United Nations troops in Kosovo who was asymptomatic. The man with the positive tick remained asymptomatic (94). A rickettsial isolate similar to *R. conorii caspia* was obtained from the eschar biopsy of a patient from Chad, in Africa. Five days before the onset of the symptoms, the patient traveled to Lake Chad where she had walked into the bush but recalled no tick bite. She presented with fever, dyspnea, a maculopapular rash, an inoculation eschar on the leg, and conjunctivitis of the right eye (94). Thus, the area of distribution of *R. conorii caspia* could be wider than initially suspected in Astrakhan and include Kosovo and Chad.

R. conorii indica (Indian Tick Typhus Rickettsia)

Indian tick typhus (ITT) is a tick-borne rickettsiosis prevalent in India. The disease was clinically described at the beginning of the century but the etiologic agent has never been isolated in patients. A spotted fever group rickettsia was isolated in 1950 from an *Rh. sanguineus* tick collected in India and assumed to be the ITT agent (95). This bacterium, classified as *R. conorii*, was considered to be the cause of ITT. However, subsequent serologic studies including cross-adsorption and microimmunofluorescence serotyping demonstrated significant differences in antibody responses of patients of ITT with the ITT rickettsia and type strains of *R. conorii* (96,97). Using molecular methods, it was recently demonstrated that these rickettsiae are closely related, although they differ as reflected in antigenic variation (78,79,98). Zhu et al. (7) have recently proposed that the agent of ITT constitutes a subspecies of *R. conorii*, different from the agent of MSF, designated *R. conorii* subsp. *indica* subsp. comb. nov.

ITT differs from MSF in that the rash is frequently purpuric and an inoculation eschar at the bite site is rarely identified (99). Cases are documented infrequently and generally using nonspecific serological methods such as the Weil–Felix test, which provides indirect evidence of possible rickettsial infection but does not allow a definitive diagnosis (100,101). In 2004, in Kerala, India, seven cases were documented for the first time by microimmuno flouresence (MIF). Patients were laborers working in tea fields and presented with fever and a generalized maculopapular rash involving palm and soles occurred in three patients (102) (Mathai and Raoult, submitted). In Thailand, two patients with spotted fever group rickettsioses, including one presenting with a rash and eschar, may have been infected with *R. conorii indica* (103). *R. conorii indica* has also been serologically identified in one patient with spotted fever in Laos (104). One case of severe infection with *R. conorii indica* in a traveler has been reported (105).

Table 1 resumes the principal characteristics of the different *R. conorii* species infections.

TREATMENT

Early empirical antibiotic therapy should be prescribed in any suspected MSF, before confirmation of the diagnosis. More than 50 years after the introduction of tetracyclines, doxycycline (200 mg/day) remains the treatment of choice for MSF (13). Although tetracyclines are contraindicated for general use in children less than nine years of age, doxycycline remains the treatment of choice for children, including young children, with MSF. In general, the risk of dental staining by doxycycline is negligible when a single, relatively short (e.g., 5–10 days) course of therapy is administered. In patients with severe hypersensitivity to tetracyclines, 50 to 75 mg/kg of body weight/day of chloramphenicol can be considered as an alternate therapy, but its use is limited by side effects, and failures and relapses have been noted (106).

TABLE 1 Ecological, Epidemiological, and Clinical Characteristics of Diseases Associated with Different Members of the *R. conorii* Complex

Rickettsia	Vector tick	Geographic repartition	Human disease name	Fever (%)	Inoculation eschar (%)	Cutaneous rash (%)	Fatal forms	References
R. conorii conorii, isolates Malish, Moroccan Kenyan	*Rhipicephalus* sp., *H. leachii*	Mediterranean area, Africa	MSF, Kenyan tick typhus, South African tick-bite fever	100	72	97	Yes	(24,56)
R. conorii israeli	*Rh. sanguineus*	Israel, Portugal	ISF	100	0–46	100	Yes	(81,86)
AFR	*Rh. sanguineus, Rh. pumilio*	Astrakhan region, Chad, Kosovo	Astrakhan spotted fever	100	23	100	No	(88)
ITTR	*Rh. sanguineus, Boophilus microplus, H. leachii*	India, Pakistan	ITT	100	0	100	No	(99)

Abbreviations: AFR, Astrakhan spotted fever rickettsial; ISF, Israeli spotted fever; ITT, Indian tick typhus; ITTR, Indian tick typhus rickettsial; MSF, Mediterranean spotted fever.

Failures and delayed apyrexia have been observed with erythromycin (107). In fact, in cell cultures, erythromycin and spiramycin are not effective. Josamycin (50 mg/kg/day) has been used with success in the treatment of MSF (13,108). In pregnant women with MSF, josamycin can be used at a dose of 3 g/day for seven days (13) and in children, 100 mg/kg/day for five days (108). Newer macrolides, such as azithromycin and clarithromycin (108,109), are also of interest. In a recent open-label controlled trial, these two drugs were compared in the treatment of children with MSF in Italy. They were equally tolerated, and no major side effects were observed. All patients recovered, and fever disappeared in less than seven days in each case. No statistical difference between the times to defervescence of the different drugs was found (63). Azithromycin seems to be of particular interest, as it is administered once a day and presents a shorter duration of therapy (three days, compared to seven days with clarithromycin). Some fluoroquinolones may have efficacy against spotted fever rickettsiae. Raoult et al. (110) cured five patients with MSF using ciprofloxacin administered intravenously. In the study of Gudiol et al. (111), apyrexia was more rapid with doxycycline than ciprofloxacin at doses of 500 mg twice daily. Ruiz Beltran and Herrero-Herrero (112) found that ciprofloxacin at doses of 750 mg every 12 hours and doxycyline were equally effective. Scarce studies have been published about efficacy of ofloxacin with conflicting results (113,114). Many classes of broad-spectrum antibiotics, including penicillin, cephalosporin, and aminoglycoside, are ineffective as therapies for rickettsial diseases. In vivo animal studies, anecdotal clinical experience, and limited evidence from small clinical trials suggest that sulfa-containing antimicrobials not only are ineffective, but may actually exacerbate MSF (115). Rifampicin failed to cure children with MSF (116). The exact duration of appropriate antibiotic therapy for SFG rickettsioses is generally related more to clinical response than to a precise number of days; however, for most of these infections, recommended therapy should continue for at least 24 hours after the patient's fever has abated. Yagupsky et al. (117) have treated children with ISF with success with doxycycline 4.4 mg/kg the first day and 2.2 mg/kg the subsequent day until the patient was afebrile for 24 hours. A single dose of 200 mg of doxycycline has been shown to be sufficient for MSF (13,118,119), although for patients with severe forms, such as malignant MSF, doxycycline should be administered intravenously up to 24 hours after apyrexia. Recommended schedule treatments are described in Table 2.

TABLE 2 Recommended Schedule Treatments

	First intention	Duration	Reference	Alternate treatment	Duration	Reference
Adults	Doxycycline 200 mg	One day or 24 hrs after apyrexia	(117,118,120)	Josamycin 3 g in three divided doses	5 days	(108)
				Ciprofloxacin 750 mg twice daily	8 days	(110, 112)
Children	Doxycycline 5 mg/kg	One day or 24 hrs after apyrexia (4.4 mg/kg the first day and then 2.2 mg/kg)	(117,118)	Josamycin 50 mg/kg/day twice daily	5 days	(108)
				Clarithromycin 15 mg/kg in two divided doses	7 days	(63)
				Azithromycin 10 mg/kg/day	3 days	(121)
Pregnante women	Josamycin 3 g/J	7 days	(13)	—	—	—
Severe forms of MSF	Intravenous vibramycine 200 mg followed by doxycycline 200 mg/J	10 days	—	—	—	—

Abbreviation: MSF, Mediterranean spotted fever.

REFERENCES

1. Conor A, Bruch A. Une fièvre éruptive observée en Tunisie. Bull Soc Pathol Exot Filial 1910; 8:492–496.
2. Olmer D. Sur une infection épidémique, avec exanthème de nature indéterminée. Mars Med 1925; 22:1291–1293.
3. Brumpt E. Longévité du virus de la fièvre boutonneuse (*Rickettsia conorii* n. sp.) chez la tique *Rhipicephalus sanguineus*. C R Soc Biol 1932; 110:1119.
4. Woese CR. Bacterial evolution. Microbiol Rev 1987; 51:222–270.
5. Stackebrandt E, Frederiksen W, Garrity GM, et al. Report of the ad hoc committee for the re-evaluation of the species definition in bacteriology. Int J Syst Evol Microbiol 2002; 52:1043–1047.
6. Vandamme P, Pot B, Gillis M, De Vos P, Kersters K, Swings J. Polyphasic taxonomy, a consensus approach to bacterial systematics. Microbiol Rev 1996; 60(2):407–438.
7. Zhu Y, Fournier PE, Eremeeva M, Raoult D. Proposal to create subspecies of *Rickettsia conorii* based on multi-locus sequence typing and an emended description of *Rickettsia conorii*. BMC Microbiol 2005; 5:1–11.
8. Parola P, Paddock C, Raoult D. Tick-borne rickettsioses around the world: emerging diseases challenging old concepts. Clin Microbiol Rev 2005; 18(4):719–756.
9. Demma LJ, Traeger MS, Nicholson WL, et al. Rocky Mountain spotted fever from an unexpected tick vector in Arizona. N Engl J Med 2005; 353(6):587–594.
10. Ogata H, Audic S, Renesto-Audiffren P, et al. Mechanisms of evolution in *Rickettsia conorii* and *R. prowazekii*. Science 2001; 293(5537):2093–2098.
11. Ogata H, Audic S, Abergel C, Fournier PE, Claverie JM. Protein coding palindromes are a unique but recurrent feature in *Rickettsia*. Genome Res 2002; 12(5):808–816.
12. Renesto P, Ogata H, Audic S, Claverie JM, Raoult D. Some lessons from Rickettsia genomics. FEMS Microbiol Lett 2005; 29:99–117.
13. Raoult D, Roux V. Rickettsioses as paradigms of new or emerging infectious diseases. Clin Microbiol Rev 1997; 10(4):694–719.
14. Tonna I, Mallia AC, Piscopo T, Cuschieri P, Fenollar F, Raoult D. Characterisation of rickettsial diseases in a hospital-based population in Malta. J Infect 2006; 53:394–402.
15. Mert A, Ozaras R, Tabak F, Bilir M, Ozturk R. Mediterranean spotted fever: a review of fifteen cases. J Dermatol 2006; 2:103–107.
16. Kuloglu F, Rolain JM, Fournier PE, Akata F, Tugrul M, Raoult D. First isolation of *Rickettsia conorii* from humans in the Trakya (European) region of Turkey. Eur J Clin Microbiol Infect Dis 2004; 23(8):609–614.
17. Psaroulaki A, Loukaidis F, Hadjichristodoulou C, Tselentis Y. Detection and identification of the aetiological agent of Mediterranean spotted fever (MSF) in two genera of ticks in Cyprus. Trans R Soc Trop Med Hyg 1999; 93(6):597–598.
18. Arnez M, Luznik-Bufon T, Avsic-Zupanc T, et al. Causes of febrile illnesses after a tick bite in Slovenian children. Pediatr Infect Dis J 2003; 22(12):1078–1083.
19. Sardelic S, Fournier PE, Punda Polic V, et al. First isolation of *Rickettsia conorii* from human blood in Croatia. Croat Med J 2003; 44(5):630–634.
20. Psaroulaki A, Spyridaki I, Ioannidis A, Babalis T, Gikas A, Tselentis Y. First isolation and identification of *Rickettsia conorii* from ticks collected in the region of Fokida in Central Greece. J Clin Microbiol 2003; 41(7):3317–3319.
21. Christova I, Van De PJ, Yazar S, Velo E, Schouls L. Identification of *Borrelia burgdorferi* sensu lato, *Anaplasma* and *Ehrlichia* species, and spotted fever group Rickettsiae in ticks from Southeastern Europe. Eur J Clin Microbiol Infect Dis 2003; 22(9):535–542.
22. Giammanco G, Vitale G, Mansueto S, Capra G, Pia Caleca M, Ammatuna P. Presence of *Rickettsia conorii* subsp. *israelensis*, the causative agent of Israeli spotted fever, in Sicily, Italy, ascertained in a retrospective study. J Clin Microbiol 2005; 43(12):6027–6031.
23. Bacellar F, De Sousa R, Santos A, Santos-Silva M, Parola P. Boutonneuse fever in Portugal: 1995–2000. Data of a state laboratory. Eur J Epidemiol 2003; 18:275–277.
24. De Sousa R, Nobrega SD, Bacellar F, Torgal J. Mediterranean spotted fever in Portugal—risk factors for fatal outcome in 105 hospitalized patients. Rickettsiology: Present and Future Directions 2003; 990:285–294.
25. De Sousa R, Bacellar F. Morbi-mortalidade por *R. conorii* em Portugal. Rev Bras Parasitol Vet 2004; 13(suppl 1):180–183.
26. Lopez Pares P, Munoz Espin T, Espejo Arenas E, Font Creus B, Segura Porta F, Martinez Vila I, et al. Mediterranean spotted fever in childhood: prospective study of 130 cases. An Esp Pediatr 1988; 28(4):293–296.
27. Turabian JL, de Lorenzo-Caceres A, Mateo S, Moreiras JL, Marcos F, Tellez A. Prospective studies on 73 cases of boutonneuse fever: validity of the clinico-epidemiological diagnosis and serology with respect to Proteus. Rev Clin Esp 1987; 181(6):300–304.

28. Tinelli M, Maccabruni A, Michelone G, Zambelli A. Mediterranean spotted fever in Lombardy: an epidemiological, clinical and laboratory study of 76 cases in the years 1977–1986. Eur J Epidemiol 1989; 5:516–520.
29. Folghera S, Fiorentini S, Martinelli F, et al. Development of a flow cytometric assay for the detection and measurement of neutralizing antibodies against human immunodeficiency virus. New Microbiol 1994; 17(1):21–28.
30. Raoult D, Lepeu G, de Micco P, et al. Recrudescence de la fièvre boutonneuse meditarraneenne dans le sud de la France. Mediterr Med 1984; 3:102–103.
31. Segura-Porta F, Font-Creus B, Espejo-Arenas E, Bella-Cueto F. New trends in Mediterranean spotted fever. Eur J Epidemiol 1989; 5:438–443.
32. Espejo-Arenas E, Font-Creus B, Bella-Cueto F, Segura-Porta F. Climatic factors in resurgence of Mediterranean spotted fever [letter]. Lancet 1986; 1:1333.
33. Raoult D, Tissot-Dupont H, Caraco P, Brouqui P, Drancourt M, Charrel C. Mediterranean spotted fever in Marseille: descriptive epidemiology and the influence climatic factors. Eur J Epidemiol 1992; 8:192–197.
34. Lambert M, Dugernier T, Bigaignon G, Rahier J, Piot P. Mediterranean spotted fever in Belgium [letter]. Lancet 1984; 2:1038.
35. Peter O, Burgdorfer W, Aeschlimann A, Chatelanat P. *Rickettsia conorii* isolated from *Rhipicephalus sanguineus* introduced into Switzerland on a pet dog. Z Parasitenkd 1984; 70:265–270.
36. Senneville E, Ajana F, Lecocq P, Chidiac C, Mouton Y. *Rickettsia conorii* isolated from ticks introduced to Northern France by a dog. Lancet 1991; 337:676.
37. Parola P, Raoult D. Ticks and tickborne bacterial diseases in humans: an emerging infectious threat. Clin Infect Dis 2001; 32(6):897–928.
38. Rolain JM, Jensenius M, Raoult D. Rickettsial infections—a threat to travellers? Curr Opin Infect Dis 2004; 17(5):433–437.
39. Jensenius M, Fournier PE, Raoult D. Rickettsioses and the international traveler. Clin Infect Dis 2004; 39(10):1493–1499.
40. Harris RL, Kaplan SL, Bradshaw MW, Williams TW Jr. Boutonneuse fever in American travelers. J Infect Dis 1986; 153(1):126–128.
41. McDonald JC, MacLean JD, McDade JE. Imported rickettsial disease: clinical and epidemiologic features. Am J Med 1988; 85:799–805.
42. Rutherford JS, Macaluso KR, Smith N, et al. Fatal spotted fever rickettsiosis, Kenya. Emerg Infect Dis 2004; 10(5):910–913.
43. Nur YA, Groen J, Yusuf MA, Osterhaus AD. IgM antibodies in hospitalized children with febrile illness during an inter-epidemic period of measles, in Somalia. J Clin Virol 1999; 12(1):21–25.
44. Kelly PJ, Mason PR, Raoult D. Spotted fever group rickettsiae in southern Africa—a review and current concepts. Cent Afr Med J 1998; 44(4):111–118.
45. Ekala MT, Gresenguet G, Belec L. Seroprevalence of rickettsial infections of the Boutonneuse fever group or its apparent group in Bangui (Central African Republic). Bull Soc Pathol Exot 1995; 88(3):126–128.
46. Williams WJ, Radulovic S, Dasch GA, et al. Identification of *Rickettsia conorii* infection by polymerase chain reaction in a soldier returning from Somalia. Clin Infect Dis 1994; 19:93–99.
47. Schroter G, Loose B, Trojan H. Serological studies on the occurrence of rickettsial infections in Togo (author's transl). Trop Med Parasitol 1975; 26:323–328.
48. Tarasevich IV, Somov GP. Comparative serological study of tick-borne typhus in northern Asia and tsutsugamushi fever. J Microb Epidemiol Immunol 1966; 1:83–86.
49. Punda-Polic V, Klismanic Z, Capkun V, Bradaric N. Demographic and epidemiologic features of Mediterranean spotted fever cases in the region of split, Croatia. Ann NY Acad Sci 2003; 990:143–148.
50. Hemmersbach-Miller M, Parola P, Raoult D, Brouqui P. A homeless man with maculopapular rash who died in Marseille, France. Clin Infect Dis 2004; 38:1498–1499.
51. Renesto P, Dehoux P, Gouin E, Touqui L, Cossart P, Raoult D. Identification and characterization of a phospholipase D-superfamily gene in rickettsiae. J Infect Dis 2003; 188(9):1276–1283.
52. Walker DH, Valbuena GA, Olano JP. Pathogenic mechanisms of disease caused by Rickettsia. Ann NY Acad Sci 2001; 990:1–11.
53. Gouin E, Egile C, Dehoux P, et al. The RickA protein of *Rickettsia conorii* activates the Arp2/3 complex. Nature 2004; 427(6973):457–461.
54. Gouin E, Gantelet H, Egile C, et al. A comparative study of the actin-based motilities of the pathogenic bacteria Listeria monocytogenes, *Shigella flexneri* and *Rickettsia conorii*. J Cell Sci 1999; 112:1697–1708.
55. Anton E, Font B, Munoz T, Sanfeliu I, Segura F. Clinical and laboratory characteristics of 144 patients with Mediterranean spotted fever. Eur J Clin Microbiol Infect Dis 2003; 22(2):126–128.
56. Raoult D, Weiller PJ, Chagnon A, Chaudet H, Gallais H, Casanova P. Mediterranean spotted fever: clinical, laboratory and epidemiological features of 199 cases. Am J Trop Med Hyg 1986; 35(4):845–850.
57. Martin Farfan A, Juarez Fernandez C, Calbo-Torrecillas F, Porras Ballesteros J, Diaz Recio M, Bermundez Recio F. Clinico-epidemiological study of 164 cases of boutonneuse fever. Rev Clin Esp 1985; 176:333–339.

58. Raoult D, Jean-Pastor MJ, Xeridat B, et al. Mediterranean boutonneuse fever: a propos of 154 recent cases. Ann Dermatol Venereol 1983; 110(11):909–914.
59. Garcia Miguel MJ, Garcia-Alix Perez A, de Jose Gomez MI, Barea Blanco I, Vidal Lopez ML, Garcia Hortelano J. Boutonneuse fever in children. An Esp Pediatr 1985; 22:353–358.
60. Moraga FA, Martinez-Roig A, Alonso JL, Boronat M, Domingo F. Boutonneuse fever. Arch Dis Child 1982; 57:149–151.
61. Cahuana A, Losada I, Galceran L, Lopez Casas JA, Pou J, Juncosa T. Mediterranean boutonneuse fever in children: study of 139 cases. An Esp Pediatr 1984; 21:642–647.
62. Cascio A, Dones P, Romano A, Titone L. Clinical and laboratory findings of boutonneuse fever in Sicilian children. Eur J Pediatr 1998; 157(6):482–486.
63. Cascio A, Colomba C, Antinori S, Paterson DL, Titone L. Clarithromycin versus azithromycin in the treatment of Mediterranean spotted fever in children: a randomized controlled trial. Clin Infect Dis 2002; 34(2):154–158.
64. Font-Creus B, Espejo-Arenas E, Munoz-Espin T, Uriz-Urzainqui S, Bella-Cueto F, Segura-Porta F. Mediterranean boutonneuse fever: study of 246 cases. Med Clin (Barc) 1991; 96:121–125.
65. Font-Creus B, Bella-Cueto F, Espejo-Arenas E, et al. Mediterranean spotted fever: a cooperative study of 227 cases. Rev Infect Dis 1985; 7:635–642.
66. Fournier PE, Gouriet F, Brouqui P, Lucht F, Raoult D. Lymphangitis associated rickettsial diseases (LARD), a new rickettsiosis caused by *Rickettsia sibirica* mongolotimonae: seven new cases of and review of the literature. Clin Infect Dis 2004; 40(10):1435–1444.
67. Raoult D, Arnolds M, Garnier JM, de Micco P, Giraud E. Fievre boutonneuse mediterraneenne de l'enfant (à propos de 41 observations). Med Hyg 1983; 41:1013–1016.
68. Pedro Pons A. Fiebre exantematica mediterranea. Med Clin (Barc) 1945; 5:1–6.
69. Omezzine-Letaief A, Yacoub S, Tissot-Dupont H, et al. Seroepidemiological survey of rickettsial infections among blood donors in central Tunisia. Trans R Soc Trop Med Hyg 1995; 89:266–268.
70. Amaro M, Bacellar F, Franca A. Report of eight cases of fatal and severe Mediterranean spotted fever in Portugal. Ann NY Acad Sci 2003; 990:331–343.
71. Raoult D, Gallais H, Ottomani A, et al. Malignant form of Mediterranean boutonneuse fever: 6 cases. Presse Med 1983; 12:2375–2378.
72. Tavares L, Botas J, Antunes F, Araujo FC. A febre escaro-nodular em Portugal. O Médico 1986; 113:836–846.
73. Carmo G, Caixeiro IS, Uva AS, Paiva JED. Febre escaro-nodular actualizaçao teorica e analise retrospectiva de 231 casos. Rer Port Doenças Infecciosas 1981; 4:13–28.
74. Soriano V, Sabria M, Davins J, Manterola JM. Complications in Mediterranean boutonneuse fever: prospective study of 78 patients. Rev Clin Esp 1989; 184:459–463.
75. Valero A. Rocky Mountain spotted fever in Palestine. Harefuah 1949; 36:99.
76. Goldwasser RA, Klingberg MA, Klingberg W, Steiman Y, Swartz TA. Laboratory and epidemiologic studies of rickettsial sotted fever in Israel. 12th Int Congr Interm Med 1974; 270–275.
77. Sekeyova Z, Roux V, Raoult D. Phylogeny of *Rickettsia* spp. inferred by comparing sequences of 'gene D', which encodes an intracytoplasmic protein. Int J Syst Evol Microbiol 2001; 51(pt 4):1353–1360.
78. Fournier PE, Roux V, Raoult D. Phylogenetic analysis of spotted fever group rickettsiae by study of the outer surface protein rOmpA. Int J Syst Bacteriol 1998; 48:839–849.
79. Roux V, Rydkina E, Eremeeva M, Raoult D. Citrate synthase gene comparison, a new tool for phylogenetic analysis, and its application for the rickettsiae. Int J Syst Bacteriol 1997; 47:252–261.
80. Zhang JZ, Fan MY, Wu YM, Fournier PE, Roux V, Raoult D. Genetic classification of *Rickettsia heilongjiangii* and *Rickettsia hulinii* two Chinese spotted fever group rickettsiae. J Clin Microbiol 2000; 38(9):3498–3501.
81. Gross EM, Yagupsky P. Israeli rickettsial spotted fever in children: a review of 54 cases. Acta Trop 1987; 44(1):91–96.
82. Shazberg G, Moise J, Terespolsky N, Hurvitz H. Family outbreak of *Rickettsia conorii* infection. Emerg Infect Dis 1999; 5(5):723–724.
83. Regev-Yochay G, Segal E, Rubinstein E. Glucose-6-phosphate dehydrogenase deficiency: possible determinant for a fulminant course of Israeli spotted fever. Isr Med Assoc J 2000; 2(10):781–782.
84. Yagupsky P, Wolach B. Fatal Israeli spotted fever in children. Clin Infect Dis 1993; 17:850–853.
85. Bacellar F, Beati L, Franca A, Pocas J, Regnery R, Filipe A. Israeli spotted fever rickettsia (*Rickettsia conorii* complex) associated with human disease in Portugal. Emerg Infect Dis 1999; 5(6):835–836.
86. De Sousa R, Ismail N, Doria-Nobrega S, et al. The presence of eschars, but not greater severity, in Portuguese patients infected with Israeli spotted Fever. Ann NY Acad Sci 2005; 1063:197–202.
87. Giammanco G, Mansueto S, Ammatuna P, Vitale G. Israeli spotted fever *Rickettsia* in Sicilian *Rhipicephalus sanguineus* ticks. Emerg Infect Dis 2003; 9(7):892–893.
88. Tarasevich IV, Makarova VA, Fetisova NF, Stepanov AV, Miskarova ED, Raoult D. Studies of a "new" rickettsiosis "Astrakhan" spotted fever. Eur J Epidemiol 1991; 7:294–298.
89. Tarasevich IV, Makarova V, Fetisova NF, et al. Astrakhan fever: new spotted fever group rickettsiosis. Lancet 1991; 337:172–173.
90. Eremeeva M, Balayeva NM, Roux V, Ignatovich V, Kotsinjan M, Raoult D. Genomic and proteinic characterization of strain S, a Rickettsia isolated from *Rhipicephalus sanguineus* ticks in Armenia. J Clin Microbiol 1995; 33:2738–2744.

91. Eremeeva ME, Balayeva NM, Ignatovich VF, Raoult D. Proteinic and genomic identification of spotted fever group rickettsiae isolated in the former USSR. J Clin Microbiol 1993; 31(10):2625–2633.
92. Drancourt M, Beati L, Tarasevich IV, Raoult D. Astrakhan fever rickettsia is identical to Israeli tick typhus rickettsia, a genotype of the *Rickettsia conorii* complex. J Infect Dis 1992; 165:1167–1168.
93. Eremeeva ME, Beati L, Makarova VA, et al. Astrakhan fever rickettsiae: antigenic and genotypic of isolates obtained from human and *Rhipicephalus pumilio* ticks. Am J Trop Med Hyg 1994; 51(5):697–706.
94. Fournier PE, Durand JP, Rolain JM, Camicas JL, Tolou H, Raoult D. Detection of Astrakhan fever rickettsia from ticks in Kosovo. Ann NY Acad Sci 2003; 990:158–161.
95. Philip CB, Hughes LE, Rao KNA, Kalra SL. Studies of Indian tick typhus and its relation to other human typhus-like rickettsiosis. 5th International Congress for Microbiology, 1950.
96. Philip RN, Casper EA, Burgdorfer W, Gerloff RK, Hugues LE, Bell EJ. Serologic typing of rickettsiae of the spotted fever group by microimmunofluorescence. J Immunol 1978; 121:1961–1968.
97. Beati L, Finidori JP, Gilot B, Raoult D. Comparison of serologic typing, sodium dodecyl sulfate–polyacrylamide gel electrophoresis protein analysis, and genetic restriction fragment length polymorphism analysis for identification of rickettsiae: characterization of two new rickettsial strains. J Clin Microbiol 1992; 30:1922–1930.
98. Roux V, Raoult D. Phylogenetic analysis of members of the genus *Rickettsia* using the gene encoding the outer-membrane protein rOmpB (ompB). Int J Syst Evol Microbiol 2000; 50(pt 4):1449–1455.
99. Jayaseelan E, Rajendran SC, Shariff S, Fishbein D, Keystone JS. Cutaneous eruptions in Indian tick typhus. Int J Dermatol 1991; 30:790–794.
100. Mathai E, LLoyd G, Cherian T, Abraham OC, Cherian AM. Serological evidence for the continued presence of human rickettsioses in southern India. Ann Trop Med Parasitol 2001; 95(4):395–398.
101. Murali N, Pillai S, Cherian T, Raghupathy P, Padmini V, Mathai E. Rickettsial infections in South India—how to spot the spotted fever. Indian Pediatr 2001; 38(12):1393–1396.
102. Sundhindra BK, Vijayakumar S, Kutty KA, et al. Rickettsial spotted fever in Kerala. Natl Med J India 2004; 17(1):51–52.
103. Parola P, Miller RS, McDaniel P, et al. Emerging rickettsioses of the Thai–Myanmar border. Emerg Infect Dis 2003; 9(5):592–595.
104. Phongmany S, Rolain JM, Phetsouvanh R, et al. Rickettsial infections and fever, Vientiane, Laos. Emerg Infect Dis 2006; 12(2):256–262.
105. Parola P, Fenollar F, Badiaga S, Brouqui P, Raoult D. First documentation of *Rickettsia conorii* infection (strain Indian tick typhus) in a traveller. Emerg Infect Dis 2001; 7(5):909–910.
106. Shaked Y, Samra Y, Maier MK, Rubinstein E. Relapse of rickettsial Mediterranean spotted fever and murine typhus after treatment with chloramphenicol. J Infect 1989; 18:35–37.
107. Munoz-Espin T, Lopez-Pares P, Espejo-Arenas E, et al. Erythromycin versus tetracycline for treatment of Mediterranean spotted fever. Arch Dis Child 1986; 61(10):1027–1029.
108. Bella F, Font B, Uriz S, et al. Randomized trial of doxycycline versus josamycin for Mediterranean spotted fever. Antimicrob Agents Chemother 1990; 34:937–938.
109. Segura F, Anton E. Clarithromycin for the treatment of Mediterranean spotted fever. Clin Infect Dis 2002; 34(4):560.
110. Raoult D, Gallais H, de Micco P, Casanova P. Ciprofloxacin therapy for Mediterranean spotted fever. Antimicrob Agents Chemother 1986; 30:606–607.
111. Gudiol F, Pallares R, Carratala J, et al. Randomized double-blind evaluation of ciprofloxacin and doxycycline for Mediterranean spotted fever. Antimicrob Agents Chemother 1989; 33:987–988.
112. Ruiz Beltran R, Herrero-Herrero JI. Evaluation of ciprofloxacin and doxycycline in the treatment of Mediterranean spotted fever. Eur J Clin Microbiol Infect Dis 1992; 11:427–431.
113. Raoult D, Drancourt M. Antimicrobial therapy of rickettsial diseases. Antimicrob Agents Chemother 1991; 35(12):2457–2462.
114. Herrero-Herrero JI, Ruiz Beltran R, Martin Sanchez AM. Naturally acquired immunity: a means of resistance to Mediterranean spotted fever? J Infect Dis 1991; 164(3):618–619.
115. Ruiz Beltran R, Herrero-Herrero JI. Deleterious effect of trimethoprim-sulfamethoxazole in Mediterranean spotted fever. Antimicrob Agents Chemother 1992; 36(6):1342–1344.
116. Bella F, Espejo-Arenas E, Uriz S, Serrano JA, Alegre MD, Tort J. Randomized trial of five-day rifampin versus one-day doxycycline therapy for Mediterranean spotted fever. J Infect Dis 1991; 164:433–434.
117. Yagupsky P, Gross EM, Alkan M, Bearman JE. Comparison of two dosage schedules of doxycycline in children with rickettsial spotted fever. J Infect Dis 1987; 155:1215–1219.
118. Bella-Cueto F, Font-Creus B, Segura-Porta F, Espejo-Arenas E, Lopez-Parez P, Munoz-Espin T. Comparative, randomized trial of one-day doxycycline versus 10-day tetracycline therapy for Mediterranean spotted fever. J Infect Dis 1987; 155:1056–1058.
119. Demartino G, Narciso P, Struglia C, Zechini F, Visco G. Therapeutic experience in the treatment of *Rickettsia conorii* infections with a single dose of doxycycline. Clin Ther 1981; 97:59–62.
120. Yebenes-Diaz G, Jimenez-Toboso J, Gonzalez-Barber A, Dorado-Pombo S. Mediterranean boutonneuse fever: effects of the duration of the treatment using doxycycline. Rev Clin Esp 1990; 186:309–310.
121. Meloni G, Meloni T. Azithromycin vs. doxycycline for Mediterranean spotted fever. Pediatr Infect Dis 2003; 15(11):1042–1044.

11 | Other Tick-Borne Rickettsioses

Oleg Medjannikov
Unité des Rickettsies, Université de la Méditerranée, Marseille, France and Laboratory of Rickettsial Ecology, Gamaleya Institute of Epidemiology and Microbiology, Gamalei, Moscow, Russia

Philippe Parola and Didier Raoult
Faculté de Médecine, Unité des Rickettsies, Université de la Méditerranée, Marseille, France

INTRODUCTION

In addition to *Rickettsia rickettsii*, *R. africae*, and *R. conorii* (including four subspecies *R. conorii* subsp. *conorii*, *R. conorii* subsp. *indica*, *R. conorii* subsp. *caspia*, and *R. conorii* subsp. *israelensis*), 14 more validated species or subspecies of tick-borne spotted fever group (SFG) rickettsiae are now considered as human pathogens. The rickettsiae designated here as human pathogens have been isolated in cell culture or have been detected by molecular methods from blood or tissues from patients with illnesses clinically compatible with spotted fever rickettsioses and who seroconverted using reference laboratory methods. In this chapter, we will describe *R. sibirica sibirica* [Siberian tick typhus (STT), North Asian tick typhus], *R. heilongjiangensis* (Far-Eastern tick-borne rickettsiosis), *R. australis* (Queensland tick typhus), *R. japonica* (Japanese or Oriental spotted fever), *R. honei* (Flinders Island spotted fever), *R. sibirica mongolitimonae* (lymphangitis-associated rickettsiosis), *R. slovaca* [tick-borne lymphadenopathy (TIBOLA)], *Dermacentor*-borne-necrosis-erythema-lymphadenopathy (DEBONEL), *R. aeschlimannii*, *R. parkeri*, *R. massiliae*, and *R. raoultii*. Furthermore, two candidatus, including "*Candidatus* Rickettsia marmionii" and "*Candidatus* Rickettsia kellyi," have been recently reported as human pathogens. Tick-borne rickettsiae possibly associated with human illnesses and other rickettsiae of undetermined pathogenicity are presented in Chapter 12.

RICKETTSIA SIBIRICA SIBIRICA (SIBERIAN TICK TYPHUS, NORTH ASIAN TICK TYPHUS)

R. sibirica is the causative agent of Siberian tick typhus (STT), an SFG rickettsiosis that was first described in the Russian Far East near the Pacific Ocean. The disease was simultaneously observed in the 1930s in two neighboring territories—Primorye (Maritime) region by Mill (1) and in Khabarovsk region by Antonov and Naishtat (2)—and was described in manuscripts published in 1936–1937. The described illness was acute and febrile; skin manifestation presented with maculopapular rash, sometimes petechial. Typical epidemiology included tick bite three to five days before the onset of the disease. On the basis of these facts, Mill proposed a name of Primorye tick-borne fever. Studying the same problem independently, Antonov and Naishtat proposed to call it Far-Eastern tick-borne typhus. Later, in between 1935 and 1939 a similar disease was found in Central Siberia (3), in the Krasnoyarsk region. The etiology of the disease remained unknown, although rickettsial origin was evident, and authors agreed that agents of "tropical tick typhus" or scrub typhus might be responsible for both the Far Eastern and Siberian disease.

Beginning in 1938, several expeditions were organized to Siberia and the Far East Russia under the leadership of Krontovskaya. The disease was disclosed in both regions and geographical distribution associated with specific tick vectors (*Dermacentor nuttali*, *D. marginatus*, *D. pictus* in Siberia; *Haemaphysalis concinna* and *D. silvarum* in Far East) and mammal reservoirs was identified (4–7).

The etiology of the disease was studied by Korshunova (8,9), who had isolated the first strains of the agent of tick-borne typhus in the Far East and Siberia using artificially avitaminotic guinea pigs. Zdrodovskii and Golinevich (10) finally proved rickettsial origin of tick-borne typhus in Siberia and the Far East in 1948–1949 and united them both in a new species, *Dermacentroxenus sibiricus*, which was later renamed *R. sibirica*. Close similarity of this rickettsia between the agents of Marseille spotted fever, epidemic typhus, and tsutsugamushi fever (scrub typhus) was evident. Accordingly, the diseases in both regions were also considered the same; amalgamated Far-Eastern and Siberian rickettsioses were named and registered at the time as STT or North Asian tick-borne rickettsiosis. Accordingly, clinical serological reactions, such as complement-binding studies and agglutination reaction, were performed with officially distributed *R. sibirica* antigen (11).

Nevertheless, the first strains isolated in humans from the Far East differed from those in Siberia. Published in 1943, the paper (9) states that immunization of guinea pigs with Siberian or Far-Eastern strains does not protect animals from the development of the disease after inoculation of heterologous strain, yet it does protect them from the homologous strain (4). Other authors stated that rickettsias from the Russian Far East and Siberia were identical (5). It should be mentioned that at that time only low-discriminative methods of bacterial identification in rickettsiology were available, such as Weil's reaction with *Proteus* OX_{19}, OX_2, and OX_K.

In 2002, an attempt was made to identify the etiology of STT in the Russian Far East by molecular biology methods. The results were surprising: none of 65 patients with clinical and serological evidences of SFG rickettsiosis had *R. sibirica*. Instead, in 13 cases another rickettsia was found, recently isolated from *D. silvarum* tick *R. heilongjiangensis* (12). Unfortunately, no old strains from patients of the Russian Far East remain in collections, so molecular identification is not possible; but based on the literature we can surmise that tick-borne rickettsial diseases in the Russian Far East were caused not by *R. sibirica*, but by *R. heilongjiangensis* [see "*R. heilongjanghensis* (Far-Eastern Tick-Borne Rickettsiosis)"]. Therefore, we have concentrated on data regarding STT from Central Siberia, a region where prototype and neotype (Netsvetayev or 232) strains of *R. sibirica* were isolated.

As with other tick-borne rickettsioses, STT is an acute zoonotic infectious disease with a geographical distribution strongly associated with distribution of its natural reservoirs. The agent, *R. sibirica*, is ecologically tied to the regions of prevalence of its natural reservoirs, ticks and small animals.

STT is well documented in the former U.S.S.R., but relatively few descriptions are available in the medical literature in English (13). Officially published data available from the Ministry of Health of Russian Federation state that annual morbidity rates in the years 1995–2004 vary from 1.5 to 2.4 per 100,000. However, in the areas where the disease is endemic, morbidity may as high as 40 or even 120 per 100,000. Active foci of the disease are widely spread in Asiatic Russia (Western, Central, and Eastern Siberia, Transbaikalia) with more than 80% of the cases observed in Altai and Krasnoyarsk regions. The disease is frequently reported during late spring and early summer. Since 1979, a constant increase of the number of cases has been observed. Between 1979 and 1997, 23,891 cases were recorded (14). Morbidity is also registered annually in the neighboring regions of Kazakhstan, Kyrgyzstan, and Mongolia (6,15). First evidence of tick-borne typhus in Inner Mongolia (China) was published in 1964 (16). Since that time, multiple studies, predominantly epidemiologic, have been performed in China.

One of the first full studies on etiology, epidemiology, natural vectors and hosts, clinics, and treatment was made by Kulagin (17). Beginning in 1942, he studied STT in the Altay region of Russia, where the morbidity rate is still among the highest. Kulagin isolated multiple strains from patients, ticks, and wild mammals (Fig. 1), precisely described the clinical picture and natural reservoirs, and made multiple pictures (17). Geographical conditions typical for STT were described as steppes and meadows (Fig. 2).

The works of Ricketts and Parker continued the study of STT in Russia. Ticks were shown as both vectors and reservoirs of STT agent. Early studies on trans-stadial and transovarial transmission of rickettsiae in tick vectors demonstrated that *D. nuttalli*, *D. pictus*, and *D. reticulatus* in Siberia and *H. concinna* in the Far East region retain *R. sibirica* in nature for months and may preserve it through molting, lay viable infected eggs, and transmit it to laboratory animals (7,17–19). The scheme of the so-called infections with natural nidality (natural foci) that were proposed by Pavlovsky (20) was applied to STT (Fig. 3). Other ticks, *H. punctata*, *Ixodes*

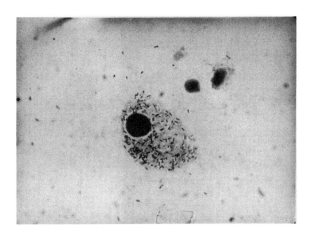

FIGURE 1 *Rickettsia sibirica* in tunica vaginalis of guinea pig after inoculation of a patient's blood, 1946 (17).

aproponophorus, and *I. plumbeus* are also claimed to be naturally infected with *R. sibirica*, but no strains from these tick species remain in collections (21).

Recent data on STT have been based on molecular detection of *R. sibirica* in ticks, which has been found in several species, and some of which have been presented as the principal vectors of STT (14). These include *D. nuttalli* in the mountainous steppe of western and eastern Siberia, *D. marginatus* in the steppe and meadow regions of western Siberia and northern Kazakhstan, *D. silvarum* in forest shrubs, and *H. concinna* in swampy tussocks of some parts of southern Siberia and the Russian Far East (14,22). Isolates obtained from these species of ticks, respectively, in 1949, 1959, 1983, and 1986 are available at the Gamaleya Research Institute of Epidemiology and Microbiology in Moscow (22). More recently, a rickettsial strain that had been isolated from *I. persucaltus* and maintained at the Omsk Research Institute of Natural Foci Infections was identified as *R. Sibirica* (23).

The rates of natural infection in ticks vary, but are usually very high. For *D. nuttalii*, the most important vector in Siberia, it may amount to as much as 64%, although for *Haemaphysalis* spp., it is not higher than 10% (21). High transovarial (up to 100%) and trans-stadial (up to 80%) transmission rates have been identified for *Dermacentor* ticks in tick models (24). *D. nuttalii* was shown as the most susceptible and stable model for infection.

Mammal hosts are considered only temporary reservoirs for *R. sibirica*. Complement-binding studies of rodents' sera showed the absence of antibodies in winter where mean temperature is below $-15°C$ and ticks are inactive, whereas first seropositive animals were captured in May. In June to July, seropositivity rates reach up to 50% (25). Larvae and nymphs of *Ixodid* ticks were infected by feeding on these animals. Dynamics of preimago ticks' numbers and quantity of seropositive animals is strongly dependent (25). The natural history of rickettsia–tick–mammal host interaction is reflected by Pavlovsky's scheme of natural nidality.

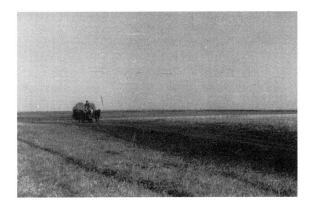

FIGURE 2 Typical landscape of Siberian tick typhus natural focus in Altay region, Russia, 1942. *Source*: Photo courtesy of Kulagin.

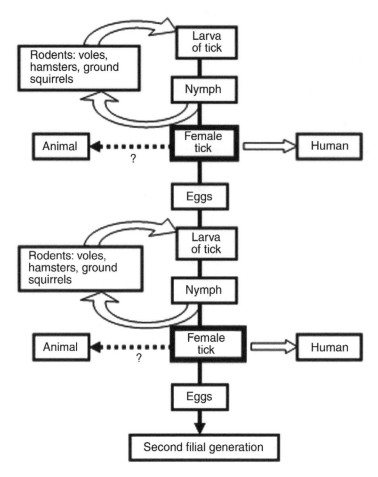

FIGURE 3 Pavlovsky's scheme of preservation of Siberian tick typhus agent in nature and transmission to humans.

Around 30 species of small mammals have been identified to be naturally infected by *R. sibirica*. They are mostly rodents, lagomorphs, and insectivores from the following genera: *Lepus, Eutamias, Marmota, Citellus, Mus, Apodemus, Rattus, Rhombomys, Meriones, Cricetus, Cricetulus, Ondatra, Arvicola, Microtus, Clethionomys,* and *Lagurus* (21).

STT is an acute infectious disease, characterized by high fever, primary affection of skin at tick-bite locus (eschar), and typical maculopapular rash. Natural transmission occurs by the bite of a tick; morbidity is seasonal with up to 80% of cases registered in May. Clinical course is benign. Incubation period varies usually from four to seven days following a tick bite. The onset is typically acute; prodrome is rare and short, in two to three days in 10% to 12% of patients. First sign is rapid increase of body temperature, up to 40°C. Classical observations describe the fever as continual or, rarely, remittent (15,17). Duration without antibiotic treatment is usually seven to nine days (Fig. 4), but may be longer, up to 20 days (17). The eschar is a typical skin lesion at the site of inoculation. Morphologically, it is an acute proliferative dermatitis with a site of wedge-shaped skin necrosis surrounded by lymphoid and epithelioid infiltration (26). Intensity of inflammatory reaction at the inoculation site significantly varies from a minimum perceptible papule to a necrotic lesion up to 40mm in diameter (Figs. 5 and 6). The frequency of eschars in STT patients varies in different reports: in most reliable sources it is around 62% to 77% (6,15). In Russian literature, the term of primary complex unites the eschar, regional lymphadenitis, and lymphangitis. Its presence is not consistent, but morphology is specific (26).

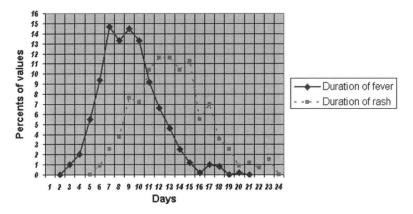

FIGURE 4 Duration of fever and rash in 345 patients with Siberian tick typhus in 1942–1947 (distribution by days of the disease). *Source*: Data of Kulagin.

The typical patient shows the following signs: the face is hyperemic, slightly puffed up, and vessels of conjunctiva are enlarged. The rash is the most persistent and characteristic sign of STT. First elements appear on the second through fourth days after the onset (Fig. 4) and morphologically resemble those in epidemic typhus. Destructive thrombotic endarteritis of the afferent arteriole results in the appearance of papules and roseolae on the skin. In STT, it rarely (in 3.6% of cases) became hemorrhagic, mostly in severe disease in elderly patients (15). In all early publications, the frequency of rash was given at 100%, and only single noneruptive cases are reported. Mild cases of STT may take their course without rash, but in those cases diagnosis should be done cautiously, because of possibility of misdiagnosis of tick-borne encephalitis, Lyme disease, human granulocytic anaplasmosis prevalent in the same territories and also transmitted also by tick bite (15,27). Myalgia and arthralgia occur in almost every patient and sometimes impede patient's self-service. Although central neurological involvement may occur, this disease is usually mild and is seldom associated with severe complications (14).

Diagnosis is based on careful clinical and epidemiological examination and laboratory diagnostic tools. Serological methods (complement-binding assay, indirect hemagglutination test, microimmunofluorescence study) can be effective, but multiple cross-reactions and late appearance of antibodies sometimes complicate the diagnosis (15,28). Isolation is often difficult and expensive, requiring high-level specialists and equipment. Quick and very sensitive polymerase chain reaction (PCR) should be performed on a regular basis, although in many cases rickettsial DNA is very hard to "catch" in patients, especially in blood. Eschars are most useful to

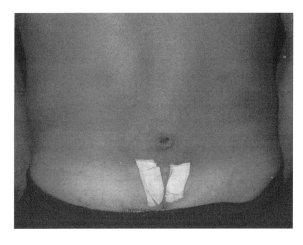

FIGURE 5 An eschar in a patient with Siberian tick typhus, general view.

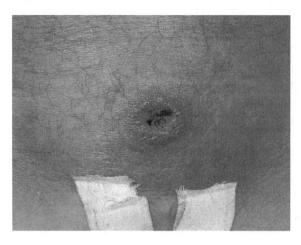

FIGURE 6 An eschar in a patient with Siberian tick typhus, close view.

assay. Treatment of STT does not differ from other SFG rickettsioses, and *R. sibirica* was shown to be susceptible to tetracyclines, chloramphenicol, fluoroquinolones, and rifampin (29,30).

R. sibirica infection was described by Russian investigators in Mongolia in 1943 (31). More recently STT has been serologically diagnosed in participants of a scientific expedition in Mongolia (32), but may have been misdiagnosed with other SFG rickettsioses (33).

Infection due to *R. sibirica* is also prevalent in China, where it has been intensively studied since its first description in 1958 (34). Since that time, more than 20 strains of *R. sibirica* have been isolated in China in Heilongjiang, Xinjiang, Beijing, Fujian provinces and Inner Mongolia (34). High seroprevalence among healthy persons and acute tick-bitten patients has been shown in endemic regions in the northern regions (35,36). The presence of antibodies against SFG rickettsiae in 76% of cattle and 58% of sheep in Inner Mongolia (37) has also been shown.

A wide variety of natural hosts and vectors were identified in China (38). Multiple studies revealed tick vectors *D. nuttalii*, *D. silvarum*, *D. niveus*, *D. sinicus*, *D. auratus*, *H. concinna*, *H. japonica*, *H. wellingtoni*, *H. longicornis*, *H. formosensis*, and *H. yeni*. Mice, voles, rats, musk rats, and hedgehogs are the mammal hosts (38).

Recently, a distinct strain of *R. sibirica*, currently considered as a subspecies [see "*R. sibirica mongolitimonae* (Lymphangitis-Associated Rickettsiosis)"], emerged as a pathogen for humans in Europe and Africa.

Rickettsial strains antigenically identical to *R. sibirica* have also been isolated from several species of ticks in Pakistan (39,40). However, because only serological methods have been used to characterize these strains, to our knowledge there is no definitive evidence of the prevalence of *R. sibirica* in Pakistan. Geographical distribution is shown in Figure 12.

RICKETTSIA HEILONGJIANGENSIS (FAR-EASTERN TICK-BORNE RICKETTSIOSIS)

The disease caused by *R. heilongjiangensis* has perhaps rightly been named "neglected rickettsiosis." Currently, it occurs in far-eastern territories of Russia (Khabarovsk territory, Amur region, Jewish autonomous republic) and northern China (Heilongjiang province). Until recently, this disease was thought to be STT. The first manuscripts to describe clinical and epidemiological features of the so-called Far-Eastern tick-borne typhus from the Khabarovsk region were published in Russia in 1936–1937 (1,2), which included the first clinical description of tick-borne typhus in Russia and China. So we may speculate that exactly that this disease was the first described tick-borne rickettsiosis in northern Asia.

The history begins in 1982, when a novel rickettsial isolate (HLJ-054) was obtained from *D. silvarum* ticks collected in Suifenhe, in the Heilongjiang Province of China. It has been molecularly characterized and recently described as a new member of SFG rickettsia, *R. heilongjiangensis* (41,42). The scientific name of the species originates from a Latinized name of the Chinese province where rickettsia was first isolated. Phylogenetically, it is grouped in a

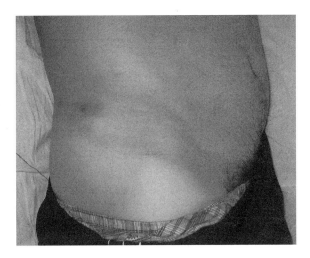

FIGURE 7 Eschar and lymphangitis in patient with Far-Eastern tick-borne rickettsiosis.

cluster with *R. japonica*. In 1992, several patients presenting with fever, headache, rash, eschar, regional lympadenopathy, and conjunctivitis following a tick bite in the same area were reported to have antibodies when tested with antigen of this rickettsia. Although complement-binding assays do not allow discrimination between spotted fever rickettsioses, Chinese investigators strongly suspected this species as a human pathogen (43).

More recently, 13 patients from the Russian Far East were shown to have an infection by *R. heilongjiangensis* (12). DNA (four fragments of three genes) was amplified from the patients' skin biopsies and blood samples, and sequencing showed 100% homology with *R. heilongjiangensis*. Further, the presence of specific antibodies against *R. heilongjiangensis* was shown when the serum samples of the same patients were tested with a panel of rickettsial antigens. This data confirmed the idea of the impossibility of distinguishing STT and *R. heilongjiangensis* infection by serology (immunofluorescence antibody). In 2006, four strains from humans were isolated (O. Mediannikov, unpublished data).

The clinical picture was similar to other SFG rickettsioses. All the patients had a history of tick bite, tick exposure, or a stay in an epidemiologically suspected location. In 12 cases a macular or maculopapular rash appeared, which was faint in most cases. Conjunctival papulae were noticed in some patients (Fig. 7). Also, 12 patients had eschars. Two patients were shown to have lymphangitis and regional lymphadenopathy (Fig. 8).

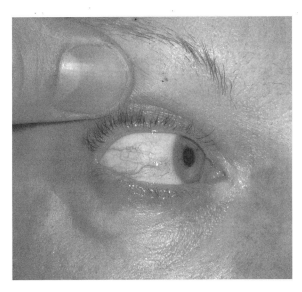

FIGURE 8 Conjunctival rash in patient with Far-Eastern tick-borne rickettsiosis.

When compared with *R. sibirica* infection based on data from Central Siberia, the disease in the Russian Far East revealed some differences. The seasonal peak of newly described rickettsiosis was from the end of June through July, when STT peaks at the end of April and through May. Further, the infection due to the variant of *R. heilongjiangensis* seemed to affect an older population (only one under 45 years), and to be relatively mild and without any reported deaths (44). The epidemiology of infections caused by the variant of *R. heilongjiangensis* remains to be further studied. Major tick vectors, at least in the Russian Far East, are *H. concinna* and *H. japonica douglasii*. DNA of *R. heilongjiangensis* was amplified from *H. concinna* female ticks and from a patient who had fallen ill after being bitten by this tick species. The same rickettsia has been found in 28% of *H. concinna* and 4.5% of *H. japonica douglasii* ticks collected from wild vegetation in endemic regions (44).

The name Far-Eastern tick-borne rickettsiosis has been proposed for this emerging infectious disease, in homage to the primary description of the disease (2) and to reflect its geographical distribution predominantly in the Russian Far East and China.

More recently, the DNA of *R. heilongjiangensis* was amplified from *H. concinna* ticks from Siberia (45). And, finally, molecular identification of old rickettsial collection from the Omsk Research Institute showed that strains of *R. heilongjiangensis*, earlier misinterpreted as *R. sibirica*, were isolated from ticks more than 30 years ago in the Russian Far East and southern Siberia (Fig. 12) (46).

To date, we have the evidence that both *R. sibirica* and *R. heilongjiangensis* may be prevalent in the Russian Far East. Strains of *R. sibirica* were isolated from *H. concinna* from Primorye region (22), although only *R. heilongjiangensis* was found in both patients and in tick vectors in the neighboring Khabarovsk region (12,22,44). As molecular identification of fastidious pathogens provided broad abilities for the study of their epidemiology, these methods should be intensively used for discrimination of geographical distribution of different SFG rickettsioses and their vectors.

RICKETTSIA AUSTRALIS (QUEENSLAND TICK TYPHUS)

Queensland tick typhus (QTT) has been recognized as a disease since 1946 when the first cases were observed among Australian troops training in the bush of northern Queensland in eastern Australia. Bacteria were isolated from 2 of 12 infected soldiers (47). This agent was found to be a new SFG rickettsia (48) by serological methods, and was named *R. australis* in 1950 (49). Thereafter, QTT has been recognized along the entire eastern coast of Australia, east of the Great Dividing Range (50–52). In the regions south of Queensland, cases were recorded in the 1990s in the eastern coastal region of New South Wales, including its capital city of Sydney (53). For a long time, QTT was thought to be the only spotted fever in Australia. Spotted fevers with slight clinical and epidemiological differences were also reported in Victoria and in Flinders Island (54). Although these cases were primarily assumed to be due to *R. australis* (51), it is now known that a different pathogenic rickettsia, *R. honei*, occurs in Flinders Island, Tasmania, and in southeastern South Australia where it was shown to be responsible for the SFG rickettsiosis cases (like that this refers to the paragraph "R.honei" p.148.). To date, *R. australis* has been definitely isolated only from patients in Queensland (Fig. 12) (47,55).

I. holocyclus, a common, human-biting tick found in Queensland, harbors *R. australis* (56). This tick also feeds on a broad range of vertebrate hosts. It is distributed primarily in coastal regions but is also prevalent in the rain forests of Queensland (54). Another vector of *R. australis* is *I. tasmani*, a species that exists along the coast as well as in the interior regions of southern and western Australia (57). This tick rarely bites humans, but may play a role in the enzootic maintenance of *R. australis* in small animals (52,56). An SFG rickettsia later identified also as *R. australis* was identified in the hemolymph of an *I. cornuatus* tick removed from a human in Victoria (58). This tick is prevalent in south coastal New South Wales, eastern Victoria, and Tasmania (57).

A number of vertebrates including bush rats, bandicoots, and domestic dogs are common hosts for all these ticks. In one study, antibodies reactive with *R. australis* were detected in 54 of 307 bandicoots and rodents trapped in northern Queensland; however, the precise role of vertebrates as reservoirs of *R. australis* is not known (59).

QTT is a notifiable disease in Australia, but it is seldom reported. A review of 62 cases of spotted fever recorded in Australia between 1946 and 1989 (50) indicated that 37 of cases that originated from Queensland and New South could be considered as infections due to *R. australis*. Most of the cases (78%) occurred between June and November. Cases were reported from both urban and suburban areas. Approximately 76% of patients recalled an antecedent tick bite. Clinically, the disease is characterized by a sudden onset with fever, headache, and myalgia. Within 10 days, maculopapular or vesicular rash appears. An inoculation eschar is identified in approximately 65% of cases, and lymphadenopathy in 71% of cases.

Treatment is usual as for other SFG rickettsioses and includes tetracycline-group antibiotics and pathogenetic treatment if needed. The disease ranges from mild to severe, but only two patients with fatal disease have been described (52,60).

RICKETTSIA JAPONICA (JAPANESE OR ORIENTAL SPOTTED FEVER)

The history of discovery of this disease emphasizes the important role of a single curious person interested by atypical cases. Between May and July 1984, the Japanese physician Mahara observed three patients with high fever and rash. All of them lived in the same rural area and had collected shoots from bamboo plantations on the same mountain. In two patients, an eschar was observed. General clinical signs resembled scrub typhus or tsutsugamushi fever. This well-known and studied zoonotic disease in Japan had always had strict geographical limitations (61). Shikoku Island, where Mahara found his patients, is not endemic for scrub typhus, and this fact, together with clinical feature not typical for *Orientia tsutsugamushi* infection, provoked his interest.

The results of the Weil–Felix test showed positive OX_2 serum agglutinins, indicating a possible SFG rickettsiosis, whereas OX_K serum agglutinins (used for the diagnosis of scrub typhus) were negative (62). Patient's sera were then shown to have antibodies reactive with SFG rickettsial antigens when tested by immunofluorescence (63,64). An evidently new rickettsiosis was called Japanese spotted fever. The causative agent was first isolated from patients on Shikoku in 1985 (65,66) and was subsequently characterized as a new rickettsia of the SFG and named *R. japonica* (67–69).

Approximately 40 cases have been reported annually since 1984, mainly along the coast of southwestern and central Japan (70,71). The disease is registered mainly from April to October. High-risk areas for acquiring the infection include bamboo plantations, crop fields, and coastal hills and forests where ticks are abundant and bites are frequent. As other SFG rickettsioses, Japanese spotted fever has an abrupt onset with headache, high fever (39–40°C), and chills. A macular rash appears after two to three days, all over the body including the palms and soles. Often it becomes petechial after three to four days and disappears in two weeks. An inoculation eschar was observed in as many as 91% of 34 patients diagnosed at Mahara Hospital in 1984–1997. The fact of a tick bite was recollected only by 38% of the patients, indicating that most bites remained unnoticed (70,71). Severe cases have been reported including patients with encephalitis, disseminated intravascular coagulopathy, multiorgan failure, and acute respiratory distress syndrome (72–75). In a series of 28 patients hospitalized during 1993–2002, six (21%) cases were classified as severe and included one fatality (74,76).

R. japonica has been detected in or isolated from six species of ticks in Japan. Of these, *H. flava, H. longicornis, D. taiwanensis*, and *I. ovatus* commonly feed on humans and are considered as the most likely vectors of the disease (71,77,78). Natural hosts of *R. japonica* in Japan are still to be identified.

For a long period, Japanese spotted fever was thought to be endemic to Japan. However, a recent report from South Korea shows that closely related rickettsia, probably another strain of *R. japonica*, may cause diseases in humans there. It was isolated from the blood of a 65-year-old farmer who presented with small eschar associated with regional lymphadenopathy, fever, erythematous and petechial rash, and confusion. ECV304 human endothelial cell line was used for the isolation. Genotypical characterization of the strain showed that it was very close to *R. japonica* prototype strain and might be considered as a regional strain (79). The vector and reservoir remain to be identified, although molecular survey of SFG rickettsiae in *H. longicornis* ticks in Korea revealed three rickettsial genovariants close to *R. japonica* (Fig. 12) (80).

RICKETTSIA HONEI (FLINDERS ISLAND SPOTTED FEVER)

An acute illness clinically resembling SFG rickettsiosis was described in 1991 by Stewart, the only medical doctor among approximately 1000 inhabitants on Flinders Island, a small island off the southeastern coast of Australia near Tasmania. Fever, headache, myalgia, slight cough, and a maculopapular rash gave the practitioner reason to suspect rickettsial infection. Serological analysis, including the Weil–Felix agglutination and rickettsial-specific immunofluorescence tests, suggested that the causative agent was a member of the SFG. At that time, the only spotted fever known in Australia was QTT, so all observed cases were considered as QTT, although clinical and epidemiological differences were noted when compared to original cases.

Twenty-six cases of a seasonal, febrile rash illness were observed over 12 years. The rash was erythematous in the majority of patients and purpuric in two patients with severe cases associated with thrombocytopenia (54). An eschar typical for SFG rickettsiosis and enlarged local nodes were observed in 25% and 55% of cases, respectively. All cases occurred in spring and summer, predominantly during December and January, which corresponded with tick activity. The usual features in Flinders Island spotted fever were a sudden onset of fever, headache, arthromyalgias with joint swelling, and slight cough. However, the rash, which appeared few days later, was maculopapular and there was no vesiculation, unlike QTT caused by *R. australis*. Although most of the reported cases of *R. australis* occurred during between June and November, and were reported from both urban and suburban areas, cases in Flinders Island spotted fever occurred predominantly during December to January (54,81). Incidence of Flinders Island spotted fever was estimated as 150 per 100,000 persons.

An isolation of the etiological agent took place in 1992, when strains were obtained from two patients with Flinders Island spotted fever (57,82). Concentrated buffy coat was applied to Vero cell monolayer by shell vial technique and on the fourth week intracellular rickettsia-like particles were found. The rickettsia was characterized by molecular methods and proposed as a new species, *R. honei* (83,84). It was named after Frank Sandland Hone, an Australian physician who was an early pioneer in Australian rickettsiology (84).

The tick vector of Flinders Island spotted fever was unknown for a long period, although *Aponomma hydrosauri* was suspected based on temporal association of bite with nine days' delayed onset of disease in a patient. A rickettsial isolate was later obtained from the same patient (58). This tick species is associated with different reptiles and rarely bites humans. During the same summer season of 1990, eight people collected the ticks that had bitten them. Six were *I. tasmanii* (the most common tick species that bites humans on Flinders Island) and two were *A. hydrosauri*. More argument of the role of this reptile tick were obtained when 63% of *A. hydrosauri* removed from 12 Australian blue-tongued lizards on Flinders Island were shown to harbor *R. honei* by molecular techniques (85,86). DNA of *R. honei* has been detected by PCR in eggs obtained from engorged female ticks of this species, suggesting transovarial transmission of *R. honei* in the tick host (85). Up to 15% of ticks collected from wild reptiles in Flinders Islands harbor *R. honei*, although neither serologic nor molecular evidence was found of this rickettsia in animals from which ticks were harvested (87). Search for a probable animal reservoir and definitive implication of *A. hydrosauri* as a vector and possibly reservoir of *R. honei* require further study, although migratory birds have been suggested to play a certain role in the introduction of the rickettsia along Asian coasts (84).

Common sense suggests that the geographical distribution of a tick species harboring pathogenic bacteria should define the disease prevalence. *A. hydrosauri* is not endemic to Flinders Island endemic; it is widespread in South Australia including the Victoria area on the mainland and in Tasmania. It has also been noted in New South Wales (88). And, predictably, in 1995, a similar rickettsiosis emerged in Tasmania, where patients were found by PCR to be infected with *R. honei* (89). *A. hydrosauri* ticks removed from Tasmanian residents were also positive by PCR. In addition, as shown in Figure 12, recent cases of rickettsiosis caused by *R. honei* were described in Schouten Island, south of the Freycinet Peninsula, Tasmania, and in South Australia (90).

Interestingly, in 1962 a rickettsia isolated in Thailand from pooled larval *Ixodes* sp. and *Rhipicephalus* sp. ticks collected on a common rat, was designated as Thai tick typhus rickettsia TT-118 (40); however, this rickettsia has been shown recently to be a strain of *R. honei* (84). This finding could easily be suggested casuistic, until more recently, DNA of *R. honei* has been recently detected in Thai *I. granulatus* ticks collected from *R. rattus* in Thailand in 1974 (91). Finally, the first case of *R. honei* rickettsiosis diagnosed by PCR and serology was reported in 2005. DNA was extracted from the serum of febrile patient from Bangkok, and amplicons showed 100% sequence similarity with the corresponding sequence of TT-118 isolate (92).

A rickettsia closely related to *R. honei* was detected by molecular tools in two *Amblyomma cajennense* adult ticks collected on cattle in south Texas in the United States (Fig. 12) (93). Sequence analysis of segments of the 17-kDa *glta* and *rompA* genes amplified from these ticks showed the highest degree of similarity to the Thai tick typhus rickettsia (homologies of 99.5%, 99.5%, and 100%, respectively). To date, no case of SFG rickettsioses has been linked to *R. honei* in the United States.

RICKETTSIA SIBIRICA MONGOLITIMONAE (LYMPHANGITIS-ASSOCIATED RICKETTSIOSIS)

This rickettsia was isolated in 1991 from *Hyalomma asiaticum* ticks collected in Inner Mongolia, in China. The isolate HA-91 differed antigenically and genotypically from other SFG rickettsiae (94). Different subspecies of *H. asiaticum* ticks are widely distributed across Asia, although to the best of our knowledge no *R. sibirica* isolates were obtained from this tick. At that time, *R. sibirica* was thought to be the only pathogenic SFG rickettsia in China.

The next appearance of this rickettsia in the scientific world occurred in 1996, when a genetically indistinguishable isolate was obtained from the blood and skin of a 63-year-old patient in southern France. The patient was hospitalized in March (an atypical month for common occurrence of Mediterranean spotted fever in this region) with a mild disease characterized by only a discrete rash and an inoculation eschar involving the groin. This patient was a resident of Marseille and had no travel history; however, the patient had collected compost from a garden where migratory birds were resting (95). That is why initial hypothesis was that the rickettsia was transmitted by tick occasionally brought with birds from Asia. The name, "*R. mongololimonae*," was then first proposed for the rickettsia to refer to the disparate sources of the isolates (i.e., Inner Mongolia and La Timone Hospital in Marseille). Using gene-sequence-based criteria to define *Rickettsia* species (42), *R. mongololimonae* was identified as a member of the *R. sibirica* species complex. Nevertheless, all strains of *R. mongolotimonae* group together in phylogenetic clusters separated from other strains of *R. sibirica*. In addition to slight serotypic differences, *R. mongololimonae* exhibits specific ecology. Classical *R. sibirica* was never found in *Hyalomma* spp. ticks. For these reasons, and in accordance with Latin nomenclature, this agent is now called *R. sibirica mongololimonae*, and the agent of North Asian tick typhus is called *R. sibirica* sensu stricto (96,97).

A second human case of infection with *R. sibirica mongolitimonae* was diagnosed in 1998 in an HIV-positive patient who had gardened in a rural area of Marseille. The patient presented with fever, headache, an eschar, lymphangitis, and painful satellite lymphadenopathy (98). Following this case, a number of patients were diagnosed with *R. sibirica mongolitimonae* infection. From January 2000 to June 2004, seven additional patients were observed in France. In three of them, the bacterium was cultivated from the inoculation eschar. The other four patients were diagnosed using PCR from the eschar (two patients) or blood (two patients), plus specific Western blot before (two patients) and after (two patients) cross-adsorption.

On the basis of evaluation of these nine cases, *R. sibirica mongolitimonae* infection differs from other tick-borne rickettsioses in the Mediterranean area. Specific characteristics include an incidence from March to early July, the occasional findings, alone or in combination, of multiple eschars, draining lymph nodes, and a lymphangitis that extends from the inoculation eschar to the draining node (Fig. 9). The unusual clinical features of this new rickettsiosis have led to the nickname, "lymphangitis-associated rickettsiosis" (LAR) (96).

It now seems that the distribution area of *R. sibirica mongolitimonae* coincides, or at least corresponds to distribution of *Hyalomma* spp. ticks worldwide. First evidence was reported in sub-Saharan Africa in 2001, when it was detected in *H. truncatum* (99). The first proven human infection with *R. sibirica mongolitimonae* was reported in a construction worker in South Africa's Northern Province. The patient presented with an eschar on his toe, lymphangitis, severe

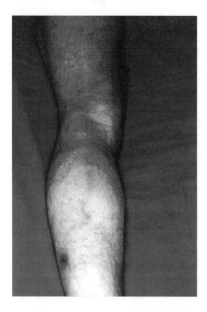

FIGURE 9 Lymphangitis extending from the inoculation eschar to the draining node in *Rickettsia sibirica mongolitimonae* infection. *Source*: From Ref. 98.

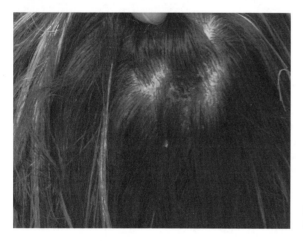

FIGURE 10 Eschar at the place of *Rickettsia slovaca* inoculation.

headache, and fever. An eschar biopsy was used for PCR amplification of the rickettsial *rOmpA* gene which showed >99% similarity with the corresponding *rOmpA* fragment of *R. sibirica mongololimonae* (100). More recently, a second African case was documented in a patient returning to France after a trip in Algeria. She presented with fever and two inoculation eschars. She had been in contact with camels, which are highly parasitized by ticks (96). Another European case has been recently reported. An isolate was recovered in 2004 from a 73-year-old Portuguese woman who suffered from acute febrile illness with maculopapular rash all over the body. Initial diagnosis was Mediterranean spotted fever and subsequent treatment with doxycycline soon improved her condition (101). Thus, LAR should be considered in the differential diagnosis of tick-borne rickettsioses in Europe, Africa, and Asia (Figs. 11 and 12).

Specific vectors and reservoirs of *R. sibirica mongolitimonae* have yet to be described, particularly in southern France. It has been hypothesized that ticks from migratory birds may have bitten French patients. The detection of *R. sibirica mongolitimonae* in *Hyalomma* spp. in Mongolia and Niger suggests a possible association of this rickettsia with ticks of this genus that are also prevalent in southern France (102). More arguments for this hypothesis have been provided recently when two cases of *R. sibirica mongolitimonae* were documented in Crete, Greece. In one patient, this rickettsia was simultaneously detected on a *H. anatolicum excavatum*

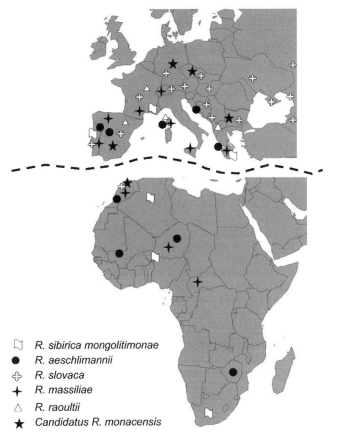

- ⌒ *R. sibirica mongolitimonae*
- ● *R. aeschlimannii*
- ✥ *R. slovaca*
- ✚ *R. massiliae*
- △ *R. raoultii*
- ★ Candidatus *R. monacensis*

FIGURE 11 Distribution of *Rickettsia* spp. recognized (by 2006) as human pathogens in Europe and Africa, except *R. conorii* and *R. africae* (see the corresponding chapters for these two rickettsiae).

tick parasitized on him (103). Recently, in Portugal, *R. sibirica mongolitimonae* has been identified in one *Rhipicephalus pusillus* tick collected on a dead Egyptian mongoose (101).

RICKETTSIA SLOVACA (TICK-BORNE LYMPHADENOPATHY AND *DERMACENTOR*-BORNE-NECROSIS-ERYTHEMA-LYMPHADENOPATHY)

A novel SFG rickettsia was isolated in 1968 from *D. marginatus* ticks collected in Slovakia (104). Based on serological studies and C + G content, two strains were found to be close but not identical to *R. sibirica* and *R. conorii* (105). Another serologically similar strain was isolated in the former U.S.S.R., present-day Armenia, in 1974 (106). Thorough studies revealed that these strains differed from all prototype strains known by that time and a new species of SFG rickettsia, *R. slovaca*, have been proposed (107). Subsequently, it has been detected or isolated from ticks in many European countries where *D. marginatus* and *D. reticulatus* have been studied for rickettsiae, including France, Switzerland, Slovakia, Russia, Ukraine, Armenia, Yugoslavia, Spain, and Portugal (Figs. 11 and 12) (108,109). Infection prevalence in ticks varies from 1% to 17% (109). These tick species are generally common throughout Europe and central Asia, but *D. marginatus* is not prevalent in northern Europe. They are active during early spring, autumn, and winter in southern Europe. Adult ticks inhabit forests and pastures and frequently bite people entering these biotopes, particularly on the scalp. These ticks may act as vectors but also as reservoirs of *R. slovaca*, which is maintained in ticks through trans-stadial and transovarial transmission (104). Eastern limits of *R. slovaca* distribution should be extended to the Ural Mountains. Anopol isolate from this area was indeed recently identified as *R. slovaca* (46).

R. slovaca is an example of a human disease–causing rickettsia that has been being considered a "nonpathogenic rickettsia" for more than 20 years following its

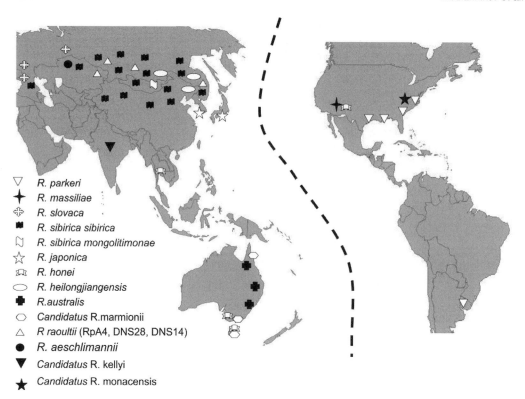

FIGURE 12 Distribution of *Rickettsia* spp. in Asia, Australia, and North and South Americas recognized (by 2006) as human pathogens, except *R. rickettsii* and *R. africae* (see corresponding chapters for these two rickettsiae).

discovery. However, in 1997, the first documented case of human infection with *R. slovaca* was reported in a woman who presented with a single eschar of the scalp and enlarged cervical lymph nodes following the bite of a *Dermacentor* sp. tick in France (Fig. 10). This case was documented by seroconversion and molecular detection of *R. slovaca* in the eschar's biopsy, and by isolation of the bacterium from the tick (110). Clinically similar but undocumented cases had been seen previously in France, Slovakia, and Hungary, where this clinical syndrome had been named TIBOLA (111).

The number of *R. slovaca* infections in Europe is still, probably, under-evaluated. From January 1996 to April 2000, its role in this syndrome was evaluated in 67 patients from France and Hungary presenting with TIBOLA (112). A total of 17 cases of *R. slovaca* infection were confirmed in this cohort by molecular methods. Recently, 14 patients were reported from southern France. It has been suggested that *R. slovaca* may be responsible for as much as 25% of SFG rickettsioses in this region (113). Infections were most likely to occur in children and in patients bitten by a tick during the colder months of the year. Fever and rash were uncommon and sequelae included localized alopecia at the bite site and chronic fatigue. Similar cases have also recently been reported in Bulgaria (114) and Spain (115). Finally, the isolation of *R. slovaca* from a patient has been recently reported, providing definitive evidence that *R. slovaca* is a human pathogen (116).

The clinical syndrome called *Dermacentor*-borne-necrosis-erythema-lymphadenopathy (DEBONEL) has been recently reported in Spain (115). In half of the cases, patients were bitten by *D. marginatus*, which contributed to the name of the syndrome. Most cases occurred between October and April, with a peak in November. The incubation period was approximately four days (range one to eight days). All patients had an eschar at the tick-bite site (86% on the scalp) associated with regional painful lymphadenopathy, and all but one complained of headache. Low-grade fever was reported in 45% of patients. After antibiotic treatment—doxycycline, except for a child who received josamycin—all patients recovered but the eschar resulted in alopecia lasting for several months for several patients. In this series, the infection was not definitely confirmed to be due to *R. slovaca*. A weak and late serological response against this rickettsia was observed in 25% of the cases analyzed. Another study from Spain showed that 16.9% of *Dermacentor*-bitten patients develop seroconversion when tested with *R. slovaca* antigen (117). All available ticks collected from patients in this study were positive for *R. slovaca*.

It is also interesting to note that in addition to *R. slovaca*, another presumably pathogenic rickettsia belonging to *R. massiliae* genogroup, *R. raoultii*, has been detected in *D. marginatus* ticks in Spain (115,118), as previously in other European countries. As *R. slovaca* seems to be involved in most cases, but not all of DEBONEL or TIBOLA, one should pay attention to other rickettsiae associated with *Dermacentor* ticks (see "*R. raoultii*").

RICKETTSIA AESCHLIMANNII

R. aeschlimannii was first isolated from *H. marginatum marginatum* ticks in Morocco in 1992 and then characterized as a new SFG rickettsia in 1997 (119). It was named after Aeschlimann, a Swiss zoologist. However, genotypical identification of similar organisms preceded its isolation, and it had previously been detected in *H. m. rufipes* in Zimbabwe and in *H. m. marginatum* in Portugal (120). It must be mentioned here that since 1950 a number of rickettsia-like organisms were observed in *Hyalomma* spp. ticks from the regions where the isolates were later recovered. Without species identification, they were considered to be *R. conorii* or similar organisms (119).

R. aeschlimannii was also later detected in *H. m. rufipes* in Niger and Mali (99). In Europe, it has been recently identified in *H. m. marginatum* in Croatia (121), from six tick species in Spain, including *H. m. marginatum* (122), and from *H. m. marginatum* in Cephalonia, the largest Ionian island of Greece (123). This rickettsia was recently isolated from *H. m. marginatum* collected on various mammals, and from *H. m. rufipes* collected on migratory birds coming from Africa and collected on Corsica (124). Latter work shows that *R. aeschlimannii* is transstadially and transovarially transmitted in ticks, indicating that *Hyalomma* may be not only vectors, but also reservoirs of *R. aeschlimannii*. Consequently, the geographic distribution of *R. aeschlimannii* in Europe would be, at least, that of *H. m. marginatum* throughout southern Europe (114). Rickettsia genotypically very close to *R. aeschlimannii* have been found in *H. punctata* in Kazakhstan (Figs. 11 and 12) (45).

The first human infection caused by *R. aeschlimannii* was reported in 2002 in a patient returning from Morocco to France. This patient presented with typical clinical signs of spotted fever: an inoculation eschar on his ankle, high fever, and a generalized maculopapular rash. MIF and Western blot assays showed that the patient's serum reacted more intensively with *R. aeschlimannii* antigens than with antigens of the other tested SFG rickettsiae. The definitive diagnosis was obtained using PCR amplification of rickettsial DNA in the patient's early serum. Sequencing of an amplified fragment showed 100% homology to the *omp*A gene of *R. aeschlimannii* (125). Another case was reported in a patient returning from a hunting and fishing trip in South Africa. An *R. appendiculatus* tick was attached to his thigh, and an eschar at the attachment site was noticed (126). He removed the tick and self-prescribed doxycycline. No further symptoms developed. A skin biopsy was, however, taken from the eschar. Molecular studies of both biopsy and tick allowed to amplify *omp*A fragments sharing >99% similarity with the *omp*A of *R. aeschlimannii*.

Hyalomma spp. ticks are actively questing and likely bite humans in Europe. Interestingly, 11 of 144 cases of spotted fever rickettsioses recently reported in Spain presented with multiple eschars (127). This feature is not typical for *R. conorii* infection, because *Rh. sanguineus*, the vector of Mediterranean spotted fever, has a low affinity to biting people and the possibility of being bitten simultaneously by several infected ticks is likely to be low (128); although very characteristically for *Hyalomma* spp. Another study shows that 3 of 170 (1.8%) *H. m. marginatum* ticks collected in Spain harbored *R. aeschlimannii* (129). Furthermore, infection rates of *H. marginatum* may be high, such as reported in Croatia (64.7%) (121).

Another important issue is in vitro proved and molecularly well-founded resistance of *R. aeschlimannii* to rifampin (29). It might present a problem of treatment because clinical or routine serological studies do not permit differentiation among multiple agents causing spotted fever rickettsioses. Moreover, therapeutic failures with rifampin administration to children with Rocky Mountain spotted fever (RMSF) have been reported in Catalonia, Spain, although *R. conorii*, the agent of RMSF, is always susceptible to rifampin (29,130). We suppose that among patients, especially those presenting with multiple eschars in southern Europe, there might be some yet unnoticed infections of *R. aeschlimannii*. Therefore, proper identification of the causal rickettsial species might be crucial to appropriate treatment.

ROCKETTSIA PARKERI

In 1939, Parker reported the isolation of the so-called "maculatum agent" from Gulf Coast ticks (*A. maculatum*) collected from cows in south Texas (131). Studies on guinea pigs showed that this bacteria causes mild febrile disease resembling spotted fever rickettsiosis. Subsequent studies characterized this bacterium as a distinct SFG rickettsia and it was named *R. parkeri* (132). It was characterized as a nonpathogenic species and received relatively little attention for the remainder of the twentieth century, although multiple speculations regarding pathogenicity of *R. parkeri* for humans followed its discovery. In 2004, Paddock et al. (133) reported the first recognized case of the infection with *R. parkeri* in a human 65 years after its initial isolation from ticks. A 40-year-old man living in suburban area in southeast Virginia presented with fever, headache, diffuse myalgias and arthralgias, and multiple eschars on his lower extremities. He recalled no arthropod bite, although he had regular contact with several household dogs and cats; he also observed multiple rodents in surrounding territories and had not traveled outside his country. Four days later, the patient noted small erythematous papules on his legs and an erythematous maculopapular rash on the trunk that spread to his extremities, including his palms and soles. The patient was initially diagnosed with infected arthropod bite and treated unsuccessfully with penicillin and cephalosporin. After routine tests, the patient was diagnosed with rickettsialpox and successfully treated with doxycycline. The rickettsia isolated from eschar biopsy on Vero cell-line bacteria was surprisingly found to be *R. parkeri* (133).

A remarkable clinical feature was the occurrence of multiple inoculation eschars, which has also been described for several other tick-borne rickettsioses, including African tick-bite fever, STT, and the rickettsiosis caused by *R. sibirica mongolitimonae* (128), but is generally an unusual clinical feature of most SFG rickettsial infections. Indeed, eschars are seldom described for patients with RMSF and it has been suggested that rare observations of eschars in patients with RMSF (134,135) could be caused by infection with *R. parkeri* rather than *R. rickettsii* (133). A 1994 report describing PCR–restriction-fragment-length polymorphism profiles of several SFG rickettsial stains isolated from patients presumably infected with *R. rickettsii* noted close similarity of one profile with that of *R. parkeri* (136). More recently, an analysis of several Western blot profiles of serum samples from patients presumed to be infected with *R. rickettsii* revealed reactivity with a 120-kDa protein of *R. parkeri*, in a pattern compatible with the profile observed from the index patient with *R. parkeri* infection (137). Collectively, these findings suggest that other likely cases of *R. parkeri* rickettsiosis were previously diagnosed as RMSF (133).

A. maculatum ticks are distributed throughout several southeastern states that border the Gulf and southern Atlantic coasts of the United States. *R. parkeri* has been identified in Gulf Coast ticks collected throughout its range (Fig. 12). Rarely, *R. parkeri* has also been detected in the lone star tick (*A. americanum*), and a study suggests that this rickettsia may be transovarially and trans-stadially transmitted in this widely distributed tick (138). Some data suggest that this tick may transmit *R. parkeri* to guinea pigs. Preliminary studies also suggest that *A. cajennense* will support the growth and survival of *R. parkeri* (139). Recent investigation has demonstrated DNA of *R. parkeri* in *A. triste* (formerly *A. maculatum*) ticks collected from humans and animals in Uruguay (140). An isolate was also recently obtained from *A. triste* in this country (141). These findings, coupled with other reports of eschar-associated spotted fever rickettsioses in patients following bites of *A. triste* in Uruguay (142,143), suggests that *R. parkeri* rickettsiosis also occurs in areas of South America. In Uruguay, it is likely that rickettsiosis caused by *R. parkeri* have been diagnosed as infection with *R. conorii* based on nonspecific serologic tests

(143). So, the occurrence and distribution of *R. parkeri* rickettsiosis could be greater than currently appreciated by the distribution of *A. maculatum*, if all these tick species are also involved in the transmission of this pathogen.

RICKETTSIA MASSILIAE

In 1992, a rickettsial agent was isolated from *Rh. sanguineus* ticks collected near Marseille. It was characterized as a distinct species within the SFG group of rickettsiae, and named *R. massiliae* (144,145). In Europe, this rickettsia has also been detected by molecular methods, in *Rh. sanguineus* in Greece (146) and *Rh. turanicus* in Portugal (147). It has also been found in *Rh. muhsamae*, *Rh. lunulatus*, and *Rh. sulcatus* in the Central African Republic (149), and in *Rh. muhsamae* collected on cattle in Mali. In 1996, a variant strain of *R. massiliae* (Bar29) was isolated in *Rh. sanguineus* tick from Catalonia (149) and identified in ticks removed from humans in Castilla, Spain (150). It has also been identified in *Rh. turanicus* parasitizing wild birds in Portugal (151). Thereafter, this species was detected in Switzerland (Fig. 11) (152). North America is the third continent where *R. massiliae* seems to be distributed. Recently, the isolate close to Bar29 was recovered from *Rh. sanguineus* ticks collected in Arizona (Fig. 12) (153). We demonstrated trans-stadial and transovarial transmission of *R. massiliae* in ticks of the *R. sanguineus* group molecularly identified as *Rh. turanicus*, which may also be considered as reservoirs (154).

R. massiliae exhibits a natural resistance to rifampin in cell cultures (29). As we have already mentioned above, the data of therapeutic failures with rifampin for the treatment of MSF in Catalonian children (130) may have an explanation in non-*R. conorii* origin of spotted fever rickettsiosis. *R. massiliae*, by the same way as *R. aeschlimannii*, may be an agent in such cases. *R. massiliae* strain has been detected in tick saliva, suggesting that the bacteria could be transmitted through the tick bite. In 2003, eight sera of 15 MSF patients in Catalonia, Spain, reacted at high titers with only *R. conorii* and *R. massiliae* Bar29 antigens, and the titers against latter rickettsia were clearly higher than that for *R. conorii* (155).

The first documented infection with *R. massiliae* in a human occurred in 2005, 20 years after the isolation of rickettsia from the patient. A spotted fever rickettsia, presumed to be *R. conorii*, was recovered in 1985 from the blood of a 45-year-old man hospitalized in Palermo, Italy, with fever, a necrotic eschar, a maculopapular rash involving palms and soles, and mild hepatomegaly. Treatment with a cephalosporin antibiotic failed, but he recovered completely after receiving a tetracycline antibiotic. His antibody titer to *R. conorii* antigens rose from 0 to 1:80 by MIF, and the patient was considered to have Mediterranean spotted fever caused by *R. conorii*. The rickettsial isolate was stored for two decades before being identified as *R. massiliae* by sequencing of portions of the *ompA* and *gltA* rickettsial genes at the Unité des Rickettsies in Marseilles (157).

RICKETTSIA RAOULTII

This is another example of rickettsia being known for a long time as a novel genotype identified in *Ixodid* ticks collected in Russia using amplification and sequencing of the *rrs* (16S rDNA), *gltA*, and *ompA* genes (157). *Rickettsia* sp. provisionally called "genotype DnS14" was initially detected from *D. nutallii* ticks collected in Siberia, whereas "genotype RpA4" was detected from *R. pumilio* ticks from the Astrakhan region. Due to their phylogenetic homogeneity, it was suggested that *Rickettsia* sp. genotypes DnS14 and RpA4 belonged to a same new species (42,157). Several years later, the isolates of this rickettsia was obtained using cell culture from *D. silvarum* ticks collected in Far-Eastern Russia and Siberia (strains identical to DnS14), and *D. reticulatus* and *D. marginatus* ticks from France and Russia (strains identical to RpA4). Genotypes identical to these isolates were also detected in *R. pumilio*, *D. reticulatus*, *D. silvarum*, *D. niveus*, *D. nuttalii*, and *D. marginatus* ticks from Central and Eastern Siberia, the European part of Russia, Kazakhstan (45,158), Spain (159), and Croatia (D. Raoult, unpublished data). Not-yet-isolated genotype DnS28 belongs evidently to the same species (157). The pathogenicity of this species has been suggested by the amplification of its DNA from the blood of patients with a clinical picture of *R. slovaca*-like infection (159,160).

A recent study demonstrated that *Dermacentor* ticks naturally infected with genotypes DnS14, DnS28, or RpA4 harbored these rickettsiae lifelong, and that transovarial and trans-stadial transmission occurred (161). Using multigene sequencing, by comparison with *R. massiliae*, the species phylogenetically validated as the closest species, this isolate was classified within a putative new spotted-fever rickettsia species. It was named after Didier Raoult (160). It also exhibited a specific multi-spacer typing genotype and a specific serotype but had the *rpoB* gene mutation conferring rifampin-resistant characteristic for *R. massiliae* group rickettsiae (160).

CANDIDATUS RICKETTSIA MARMIONII

During 2003–2005, six patients from Australian states of Queensland (four cases), Tasmania, and South Australia were diagnosed with an SFG rickettsiosis characterized by fever (all patients), headache (83%), arthralgia (50%), cough (50%), maculopapular rash (33%), and pharyngitis (33%) (Fig. 12). An eschar was reported in only one patient. Genetic analysis of an isolate obtained from a patient showed close similarity to, but distinction from, *R. honei*, with 99.0%, 99.7%, and 99.6% homology of the 17-kDa antigen, gltA, and 16S rRNA genes, respectively. Investigators have proposed the name "*R. marmionii*" to describe this rickettsia and "Australian spotted fever" to describe the rickettsiosis it causes. The definitive status of *R. marmionii* as a distinct species or as a subspecies of *R. honei* remains to be determined. Potential vectors include *H. novaeguineae* and *I. holocyclus* (162).

CANDIDATUS RICKETTSIA KELLYI

A group of scientists recently reported the first laboratory-confirmed human infection due to a new rickettsial genotype in India, "*Candidatus Rickettsia kellyi*," in a one-year-old boy with fever and maculopapular rash (Fig. 12) (163). The diagnosis was made by serologic testing, PCR detection, and immunohistochemical testing of the organism from a skin biopsy specimen. To date, the strain has not yet been isolated from either a patient or from any arthropod vector. The described case is the first and the only case of infection due to this new rickettsia species and further investigations are required for the clarification of its role in human pathology.

CANDIDATUS RICKETTSIA MONACENSIS

A rickettsia that has been published under the provisory name *R. monacensis* was first isolated from *I. ricinus* ticks collected in 1998 in a city park in Munich, Germany (164). No isolate is available in any of two official collections. The name *R. monacensis* has not been validly published and *Candidatus* status is appropriate (165). More recently, it was identified in *I. ricinus* in Hungary (166). *R. monacensis* can be cultivated in mammalian (L929, Vero) and tick (ISE6, DAE100, IRE11) and shows cytopathogenic effect in several cell lines. Hamsters appear refractory to infection with *R. monacensis* (164). Phylogenetically, it is closely related to rickettsiae previously detected in *I. ricinus*, including "the Cadiz agent" in Spain (167), IRS3 and IRS4 in Slovakia and Bulgaria (168,169), and *I. scapularis* ticks from New York, in the United States. (170). Transposon-based transformation vectors with fluorescent proteins as reporter genes have been developed for this species (171). *R. monacensis* was shown to be significantly less susceptible than typical extracellular bacteria to antimicrobial peptides including cecropin A, ceratotoxin A, and lysozyme (172). Recently, the first cases of human infection due to *R. monacensis* have been reported (173). Authors succeeded in isolation of a strain from an MSF-like patient, and identification of rickettsial DNA in blood of two acute patients. Recently, two human cases of infection due to *R. monacensis* have been documented in Spain. The first case was an 84-year-old man from La Rioja, who consulted for fever and a maculopapular rash, without any inoculation eschar. The second case was a 59-year-old woman from Basque country. She presented with a history of tick bite, fever, and a rash at the tick-bite site. Both cases were documented by culture of rickettsiae from blood (J.A. Otéo, personal communication).

CONCLUSION

It must be noted again that many of the rickettsias presented in this chapter were first identified in ticks several years or even decades before a conclusive association with human disease was demonstrated, up to 60 years after their identification in ticks. Many other rickettsias that have been detected in ticks only satisfy the first component necessary as a potential tick-borne pathogen, i.e., they have been detected in ticks with a natural proclivity to bite humans. Some of them might be reconsidered as human pathogens in years to come (Chapter 12).

REFERENCES

1. Mill EI. Tick-borne fever in Maritime Region [in Russian]. Far Eastern Med J 1936; 3:34–36.
2. Antonov NI, Naishtat AG. Far-Eastern tick-borne typhus [in Russian]. Meditsinskaya Parazitologia i Parazitarnye Bolezni 1937; 6:73–81.
3. Shmatikov MD, Velik MA. Tick-borne spotted fever [in Russian]. Klin Med (Mosk) 1939; 7:124–128.
4. Krontovskaya MK, Savitskaya EP. Tick-borne typhus in the east of USSR [in Russian]. Sov Med 1946; 12:15–16.
5. Savitskaya EP. To the etiology of tick typus in Khabarovsk region [in Russian]. Zh Mikrobiol Epidemiol Immunobiol 1943; 87:10–11.
6. Lyskovtsev MM. Tickborne rickettsiosis. Misc Publ Entomol Soc Am 1968; 42–140.
7. Alfeev NI, Kulagin SM. Studies on ticks *Dermacentor marginatus* and *Dermacentor pictus* as vectors of tick-borne rickettsiosis [in Russian]. In: Pavlovsky EN, ed. Voprosy Kraevoy, Obschey i Experimentalnoy Parazitologii i Meditsinskoy Zoologii. Moscow: Medgiz, 1953:41–48.
8. Korshunova OS. Etiology of tick-borne typhus in Krasnoyarsk region [in Russian]. Zh Mikrobiol Epidemiol Immunobiol 1943; 1–2:59–64.
9. Korshunova OS. About etiology of Far Eastern tick-borne typhus. Part I [in Russian]. Zh Mikrobiol Epidemiol Immunobiol 1943; 1–2:51–55.
10. Zdrodovskii PF, Golinevich EM. The Rickettsial Diseases. English edn. London: Pergamon Press, 1960.
11. Kireeva RIA. Clinical characteristic of North Asian tick-borne typhus [in Russian]. Zh Mikrobiol Epidemiol Immunobiol 1956; 9:73–76.
12. Mediannikov OY, Sidelnikov Y, Ivanov L, et al. Acute tick-borne Rickettsiosis caused by *Rickettsia heilongjiangensis* in Russian Far East. Emerg Infect Dis 2004; 10:810–817.
13. Rehacek J, Tarasevich IV. Acari-Borne Rickettsiae and Rickettsioses in Eurasia. Veda, Bratislava: Publishing House of the Slovak Academy of Sciences, 1988.
14. Rudakov NV, Samoilenko IE, Yakimenko VV, et al. The re-emergence of Siberian tick typhus: field and experimental observations. In: Raoult D, Brouqui P, eds. Rickettsiae and Rickettsial Diseases at the Turn of the Third Millennium. Paris: Elsevier, 1999:269–273.
15. Lyskovtsev MM. Tick-borne Rickettsiosis [in Russian]. Moscow: Medgiz, 1963.
16. Fan MY, Zhao SX, Zhang WH, et al. A serosurvey for typhus, North Asian tick-borne spotted fever, rickettsialpox and Q fever in Abagnar Qi (county), Inner Mongolia [in Chinese]. Chin J Hyg 1964; 9:46–48.
17. Kulagin SM. Tick-borne Typhus in Altay Territory [in Russian]. Publications of Gamaleya Institute of Epidemiology and Microbiology, 1953.
18. Zhmaeva ZM, Pchelkina AA, Bedryev AB. *Ixodid* ticks—reservoirs and vectors of mixed infections. Med Parazitol (Mosk) 1969; 38:405–410.
19. Zhmaeva ZM, Korshunova OS. Preservation of the virus of Far Eastern spotted typhus fever in tick *Haemaphysalis concinna* [in Russian]. In: Pavlovsky EN, ed. Voprosy Kraevoy, Obschey i Experimentalnoy Parasitologii. Moscow: Medgiz, 1948:37–38.
20. Pavlovsky EN. Natural nidality and idea of landscape epidemiology of transmissive diseases of human. Meditsinskaya Parazitologia i Parazitarnye Bolezni 1944; 6:29–38.
21. Balashov YS, Daiter AB. Blood-feeding arthropods and rickettsiae [in Russian]. Leningrad: Nauka, 1973.
22. Balayeva NM, Eremeeva ME, Ignatovich VF, et al. Biological and genetic characterization of *Rickettsia sibirica* strains isolated in the endemic area of the North Asian tick typhus. Am J Trop Med Hyg 1996; 55:685–692.
23. Shpynov SN, Fournier PE, Rudakov NV, et al. Book of abstracts of 4th International Conference on Rickettsiae and Rickettsial Diseases, Logrono, Spain, June 18–21, 2005. Logrono, Spain: Trama Impressores S.A.L., 2005:179.
24. Samoilenko IE, Rudakov NV, Yakimenko VV, et al. Results of experimental studies of *Rickettsia sibirica* interactions with tick vectors [in Russian]. In: Rudakov NV, ed. Human Infections in Natural Foci. Omsk: Omsk Research Institute of Natural Foci Infections Publishing House, 1996:204–208.
25. Somov GP. Studies of rodents as reservoirs of North Asian tick-borne rickettsiosis [in Russian]. Zh Mikrobiol Epidemiol Immunobiol 1965; 4:6–11.

26. Davydovsky IV. Pathohistology of skin lesions in tick-borne typhus [in Russian]. Archiv Patologicheskoy Anatomii i Patologicheskoy Physiologii 1940; 6:12–24.
27. Mediannikov OY, Sidel'nikov I. The onset of chronic Lyme-borreliosis after the cure of tick-borne rickettsia infection in simultaneous infection [in Russian]. Klin Med (Mosk) 2002; 80:64–66.
28. Raoult D, Roux V. Rickettsioses as paradigms of new or emerging infectious diseases. Clin Microbiol Rev 1997; 10:694–719.
29. Rolain JM, Maurin M, Vestris G, Raoult D. In vitro susceptibilities of 27 rickettsiae to 13 antimicrobials. Antimicrob Agents Chemother 1998; 42:1537–1541.
30. Loban KM, Tarasevich IV. Rickettsioses [in Russian]. In: Pokrovsky VI, ed. Handbook of Zoonoses. Leningrad: Meditsina, 1983:94–125.
31. Baydin MN. Endemical Nidus of Tick-borne Typhus in Mongolian People's Republic [in Russian]. Publications of Gamaleya Institute of Epidemiology and Microbiology, 1943.
32. Lewin MR, Bouyer DH, Walker DH, et al. *Rickettsia sibirica* infection in members of scientific expeditions to northern Asia. Lancet 2003; 362:1201–1202.
33. Rolain JM, Shpynov S, Raoult D. Spotted-fever-group rickettsioses in north Asia. Lancet 2003; 362:1939.
34. Fan MY, Zhang JZ, Chen M, et al. Spotted fever group rickettsioses in China. In: Raoult D, Brouqui P, eds. Rickettsiae and Rickettsial Diseases at the Turn of the Third Millennium. Paris: Elsevier, 1999:247–257.
35. Ai CX, Chen GC, Zhang YF, et al. Investigation of natural foci of spotted fever group rickettsiae in Jinghe County, Xingjiang [in Chinese]. Chin J Epidemiol 1979; 3:230.
36. Ai CX. Survey of natural infection of ticks with *Rickettsia* of the spotted fever group in the northwestern section of Xinjiang Province [in Chinese]. Chung Hua Liu Hsing Ping Hsueh Tsa Chih 1983; 4:103–104.
37. Fan MY, Walker DH, Liu QH, et al. Rickettsial and serologic evidence for prevalent spotted fever rickettsiosis in Inner Mongolia. Am J Trop Med Hyg 1987; 36:615–620.
38. Chen M, Fan MY, Bi DZ, et al. Detection of *Rickettsia sibirica* in ticks and small mammals collected in three different regions of China. Acta Virol 1998; 42:61–64.
39. Robertson RG, Wiseman CL Jr, Traub R. Tick-borne rickettsiae of the spotted fever group in west Pakistan. I. Isolation of strains from ticks in different habitats. Am J Epidemiol 1970; 92:382–394.
40. Robertson RG, Wisseman CL Jr. Tick-borne rickettsiae of the spotted fever group in west Pakistan. II. Serological classification of isolates from west Pakistan and Thailand: evidence for two new species. Am J Epidemiol 1973; 97:55–64.
41. Zhang JZ, Fan MY, Wu YM, et al. Genetic classification of *Rickettsia heilongjiangii* and *Rickettsia hulinii*, two Chinese spotted fever group rickettsiae. J Clin Microbiol 2000; 38:3498–3501.
42. Fournier PE, Dumler JS, Greub G, et al. Gene sequence-based criteria for identification of new rickettsia isolates and description of *Rickettsia heilongjiangensis* sp. nov. J Clin Microbiol 2003; 41:5456–5465.
43. Lou D, Wu YM, Wang B, et al. Confirmation of patients with tick-borne spotted fever caused by *Rickettsia heilongjiangi* [in Chinese]. Chin J Epidemiol 1989; 10:128–132.
44. Mediannikov OY, Sidelnikov YN, Ivanov LI, et al. Book of abstracts of 4th International Conference on Rickettsiae and Rickettsial Diseases, Logrono, Spain, June 18–21, 2005. Logrono, Spain: Trama Impressores S.A.L., 2005:O-52.
45. Shpynov SN, Fournier PE, Rudakov NV, et al. Detection of a rickettsia closely related to *Rickettsia aeschlimannii*, "*Rickettsia heilongjiangensis*," *Rickettsia* sp. strain RpA4, and *Ehrlichia muris* in ticks collected in Russia and Kazakhstan. J Clin Microbiol 2004; 42:2221–2223.
46. Shpynov SN, Fournier PE, Rudakov NV, Samoilenko IE, Reshetnikova TA, Yastrebov VK, Schaiman MS, Tarasevich IV, Raoult D. Molecular identification of a collection of spotted fever group rickettsiae obtained from patients and ticks from Russia. Am J Trop Med Hyg 2006; 74(3):440–443.
47. Andrew R, Bonnin JM, Williams S. Tick typhus in North Queensland. Med J Aust 1946; II:253.
48. Plotz H, Smadel JE, Bennet BI. North Queensland tick typhus: studies of the aetiological agent and its relation to other rickettsial diseases. Med J Aust 1946; 263–268.
49. Philip CB. Miscellaneous human rickettsioses. In: Pullen RL, ed. Communicable Diseases. Philadelphia: Lea & Febiger, 1950:781–788.
50. Sexton DJ, Banks J, Graves S, et al. Prevalence of antibodies to spotted fever group rickettsiae in dogs from southeastern Australia. Am J Trop Med Hyg 1991; 45:243–248.
51. Sexton DJ, Dwyer BW, Kemp R, et al. Spotted fever group rickettsial infections in Australia. Rev Infect Dis 1991; 13:876–886.
52. Graves S, Stenos J. Rickettsioses in Australia. In: Raoult D, Brouqui P, eds. Rickettsiae and Rickettsial Diseases at the Turn of the Third Millennium. Paris: Elsevier, 2003:244–246.
53. Dwyer BW, Graves SR, McDonald MI, et al. Spotted fever in East Gippsland, Victoria: a previously unrecognized focus of rickettsial infection. Med J Aust 1991; 154:121–125.
54. Stewart RS. Flinders Island spotted fever: a newly recognized endemic focus of tick typhus in Bass Strait. Part 1. Clinical and epidemiological features. Med J Australia 1991, 154, 94–99.

55. Pope JH. The isolation or rickettsia resembling *Rickettsia australis* in South-East Queensland. Med J Aust 1955; 1:763.
56. Campbell RW, Domrow R. Rickettsioses in Australia: isolation of *Rickettsia tsutsugamushi* and *R. australis* from naturally infected arthropods. Trans R Soc Trop Med Hyg 1974; 68:397–402.
57. Roberts FHS. A systematic study of the Australian species of the genus *Ixodes* (Acarinae: Ixodidae). Aust J Zool 1960; 8:392–485.
58. Graves SR, Stewart L, Stenos J, et al. Spotted fever group rickettsial infection in South-Eastern Australia: isolation of rickettsiae. Comp Immun Microbiol Infect Dis 1993; 16:223–233.
59. Cook I, Campbell RW. Rickettsiosis—North Queensland tick typhus. Rep Qld Inst Med Res 1965; 20:4.
60. Sexton DJ, King G, Dwyer BW. Fatal Queensland tick typhus [letter]. J Infect Dis 1990; 162:779–780.
61. Watt G, Parola P. Scrub typhus and tropical rickettsioses. Curr Opin Infect Dis 2003; 16:429–436.
62. Mahara F. Three Weil–Felix reaction OX2 positive cases with skin eruptions and high fever. J Anan Med Assoc 1984; 68:4–7.
63. Mahara F, Koga K, Sawada S, et al. The first report of the rickettsial infections of spotted fever group in Japan: three clinical cases. Jpn J Assoc Infect Dis 1985; 59:1165–1172.
64. Uchida T, Tashiro F, Funato T, et al. Immunofluorescence test with *Rickettsia montana* for serologic diagnosis of rickettsial infection of the spotted fever group in Shikoku, Japan. Microbiol Immunol 1986; 30:1061–1066.
65. Uchida T, Tashiro F, Funato T, et al. Isolation of a spotted fever group Rickettsia from a patient with febrile exanthematous illness in Shikoku, Japan. Microbiol Immunol 1986; 30:1323–1326.
66. Uchida T, Uchiyama T, Koyama AH. Isolation of spotted fever group rickettsiae from humans in Japan [letter]. J Infect Dis 1988; 158:664–665.
67. Uchida T, Yu XJ, Uchiyama T, et al. Identification of a unique spotted fever group rickettsia from humans in Japan. J Infect Dis 1989; 159:1122–1126.
68. Uchida T, Uchiyama T, Kumano K, et al. *Rickettsia japonica* sp. nov., the etiological agent of spotted fever group rickettsiosis in Japan. Int J Syst Bacteriol 1992; 42:303–305.
69. Uchida T. *Rickettsia japonica*, the etiologic agent of oriental spotted fever. Microbiol Immunol 1993; 37:91–102.
70. Mahara F. Japanese spotted fever: report of 31 cases and review of the literature. Emerg Infect Dis 1997; 3:105–111.
71. Mahara F. Rickettsioses in Japan. In: Raoult D, Brouqui P, eds. Rickettsiae and Rickettsial Diseases at the Turn of the Third Millennium. Paris: Elsevier, 1999:233–239.
72. Kodama K, Senba T, Yamauchi H, et al. Japanese spotted fever associated with multiorgan failure. J Infect Chemother 2001; 7:247–250.
73. Kodama K, Senba T, Yamauchi H, et al. A patient with Japanese spotted fever complicated by meningoencephalitis. Kansenshogaku Zasshi 2001; 75:812–814.
74. Kodama K, Senba T, Yamauchi H, et al. Clinical study of Japanese spotted fever and its aggravating factors. J Infect Chemother 2003; 8:83–87.
75. Araki M, Takatsuka K, Kawamura J, et al. Japanese spotted fever involving the central nervous system: two case reports and a literature review. J Clin Microbiol 2002; 40:3874–3876.
76. Kodama K, Senba T, Yamauchi H, et al. Japanese spotted fever definitively diagnosed by the polymerase chain reaction method. J Infect Chemother 2002; 8:266–268.
77. Fournier PE, Fujita H, Takada N, et al. Genetic identification of rickettsiae isolated from ticks in Japan. J Clin Microbiol 2002; 40:2176–2181.
78. Katayama T, Furuya Y, Yoshida Y, et al. Spotted fever group rickettsiosis and vectors in Kamagawa prefecture. Kansenshogaku Zasshi 1996; 70:561–568.
79. Chung M-H, Lee S-H, Kim M-J, Lee J-H, Kim E-S, Lee J-S, Kim M-K, Park M-Y, Kang J-S. Japanese spotted fever. South Korea Emerg Infect Dis 2006; 12(7).
80. Lee JH, Park H, Jung KD, Jang WJ, Koh ES, Kang SS, et al. Identification of the spotted fever group rickettsiae detected from *Haemaphysalis longicornis* in Korea. Microbiol Immunol 2003; 47:301–304.
81. Graves SR, Dwyer BW, McColl D, et al. Flinders island spotted fever: a newly recognised endemic focus of tick typhus in Bass Strait. Part 2. Serological investigations. Med J Aust 1991; 154:99–104.
82. Baird RW, Lloyd M, Stenos J, et al. Characterization and comparison of Australian human spotted fever group rickettsiae. J Clin Microbiol 1992; 30:2896–2902.
83. Baird RW, Stenos J, Stewart R, et al. Genetic variation in Australian spotted fever group rickettsiae. J Clin Microbiol 1996; 34:1526–1530.
84. Stenos J, Roux V, Walker DH, et al. *Rickettsia honei* sp. nov., the aetiological agent of Flinders Island spotted fever in Australia. Int J Syst Bacteriol 1998; 48:1399–1404.
85. Graves S, Stenos J. *Rickettsia honei*—a spotted fever group rickettsia on three continents. Rickettsiology: Present and Future Directions 2003; 990:62–66.
86. Whitworth T, Popov V, Han V, et al. Ultrastructural and genetic evidence of a reptilian tick, *Aponomma hydrosauri*, as a host of *Rickettsia honei* in Australia—possible transovarial transmission. Rickettsiology: Present and Future Directions 2003; 990:67–74.
87. Stenos J, Graves S, Popov VL, et al. *Aponomma hydrosauri*, the reptile-associated tick reservoir of *Rickettsia honei* on Flinders Island, Australia. Am J Trop Med Hyg 2003; 69:314–317.

88. Roberts FHS. Australian ticks. Melbourne, Australia: Commonwealth Scientific and Industrial Research Organisation, 1970.
89. Chin RH, Jennens ID. Rickettsial spotted fever in Tasmania. Med J Aust 1995; 162:669.
90. Unsworth NB, Stenos J, McGregor AR, Dyer JR, Graves SR. Not only 'Flinders Island' spotted fever. Pathology 2005; 37(3):242–245.
91. Kollars TM, Tippayachai B, Bodhidatta D. Thai tick typhus, *Rickettsia honei*, and a unique rickettsia detected in *Ixodes granulatus* (Ixodidae: Acari). Am J Trop Med Hyg 2001; 65:535–537.
92. Jiang J, Sangkasuwan V, Lerdthusnee K, Sukwit S, Chuenchitra T, Rozmajzl PJ, Eamsila C, Jones JW, Richards AL. Human infection with *Rickettsia honei*, Thailand. Emerg Infect Dis 2005; 11(9):1473–1475.
93. Billings AN, Yu XJ, Teel FD, et al. Detection of a spotted fever group rickettsia in *Ambliomma cajennense* (Acari: Ixodidae) in south Texas. J Med Entomol 1998; 35:474–478.
94. Yu X, Jin Y, Fan MY, et al. Genotypic and antigenic identification of two new strains of spotted fever group rickettsiae isolated from China. J Clin Microbiol 1993; 31:83–88.
95. Raoult D, Brouqui P, Roux V. A new spotted-fever-group rickettsiosis. Lancet 1996; 348:412.
96. Fournier PE, Gouriet F, Brouqui P, et al. Lymphangitis-associated rickettsiosis, a new rickettsiosis caused by *Rickettsia sibirica mongolotimonae*: Seven new cases and review of the literature. Clin Infect Dis 2005; 40:1435–1444.
97. Fournier PE, Zhu Y, Raoult D. Book of abstracts of 4th International Conference on Rickettsiae and Rickettsial Diseases, Logrono, Spain, June 18–21, 2005. Logrono, Spain: Trama Impressores S.A.L., 2005:180.
98. Fournier PE, Tissot-Dupont H, Gallais H, et al. *Rickettsia mongolotimonae*: a rare pathogen in France. Emerg Infect Dis 2000; 6:290–292.
99. Parola P, Inokuma H, Camicas JL, et al. Detection and identification of spotted fever group *Rickettsiae* and *Ehrlichiae* in African ticks. Emerg Infect Dis 2001; 7:1014–1017.
100. Pretorius AM, Jensenius M, Birtles RJ. Update on spotted fever group Rickettsiae in South Africa. Vector Borne Zoonotic Dis 2004; 4:249–260.
101. de Sousa R, Barata C, Vitorino L, Santos-Silva M, Carrapato C, Torgal J, Walker D, Bacellar F. *Rickettsia sibirica* isolation from a patient and detection in ticks. Portugal Emerg Infect Dis 2006; 12(7).
102. Morel PC. Les *Hyalomma* (Acariens: Ixodidae) de France. Ann Parasitol 1959; 34:552–555.
103. Psaroulaki A, Germanakis A, Gikas A, et al. Simultaneous detection of "*Rickettsia mongolotimonae*" in a patient and in a tick in Greece. J Clin Microbiol 2005; 43:3558–3559.
104. Rehacek J. *Rickettsia slovaca*, the organism and its ecology. Acta Sci Nat Brno 1984; 18:1–50.
105. Schramek S. Deoxyribonucleic acid–base composition of rickettsiae belonging to the Rocky Mountain Spotted Fever group isolated in Czechoslovakia. Acta Virol 1974; 18:173–174.
106. Makarova VA. Antigenic structure of spotted fever group rickettsiae isolated in Armenian SSR. Zh Microbiol Epidemiol Immunol 1978; 4:112–116.
107. Urvolgyi J, Brezina R. *Rickettsia slovaca*: a new member of spotted fever group rickettsiae. In: Kazar J, Ormsbee RM, Tarasevich IV, eds. Proceedings of the 2nd International Symposium on Rickettsiae and Rickettsial Diseases, Veda, Bratislava. Veda, Bratislava: Slovak Academy of Science, 1978:299–305.
108. Eremeeva ME, Balayeva NM, Ignatovich VF, Raoult D. Proteinic and genomic identification of spotted fever group rickettsiae isolated in the former USSR. J Clin Microbiol 1993; 31(10):2625–2633.
109. Sekeyova Z, Roux V, Xu W, et al. *Rickettsia slovaca* sp. nov., a member of the spotted fever group rickettsiae. Int J Syst Bacteriol 1998; 48:1455–1462.
110. Raoult D, Berbis P, Roux V, et al. A new tick-transmitted disease due to *Rickettsia slovaca*. Lancet 1997; 350:112–113.
111. Lakos A. Tick-borne lymphadenopathy (TIBOLA)—a new, probably rickettsial infection. Inf Dis Rev 1999; 1:114–116.
112. Raoult D, Lakos A, Fenollar F, et al. Spotless rickettsiosis caused by *Rickettsia slovaca* and associated with *Dermacentor* ticks. Clin Infect Dis 2002; 34:1331–1336.
113. Gouriet F, Rolain J-M, Raoult D. *Rickettsia slovaca* infection, France. Emerg Infect Dis 2006; 12(3):521–523.
114. Komitova R, Lakos A, Aleksandrov A, et al. A case of tick-transmitted lymphadenopathy in Bulgaria associated with *Rickettsia slovaca*. Scand J Infect Dis 2003; 35:213.
115. Oteo JA, Ibarra V, Blanco JR, et al. *Dermacentor*-borne necrosis erythema and lymphadenopathy: clinical and epidemiological features of a new tick-borne disease. Clin Microbiol Infect 2004; 10:327–331.
116. Cazorla C, Enea M, Lucht F, et al. First isolation of *Rickettsia slovaca* from a patient, France. Emerg Infect Dis 2003; 9:135.
117. Lledo L, Gegundez MI, Fernandes N, Sousa R, Vicente J, Alamo R, Fernandez-Soto P, Perez-Sanchez R, Bacellar F. The seroprevalence of human infection with *Rickettsia slovaca*, in an area of northern Spain. Ann Trop Med Parasitol 2006; 100(4):337–343.
118. Marquez FJ, Ibarra V, Oteo JA, et al. Which spotted fever group rickettsia are present in *Dermacentor marginatus* ticks in Spain? Rickettsiology: Present and Future Directions 2003; 990:141–142.

119. Beati L, Meskini M, Thiers B, et al. *Rickettsia aeschlimannii* sp. nov., a new spotted fever group rickettsia associated with *Hyalomma marginatum* ticks. Int J Syst Bacteriol 1997; 47:548–554.
120. Beati L, Kelly PJ, Matthewman LA, et al. Prevalence of *Rickettsia*-like organisms and spotted fever group Rickettsiae in ticks (Acari: Ixodidae) from Zimbabwe. J Med Entomol 1995; 32:787–792.
121. Punda-Polic V, Petrovec M, Trilar T, et al. Detection and identification of spotted fever group rickettsiae in ticks collected in southern Croatia. Exp Appl Acarol 2002; 28:169–176.
122. Fernandez-Soto P, Encinas-Grandes A, Perez-Sanchez R. *Rickettsia aeschlimannii* in Spain: molecular evidence in *Hyalomma marginatum* and five other tick species that feed on humans. Emerg Infect Dis 2003; 9:889–890.
123. Psaroulaki A, Ragiadakou D, Kouris G, et al. Ticks and tick-borne rickettsiae in the Greek island of Cephalonia. Book of Abstracts of 4th International Conference on Rickettsiae and Rickettsial Diseases, Logrono, Spain, June 18–21, 2005. Logrono, Spain: Trama Impressores S.A.L., 2005:208.
124. Matsumoto K, Parola P, Brouqui P, et al. *Rickettsia aeschlimannii* in *Hyalomma* ticks from Corsica. Eur J Clin Microbiol Infect Dis 2004; 23:732–734.
125. Raoult D, Fournier PE, Abboud P, et al. First documented human *Rickettsia aeschlimannii* infection. Emerg Infect Dis 2002; 8:748–749.
126. Pretorius AM, Birtles RJ. *Rickettsia aeschlimannii*: a new pathogenetic spotted fever group Rickettsia, South Africa. Emerg Infect Dis 2002; 8:874.
127. Anton E, Font B, Munoz T, et al. Clinical and laboratory characteristics of 144 patients with Mediterranean spotted fever. Eur J Clin Microbiol Infect Dis 2003; 22:126–128.
128. Parola P, Raoult D. Ticks and tickborne bacterial diseases in humans: an emerging infectious threat. Clin Infect Dis 2001; 32:897–928.
129. Oteo Revuelta JA, Portillo A, Santibanez S, et al. Book of Abstracts of 4th International Conference on Rickettsiae and Rickettsial Diseases, Logrono, Spain, June 18–21, 2005. Logrono, Spain: Trama Impressores S.A.L., 2005:92.
130. Bella F, Espejo-Arenas E, Uriz S, et al. Randomized trial of five-day rifampin versus one-day doxycycline therapy for Mediterranean spotted fever. J Infect Dis 1991; 164:433–434.
131. Parker RR, Kohls GM, Cox GW, et al. Observations on an infectious agent from *Amblyomma maculatum*. Public Health Rep 1939; 54:1482–1484.
132. Lackman DB, Bell EJ, Stoenner HG, et al. The Rocky Mountain spotted fever group rickettsias. Health Lab Sci 1955; 2:135–141.
133. Paddock CD, Sumner JW, Comer JA, et al. *Rickettsia parkeri*: a newly recognized cause of spotted fever rickettsiosis in the United States. Clin Infect Dis 2004; 38:805–811.
134. Cox GM, Sexton DJ. Photo quiz: Rocky Mountain spotted fever. Clin Infect Dis 1995; 21:315, 429.
135. Walker DH, Gay RM, Valdes-Dapena M. The occurrence of eschars in Rocky Mountain spotted fever. J Am Acad Dermatol 1981; 4:571–576.
136. Ralph D, Pretzman C, Daugherty N, et al. Genetic relationships among the members of the family *Rickettsiaceae* as shown by DNA restriction fragment polymorphism analysis. Ann NY Acad Sci 1990; 590:541–552.
137. Raoult D, Paddock CD. *Rickettsia parkeri* infection and other spotted fevers in the United States. N Engl J Med 2005; 353:626–627.
138. Goddard J. Experimental infection of lone star ticks, *Amblyomma americanum* (L.), with *Rickettsia parkeri* and exposure of guinea pigs to the agent. J Med Entomol 2003; 40:686–689.
139. Sanguioni LA, Horta MC, Vianna MC, et al. Rickettsial infections in animals and Brazilian spotted fever endemicity. Emerg Infect Dis 2005; 11:265–270.
140. Venzal JM, Portillo A, Estrada-Pena A, et al. *Rickettsia parkeri* in *Amblyomma triste* from Uruguay. Emerg Infect Dis 2004; 10:1493–1495.
141. Pacheco RC, Venzal JM, Richtzenhain LJ, Labruna MB. *Rickettsia parkeri* in Uruguay. Emerg Infect Dis 2006; 11:1804–1805.
142. Conti-Diaz IA, Rubio I, Somma Moreira RE, et al. Cutaneous-ganglionar rickettsiosis by *Rickettsia conorii* in Uruguay. Rev Inst Med Trop Sao Paulo 1990; 32:313–318.
143. Diaz IA. Rickettsiosis caused by *Rickettsia conorii* in Uruguay. Ann NY Acad Sci 2003; 990:264–266.
144. Beati L, Finidori JP, Gilot B, et al. Comparison of serologic typing, sodium dodecyl sulfate–polyacrylamide gel electrophoresis protein analysis, and genetic restriction fragment length polymorphism analysis for identification of rickettsiae: characterization of two new rickettsial strains. J Clin Microbiol 1992; 30:1922–1930.
145. Beati L, Raoult D. *Rickettsia massiliae* sp. nov., a new spotted fever group rickettsia. Int J Syst Bacteriol 1993; 43:839–840.
146. Babalis T, Tselentis Y, Roux V, et al. Isolation and identification of a rickettsial strain related to *Rickettsia massiliae* in Greek ticks. Am J Trop Med Hyg 1994; 50:365–372.
147. Bacellar F, Regnery RL, Nuncio MS, et al. Genotypic evaluation of rickettsial isolates recovered from various species of ticks in Portugal. Epidemiol Infect 1995; 114:169–178.
148. Dupont HT, Cornet JP, Raoult D. Identification of rickettsiae from ticks collected in the Central African Republic using the polymerase chain reaction. Am J Trop Med Hyg 1994; 50:373–380.

149. Beati L, Roux V, Ortuno A, et al. Phenotypic and genotypic characterization of spotted fever group rickettsiae isolated from Catalan *Rhipicephalus sanguineus* ticks. J Clin Microbiol 1996; 34:2688–2694.
150. Fernandez-Soto P, Perez-Sanchez R, Diaz Martin V, Encinas-Grandes A, Alamo Sanz R. *Rickettsia massiliae* in ticks removed from humans in Castilla y Leon, Spain. Eur J Clin Microbiol Infect Dis 2006 [Epub ahead of print].
151. Santos-Silva MM, Sousa R, Santos AS, Melo P, Encarnacao V, Bacellar F. Ticks parasitizing wild birds in Portugal: detection of *Rickettsia aeschlimannii, R. helvetica* and *R. massiliae.* Exp Appl Acarol 2006; 39(3–4):331–338.
152. Bernasconi MV, Casati S, Peter O, et al. *Rhipicephalus* ticks infected with *Rickettsia* and *Coxiella* in Southern Switzerland (Canton Ticino). Infect Genet Evol 2002; 2:111–120.
153. Eremeeva ME, Bosserman EA, Demma LJ, Zambrano ML, Blau DM, Dasch GA. Isolation and identification of *Rickettsia massiliae* from *Rhipicephalus sanguineus* ticks collected in Arizona. Appl Environ Microbiol 2006; 72(8):5569–5577.
154. Matsumoto K, Ogawa M, Brouqui P, et al. Transmission of *Rickettsia massiliae* in the tick, *Rhipicephalus turanicus.* Med Vet Entomol 2005; 19:263–270.
155. Cardenosa N, Segura F, Raoult D. Serosurvey among Mediterranean spotted fever patients of a new spotted fever group rickettsial strain (Bar29). Eur J Epidemiol 2003; 18:351–356.
156. Vitale G, Mansueto S, Rolain JM, et al. *Rickettsia massiliae* human isolation. Emerg Infect Dis 2005; 12:174–175.
157. Rydkina E, Roux V, Fetisova N, Rudakov N, Gafarova M, Tarasevich I, Raoult D. New rickettsiae in ticks collected in territories of the former Soviet Union. Emerg Infect Dis 1999; 5:811–814.
158. Shpynov S, Parola P, Rudakov N, Samoilenko I, Tankibaev M, Tarasevich I, et al. Detection and identification of spotted fever group rickettsiae in *Dermacentor* ticks from Russia and central Kazakhstan. Eur J Clin Microbiol Infect Dis 2001; 20:903–905.
159. Ibarra V, Blanco JR, Portillo A, Eiros JM, Oteo JA. *Rickettsia slovaca* infection: DEBONEL/TIBOLA. Ann NY Acad Sci 2006; 1078:206–214.
160. Mediannikov O, Matsumoto K, Samoylenko I, Drancourt M, Roux V, Rydkina E, Davoust B, Tarasevich I, Brouqui P, Fournier PE. *Rickettsia raoultii* sp. nov., a new pathogenic spotted fever group rickettsia associated with tick-borne lymphadenitis. Submitted.
161. Samoilenko IE, Rudakov NV, Shpynov SN, Tankibaev MA, Yakimenko VV, Kumpan LV. Study of biological characteristics of spotted fever group rickettsial genotypes RpA4, DnS14, and DnS28. Ann NY Acad Sci 2003; 990:612–626.
162. Graves S, Unsworth N, Stenos J. Rickettsioses in Australia. Ann NY Acad Sc 2006; 1078:74–79.
163. Rolain JM, Mathai E, Lepidi H, Somashekar HR, Mathew LG, Prakash JAJ, Raoult D. "*Candidatus* Rickettsia kellyi," India. Emerg Infect Dis 2006; 12(3):483–485.
164. Simser JA, Palmer AT, Fingerle V, Wilske B, Kurtti TJ, Munderloh UG. *Rickettsia monacensis* sp. nov., a spotted fever group Rickettsia, from ticks (*Ixodes ricinus*) collected in a European city park. Appl Environ Microbiol 2002; 68:4559–4566.
165. Raoult D, Fournier PE, Eremeeva M, Graves S, Kelly PJ, Oteo JA, Sekeyova Z, Tamura A, Tarasevich I, Zhang L. Naming of rickettsiae and rickettsial diseases. Ann NY Acad Sci 2005; 1063:1–12.
166. Sreter-Lancz Z, Sreter T, Szell Z, Egyed L. Molecular evidence of *Rickettsia helvetica* and *R. monacensis* infections in *Ixodes ricinus* from Hungary. Ann Trop Med Parasitol 2005; 99:325–330.
167. Marquez FJ, Muniain MA, Soriguer RC, Izquierdo G, Rodriguez-Bano J, Borobio MV. Genotypic identification of an undescribed spotted fever group rickettsia in *Ixodes ricinus* from southwestern Spain. Am J Trop Med Hyg 1998; 58:570–577.
168. Christova I, Van De PJ, Yazar S, Velo E, Schouls L. Identification of *Borrelia burgdorferi* sensu lato, *Anaplasma* and *Ehrlichia* species, and spotted fever group Rickettsiae in ticks from Southeastern Europe. Eur J Clin Microbiol Infect Dis 2003; 22:535–542.
169. Sekeyova Z, Fournier PE, Rehacek J, Raoult D. Characterization of a new spotted fever group Rickettsia detected in *Ixodes ricinus* (Acari: Ixodidae) collected in Slovakia. J Med Entomol 2000; 37:707–713.
170. Moreno CX, Moy F, Daniels TJ, Godfrey HP, Cabello FC. Molecular analysis of microbial communities identified in different developmental stages of *Ixodes scapularis* ticks from Westchester and Dutchess Counties, New York. Environ Microbiol 2006; 8:761–772.
171. Baldridge GD, Burkhardt N, Herron MJ, Kurtti TJ, Munderloh UG. Analysis of fluorescent protein expression in transformants of *Rickettsia monacensis*, an obligate intracellular tick symbiont. Appl Environ Microbiol 2005; 71:2095–2105.
172. Baldridge GD, Kurtti TJ, Munderloh UG. Susceptibility of *Rickettsia monacensis* and *Rickettsia peacockii* to Cecropin A, Ceratotoxin A, and lysozyme. Curr Microbiol 2005; 51:233–238.
173. Jado I, Oteo JA, Aldamiz M, et al. *R. monacensis* a new rickettsia species causing human diseases. Submitted.

12 | Other Rickettsiae of Possible or Undetermined Pathogenicity

Oleg Mediannikov
Unité des Rickettsies, Université de la Méditerranée, Marseille, France, and Laboratory of Rickettsial Ecology, Gamaleya Institute of Epidemiology and Microbiology, Moscow, Russia

Christopher D. Paddock
Infectious Disease Pathology Activity, Division of Viral and Rickettsial Diseases, Centers for Disease Control and Prevention, Atlanta, Georgia, U.S.A.

Philippe Parola
Faculté de Médecine, Unité des Rickettsies, Université de la Méditerranée, Marseille, France

INTRODUCTION

Rickettsiae are a large and diverse group of bacteria that have been classically associated with various hematophagous arthropods that may inoculate these bacteria into humans and animals to initiate infection in the vertebrate host (1). The factors responsible for pathogenicity to humans may be direct (i.e., the particular rickettsia is able to survive in a human host and elicit disease) or indirect (i.e., the rickettsia is associated with an arthropod that feeds on humans and places the rickettsia in proximity to a host, and the agent resides in a particular area of the arthropod that affords transport into a human host). To be considered as a human pathogen, a rickettsia should be isolated in cell culture from blood or tissue of patients, or be detected by molecular methods from blood or tissue from patients with illnesses clinically compatible with spotted fever rickettsioses and who have seroconverted using standard reference laboratory methods (2). We refer the reader to Chapters 8 through 11 for the description of these recognized pathogens and the related diseases.

Many other rickettsiae, not fulfilling these criteria, have been identified in ticks and other biological niches. Some of these agents were isolated in culture many years ago and others have been detected only recently using molecular tools. We can distinguish three categories (3). The first includes recognized species with valid names. However, as with other bacteria, rickettsiae must fulfill certain requirements to be officially validated as a new species or subspecies. These criteria include: isolation of the agent as a pure culture; demonstration that the agent possesses unique genomic and phenotypic characteristics; availability of the isolate to the scientific community through at least two independent official culture collections; and the new name should appear in the approved lists of bacterial names. The American type culture collection (ATCC) was the only official culture collection that accepted rickettsiae until the Unité des Rickettsies in Marseille, France, was recently recognized as an official collection site by the World Data Centre for Microorganisms. Some rickettsiae fulfill the genomic criteria but are yet to be cultured or completely described. For this group, the *Candidatus* status is quite applicable. The third group includes many rickettsiae that have been incompletely described—based on genomic criteria only—and have been designated by strain names or numbers (refer to Fig. 2 from Chapter 1). Among these described and incompletely described rickettsiae are several potential pathogens. Some newly reported *Rickettsia* and *Rickettsia*-like bacteria have been described in various ecologic niches that do not involve blood-feeding insects or arachnids. Some recent examples include male-killing *Rickettsia* species in coccinellid beetles (4), *Rickettsia* species in hematophagous leeches (5,6), *Candidatus* Xenohaliotis californiensis, a newly described rickettsial pathogen of abalone in North America (7), and many others. Under normal circumstances, these rickettsiae are unlikely to gain access to a human host; if this were to occur, however, it is possible

VALIDATED SPECIES

A detailed list of rickettsial species of possible or undetermined pathogenicity in humans is provided in Table 1.

Rickettsia asiatica

In June 1993, a rickettsial isolate named IO-1 was obtained from *Ixodes ovatus* ticks in Fukushima. Since that time, 32 additional strains with identical *gltA* sequences IO-1 have been obtained from *I. ovatus* ticks in Japan (8,9). Preliminary results of mouse serotyping and sequencing of the entire 16S rRNA and *gltA* genes demonstrated that strain IO-1 exhibited unique serotypic and genotypic characteristics (10,11). More recently, using multilocus sequence comparison, five rickettsial isolates from *I. ovatus* collected at various locations in Japan were found to be identical to each other and represent a novel species that was named *R. asiatica* (12). The type strain of *R. asiatica* sp. nov. is IO-1. Phylogenetically this species is close to *R. helvetica*, a possible human pathogen (see below). No information is currently available about the possible pathogenicity of R. asiatica for vertebrate hosts. The currently known geographical distribution is restricted to Japan (12).

Rickettsia bellii

In 1966, a rickettsial agent was isolated in embryonated chicken eggs from a triturated pool of *Dermacentor variabilis* ticks collected from vegetation in Arkansas. The isolate was identified as a unique species and named *R. bellii* (13). Rickettsial isolates, characterized as *R. bellii* y using immunofluorescence typing, have been recovered from various *Ixodid* and *Argasid* tick species, including *D. andersoni*, *D. occidentalis*, *D. albopictus*, *Haemaphysalis leporispalustris*, *Ornithodoros concanensis*, and *Argas cooleyi* (13–15). Recent molecular studies have shown that *R. bellii* represents a distinct group within rickettsiae (16). Although further investigations are necessary, it is likely that *R. bellii* is one of the most abundant and broadly distributed rickettsiae infecting ticks in the U.S.A. (17). Recent investigation have isolated *R. bellii* in 16 of 40 *A. cooperi* ticks collected in the state of São Paulo in Brazil (18), suggesting that the distribution of this rickettsia includes many regions of the Western Hemisphere.

Recently, the genome sequence of *R. bellii*, presented as the earliest diverging species of known rickettsiae, was obtained (19). The 1,552,076-bp chromosome does not exhibit the colinearity observed in other rickettsia genomes, and encodes a complete set of putative conjugal DNA transfer genes most similar to homologs found in *Protochlamydia amoebophila* UWE25, an obligate symbiont of amebae. The genome exhibits many other genes highly similar to homologs in intracellular bacteria of amebae. Microscopic analyses reveal bacterial mating through sex pili-like cell surface appendages. *R. bellii* efficiently multiplies in the nucleus of eukaryotic cells and can survive in an ameba for long periods. These results suggest that ameba-like ancestral protozoa could have served as a genetic "melting pot" where the ancestors of rickettsiae and other bacteria promiscuously exchanged genes, eventually leading to their adaptation to the intracellular lifestyle within eukaryotic cells.

There are no studies to suggest that *R. belli* causes disease in humans; however, the pathogenicity of *R. bellii* by bacterial inoculation in guinea pigs and rabbits has been recently evaluated. The characteristics of the lesions obtained in these animal models suggest bacterial multiplication: (*i*) intact bacteria were detected after two weeks by immunohistochemistry in the tissues; (*ii*) an eschar was present; and (*iii*) the appearance of the inflammatory lesions and eschar were not immediate. Animal models do not definitely predict the pathogenicity of rickettsiae in humans (20), however, these findings suggest that the role of *R. bellii* as a potential human pathogen deserves further investigation (19).

TABLE 1 Rickettsial Species of Possible or Undetermined Pathogenicity in Humans

Rickettsial species	Geographic location	Year of discovery/ publication	Vector/host	Current evidence to suggest a pathogenic role in human hosts
Validated species				
R. asiatica	Japan	1993	Ioxdes ovatus	None
R. bellii	U.S.A.	1966	Dermacentor variabilis, D. andersoni, D. occidentalis, D. albopictus, Haemaphysalis leporispalustris, O. concanensis, A. cooleyi	None
	Brazil	2004	Amblyomma cooperi	
R. canadensis	Canada, U.S.A.	1967	H. leporispalustris, D. andersoni, D. variabilis, A. americanum	Spotted fever in U.S.A. (?)
	Japan	2005	Haemaphysalis sp.	Cerebral vasculitis in U.S.A. (?)
R. helvetica	Europe (Switzerland, France, Germany, Sweden, Hungary, Slovenia, Portugal, Spain, Italy, Bulgaria)	1979	I. ricinus	Perimyocarditis (?) Cardiac valve pathology (?) Sarcoidosis (?) Febrile illness in Europe (?)
	Japan	2002	I. ovatus, I. persulcatus, I. monospinosus	Spotted fever in Thailand and Laos (?)
R. montanensis	U.S.A.	1963	D. variabilis, D. andersoni	None
R. peacockii	U.S.A.	1925	D. andersoni	None
R. rhipicephali	U.S.A.	1975	Rhipicephali sanguineus, D. occidentalis, D. andersoni, D. variabilis	None
	Europe (France, Portugal, Greece, Croatia)	1992	Rh. sanguineus	
	Africa (Central African Republic)	1994	Rh. sanguineus	
R. tamurae	Asia (Japan, Thailand)	1993	A. testudinarium	Spotted fever in Thailand (?)
Rickettsiae classified as Candidatus species				
Candidatus Rickettsia amblyommii	U.S.A.	1974	A. americanum	Febrile illness in Arkansas and Virginia (?)
	Brazil	2004	A. cajennense, A. coelebs, A. longirostre	Bullis fever in Texas (?)
Candidatus Rickettsia andeanae	Peru	2002	A. maculatum, I. boliviensis	None
Candidatus Rickettsia tarasevichiae	European and Asian Russia	2002	I. persulcatus	None
	Japan	2005	Ixodes sp.	
Candidatus Rickettsia uilenbergi	Africa	2006	A. tholloni	None

(Continued)

TABLE 1 Rickettsial Species of Possible or Undetermined Pathogenicity in Humans (*Continued*)

Rickettsial species	Geographic location	Year of discovery/ publication	Vector/host	Current evidence to suggest a pathogenic role in human hosts
Candidatus Rickettsia davousti	Africa	2006	*A. tholloni*	
Candidatus Rickettsia principis	Russia (Far Eastern)	2004	*H. japonica douglasii*	
Candidatus Rickettsia rara	Russia (Far Eastern)	2006	*H. concinna*	
Other incompletely described and unnamed rickettsias				
Rickettsia sp. strain 364D	U.S.A. (California)	1973	*D. occidentalis*	Spotted fever in U.S.A. (?)
Rickettsia sp. strains Cooleyi and ISS	U.S.A.	1998	*I. scapularis*	None
Rickettsia sp. strain COOPERI	Brazil	2004	*A. cooperi*	None
Rickettsia sp. strain parumapertus	U.S.A.	1951	*D. parumapertus*	None
Rickettsia sp. strain Tillamook	U.S.A.	1976	*I. pacificus*	None
Other rickettsial genotypes detected in ticks				
Rickettsia sp. RDla420	Thailand	2003	*D. auratus*	None
Rickettsia sp. RDla440	Thailand	2003	*Dermacentor* sp.	
Rickettsia sp. ATT	Thailand	2003	*A. testudinarium*	
Rickettsia sp. HOT1,2	Thailand	2003	*H. ornithophila*	
Rickettsia sp. S	Armenia	1955	*Rh. sanguineus*	
Rickettsia sp. R300	Brazil	2005	*H. juxtakochi*	
R. midichlorii	U.S.A.	2003	*I. scapularis*	
Rickettsia sp. AaR/SoCarolina	U.S.A.	2001	*A. americanum*	
R. moreli	Spain	1996	*I. ricinus*	
Rickettsiae sp. MK37, IM32a	East Africa	2005	*Ornithodoros moubata*	
R. kulagini	Ukraine	2006	*Rh. sanguineus*	

Rickettsia canadensis

R. canadensis (formerly *canada*) was first isolated from the pool of *H. leporispalustris* ticks collected from rabbits in the Richmond area of Ottawa, Canada (21). Later, identical strain was isolated in California from the same tick species (22). Until recently, this rickettsia was found only in North America, but in 2005, molecular methods were used to demonstrate the occurrence of *R. canadensis* in *Haemaphysalis* sp. ticks in Fukuoka, Japan (23). It has also been found in various species of ticks, including *D. andersoni*, *D. variabilis*, and *Amblyomma americanum* (24–26). Experimentally, the ability of *R. canadensis* to induce long-term rickettsiemia in birds (chickens) and mice (*Microtus pennsylvanicus*) has been proved, although Leporids (*Lepus americanus* and *Oryctolagus cuniculus*) were shown to resist rickettsial infection (26).

R. canadensis was initially considered to be a member of the typhus group rickettsiae on the basis of its antigenic characteristics (27). However, recent molecular studies (16,28–30) indicate that it is distinct from the typhus and spotted fever groups (SFGs) (31). In spite of its unique phylogenetic position, *R. canadensis* exhibit typical morphological traits of the both typhus and SFG rickettsiae. *R. canadensis* has been reported to be transstadially and transovarially passaged in ticks. It has both rompA and rompB proteins similar with SFG rickettsiae. Interestingly, intranuclear growth (a morphological trait traditionally used in taxonomy to separate SFG and typhus group rickettsiae) is observed in tick gut epithelium cells, hypodermal tissues, and, occasionally, in hemocytes (25,26).

The role of *R. canadensis* as a human pathogen has not been definitively established. Serologic evidence of human infection has been reported in four patients presenting with a Rocky Mountain spotted fever (RMSF)-like disease in California and Texas (32). A role for *R. canadensis* in acute cerebral vasculitis was also suspected in a patient from southwestern Ohio, based on serological studies that included immunoblot analysis (33,34).

Rickettsia helvetica

R. helvetica was first isolated in *I. ricinus* (the vector of Lyme borreliosis) in Switzerland in 1979 (35,36). Because transstadial and transovarial transmission of this rickettsia has been demonstrated in *I. ricinus*, this tick represents both a potential vector and natural reservoir of *R. helvetica*. No animal reservoirs were found, although wild deer were intensively studied (37). *R. helvetica* has been identified in *I. ricinus* in many European countries, including France, Germany, Sweden, Hungary, Slovenia, Portugal, Spain, Italy, and Bulgaria (38–43) where the average infection rate is approximately 10%. Recently, it has been shown that the distribution of *R. helvetica* is not limited to Europe, but extends to Asia. Rickettsiae identical with or closely related to *R. helvetica* have been isolated from *I. ovatus*, *I. persulcatus*, and *I. monospinosus* ticks collected in Japan (8,11). By polymerase chain reaction (PCR), it has also been found in *H. japonica* (8). *R. helvetica* has also recently been detected in Morocco in North Africa (Parola, Unpublished).

R. helvetica was considered a "nonpathogenic rickettsia" during approximately 20 years after its discovery. However, in 1999 it was implicated in fatal perimyocarditis in several patients in Sweden. Infection was documented by electron microscopy, PCR, and serology (44). These researchers subsequently reported a controversial association between *R. helvetica* and sarcoidosis in Sweden (45) and finding of *R. helvetica* DNA in pathological human aortic valves (46). However, the validity of these associations has been questioned by some rickettsiologists (47) and additional studies did not reveal antirickettsial antibodies in a group of Scandinavian sarcoidosis patients (48).

In 2000, seroconversion to *R. helvetica* was described for a French patient with a nonspecific febrile illness (49). Strong serologic data, including cross-absorption and Western blotting, supported *R. helvetica* etiology of the disease. In 2003, serological findings in tick-bite patients from Switzerland were suggestive of acute or past *R. helvetica* infection (50). More recently, a patient from France and three patients from Italy were also diagnosed using serological criteria that included microimmuno flourescence (MIF), Western blotting, and cross-absorption methods. All four reported tick bites and one developed an eschar (51). Recently, five cases of SFG rickettsiosis, possibly caused by *R. helvetica*, were reported in patients living along the central Thai–Myanmar border. Two patients reported a tick bite, one presented with an eschar, and another patient presented with rash. Infections were documented by MIF and Western blot assays (52). Three more cases were serologically documented in patients from eastern Thailand with undifferentiated febrile illnesses. Although no vector of *R. helvetica* has been identified in Thailand, it is known that *I. ovatus*, which has been shown to carry *R. helvetica* at least in Japan, is also prevalent in Thailand (53). Further evidence of *R. helvetica* infections in the Far East is supported by a recent report of a Japanese traveler returning from Australia with tick paralysis due to *I. holocyclus* who subsequently seroconverted to *R. helvetica* (54). Eight from 11 patients in Laos with serologically diagnosed rickettsial infection had the highest titers against *R. helvetica* in immunofluorescence. One patient developed rash, unlike European cases (55).

These data suggest that *R. helvetica* occurs across a much larger geographical area than previously known and is associated with *Ixodes* spp. ticks. The few patients for whom serology-based diagnosis exist had relatively mild, self-limited illnesses associated with headache and myalgias, and less frequently with rash and or an eschar (51). Additional evaluation and isolation of the bacterium from clinical samples are, however, definitely needed to confirm the pathogenicity of *R. helvetica*.

Rickettsia montanensis

R. montanensis (formerly *R. montana*) was first isolated from *D. variabilis* and *D. andersoni* ticks collected in Montana in 1963 (56). This rickettsia is distributed extensively in *Dermacentor* sp.

ticks in the U.S.A. In North Carolina, the state with the highest incidence of RMSF, 71 of 72 rickettsiae isolated from *D. variabilis* were *R. montanensis*, and only one was *R. rickettsii*. On Long Island, New York, all isolates from adults *D. variabilis* were *R. montanensis* (17). In Maryland, 15 (3.8%) of 392 adult *D. variabilis* collected from several counties during 2002 tested positive for SFG rickettsiae by molecular methods, and all were identified as *R. montanenesis* (57). *R. montanensis* has also been detected as the predominant rickettsial species, infecting *D. variabilis* ticks collected from some areas of Massachusetts, Connecticut, and Ohio (58–60). Transovarial transmission of *R. montanensis* has been demonstrated in *D. variabilis* (61) and its geographic distribution may also parallel the distribution of this tick. There are no data to indicate that *R. montanensis* causes human illness.

Rickettsia peacockii

During a survey conducted in 1925, Parker and Spencer (62) determined that 36% of *D. andersoni* ticks collected in the eastern side of the Bitterroot Valley, Montana, harbored a rickettsia localized predominantly to acarine ovaries. In 1981, Burgdorfer et al. (63) found as many as 80% of wood ticks collected from the Sapphire Mountain range of the valley were infected with a rickettsia provisionally named the "East Side agent" that was transstadially and transovarially transmitted in *D. andersoni*. The East Side agent was subsequently characterized as a new species of SFG rickettsiae and named *R. peacockii*. Sequencing of 16S rRNA- and rompA-encoding genes showed close similarity with, but distinct from, *R. rickettsii* (64). Interestingly, the presence of *R. peacockii* within ovaries of *D. andersoni* interferes with the ability of virulent *R. rickettsii* to infect the ovarian tissues and to be transovarially transmitted to progeny (63).

In 2001, *R. peacockii* was successfully maintained in a continuous culture of an embryonic cell line (DAE100) of *D. andersoni*, without apparent adverse effects on the host cells (65). *R. peacockii* apparently does not invade tick hemocytes or salivary gland tissue (64), precluding a formal route of invasion into a vertebrate host. The molecular basis for the apparent "nonpathogenicity" of *R. peacockii* has been explored recently and its inability to express rompA has been suggested as one reason for its apparent lack of virulence in vertebrates (66). Other studies have identified a naturally occurring transposon (ISRpel) that disrupts the *rickA* gene involved in actin-based motility of *R. peacockii* (67). In this context, it seems quite possible that *R. peackockii* is in fact a nonpathogen, although there are no direct studies that prove or disprove this possibility. To our knowledge, this rickettsia is not available in either of the two official collections.

Rickettsia rhipicephali

During a survey for tick-borne rickettsiae in Mississippi in 1975, an SFG rickettsia distinct from *R. rickettsii* was isolated from *Rhipicephalus sanguineus* ticks collected on dogs (68). This rickettsia was named *R. rhipicephali* and ultrastrucural studies showed that it invades both salivary glands and ovaries of the tick (69). *R. rhipicephali* has also been detected in *D. occidentalis* in California (70), *D. andersoni* in Montana (71), and *D. variabilis* in South Carolina (68). However, it has recently been shown that *D. variabilis* ticks are unable to maintain *R. rhipicephali* transovarially for more than one generation, suggesting that *D. variabilis* is not an efficient host for this rickettsia in nature (61). *R. rhipicephali* has also been found in *Rh. sanguineus* ticks from France, Portugal, Greece, Croatia, and the Central African Republic (72–76).

Meadow voles inoculated with *R. rhipcephali* develop scrotal swelling and splenomegaly, and some animals die from the infection (77). Furthermore, adult and immature stages of *Rh. sanguineus* occasionally bite humans, suggesting a potential route for transmission of *R. rhipicephali* to humans. However, *Rh. sanguineus* ticks also harbor or transmit many other species of SFG rickettsiae, including known pathogens such as *R. conorii* (78), *R. rickettsii* (79), and *R. massiliae* (80,81) that could confound attempts to definitively associate *R. rhipicephali* with a specific disease manifestation. Further work will be needed to confirm or refute the ability of this rickettsia to cause symptomatic infection in humans.

Rickettsia tamurae

In 1993, in Tokushima prefecture of Japan, a rickettsial strain initially named "AT-1" was isolated from *A. testudinarium* ticks (9,82). Thereafter, a total of 45 isolates were obtained from the same tick species in Japan and were demonstrated to be genetically highly similar to AT-1 (11).

This rickettsia is phylogenetically similar to, but distinct from, *Candidatus* Rickettsia monacencis (8,11) and the related strains IRS3 and IRS4 detected in *I. ricinus* ticks in Europe (83). Rickettsial DNA identical to this species was also found in *A. testudinarium* ticks in Thailand (84).

Recently, using comparative analysis of sequences obtained from 16S *rRNA*, *gltA*, *ompA*, *ompB*, *sca4* gene fragments, as well as mouse serotyping, it was demonstrated that "strain AT-1" represents a new species within the genus *Rickettsia*, and it was named *R. tamurae* (85). Because *A. testudinarium* frequently bites humans, it may serve as a potential vector of *R. tamurae* in the Far East. A recent serological survey of acutely ill patients in Laos revealed a case of possible infection with this species in patient (55).

RICKETTSIAE CLASSIFIED AS *CANDIDATUS* SPECIES
Candidatus Rickettsia amblyommii

"*R. amblyommii*," as found in the literature, and also referred to as strains 85-1034, WB-8-2, and MOAa, was first isolated from lone star ticks (*A. americanum*) collected in Tennessee in 1974 and subsequently identified throughout the range of the lone star tick (86–88). Lone star ticks are especially abundant in the southern and Midwestern U.S.A., and all three stages of *A. americanum* readily bite humans. In some areas of the U.S.A., 40% or more of *A. americanum* may be infected with this rickettsia (89,90). *R. amblyommii* has also been recently detected in *A. cajennense* and *A. coelebs* ticks collected from the western Amazon forest of Brazil (91). Recent investigations have also identified an SFG rickettsia (strain "Aranha") in *A. longirostre* ticks collected on Brazilian porcupine that shows very close phylogenetic relationship with *R. amblyommii* (92). A closely related rickettsia has also been recently detected in tick from French Guyana, South America (93).

At the present, it appears that this species is strictly *Amblyomma*-associated. Morphologically, it does not differ from other SFG rickettsiae when grown on tick cell lines and reacts with *R. rickettsii*-specific monoclonal antibodies. Phylogenetic analyses group *R. amblyommii* with *R. montanensis* and *Rickettsia* sp. strains ISS and Cooleyi (88).

The role of *R. amblyommii* as an agent of human disease has been suggested by a study that examined Western blot profiles of 12 members of a military unit that developed mild illnesses and antibodies reactive with SFG rickettsiae following field maneuvers in tick-infested habitats in Arkansas and Virginia. Investigators determined that five of these patients exhibited specific profiles of reactivity to major surface proteins antigens of strain 85-1034 suggesting infection with this agent (94).

Some investigators have speculated that *R. amblyommii* may be the same agent as *R. texiana*, a putative rickettsial pathogen associated with an epidemic of febrile, presumably tick-borne, infectious disease known as Bullis fever that afflicted more than 1000 soldiers participating in field training exercises at Camp Bullis, Texas, during the spring and summer months of 1942 and 1943 (95). Considerable epidemiologic and entomologic evidence collected during the outbreak implicated an infectious agent transmitted by the bite of lone star ticks (96). Because all patients reported a history of tick bites, most notably bites from *A. americanum*, the disease was also initially referred to as "Texas tick fever" and "lone star fever." Clinical features included fever, chills, orbital and postoccipital headache, weakness, weight loss, and leucopenia. All patients demonstrated enlargement of at least some lymph nodes and many had a generalized lymphadenopathy. A maculopapular rash involving the trunk was noted in 10% of cases. The illnesses varied from a mild febrile syndrome of short duration to severe disease and included one death (97). Impression smears made from biopsied lymph nodes stained by the Machiavello technique showed small intracellular fuchsinophilic rods, morphologically similar to rickettsiae (98). Rickettsia-like organisms were also isolated from blood and lymph nodes of patients and from *A. americanum* ticks collected in the area (99). Isolates from humans and ticks, passaged in chick embryo culture and in animals, subsequently produced clinical features compatible with Bullis fever when inoculated in human volunteers. The name *R. texiana* was proposed for this agent (95). Because *A. americanum* frequently harbor SFG rickettsiae (89), most notably *R. amblyommii*, it has been suggested that *R. texiana* may have been represented by a strain of this rickettsia; however, no isolate of *R. texiana* is known to exist today, precluding analyses by contemporary molecular tools (Table 1).

Candidatus Rickettsia andeanae

During a survey for ectoparasites that followed an outbreak of an apparent spotted fever rickettsiosis in northern Peru in 2002, a unique SFG rickettsia was detected in *A. maculatum* and *I. boliviensis* ticks that showed 97% homology with the most closely related rickettsial *rompB* sequences for *R. aeschlimannii* and *R. rhipicephali* (100). Phylogenetic analyses of four additional rickettsial genes (*gltA*, *ompA*, *sca4*, and the 17-kDa gene) confirmed the uniqueness of this rickettsia from other known SFG rickettsiae and the name "*R. andeanae*" was proposed (101). No isolate of this agent has been obtained in cell culture and the pathogenic potential of *R. andeanae* remains to be determined.

Candidatus Rickettsia tarasevichiae

A novel rickettsial agent, provisionally called "*R. tarasevichiae*" was first identified (102) and subsequently isolated (103) in *I. persulcatus* in different regions of Russia. Prevalence varied from 10% to 50% and more. Interesting observation was made on its prevalence, which rises from Western Siberia regions toward Far East where it reaches 95% (O. Mediannikov, unpublished data). Phylogenetically, this rickettsia is distant from other rickettsiae and the most similar species, although quite remote, is *R. canadensis*. In a similar manner, *ompA* gene was not found in this rickettsia. This rickettsia was also identified recently in an *Ixodes* sp. tick collected from a dog in Northern Japan (23). No evidence for infection with this agent in humans has been demonstrated.

OTHER CANDIDATI

Two distinct rickettsias have been recently identified in *A. tholloni* ticks from elephants in Africa. The names "*Candidatus* Rickettsia uilenbergi" (DQ402515) and "*Candidatus* Rickettsia davousti" (DQ402517) have been proposed (104). *Candidatus* Rickettsia midichlorii has been detected in *I. scapularis* ticks in Wisconsin (Accession No. AY348295) and *Candidatus* Rickettsia moreli in *I. ricinus* ticks from Spain (Accession Nos. Y08784 and Y08785).

Candidatus Rickettsia principis (AY578115) was identified in human-biting tick, *H. japonica douglasii*, in Far Eastern regions of Russia (105). In the same region, *Candidatus* Rickettsia rara (DQ365805) was identified in another tick species *H. concinna*, a vector of Far Eastern tick-borne rickettsiosis (Table 1).

OTHER INCOMPLETELY DESCRIBED AND UNNAMED RICKETTSIAE
Rickettsia sp. Strain 364D

In 1973, Cory et al. (106) reported the isolation of an SFG rickettsia from pools of Pacific Coast ticks (*D. occidentalis*) collected in Mendicino County, California. The isolate, and another strain obtained from *D. occidentalis* ticks collected in southern California in 1966 (designated as strain 364D), were later determined by microimmunofluorescence to represent a distinct rickettsial serotype that was related to, but distinguishable from, *R. rickettsii* (107). Contemporary molecular analyses evaluating variable number tandem repeat loci corroborate the serotyping data and suggest that strain 364D may represent a distinct rickettsial species (108). Isolates of the 364D serotype elicit minimal-to-moderate scrotal reactions when inoculated into guinea pigs, and convalescing animals develop robust antibody titers to this agent (109). Nymphal and adult stages of the Pacific Coast tick are relatively indiscriminant feeders and will readily bite humans (110). In this context, it seems quite possible that strain 364D causes infection in humans (111). Indeed, some antibody adsorption results of convalescent-phase serum specimens of patients in northern California with confirmed RMSF suggest infection with strain 364D (70).

Rickettsia sp. Strains Cooleyi and ISS

In 1998, a novel SFG rickettsia provisionally designated genotype "Cooleyi," was described from *I. scapularis* ticks collected in Texas. Analyses of 17-kDa gene, *gltA*, and *rompA* sequences amplified from this tick revealed distinct differences between the *I. scapularis* rickettsia and other described SFG rickettsiae. The identity of this rickettsia awaits further characterization, although preliminary evaluation shows similarities of some sequence with other *Ixodes*-associated rickettsiae, including *R. australis* and *R. helvetica* (112). At the same time, almost identical rickettsia (encoded as ISS, *I. scapularis* symbiont) has been identified in laboratory population of *I. scapularis* ticks collected in 1988 from white-tailed deer in Minnesota (88,113). Because *I. scapularis* ticks readily bite humans, the role of strain Cooleyi as a potential pathogen deserves further attention.

Rickettsia sp. Strain COOPERI

A unique spotted fever rickettsia, strain COOPERI, was recently isolated from 3 of 40 *A. cooperi* collected in the state of Sao Paulo, Brazil. By phylogenetic analysis based on *rompA*, *gltA*, and gene D, this rickettsia was found to be closely related to, but distinct from, *R. parkeri*, *R. africae*, and *R. sibirica* (18). Recent cross-adsorption studies of serum specimens of dogs from a spotted fever-endemic region of São Paulo indicate the occurrence of infection with an SFG rickettsia other than *R. rickettsii*. Because strain COOPERI has been collected from the same area, it has been proposed that this rickettsia may be a potential pathogen (114).

Rickettsia sp. Strain Parumapertus

An SFG rickettsia, related to, but distinct from, *R. rickettsii* was isolated from *D. parumapertus* ticks collected in Nevada in 1951 (115), and in the Great Salt Lake desert region of Utah during 1954–1957 (116). Yolk sac cultures of these strains caused mild fever and scrotal swelling in guinea pigs but the animals routinely recovered from the infection. By microimmunofluorescence serotyping, the parumapertus strain is included in a minor subgroup of SFG that also contains *R. conorii*, *R. parkeri*, and *R. sibirica* (107). Because the latter three agents are recognized pathogens, it is reasonable to postulate that the parumapertus strain would also cause disease if introduced into a susceptible human host. *D. parumapertus* ticks are generally host-specific and seldom feed on animals other than rabbits (110); nonetheless, this rickettsia deserves further attention as a potential agent of sporadic rickettsial disease in the western U.S.A.

Rickettsia sp. Strain Tillamook

In 1976, Hughes et al. (117) described a unique SFG rickettsia isolated from *I. pacificus* ticks in Tillamook County in western Oregon. The Tillamook strain elicited mild scrotal swelling and low fever in guinea pigs inoculated intraperitoneally with the agent and was lethal to mice injected intravenously with a 20% yolk sac suspension of the agent (117). Isolates similar or identical to the Tillamook strain were subsequently obtained from *I. pacificus* ticks in Sonoma and Monterey counties in northern California (70,109). *I. pacificus* is a commonly encountered tick in the western U.S.A., and adult and immature stages ticks are avid biters of humans (110). In this context, the possibility that the Tillamook strain causes disease in humans warrants further investigation (Table 1) (70,111).

OTHER RICKETTSIAL GENOTYPES DETECTED IN TICKS

Many other nonclassified or incompletely characterized SFG rickettsiae have been detected in or isolated from various species of *Ixodid* ticks around the world. Two *Rickettsia* spp. were recently detected in Thailand near the central Thai–Myanmar border. These include *Rickettsia* strain RDla420, detected in *D. auratus* ticks collected from a bear, and *Rickettsia* strain RDla440, identified from pools of *Dermacentor* larvae collected from a wild pig nest. Strain RDla440 appears most closely related to *Rickettsia* sp. strain DnS14 and *Rickettsia* sp. strain RpA4, previously detected in Russia (118,119). DNA sequences of unknown *Rickettsia* spp. have been detected in human-biting ticks collected in central Thailand including ATT, detected in *A. testudinarium* ticks and HOT1 and HOT2, detected from *H. ornithophila* ticks (84).

In Europe, *Rickettsia* sp. "strain S" has been isolated from *Rh. sanguineus* in Armenia. Surprisingly, this strain appears related to *R. africae* (120). *Rickettsia* strain R300 was recently detected from *H. juxtakochi* ticks in Brazil; genetic analyses show that strain R300 is closely related to *R. rhipicephali* (121). Almost identical, but novel rickettsial species were identified in *H. ornithophila* in Thailand (84) and in *Ixodes* sp. in Japan (23).

Other rickettsial genomic fragments detected from ticks have been deposited in GenBank, without further documentation. These include *Rickettsia* strain AaR/So Carolina (that appears to be closely related to *Candidatus* Rickettsia amblyommii) in *A. americanum* ticks (Accession No. AF453408). Two *gltA* genotypes (MK37 and IM32a, Accession Nos. DQ092216 and DQ0922165) were identified in argasid soft ticks (*O. moubata*), and both are phylogenetically distant and the closest relation is with *R. felis*. A species close to *R. massiliae* was found in *Rh. sanguineus* ticks in Crimea, Ukraine (DQ365806).

In addition, some novel alpha-proteobacteria that phylogenetically belong to the order *Rickettsiales*, but, not definitely to the family *Rickettsiaceae*, were identified in *Ixodid* ticks. Among these are the "Montezuma" agent (122) widely distributed in *I. persulcatus*, "*Nicolleia massiliensis*" (GenBank Accession No. DQ788562) from European *I. ricinus* and unnamed bacteria from *H. wellingtoni* (118). These rickettsiae have not yet been isolated in cell culture, but are widely distributed in *Ixodid* ticks and deserve further investigation (Table 1).

CONCLUSION

Many of the rickettsiae we now know as human pathogens were first identified in ticks several years or even decades before a conclusive association with human disease was demonstrated. This is the case for eight of the 13 species or subspecies of tick-borne SFG rickettsiae confirmed as pathogens since 1984 (2,123). In the case of *R. parkeri* (see Chapter 11 "Other Tick-Borne Rickettsioses"), the wait was as long as 65 years (124). Most of the rickettsiae listed in this chapter satisfy the first component necessary of a potential tick-borne pathogen, that is, they have been detected in ticks with a natural proclivity to bite humans. It is quite likely that one or more of these will be reconsidered as human pathogens in years to come. High levels of awareness, including careful history-taking and thorough physical and laboratory examinations by primary physicians along with the use of contemporary methods based on molecular biology techniques, have facilitated the discovery and description of all emerging human rickettsioses and will undoubtedly lead to the discovery of new tick-borne rickettsial diseases around the world.

REFERENCES

1. Perlman SJ, Hunter MS, Zchori-Fein E. The emerging diversity of Rickettsia. Proc Biol Sci 2006; 273:2097–2106.
2. Parola P, Paddock CD, Raoult D. Tick-borne rickettsioses around the world: emerging diseases challenging old concepts. Clin Microbiol Rev 2005; 18:719–756.
3. Raoult D, Fournier PE, Eremeeva M, et al. Naming of Rickettsiae and rickettsial diseases. Ann NY Acad Sci 2005; 1063:1–12.
4. von der Schulenburg JHG, Habib M, Sloggett JJ, et al. Incidence of male-killing *Rickettsia* spp. (a-Proteobacteria) in the ten-spot ladybird beetle *Adalia decempunctata* L. (Coleoptera: coccinellidae). Appl Environ Microbiol 2001; 67:270–277.
5. Kikuchi Y, Sameshima S, Kitade O, Kojima J, Fukatsu T. Novel clade of *Rickettsia* spp. from leeches. Appl Environ Microbiol 2002; 68:999–1004.
6. Kikuchi Y, Fukatsu T. Rickettsia infection in natural leech populations. Microb Ecol 2005; 49:265–271.
7. Friedman CS, Andree KB, Beauchamp KA, et al. '*Candidatus* Xenohaliotis californiensis', a newly described pathogen of abalone, *Haliotis* spp., along the west coast of North America. Int J Syst Evol Microbiol 2000; 50(Pt 2):847–855.
8. Ishikura M, Fujita H, Ando S, Matsuura K, Watanabe M. Phylogenetic analysis of spotted fever group Rickettsiae isolated from ticks in Japan. Microbiol Immunol 2002; 46:241–247.
9. Fujita H, Watanabe Y, Ishikura M, Takada N. List of all isolates of spotted fever group rickettsiae from ticks in Japan 1993–1998. Ann Rep Ohara Hosp 1999; 42:45–50.
10. Takada N, Fujita H, Yano Y, Ishiguro F, Iwasaki H, Masuzawa T. First records of tick-borne pathogens, *Borrelia*, and spotted fever group Rickettsiae in Okinawajima Island, Japan. Microbiol Immunol 2001; 45:163–165.

11. Fournier PE, Fujita H, Takada N, Raoult D. Genetic identification of rickettsiae isolated from ticks in Japan. J Clin Microbiol 2002; 40:2176–2181.
12. Fujita H, Fournier PE, Takada N, Saito T, Raoult D. *Rickettsia asiatica* sp. nov., isolated in Japan. Int J Syst Evol Microbiol 2006; 56:2365–2368.
13. Philip RN, Casper EA, Anacker RL, et al. *Rickettsia bellii* sp. nov.: a tick-borne rickettsia, widely distributed in the United States, that is distinct from the spotted fever and typhus biogroups. Int J Syst Bacteriol 1983; 33:94–106.
14. Gage KL, Schrumpf ME, Karstens RH, Burgdorfer W, Schwan TG. DNA typing of rickettsiae in naturally infected ticks using a polymerase chain reaction/restriction fragment length polymorphism system. Am J Trop Med Hyg 1994; 50:247–260.
15. Azad AF, Beard CB. Rickettsial pathogens and their arthropod vectors. Emerg Infect Dis 1998; 4:179–186.
16. Fournier PE, Dumler JS, Greub G, Zhang J, Wu Y, Raoult D. Gene sequence-based criteria for identification of new rickettsia isolates and description of *Rickettsia heilongjiangensis* sp. nov. J Clin Microbiol 2003; 41:5456–5465.
17. Walker DH, Fishbein DB. Epidemiology of rickettsial diseases. Eur J Epidemiol 1991; 7:237–245.
18. Labruna MB, Whitworth T, Horta MC, et al. Rickettsia species infecting *Amblyomma cooperi* ticks from an area in the state of Sao Paulo, Brazil, where Brazilian spotted fever is endemic. J Clin Microbiol 2004; 42:90–98.
19. Ogata H, La Scola B, Audic S, et al. Genome sequence of *Rickettsia bellii* illuminates the role of amoebae in gene exchanges between intracellular pathogens. PLoS Genet 2006; 2:e76.
20. Parola P, Raoult D. Ticks and tickborne bacterial diseases in humans: an emerging infectious threat. Clin Infect Dis 2001; 32:897–928.
21. McKiel YA, Bell EJ, Lackman DB. *Rickettsia canada*: a new member of the typhus group of rickettsiae isolated from *Haemaphysalis leporispalustris* ticks in Canada. Can J Microbiol 1967; 13:503–510.
22. Philip RN, Casper EA, Anacker RL, Peacock MG, Hayes SF, Lane RS. Identification of an isolate of *Rickettsia canada* from California. Am J Trop Med Hyg 1982; 31:1216–1221.
23. Hiraoka H, Shimada Y, Sakata Y, et al. Detection of rickettsial DNA in *Ixodid* ticks recovered from dogs and cats in Japan. J Vet Med Sci 2005; 67:1217–1222.
24. Brinton LP, Burgdorfer W. Fine structure of *Rickettsia canada* in tissues of *Dermacentor andersoni* Stiles. J Bacteriol 1971; 105:1149–1159.
25. Burgdorfer W, Brinton LP. Intranuclear growth of *Rickettsia canada*, a member of the typhus group. Infect Immun 1970; 2:112–114.
26. Burgdorfer W. Observations on *Rickettsia canada*: a recently described member of the typhus group rickettsiae. J Hyg Epidemiol Microbiol Immunol 1968; 12:26–31.
27. Ignatovich VF. Antigenic relations of *Rickettsia prowazekii* and *Rickettsia canada*, established in the study of sera of patients with Brill's disease. J Hyg Epidemiol Microbiol Immunol 1977; 21:55–60.
28. Roux V, Rydkina E, Eremeeva M, Raoult D. Citrate synthase gene comparison, a new tool for phylogenetic analysis, and its application for the rickettsiae. Int J Syst Bacteriol 1997; 47:252–261.
29. Roux V, Raoult D. Phylogenetic analysis of the genus *Rickettsia* by 16S rDNA sequencing. Res Microbiol 1995; 146:385–396.
30. Sekeyova Z, Roux V, Raoult D. Phylogeny of *Rickettsia* spp. inferred by comparing sequences of 'gene D', which encodes an intracytoplasmic protein. Int J Syst Evol Microbiol 2001; 51:1353–1360.
31. Eremeeva ME, Madan A, Shaw CD, Tang K, Dasch GA. New perspectives on rickettsial evolution from new genome sequences of rickettsia, particularly *R. canadensis*, and *Orientia tsutsugamushi*. Ann NY Acad Sci 2005; 1063:47–63.
32. Bozeman FM, Elisberg BL, Humphries JW, Runcik K, Palmer DB, Jr. Serologic evidence of *Rickettsia canada* infection of man. J Infect Dis 1970; 121:367–371.
33. Linnemann CC, Pretzman CI, Peterson ED. Acute febrile cerebrovasculitis—a non-spotted fever group rickettsial disease. Arch Intern Med 1989; 149:1682–1684.
34. Hechemy KE, Fox JA, Groschel DHM, Fayden FG, Wenzel RP. Immunoblot studies to analyse antibody to the *Rickettsia typhi* group antigen in sera from patients with acute febrile cerebrovasculitis. Microbiol Cell Biol 1991; 29:2559–2565.
35. Beati L, Peter O, Burgdorfer W, Aeschlimann A, Raoult D. Confirmation that *Rickettsia helvetica* sp. nov. is a distinct species of the spotted fever group of rickettsiae. Int J Syst Bacteriol 1993; 43:521–526.
36. Burgdorfer W, Aeschlimann A, Peter O, Hayes SF, Philip RN. *Ixodes ricinus*: vector of a hitherto undescribed spotted fever group agent in Switzerland. Acta Trop 1979; 36:357–367.
37. Skarphedinsson S, Jensen PM, Kristiansen K. Survey of tickborne infections in Denmark. Emerg Infect Dis 2005; 11:1055–1061.
38. Beninati T, Lo N, Noda H, et al. First detection of spotted fever group Rickettsiae in *Ixodes ricinus* from Italy. Emerg Infect Dis 2002; 8:983–986.
39. Christova I, Van De PJ, Yazar S, Velo E, Schouls L. Identification of *Borrelia burgdorferi* sensu lato, *Anaplasma* and *Ehrlichia* species, and spotted fever group Rickettsiae in ticks from Southeastern Europe. Eur J Clin Microbiol Infect Dis 2003; 22:535–542.
40. Nilsson K, Lindquist O, Liu A, Jaenson TGT, Friman G, Pahlson C. *Rickettsia helvetica* in *Ixodes ricinus* ticks in Sweden. J Clin Microbiol 1999; 37:400–403.

41. Parola P, Beati L, Cambon M, Raoult D. First isolation of *Rickettsia helvetica* from *Ixodes ricinus* ticks in France. Eur J Clin Microbiol Infect Dis 1998; 17:95–100.
42. Sanogo YO, Parola P, Shpynov SN, et al. Genetic diversity of bacterial agents detected in ticks removed from asymptomatic patients in northeastern Italy. Ann NY Acad Sci 2003; 990:182–190.
43. Hartelt K, Oehme R, Frank H, Brockmann SO, Hassler D, Kimmig P. Pathogens and symbionts in ticks: prevalence of *Anaplasma phagocytophilum* (*Ehrlichia* sp.), *Wolbachia* sp., *Rickettsia* sp., and *Babesia* sp. in Southern Germany. Int J Med Microbiol 2004; 293(suppl 37):86–92.
44. Nilsson K, Lindquist O, Pahlson C. Association of *Rickettsia helvetica* with chronic perimyocarditis in sudden cardiac death. Lancet 1999; 354:1169–1173.
45. Nilsson K, Pahlson C, Lukinius A, Eriksson L, Nilsson L, Lindquist O. Presence of *Rickettsia helvetica* in granulomatous tissue from patients with sarcoidosis. J Infect Dis 2002; 185:1128–1138.
46. Nilsson K, Liu A, Pahlson C, Lindquist O. Demonstration of intracellular microorganisms (*Rickettsia* spp., *Chlamydia pneumoniae*, *Bartonella* spp.) in pathological human aortic valves by PCR. J Infect 2005; 50:46–52.
47. Walker DH, Valbuena GA, Olano JP. Pathogenic mechanisms of diseases caused by *Rickettsia*. Ann NY Acad Sci. In press.
48. Planck A, Eklund A, Grunewald J, Vene S. No serological evidence of *Rickettsia helvetica* infection in Scandinavian sarcoidosis patients. Eur Respir J 2004; 24:811–813.
49. Fournier PE, Gunnenberger F, Jaulhac B, Gastinger G, Raoult D. Evidence of *Rickettsia helvetica* infection in humans, Eastern France. Emerg Infect Dis 2000; 6:389–392.
50. Baumann D, Pusterla N, Peter O, et al. Fever after a tick bite: clinical manifestations and diagnosis of acute tick bite-associated infections in northeastern Switzerland. Dtsch Med Wochenschr 2003; 128:1042–1047.
51. Fournier PE, Allombert C, Supputamongkol Y, Caruso G, Brouqui P, Raoult D. Aneruptive fever associated with antibodies to *Rickettsia helvetica* in Europe and Thailand. J Clin Microbiol 2004; 42:816–818.
52. Parola P, Miller RS, McDaniel P, et al. Emerging rickettsioses of the Thai–Myanmar border. Emerg Infect Dis 2003; 9:592–595.
53. Tanskul P, Stark HE, Inlao I. A checklist of ticks of Thailand (Acari: Metastigmata: Ixodoidea). J Med Entomol 1983; 20:330–341.
54. Inokuma H, Takahata H, Fournier PE, et al. Tick paralysis by *Ixodes holocyclus* in a Japanese traveler returning from Australia associated with *Rickettsia helvetica* infection. J Travel Med 2003; 10:61–63.
55. Phongmany S, Rolain JM, Phetsouvanh R, et al. Rickettsial infections and fever, Vientiane, Laos. Emerg Infect Dis 2006; 12:256–262.
56. Bell EJ, Kohls GM, Stoenner HG, Lackman DB. Nonpathogenic rickettsias related to the spotted fever group isolated from ticks, *Dermacentor variabilis* and *Dermacentor Andersoni* from Eastern Montana. J Immunol 1963; 90:770–781.
57. Ammerman NC, Swanson KI, Anderson JM, et al. Spotted-fever group Rickettsia in *Dermacentor variabilis*, Maryland. Emerg Infect Dis 2004; 10:1478–1481.
58. Anderson JF, Magnarelli LA, Philip RN, Burgdorfer W. *Rickettsia rickettsii* and *Rickettsia montana* from *Ixodid* ticks in Connecticut. Am J Trop Med Hyg 1986; 35:187–191.
59. Feng WC, Murray ES, Burgdorfer W, et al. Spotted fever group rickettsiae in *Dermacentor variabilis* from Cape Cod, Massachusetts. Am J Trop Med Hyg 1980; 29:691–694.
60. Pretzman C, Daugherty N, Poetter K, Ralph D. The distribution and dynamics of Rickettsia in the tick population of Ohio. Ann NY Acad Sci 1990; 590:227–236.
61. Macaluso KR, Sonenshine DE, Ceraul SM, Azad AF. Rickettsial infection in *Dermacentor variabilis* (Acari: Ixodidae) inhibits transovarial transmission of a second *Rickettsia*. J Med Entomol 2002; 39:809–813.
62. Parker RR, Spencer RR. Rocky mountain spotted fever: a study of the relationship between the presence of rickettsia-like organisms in tick smears and the infectiveness of the same ticks. Public Health Rep 1926; 41:461–469.
63. Burgdorfer W, Hayes SF, Mavros AJ. Nonpathogenic rickettsiae in *Dermacentor andersoni*: a limiting factor for the distribution of *Rickettsia rickettsii*. In: Brugdorfer W, Anacker RL, eds. Rickettsiae and Rickettsial Diseases. New York: Academic Press, 1981:585–594.
64. Niebylski ML, Schrumpf ME, Burgdorfer W, Fischer ER, Gage KL, Schwan TG. *Rickettsia peacockii* sp. nov., a new species infecting wood ticks, *Dermacentor andersoni*, in Western Montana. Int J Syst Bacteriol 1997; 47:446–452.
65. Simser JA, Palmer AT, Munderloh UG, Kurtti TJ. Isolation of a spotted fever group Rickettsia, *Rickettsia peacockii*, in a Rocky Mountain wood tick, *Dermacentor andersoni*, cell line. Appl Environ Microbiol 2001; 67:546–552.
66. Baldridge GD, Burkhardt NY, Simser JA, Kurtti TJ, Munderloh UG. Sequence and expression analysis of the *ompA* gene of *Rickettsia peacockii*, an endosymbiont of the Rocky Mountain wood tick, *Dermacentor andersoni*. Appl Environ Microbiol 2004; 70:6628–6636.
67. Simser JA, Rahman MS, Dreher-Lesnick SM, Azad AF. A novel and naturally occurring transposon, ISRpe1 in the *Rickettsia peacockii* genome disrupting the *rickA* gene involved in actin-based motility. Mol Microbiol 2005; 58:71–79.

68. Burgdorfer W, Brinton LP, Krinsky WL, Philip RN. *Rickettsia rhipicephali*: a new spotted fever group rickettsia from the brown dog tick *Rhipicephalus sanguineus*. In: Kazar J, Ormsbee RA, Tarasevich IV, eds. Rickettsiae and Rickettsial Diseases. Bratislava: House of the Slovak Academy of Sciences, 1978:307–316.
69. Hayes SF, Burgdorfer W. Ultrastructure of *Rickettsia rhipicephali*, a new member of the spotted fever group rickettsiae in tissues of the host vector *Rhipicephalus sanguineus*. J Bacteriol 1979; 137:605–613.
70. Lane RS, Emmons RW, Dondero DV, Nelson BC. Ecology of tick borne agents in California: further observations on rickettsiae. In: Burgdorfer W, Anacker RL, eds. Rickettsiae and Rickettsial Diseases. New York: Academic Press, 1981:575–584.
71. Philip RN, Casper EA. Serotypes of spotted fever group rickettsiae isolated from *Dermacentor andersoni* (Stiles) ticks in western Montana. Am J Trop Med Hyg 1981; 30:230–238.
72. Bacellar F, Regnery RL, Nuncio MS, Filipe AR. Genotypic evaluation of rickettsial isolates recovered from various species of ticks in Portugal. Epidemiol Infect 1995; 114:169–178.
73. Drancourt M, Kelly PJ, Regnery RL, Raoult D. Identification of spotted fever group rickettsiae using polymerase chain reaction and restriction-endonuclease length polymorphism analysis. Acta Virol 1992; 36:1–6.
74. Duh D, Petrovec M, Trilar T, et al. A follow-up study on newly recognized spotted fever group rickettsiae in ticks collected in southern Croatia. Ann NY Acad Sci 2003; 990:149–151.
75. Dupont HT, Cornet JP, Raoult D. Identification of rickettsiae from ticks collected in the Central African Republic using the polymerase chain reaction. Am J Trop Med Hyg 1994; 50:373–380.
76. Psaroulaki A, Spyridaki I, Ioannidis A, Babalis T, Gikas A, Tselentis Y. First isolation and identification of *Rickettsia conorii* from ticks collected in the region of Fokida in Central Greece. J Clin Microbiol 2003; 41:3317–3319.
77. Burgdorfer W, Sexton DJ, Gerloff RK, Anacker RL, Philip RN, Thomas LA. *Rhipicephalus sanguineus*: vector of a new spotted fever group rickettsia in the United States. Infect Immun 1975; 12:205–210.
78. Brumpt E. Longevite du virus de la fièvre boutonneuse (*Rickettsia conorii*, n. sp.) chez fa tique *Rhipicephalus sanguineus*. C R Soc Biol 1932; 110:1119.
79. Demma LJ, Traeger MS, Nicholson WL, Paddock CD, Blau DM, Eremeeva ME, Dasch GA, Levin ML, Singleton J, Jr, Zaki SR, Cheek JE, Swerdlow DL, McQuiston JH. Rocky Mountain spotted fever from an unexpected tick vector in Arizona. N Engl J Med 2005; 353:587–594.
80. Vitale G, Mansueto S, Rolain JM, Raoult D. *Rickettsia massiliae* human isolation. Emerg Infect Dis 2005; 12:174–175.
81. Eremeeva ME, Bosserman EA, Demma LJ, Zambrano ML, Blau DM, Dasch GA. Isolation and identification of *Rickettsia massiliae* from *Rhipicephalus sanguineus* ticks collected in Arizona. Appl Environ Microbiol 2006; 72:5569–5577.
82. Yano Y, Takada N, Fujita H. Ultrastructure of spotted fever group Rickettsiae in tissues of larval *Amblyomma testudinarium* (Acari: Ixodidae). J Acarol Soc Jpn 2000; 9:181–184.
83. Sekeyova Z, Fournier PE, Rehacek J, Raoult D. Characterization of a new spotted fever group Rickettsia detected in *Ixodes ricinus* (Acari: Ixodidae) collected in Slovakia. J Med Entomol 2000; 37:707–713.
84. Hirunkanokpun S, Kittayapong P, Cornet JP, Gonzalez JP. Molecular evidence for novel tick-associated spotted fever group rickettsiae from Thailand. J Med Entomol 2003; 40:230–237.
85. Fournier PE, Takada N, Fujita H, Raoult D. *Rickettsia tamurae* sp. nov., isolated from *Amblyomma testudinarium* ticks. Int J Syst Evol Microbiol 2006; 56:1673–1675.
86. Burgdorfer W, Hayes SF, Thomas LA, Lancaster JL. A new spotted fever group rickettsia from the lone star tick, *Amblyomma americanum*. In: Burgdorfer W, Anacker RL, eds. Rickettsiae and Rickettsial Diseases. New York: Academic Press, 1981:595–602.
87. Pretzman C, Stothard DR, Ralph D, Fuerst A. A new Rickettsia isolated from the lone star tick, *Amblyomma americanum* (Ixodidae). 11th Sesqui-annual Meeting of the American Society for Rickettsiology and Rickettsial Diseases, St. Simons Island, GA, 1994:24.
88. Weller SJ, Baldridge GD, Munderloh UG, Noda H, Simser J, Kurtti TJ. Phylogenetic placement of rickettsiae from the ticks *Amblyomma americanum* and *Ixodes scapularis*. J Clin Microbiol 1998; 36:1305–1317.
89. Goddard J, Norment BR. Spotted fever group rickettsiae in the lone star tick, *Amblyomma americanum* (Acari: Ixodidae). J Med Entomol 1986; 23:465–472.
90. Kelly DJ, Carmichael JR, Booton GC, Poetter KF, Fuerst PA. Novel spotted fever group Rickettsiae (SFGR) infecting *Amblyomma americanum* ticks in Ohio, USA. Ann NY Acad Sci 2005; 1063:352–355.
91. Labruna MB, Whitworth T, Bouyer DH, et al. *Rickettsia bellii* and *Rickettsia amblyommii* in *Amblyomma* ticks from the State of Rondonia, Western Amazon, Brazil. J Med Entomol 2004; 41:1073–1081.
92. Labruna MB, McBride JW, Bouyer DH, Camargo LM, Camargo EP, Walker DH. Molecular evidence for a spotted fever group *Rickettsia* species in the tick *Amblyomma longirostre* in Brazil. J Med Entomol 2004; 41:533–537.
93. Parola P, Matsumoto K, Socolovski C, Brouqui P, Parzy D, Raoult D. A tick-borne spotted fever group rickettsia similar to *Rickettsia amblyommii* in French Guyana. Ann Trop Med Parasitol. In press.

94. Dasch GA, Kelly DJ, Richards AL, Sanchez JL, Rives CC. Program and abstracts of the Joint Annual Meeting of the American Society of Tropical Medicine and Hygiene and the American Society of Parasitologists, Atlanta, USA. Am J Trop Med Hyg 2003; 49(suppl):220.
95. Anigstein L, Anigstein D. A review of the evidence in retrospect for a rickettsial etiology in Bullis fever. Tex Rep Biol Med 1975; 33:201–211.
96. Brennan JM. Field investigations pertinent to Bullis fever, Texas. Rep Biol Med 1945; 3:204–226.
97. Woodland JC, McDowell MM, Richards JT. Bullis fever (lone star fever-tick fever). J Am Med Assoc 1943; 22:1156–1160.
98. Livesey HR, Pollard M. Laboratory report on a clinical syndrome referred to as "Bullis fever." Am J Trop Med 1943; 23:475–479.
99. Anigstein L, Bader MN. Investigations on rickettsial diseases in Texas. Part 4. Experimental study of Bullis fever, Texas. Tex Rep Biol Med 1943; 1:389–409.
100. Blair PJ, Jiang J, Schoeler GB, et al. Characterization of spotted fever group rickettsiae in flea and tick specimens from northern Peru. J Clin Microbiol 2004; 42:4961–4967.
101. Jiang J, Blair PJ, Felices V, et al. Phylogenetic analysis of a novel molecular isolate of spotted fever group Rickettsiae from northern Peru: *Candidatus* Rickettsia andeanae. Ann NY Acad Sci 2005; 1063:337–342.
102. Shpynov SN, Fournier PE, Rudakov NV, Raoult D. "*Candidatus* Rickettsia tarasevichiae" in *Ixodes persulcatus* ticks collected in Russia. Ann NY Acad Sci 2003; 990:162–172.
103. Shpynov SN, Rudakov NV, Fournier PE, Raoult D. Detection of a new species of Ricketssiae in the ticks *Ixodes persulcatus* in Russia. Med Parazitol (Mosk) 2005; 2:6–9.
104. Matsumoto K, Parola P, Rolain JM, Jeffrey I, Raoult D. Detection of "*Candidatus* Rickettsia uilenbergi" and "*Candidatus* Rickettsia davousti" in *Amblyomma tholloni* ticks from elephants in Africa. Submitted.
105. Mediannikov O, Sidelnikov Y, Ivanov L, Fournier PE, Tarasevich I, Raoult D. Far eastern tick-borne rickettsiosis: identification of two new cases and tick vector. Ann NY Acad Sci 2006; 1078:80–88.
106. Cory J, Yunker CE, Howarth JA, et al. Isolation of spotted fever group and *Wolbachia*-like agents from field-collected materials by means of plaque formation in mammalian and mosquito cells. Acta Virol 1975; 19:443–445.
107. Philip RN, Casper EA, Burgdorfer W, Gerloff RK, Hugues LE, Bell EJ. Serologic typing of rickettsiae of the spotted fever group by micro immunofluorescence. J Immunol 1978; 121:1961–1968.
108. Eremeeva ME, Erdman D, Tioleco N. Utility of variable number tandem repeat (VNTR) loci for genetic subtyping of isolates of *Rickettsia rickettsii*. Abstract 151. 20th Meeting of the American Society for Rickettsiology, Asilomar, USA, Sept. 2, 2006.
109. Philip RN, Lane RS, Casper EA. Serotypes of tick-borne spotted fever group rickettsiae from western California. Am J Trop Med Hyg 1981; 30:722–727.
110. Furman DP, Loomis EC. The Ticks of California (Acari: Ixodida). Berkeley, CA: University of California Press, 1984.
111. Paddock CD. *Rickettsia parkeri* as a paradigm for multiple causes of tick-borne spotted fever in the western hemisphere. Ann NY Acad Sci 2005; 1063:315–326.
112. Billings AN, Teltow GJ, Weaver SC, Walker DH. Molecular characterization of a novel rickettsia species from *Ixodes scapularis* in Texas. Emerg Infect Dis 1998; 4:305–309.
113. Noda H, Munderloh UG, Kurtti TJ. Endosymbionts of ticks and their relationship to *Wolbachia* spp. and tick-borne pathogens of humans and animals. Appl Environ Microbiol 1997; 63:3926–3932.
114. Horta MC, Labruna MB, Sangioni LA, et al. Walker DH. Prevalence of antibodies to spotted fever group Rickettsiae in humans and domestic animals in a Brazilian spotted fever-endemic area in the state of Sao Paulo, Brazil: serologic evidence for infection by *Rickettsia rickettsii* and another spotted fever group Rickettsiae. Am J Trop Med Hyg 2004; 71:93–97.
115. Philip CB, Hughes LE. Disease agents found in the rabbit tick, *Dermacentor parumapertus*, in the southwestern United States. Atti del VI Congresso Internazionale di Microbiologia Roma, 1953:541.
116. Stoenner HG, Holdenried R, Orsborn JS. Jr. The occurrence of *Coxiella burnetii*, *Brucella*, and other pathogens among fauna of the Great Salt Lake Desert in Utah. Am J Trop Med Hyg 1959; 8:590–596.
117. Hughes LE, Clifford CM, Gresbrink R, Thomas LA, Keirans JE. Isolation of a spotted fever group rickettsia from the Pacific Coast tick, *Ixodes pacificus*, in Oregon. Am J Trop Med Hyg 1976; 25:513–516.
118. Parola P, Cornet JP, Sanogo YO, et al. Detection of *Ehrlichia* spp., *Anaplasma* spp., *Rickettsia* spp., and other eubacteria in ticks from the Thai–Myanmar border and Vietnam. J Clin Microbiol 2003; 41:1600–1608.
119. Rydkina E, Roux V, Fetisova NF, et al. New *Rickettsiae* in ticks collected in territories of the former Soviet Union. Emerg Infect Dis 1999; 5:811–814.
120. Eremeeva M, Balayeva NM, Roux V, Ignatovich V, Kotsinjan M, Raoult D. Genomic and proteinic characterization of strain S, a Rickettsia isolated from *Rhipicephalus sanguineus* ticks in Armenia. J Clin Microbiol 1995; 33:2738–2744.
121. Labruna MB, Camargo LM, Camargo EP, Walker DH. Detection of a spotted fever group Rickettsia in the tick *Haemaphysalis juxtakochi* in Rondonia, Brazil. Vet Parasitol 2005; 127:169–174.

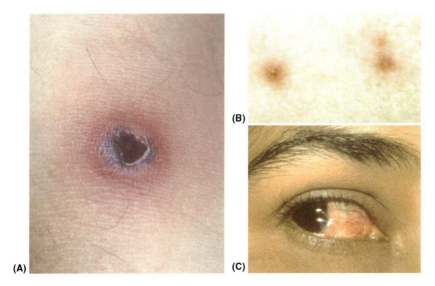

FIGURE 6.5 (**A**) Eschar on the arm of a New York City patient with rickettsialpox. *R. akari* was subsequently isolated in cell culture from this lesion (20). (**B**) Papulovesicular rash on the upper back of a New York City patient with rickettsialpox. The patient had approximately 20 to 30 similar lesions on her back and face, and first noted the rash three days after the appearance of an eschar. (**C**) Conjunctival injection in a patient with rickettsialpox. (*See text p. 75.*)

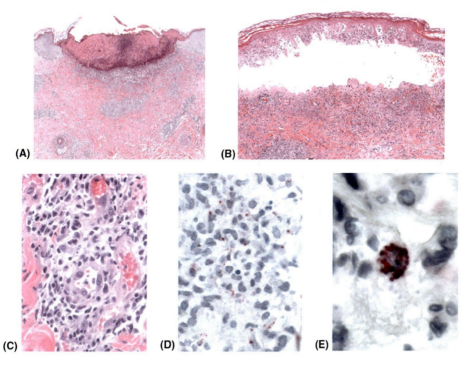

FIGURE 6.6 Cutaneous histopathology of rickettsialpox and immunohistochemical localization of *R. akari*. (**A**) A primary lesion (eschar), demonstrating extensive epidermal and dermal necrosis, with perivascular and periadnexal inflammation (original magnification: ×12.5, hematoxylin and eosin stain). (**B**) Papulovesicular lesion showing prominent subepidermal vesicle (original magnification: ×25, hematoxylin and eosin stain). (**C**) Perivascular inflammatory cell infiltrate, comprised predominantly of lymphocytes and macrophages, with swelling of vascular endothelium of involved vessel (original magnification: ×100, hematoxylin and eosin stain). (**D**) *R. akari* distributed in a perivascular inflammatory cell focus in an eschar (original magnification: ×100, immunoalkaline phosphatase with rabbit anti-*R. rickettsii* antibody and naphthol fast-red, with hematoxylin counterstain). (**E**) Coccoid intracellular *R. akari* in a macrophage in the perivascular infiltrate of an eschar (original magnification: ×158, immunoalkaline phosphatase with rabbit anti-*R. rickettsii* antibody and naphthol fast-red, with hematoxylin counterstain). (*See text p. 80.*)

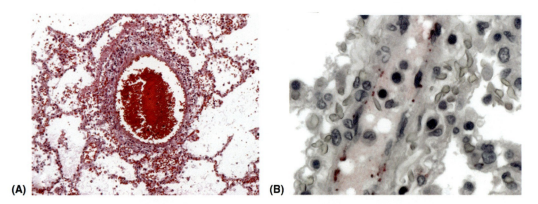

FIGURE 8.5 Histopathology and immunohistochemical localization of *R. rickettsii* in the tissues of a Brazilian patient with fatal RMSF. (**A**) Arteriole in the lung showing transmural lymphohistiocytic inflammatory infiltrate (original magnification: ×50, hematoxylin and eosin stain). (**B**) Intracellular rickettsiae in endothelial cells and intravascular mononuclear cells in a pulmonary arteriole (original magnification: ×158, polyclonal rabbit anti-*R. rickettsii* antibody, immunoalkaline phosphatase with naphthol fast-red and hematoxylin counterstain). *Abbreviation*: RMSF, Rocky Mountain spotted fever. (*See text p. 102.*)

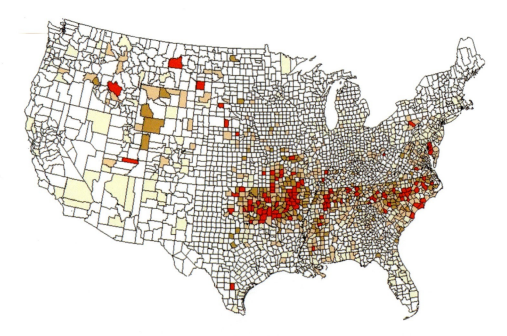

FIGURE 8.6 Annual incidence of RMSF in the United States, 1997–2002, by county of occurrence (cases per million population: *tan* = 0.01–5; *pink* = 5–15; *brown* = 15–30; *red* = 30–511). The annual incidence was computed by case reports submitted to CDC through mandated reporting to the National Electronic Telecommunications Surveillance System and census data on residents per county. *Abbreviations*: RMSF, Rocky Mountain spotted fever; CDC, Centers for Disease Control and Prevention. *Source*: From Ref. 86. (*See text p. 104.*)

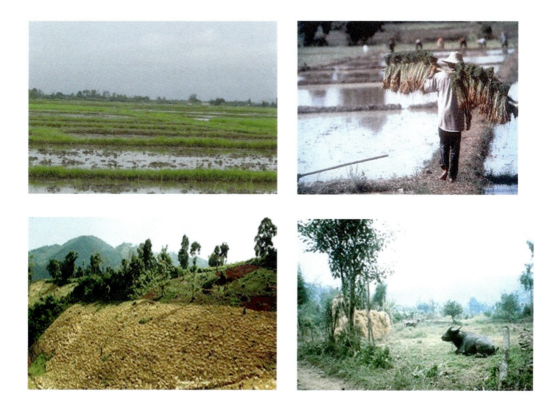

FIGURE 17.3 Scrub typhus habitats. Transmission occurs in active rice fields (*top left*). Farmers intrude on the chigger-rodent cycle taking place on walkways between flooded fields (*top right*). Typical "scrub" or secondary vegetation in Thailand (*bottom panels*). *Source*: Top left photo courtesy of Dr. Kriangkrai Lerdthusnee, Department of Entomology, AFRIMS. (*See text p. 240.*)

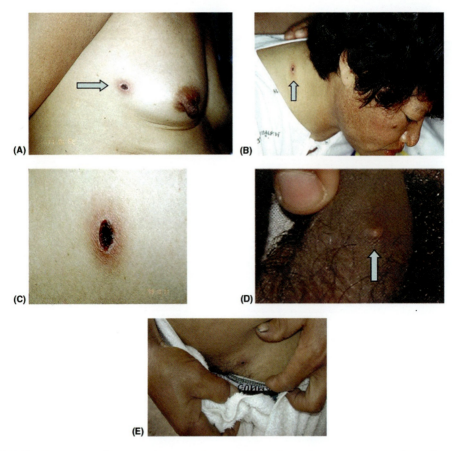

FIGURE 17.7 Two eschars (*blue arrows*) in exposed areas (**A**, **B**). Eschars (**C**) may be atypical and lose their crust in moist locations such as the scrotum (**D**). Typical eschars may be missed because they are located in difficult to examine areas (**E**). *Source*: Photos courtesy of Dr. Kriangkrai Lerdthushee. (*See text p. 245*.)

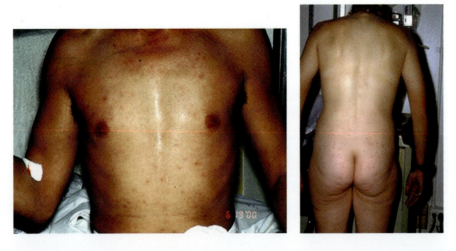

FIGURE 17.8 Scrub typhus rash. The subtle rash seen in *O. tsutsugamushi* infection is fleeting and predominates on the trunk. (*See text p. 246*.)

122. Mediannikov OY, Ivanov LI, Nishikawa M, et al. Microorganism "Montezuma" of the order Rickettsiales: the potential causative agent of tick-borne disease in the Far East of Russia. Zh Mikrobiol Epidemiol Immunobiol 2004; 1:7–13.
123. Mediannikov O, Matsumoto K, Samoilenko IE, et al. *Rickettsia raoultii* sp. nov., a new pathogenic spotted fever group rickettsia associated with tick-borne lymphadenitis. Submitted.
124. Paddock CD, Sumner JW, Comer JA, et al. *Rickettsia parkeri*: a newly recognized cause of spotted fever rickettsiosis in the United States. Clin Infect Dis 2004; 38:805–811.

Section III: ANAPLASMATACEAE AND HUMAN ANAPLASMOSIS AND EHRLICHIOSES

13 | Bacteriology and Phylogeny of Anaplasmataceae

Philippe Brouqui and Kotaro Matsumoto
Faculté de Médecine, Unité des Rickettsies, Université de la Méditerranée, Marseille, France

INTRODUCTION

Anaplasmataceae comprise a group of intracellular alpha proteobacteria that are pathogenic for certain mammals, including humans and cattle, for which the host cells are of bone marrow or hematopoietic origin including erythrocytes, monocytes or macrophages, neutrophils, and platelets. Members of this family share a high degree of nucleotide sequence similarity with respect to several chromosomal genes, such as *rrs*, *groESL* operon, citrate synthase *gltA*, ribosomal polymerase *RpoB*, and the ankyrin *Ank* gene (1). The organisms grow within a cytoplasmic vacuole containing one to many individual organisms; such structures resembled mulberries when observed by light microscopy, leading to the term "morulae." The first discovered agent was named *Anaplasma marginale* by Theiler in 1910. Since that time, several other members of the family have been described from animals and humans. Recent improvements in molecular phylogenetic methods led to a modification of the taxonomy of the Anaplasmataceae in 2001 (2). This reorganization of the genera within the family was based on comparison of sequences obtained from *rrs* (16S rRNA encoding gene) and the *groESL* operon, which contains a spacer region between *groES* and the *groEL* heat shock protein genes and is thought to be more phylogenetically informative than the coding regions (3,4). Multiple alignment and analysis of the *rrs* gene sequences as well as that of the *groESL* operon gene identified four clades: *Anaplasma*, *Ehrlichia*, *Neorickettsia*, and *Wolbachia*. Although the nomenclature largely remained unchanged, some taxa, such as *Cowdria ruminantium*, were reclassified (2). Analysis of other gene sequences as well as the complete genome sequencing of several species of the family such as *A. phagocytophilum*, *Ehrlichia chaffeensis*, *E. ruminantium*, *Neorickettsia sennetsu*, and *Wolbachia pipientis* further confirm the new organization of the family Anaplasmataceae and will be discussed in detail in this review (5). The Anaplasmataceae now include four genera: the genus *Anaplasma*, the genus *Ehrlichia*, the genus *Neorickettsia*, and the genus *Wolbachia*.

THE GENUS NEORICKETTSIA (1953)
Taxonomy and Phylogeny

The genus *Neorickettsia* was previously classified as *Ehrlichia* spp. Such a classification stimulated many unsuccessful searches for tick vectors. We now know that perpetuation depends on trematodes, as described for the first reported member of this genus, the agent of salmonid fluke poisoning. *N. helminthoeca* causes a febrile illness of western North American dogs and bears that ingest salmon infected by the fluke *Nanophyetus salmincola*. *N. sennetsu* (formerly *E. sennetsu*) is the agent of glandular (Sennetsu) fever, a mononucleosis-like illness described only in residents of Japan and Malaysia (6). Early epidemiological studies suggested that individuals that consumed uncooked fish from certain areas in Japan were at risk, which at the time seemed illogical given the ehrlichial nature of the infection (and thus implying tick transmission) but now suggesting the possibility of exposure by ingesting fish contaminated with infected flukes. *N. risticii* (formerly *E. risticii*) is the agent of Potomac horse fever in the United States, a disease that causes watery diarrhea in horses after the feed upon snail-ridden grass or ingest metacercaria-containing aquatic insects (7,8). The *Stellanantchasmus falcatus* agent was discovered in the fluke *Stellantchasmus falcatus*; no mammalian infections have been reported (9).

All four microorganisms share between 94.9% and 100% similarity in *rrs* sequences (2). Analysis and comparison of the citrate synthase gene (*gltA*) sequences of *N. risticii*, *N. sennetsu*, and *N. helminthoeca* and the β-subunit of the RNA polymerase encoding gene (*rpoB*) of *N. risticii* and *N. sennetsu* confirmed their close relationship (10,11). A phylogenetic tree based on concatenated sequences of the *groEL*, *rrs*, and *gltA* gene sequences clearly demonstrates a natural grouping of the *Neorickettsia* genus (Fig. 1).

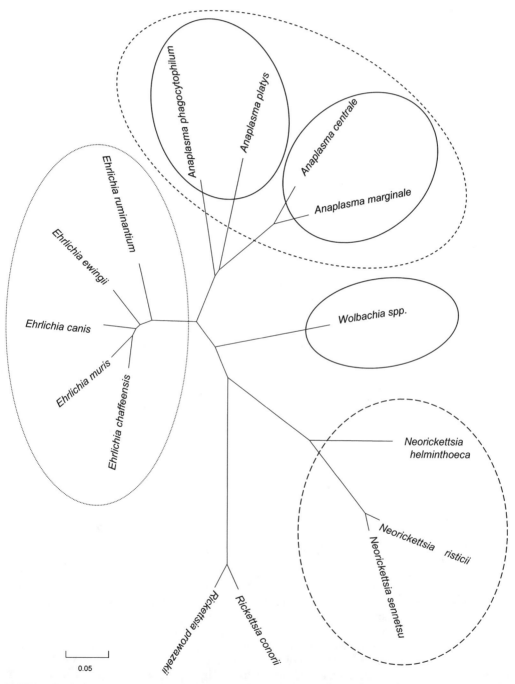

FIGURE 1 Phylogenetic tree of the Anaplasmataceae based on concatenated sequences of *rrs*, *gltA*, and *groEL* genes (3504-3566bp) using the Neighbor–Joining method.

Morphology

Neorickettsia species are coccoid or pleomorphic cells that reside in cytoplasmic vacuoles within monocytes and macrophages of dogs, horses, bats, and humans. They are gram-negative and nonmotile. These bacteria form aggregates within the vacuoles and thus present morphologically within the characteristic morulae. The morulae are less compact, however, and are smaller than those of *Ehrlichia* spp. in DH82 cells (Fig. 2) (12). By electron microscopy, they demonstrate small (0.2–0.4 μm) electron-dense forms, but relatively large (0.8–1.5 μm) lighter forms may be observed (13,14). *Neorickettsia* multiply by binary fission and are found in early endosomes enriched with transferrin receptors in the cytoplasm (15). The endosomal membrane tightly envelops individual organisms or groups of organisms.

Antigenic Characterization

Indirect fluorescent antibody tests and western immunoblot of purified cells of *N. helminthoeca*, *N. sennetsu*, and *N. risticii* using antisera from infected animals have shown that the surface antigens of these organisms are highly cross-reactive (16,17). The cross-reactive antigens detected by western blot are numerous and include a 51 to 55 kDa which should be the 55-kDa *groEL* homolog that cross-reacts with other members of the Anaplasmataceae and the Rickettsiaceae, but not *Escherichia coli* (18). Alternatively, these antigens represent a 51-kDa putative outer membrane protein (19).

Metabolism

Members of the genus *Neorickettsia* possess an aerobic type of metabolism and are asaccharolytic. *Neorickettsia* can utilize glutamine and glutamate and can generate adenosine triphosphate (20,21) but prefer to use glutamine rather than glutamate. This may be explained by the fact that the organisms are enveloped by the host membrane and that the glutamine enters endosomes more readily than glutamate. *Neorickettsia* cannot utilize glucose-6-phosphate or glucose. Their greatest metabolic activities are observed at pH 7.2 to 8.0 and decline rapidly below pH 7 (20).

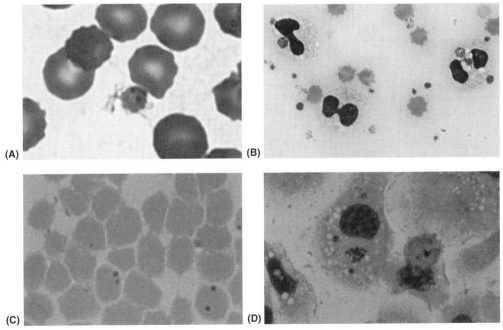

FIGURE 2 Morphology of Anaplasmataceae. (**A**) *A. platys* inclusions in infected thrombocyte (smear from naturally infected dog), (**B**) *A. phagocytophilum* in circulating neutrophils (smear from a naturally infected horse), (**C**) *A. marginale* in erythrocytes (smear from experimentally infected cow), and (**D**) *E. canis* in DH82 monocytic cell line from in vitro culture. *Source*: Figures (**A**) and (**C**) courtesy of Pr Inokuma.

Recently, the comparative genomics of *Neorickettsia* with other members of the Anaplasmataceae and the Rickettsiaceae demonstrated that *Neorickettsia*, as well as other Anaplasmataceae, have the ability to synthesize all nucleotides and most vitamins and cofactors (5). This ability is different from that of the Rickettsiaceae that cannot make purines or pyrimidines and therefore must rely on nucleotide translocases and interconversion of the bases to obtain the full complement of nucleotides (22). The presence of nucleotide, vitamin, and cofactor biosynthetic pathways in Anaplasmataceae suggest that they do not need to compete with the host cell and may even supply host cells with essential vitamins and nucleotides. In addition, genomic analyses of the Anaplasmataceae suggest that *Neorickettsia* as well as other members of the family have the ability to make glycine and aspartate.

Host–Parasite Interaction

Neorickettsia are transmitted and maintained in trematodes found in snails of the family Pleuroceridae (23). Infection of mammals is required for completion of the life cycle of the trematodes, but it is not directly required for the maintenance of *Neorickettsia*. Dogs, horses, bats, and humans accidentally acquire *Neorickettsia* by ingestion of the metacercaria stage of the trematodes in fish or adult aquatic insects. *N. helminthoeca* infects neither the fish nor the snails carrying the trematode.

Physiopathology and Immune Response

Neorickettsia enter macrophages by receptor-mediated endocytosis, not by phagocytosis, and reside in early endosomes that do not fuse with lysosomes (24). Internalization and proliferation are dependant on Ca^{2+}-calmodulin-signalin and protein tyrosine phosphorylation (25). Release of *Neorickettsia*, with *Ehrlichia*, appears to occur not only by cell lysis, but also through exocytosis by fusion of the inclusion membrane with the plasma membrane (13,26). Both humoral and cell-mediated immune responses appear to play significant roles in protection. The presence of neutralizing antibodies and antibody-dependent cellular toxicity has been demonstrated using a cell culture system and a murine model (27). Polyclonal antiserum to *N. risticii*, for example, does not inhibit binding of *N. risticii* cells to P388D1 macrophages or their internalization, but internalized antibody-coated *N. risticii* fails to survive (28).

THE GENUS *ANAPLASMA* (1910)
Taxonomy and Phylogeny

The genus *Anaplasma* includes three species that infect circulating erythrocytes, one species that infects platelets, and two species that infect circulating white blood cells. *A. marginale* is responsible for bovine anaplasmosis, a severe febrile hemolytic anemia of cattle that occurs after bites of several different tick species such as *Dermacentor andersoni* in Northern America and *Boophilus microplus* in Africa; the infection occurs worldwide. *A. centrale* causes a similar but usually mild disease in cattle, and *A. ovis* does so in sheep and goats. *A. platys* is the causative agent of infectious cyclic thrombocytopenia in dogs and cats, a disease that manifests as progressively diminishing episodes of fever and thrombocytopenia. The bacterium is transmitted to animal by the bite of *Rhipicephalus sanguineus* or *Amblyomma* sp. ticks. *A. bovis* is the causative agent of bovine ehrlichiosis of Africa, the Middle East, India, and Sri Lanka, a disease that is clinically characterized by fluctuating fever lymphadenopathy, depression, and occasionally death (29). *A. bovis* infects circulating monocytes of cattle. The principal manifestations include fever, anorexia, diarrhea, and infrequently, involvement of the central nervous system. Leucopenia and thrombocytopenia may occur. *A. bovis* is transmitted by ticks including *Rh. appendiculatus* and *Amblyomma variegatum* in Africa (29) and possibly by *A. cajennense* in Guadaloupe and Brazil. *A. bovis* has also been detected in the Americas, and *A. bovis*-like *rrs* gene sequence has been detected in rabbits from Nantucket Island in the United States.

The human granulocytic *Ehrlichia*—*E. equi*—*E. phagocytophila* are granulocytic agents that infect ruminants such as cattle, sheep, and goats causing "Pasture fever" or "tick-borne fever" (30). Infection of horses is referred to as equine granulocytic ehrlichiosis (31), and that of humans is referred to as human granulocytic ehrlichiosis (HGE) (32). Rodents are commonly infected. This species is transmitted by hard ticks of the genus *Ixodes* such as *Ixodes dammini* and *I. pacificus* in the United States and *I. ricinus* and *I. trianguliceps* in Europe (33). The cell targets of this *Ehrlichia* are granulocytes. Main clinical features are fever, leucopenia, and thrombocytopenia. Liver damage has been reported in humans.

The agents known as *E. equi*, *E. phagocytophila*, and HGE share at least 99.1% nucleotide sequence similarity in their *rrs* genes and have identical *GroEL* amino acid sequences (2). Similar findings have been reported with the *gltA* gene. These microorganisms also share the same tick vectors, the target cell, and ecology, and they are virtually indistinguishable by their antigenic properties. Consequently, all three were merged into *A. phagocytophilum* (2), a new combination name for the agent first described in 1949 as *Cytoecetes phagocytophila*. The new combination name was given in reference to the historical precedence of *Anaplasma* (Theiler 1910) and its validity has been debated among ehrlichial scientific experts. In fact, some of them have proposed to separate this group from the genus *Anaplasma* and to return it to the genus *Cytoecetes* in reference to the previously described "*Cytoecetes microti*" (Tyzzer 1938) which clearly demonstrated phenotypic similarity to *A. phagocytophilum* (34). From 1949 to the mid-1990s, European veterinary literature referred to the agent of tick-borne fever as *C. phagocytophila*. In fact, *A. marginale* and *A. phagocytophilum* differ with respect to tick vectors (metastriate vs. prostriate ticks, respectively), mammalian host, cell target, epidemiology, and clinical presentation. This renders confusing the practice by some authors to refer to the erythrocytic infection as animal anaplasmosis and the granulocytic infection as human anaplasmosis. Such a change in the common name for the infection (all variants of tick-borne fever) is not supported by established data (35). When using more variable gene sequence comparisons such as the *gltA* gene or *GroESL*, the erythrocytic *A. marginale* and *A. centrale* cluster together and apart from the granulocytic *A. phagocytophilum* and the thrombocytic *A. platys* (10,35,36) supporting the interpretation that they are within distinct genera. This is shown by a phylogeny based on concatenated (3504–3566 bp) sequences of the *rrs*, *gltA*, and *groEL* genes shown in Figure 1. Moreover, the estimated G+C content of the DNA of *Anaplasma* spp. varies between approximately 30 and 56 mol.% (2). Microorganisms that show more than 10 mol.% differences in DNA G+C content are considered to be within different genera (37,38). The G+C mol.% content of *A. phagocytophilum* is 43.8 and that of *A. marginale* is 56, suggesting that these two bacteria should not be classified within the same genus. The name "*Cytoecetes*" was arbitrarily omitted from the Approved List of Bacterial Names when that list was developed. However, as more data are accumulated, it seems that the granulocytic *Anaplasma* will eventually be reclassified as distinct from the erythrocytic *Anaplasma*, and returned to the previously validly published genus *Cytoecetes*.

Morphology

Small, often pleomorphic or coccoid cells ranging from 0.3 to 0.4 μm in diameter are found in cytoplasmic inclusion bodies (morulae) in mature or immature hematopoietic mammalian cells. Morulae are suspended in a nonfibrillar matrix, ranging in size up to 4 μm in diameter and appearing more compact and bigger than those of *Neorickettsia* in DH82 cells (12). No spore formation has been reported. In blood, the organisms appear as intracellular round inclusions in the target cells and stainbluish-purple by Romanowsky methods. *Anaplasma* are Gram-negative and nonmotile. No lipopolysaccharide and lipooligosaccharide have been detected in the cell wall of *Anaplasma* and no information is available on whether it contains peptidoglycan. By electron microscopy, *A. phagocytophilum* can be seen to reside within membrane-bound vacuoles that are very early endosomes (39). The ultrastructure of the cell envelope reveals simple inner and outer leaflets similar to those of gram-negative bacteria (40). The internal structures consisting of chromatin strands and ribosomes are readily visualized. Two morphologic forms are described: a large reticulate cell and a smaller "dense core" form. Both undergo binary fission. Interestingly, and similar to members of the genus *Ehrlichia*, *Anaplasma* lack genes for lipid A biosynthesis. They also incorporate cholesterol for their survival, as other fastidious and pleomorphic bacteria do (41).

Antigenic Characterization—Antigenic Variability

All *Anaplasma* species contain a multigene family encoding major surface proteins that are the immunodominant antigen of the genus. The genes are generally characterized by the presence of highly conserved 5′ and 3′ sequences that flank a hypervariable core region (42,43). One or several of these genes may be transcriptionally active to produce protein antigens of various molecular sizes ranging from 36 to 49 kDa (44).

Like the bacteria from the genus *Ehrlichia*, *Anaplasma* have the ability to escape mammalian immune system. This phenomenon was first identified in *A. marginale*, which parasites the erythrocytes of ruminants. The bacteria possess a major surface protein of 36 kDa named MSP2. This protein is encoded by the *MSP2* multigene family (45). In infected ruminants, *A. marginale* may persist several years (up to seven years) due to cyclic variation of the MSP2 (46). Each *A. marginale* bacteremia is associated with an MSP2 variant. Ticks ingest with their blood meal a heterogeneous population of *A. marginale* MSP2 variants and this heterogeneity seems restricted when the *A. marginale* multiplies within salivary gland of the tick (46). Other members of the genus *Anaplasma* such as *A. phagocytophilum* possess the same multigene family suggesting that this phenomenon may support the persistence of these pathogens in their infected host (46,47). Moreover, *MSP2* is considered an adhesion protein and its diversity would be important for adaptation to new mammalian niches (48,49).

Host–Parasite Interaction

To date, Ixodid ticks (*Ixodes ricinus*) are the only known vectors for all *Anaplasma* species. *D. andersoni*, *B. microplus*, *I. dammini*, *I. pacificus*, and *I. ricinus*, among others, are important biological vectors. Mechanical vectors such as male ticks and biting flies may also contribute to the transmission of *A. marginale*. The bacteria are maintained in the tick by transstadial, but not transovarial transmission, thus, emergent larval ticks are not infectious. Ticks are consequently vectors but not reservoirs. Domestic and wild ruminants, especially cervids, are considered as the main amplifying hosts for bacteria of the *Anaplasma* genus, but small mammals such as mice or other rodents may serve in that capacity for *A. phagocytophilum*.

Target Cells

Anaplasma species are found in cytoplasmic vacuoles of hematopoietic cells, in the peripheral blood, or in tissues containing mononuclear phagocytes such as spleen, liver, and bone marrow. The target cells depend on the species involved. *A. marginale*, *A. centrale*, *A. ovis* parasites the erythrocytes, *A. phagocytophilum* the polymorphonuclear cells, *A. bovis* the mononuclear cells, and *A. platys* the platelets. Invasion and survival strategies of *A. phagocytophilum* have been well described and recently reviewed (50). *A. phagocytophilum* binds to P-selectin glycoprotein ligand-1 (PSGL-1) of human neutrophils, thereby explaining its tropism for this target cell (51). Like members of the genus *Neorickettsia*, *A. phagocytophilum* resides within a vacuole that does not fuse with lysosomes. It specifically blocks lysosome fusion with the protective phagosome in which it resides. Similar to what has been reported in *Neorickettsia*, this inhibition is dependant on bacterial protein synthesis as oxytetracycline treatment results in maturation of the *A. phagocytophilum*-containing vacuoles (52). *A. phagocytophilum* escape from cell-dependent killing by repression of nicotinamide adenine dinucleotide phosphate (NADPH) oxidase and consequent inhibition of superoxide anion (O_2^-) production. It also delays neutrophil apoptosis, which in addition to partially compensating for *A. phagocytophilum*'s long doubling time, probably extends its host cell life such that it can successfully execute the aforementioned strategies (50,53).

THE GENUS *EHRLICHIA* (1945)
Taxonomy and Phylogeny

This genus includes several species recognized to be pathogenic in humans or in animals: *E. canis*, *E. chaffeensis*, *E. ewingii*, *E. ruminantium* (formerly *C. ruminantium*), and *E. muris* (2). *E. canis* parasites the circulating monocytes and is transmitted to dogs, coyotes, foxes, and wolves by the tick *Rh. sanguineus* and cause canine monocytic ehrlichiosis or "tropical canine pancytopenia," which is a severe febrile infection distributed worldwide. Asymptomatic and more recently symptomatic infection by *E. canis* has been reported in humans (54). *E. chaffeensis* infects mainly human monocytes causing human monocytic ehrlichiosis. Infection in deer, goats, and dogs may be persistent; deer appear to be the main amplifying host. Transmission occurs mainly by the bite of the Lone Star tick, *A. Americanum*, although limited data suggest that the American dog ticks *D. variabilis* may also play a role in transmission (55). Human monocytic ehrlichiosis can result in severe illness with fever, pancytopenia, and occasionally other manifestations such as meningitis. The distribution seems limited to North America, reflecting the distribution of the Lone Star tick vector. *E. ewingii* has been regarded as solely a dog pathogen but has recently been reported to cause disease in humans (56). *E. ewingii* causes a granulocytic ehrlichiosis by infecting peripheral circulating neutrophils of dogs and humans and cause mild to moderate illness with fever and pancytopenia. The disease seems restricted to the United States reflecting the distribution of its vector, again the Lone Star tick. *E. ruminantium* has recently been renamed (formerly *C. ruminantium*) because it shared many biological characteristics with members of the genus *Ehrlichia* (2). *E. ruminantium* is the causative agent of heartwater or cowdriosis, a severe infection of ruminants that occurs after bites of ticks of the genus *Amblyomma*, particularly *A. variegatum* and *A. haebreum*. The disease is limited to sub-Saharan Africa and the Caribbean, paralleling the distribution of the tick vector (57). *E. ruminantium* infects primarily the endothelial cells of the mammal host, and when the cells of the capillaries of the brain become infected, causes encephalitis. The pathophysiology of the pathognomonic lesion of hydropericardium (thus, "heartwater") remains poorly described. Recently, *E. ruminantium* DNA has been detected in young patients with encephalitis in South Africa (58). *E. ruminantium* forms a distinct clade in the genus *Ehrlichia* but differs from other species of the same genus by only 0.2% to 0.5% in the *rrs* sequence, and by 12.4% from *E. canis groESL* gene sequence (3). *E. muris*, an infection of Asian rodents, has not been reported yet as a human pathogen. *E. muris* causes mild to severe infection in wild mice including splenomegaly and lymphadenopathy. In Japan under natural conditions, *Haemaphysalis flava* ticks transmit *E. muris*. *E. muris* occupies a distinct clade in the genus *Ehrlichia* but shares at least 99.7% sequence similarity in the *rrs* gene and 80.2% in the *gltA* gene with *Ehrlichia* spp. (Table 1) (10). Although members of this genus display several differences in cell target, epidemiology, antibiotic sensitivity, and clinical presentation, they share numerous serological cross-reactions. Their genetic relatedness and DNA G+C mol.% content comprise less than 5% difference between each member, confirming that they belong to the same genus (Table 2).

Morphology

Cell morphology of *Ehrlichia* is very similar to that of *Anaplasma*. *Ehrlichia* occur in membrane-bound vacuoles forming morulae in cells of hematopoietic origin, and for one species within endothelial cells. As do *Anaplasma*, they lack genes for lipid A biosynthesis explaining why lipopolysaccharide has not yet been detected in *Ehrlichia* (41). By electron microscopy, the cell envelope reveals simple inner and outer leaflets similar to those of Gram-negative bacteria. *Ehrlichia* undergo binary fission and present as both dense-core and reticulate bodies. They may also produce an abundant membrane that on occasion wraps around individual *Ehrlichia* or invaginates into the ehrlichial cells and occasionally forms tubule and vesicle profiles in the vacuolar space. Unlike the genus *Anaplasma*, *Ehrlichia* possess a fibrillar matrix within the vacuolar space (40).

Antigenic Characterization

Among sequences that have been characterized in *Ehrlichia*, some genes encode immunoreactive proteins such as the *E. chaffeensis* 120 kDa, the variable-length PCR target protein (VLPT) and the p28 multigene family, as well as homologs such as the *map1* multifamily gene of *E. ruminantium*. The *E. chaffeensis* 120-kDa gene encodes a heavily glycosylated, immunodominant surface protein that is mainly expressed on dense-core forms and as a component on the intracellular matrix of *E. chaffeensis*. This gene demonstrates interstrain variation, and the p120 protein expressed by different isolates of *E. chaffeensis* vary in molecular weight although immune sera from patients with human monocytic ehrlichiosis (HME) react with p120 antigens from various strains regardless of variations in the number of repeated units (59). The VLPT gene demonstrates even greater interstrain diversity. The 28-kDa multigene family of *E. chaffeensis* (Arkansas strain) comprises at least 22 complete paralogous genes from 813 to 900 kb distributed along a 27-kb segment of the genome (60). None of the 26- to 32-kDa proteins encoded are identical, and the amino acid sequence identity varies from approximately 20% to

(Text continues on page 189.)

TABLE 1 Levels of Similarity Between gltA Sequences, Citrate Synthase Amino Acid Sequences, and 16S rRNA Gene Sequences of the Members of the *Anaplasmataceae*

Organism	C+G (mol%)[a]	1	2	3	4	5	6	7	8	9	10	11	12	13
E. muris	38.5		94.7 (94.1)	87.1 (85.6)	85.4 (84.9)	80.2 (79.0)	60.8 (59.8)	57.8 (58.7)	58.0 (57.2)	53.8 (44.4)	54.6 (45.4)	53.4 (47.5)	60.8 (51.9)	57.4 (51.6)
IOE[b]	NA	98.7		87.1 (86.8)	85.7 (86.1)	79.7 (78.6)	60.8 (58.5)	57.1 (58.3)	57.7 (57.1)	53.4 (45.9)	54.6 (46.0)	54.8 (48.8)	60.6 (52.1)	57.8 (52.5)
E. chaffeensis	33.9	98.1	98.7		85.1 (84.6)	79.0 (76.6)	63.1 (59.5)	57.8 (58.5)	58.1 (58.5)	53.5 (46.2)	53.7 (46.2)	53.2 (48.7)	61.6 (50.7)	58.2 (52.8)
E. canis	35.3	97.3	97.8	98.2 (92.4)		79.5 (77.8)	61.1 (58.8)	58.2 (58.0)	58.3 (58.0)	53.1 (45.4)	53.8 (45.9)	54.6 (49.7)	62.2 (53.9)	58.5 (54.7)
E. ruminantium	32.2	97.2	97.3	97.6 (88.2)	97.2 (87.6)		63.3 (61.3)	58.5 (58.8)	58.3 (58.4)	54.2 (46.1)	54.4 (47.3)	55.3 (49.6)	60.8 (51.4)	57.8 (51.7)
A. phagocytophilum	43.8	92.4	92.5	92.7 (76.4)	92.3 (76.7)	92.5 (75.7)		63.8 (65.5)	63.8 (64.0)	50.6 (46.2)	50.5 (46.7)	53.5 (49.7)	55.8 (51.5)	53.3 (50.6)
A. marginale	56	92.2	92.4	92.2	92.2	92.2	96.4		74.6 (78.9)	50.1 (44.9)	50.3 (45.4)	53.1 (49.2)	53.9 (49.4)	55.3 (50.2)
A. centrale	NA	92.0	92.2	92.0	91.9	91.7	96.1	98.1		50.3 (44.9)	49.7 (44.7)	53.1 (46.2)	53.8 (49.4)	52.7 (49.8)
N. sennetsu	42	84.0	83.8	84.0	83.9	84.2	85.0	84.7	84.4		94.9 (95.0)	63.9 (64.3)	52.8 (47.2)	54.2 (46.9)
N. risticii	42	83.7	83.5	83.8 (60.7)	83.6 (60.9)	83.8 (59.1)	84.8 (59.4)	84.7	84.3	99.0		65.3 (66.1)	53.3 (48.2)	54.7 (47.1)
N. helmintoeca	42	84.2	84.5	84.5	84.5	84.2	84.6	84.3	83.9	94.3	94.8		53.6 (47.6)	52.7 (50.5)
R. prowazekii		82.7	82.4	82.8	82.7	83.2	83.9	83.4	83.6	82.4	82.2	81.9		64.2 (61.1)
B. henselae		82.5	82.5	82.8 (60.1)	82.6 (60.1)	82.7 (58.5)	83.4 (58.5)	82.7	83.2	81.3	81.0 (60.6)	81.1	85.2	

The values on the upper right are the levels of similarity between 16S rRNA gene sequences and (in parentheses) between groEL sequences. C+G mol% content among *Anaplasmataceae* evaluated by genome sequencing or by gene sampling.
[a]C+G mol% content among *Anaplasmataceae*
[b]IOE: *Ixodes Ovatus* Ehrlichia (*Ehrlichia* sp. HF strains).
Source: From Ref. 3.

The values on the upper right are the levels of similarity between gltA sequences and (in parentheses) between citrate synthase amino acid sequences, and the values on the lower left are the levels of similarity between 16S rRNA gene sequences and (in parentheses) between groEL sequences.

TABLE 2 List of all microorganisms closely related to Anaplasmataceae based on comparison of the *rrs* gene sequence and listed in GenBank® at July 2006 with accession number and for which the *rrs* gene is more than 98% similar to that of representative bacterium (type strain or established species)

Microorganisms placed in the tree and considered as type strain of the species	Microorganisms for which difference of *rrs* genes are less than 2% with type strain and should be considered as isolates or strains
*1 *N. risticii* Shasta-CDMP strain, AF206300	*N. risticii* Illinois, M21290
	N. risticii S22, AY005439
	N. risticii horse2, AF380258
	N. risticii horse1, AF380257
	N. risticii SHSN-1, AF037210
	N. risticii SHSN-2, AF037211
	N. risticii, AF036654
	N. risticii, AF036653
	N. risticii S6, AY005441
	N. risticii, AF036649
	Ehrlichia sp. SF agent, U34280
*2 *N. sennetsu* Miyayama, CP000237	*N. sennetsu*, M73225
*3 *E. canis* Jake, CP000107	*E. canis* Gzh982, AF162860
	E. canis Oklahoma, M73221
	E. canis Florida, M73226
	E. canis Madrid, AY394465
	E. canis VDE, AF373613
	E. canis VHE, AF373612
	E. canis Kagoshima 1, AF536827
	E. canis 611, U26740
	Ehrlichia sp. Tibet, AF414399
	Ehrlichia sp. ERm58, AF311967
	E. ovina Turkey, AF318946
	Ehrlichia sp. Germishuys, U54805
	Ehrlichia sp. EBm52, AF497581
	Ehrlichia sp. EHt224, AF311968
*4 *Ehrlichia* sp. EHf699, AY309969	*Ehrlichia* sp. EH1087, AY309971
	Ehrlichia sp. EH727, AY309970
*5 *E. chaffeensis* Arkansas, CP000236	*E. chaffeensis*, AF147752
	E. chaffeensis 91HE17, U23503
	E. chaffeensis St. Vincent, U86665
	E. chaffeensis Jax, U86664
	E. chaffeensis Sapulpa, U60476
*6 *Ehrlichia* sp. HF565, AB024928	*Ehrlichia* sp. Shizuoka-36, AB178793
	Ehrlichia sp. FN147, AB196303
	Ehrlichia sp. HI-2000, AF260591
	Ehrlichia sp. Anan, AB028319
*7 *E. muris* AS145, U15527	*E. muris* FN2619, AB196302
	E. muris NA1, AB013009
	E. muris I268, AB013008
*8 *Ehrlichia* sp. TS37, AB074459	*Ehrlichia* sp. SS15-E-L, AB211162
*9 *E. ewingii* 95E9-TS, U96436	*E. ewingii*, M73227
*10 *E. ruminantium* Welgevonden, CR925678	*E. ruminantium* Ball3, U03777
	E. ruminantium BelaVista, AF318022
	E. ruminantium Gardel, CR925677
	E. ruminantium Mara87/7, AF069758
	E. ruminantium Omatjenne, U03776
	E. ruminantium Porto Henrique, AF318021
	E. ruminantium Senegal stock, X62432
	E. ruminantium, X61659
	Ehrlichia sp. South African canine, AF325175
*11 *Candidatus* Neoehrlichia mikurensis Nagano21, AB196305	*Candidatus* Neoehrlichia mikurensis IS58, AB074460
	Candidatus Neoehrlichia mikurensis TK4456, AB084582
	Candidatus Neoehrlichia mikurensis FIN686, AB196304
	Candidatus Neoehrlichia mikurensis TJ43, AB213021
	Candidatus Neoehrlichia mikurensis Rattus, AY135531
	Ehrlichia-like sp. Schotti variant, AF104680

(*Continued*)

TABLE 2 List of all microorganisms closely related to Anaplasmataceae based on comparison of the *rrs* gene sequence and listed in GenBank® at July 2006 with accession number and for which the *rrs* gene is more than 98% similar to that of representative bacterium (type strain or established species) (*Continued*)

Microorganisms placed in the tree and considered as type strain of the species	Microorganisms for which difference of *rrs* genes are less than 2% with type strain and should be considered as isolates or strains
*12 *A. marginale* 2:3, AF414878	*A. marginale* Eland, AF414872
	A. marginale F12, AF414874
	A. marginale Florida, AF309867
	A. marginale Hongan, DQ341369
	A. marginale Lushi, AJ633048
	A. marginale, M60313
	A. marginale Macheng, DQ341370
	A. marginale non-tailed, AF414875
	A. marginale tailed, AF414876
	A. marginale South Africa, AF414871
	A. marginale South Idaho, AF309868
	A. marginale St. Maries, AY048816
	A. marginale Uruguay, AF414877
	A. marginale Veld, AF414873
	A. marginale Virginia, AF309866
	A. marginale Virginia, AF311303
*13 *A. ovis* OVI, AF414870	*A. ovis*, AF318945
	A. ovis, AY262124
	A. ovis Chende, AJ633052
	A. ovis G2.12.2, AY837735
	A. ovis G2.12.25, AY837736
	A. ovis G2.12.46, AY837737
	A. ovis Idaho, AF309865
	A. ovis Jingtai, AJ633049
	A. ovis Yuzhong, AJ633050
	A. ovis Zhangjiachuan, AJ633051
*14 *A. centrale* South Africa, AF414869	*A. centrale*, AB211164
	A. centrale, AF283007
	A. centrale Israel vaccine, AF309869
	A. centrale vaccine, AF318944
	A. centrale vaccine, AF414868
*15 *A. bovis*, U03775	*A. bovis*, AB211163
	A. bovis, AY144729
	A. bovis NR07, AB196475
	Anaplasma sp. AnHl446, AF497579
*16 *Anaplasma* sp. S Africa dog-1076, AY570539	*Anaplasma* sp. S Africa dog-1108, AY570538
	Anaplasma sp. S Africa dog-1245, AY570540
*17 *A. platys* Gzh981, AF156784	*A. platys*, AF286699
	A. platys, AF287153
	A. platys, AY530806
	A. platys, M82801
	A. platys Okinawa 1, AF536828
	A. platys Okinawa, AY077619
	A. platys Sommieres, AF303467
	A. platys Venezuela-Lara, AF399917
	Anaplasma sp. AnDa465, AF497576
	Ehrlichia sp. Omatjenne, U54806
	Ehrlichia sp. Bom Pastor, AF318023
	Uncultured *Anaplasma* sp. G2.12.31, AY837739
	Uncultured *Anaplasma* sp. G2.12.35, AY837740
	Uncultured *Anaplasma* sp. G2.12.7B, AY837738
*18 *Ehrlichia*-like sp., U52514	*Ehrlichia* sp. GA No. 2, U27103
	Ehrlichia sp. GA No. 4, U27104
	Ehrlichia sp. OK No. 1, U27102
	Ehrlichia sp. OK No. 3, U27101

TABLE 2 List of all microorganisms closely related to Anaplasmataceae based on comparison of the *rrs* gene sequence and listed in GenBank® at July 2006 with accession number and for which the *rrs* gene is more than 98% similar to that of representative bacterium (type strain or established species) (*Continued*)

Microorganisms placed in the tree and considered as type strain of the species	Microorganisms for which difference of *rrs* genes are less than 2% with type strain and should be considered as isolates or strains
*19 *A. phagocytophilum* HZ, CP000235	*A. phagocytophilum* FG, M73224
	A. phagocytophilum OS, M73220
	A. phagocytophilum CAHU-HGE1, AF093788
	A. phagocytophilum CAHU-HGE2, AF093789
	A. phagocytophilum CAMAWI, AF172167
	A. phagocytophilum CAMEBS, AF172165
	A. phagocytophilum CASITL, AF172166
	A. phagocytophilum CASOLJ, AF172164
	A. phagocytophilum ES34, AB196720
	A. phagocytophilum J4-3-1, AY969010
	A. phagocytophilum J4-3-2, AY969011
	A. phagocytophilum J4-3-4, AY969012
	A. phagocytophilum J4-3-5, AY969013
	A. phagocytophilum J4-3-6, AY969014
	A. phagocytophilum J4-3-7, AY969015
	A. phagocytophilum Jilin-1, DQ342324
	A. phagocytophilum, M73223
	A. phagocytophilum NCH-1/530-N8, U23039
	A. phagocytophilum NCH-1, U23038
	A. phagocytophilum SS33P-L, AB196721
	A. phagocytophilum Strong, AY527214
	A. phagocytophilum Susy, AY527213
	A. phagocytophilum, U02521
	A. phagocytophilum USG3, AY055469
	Ehrlichia sp. LGE agent, AF241532
	Ehrlichia sp., AF057707
	Ehrlichia sp., AF084907
	Ehrlichia sp. Ia, AJ242785
	Ehrlichia sp. Ib, AJ242783
	Ehrlichia sp. Jena 14, AJ312941
	Ehrlichia sp. Jena 16, AJ313512
	Ehrlichia sp. Jena 22, AJ312939
	Ehrlichia sp. Jena 238, AJ313511
	Ehrlichia sp. Jena 72, AJ312940
	Ehrlichia sp. Jena 8, AJ313513
	Ehrlichia sp. Jena 84, AJ312942
	Ehrlichia sp. RND-1, AF469005
	Ehrlichia sp. rosa, U10873
	Ehrlichia sp. Swiss horse 1, U77389
	Ehrlichia sp. type IIb, AJ242784

80% (61). A very similar system has been identified in *E. canis* and *E. ruminantium* (62). Variations in reactivity among different isolates of *E. chaffeensis* have also been demonstrated with monoclonal antibodies reflecting the diversity of p28 proteins.

Host–Parasite Interaction

Ticks are the only known vectors for *Ehrlichia* species. Although the organisms are passed transstadially in ticks, definite transovarial transmission of identified *Ehrlichia* has not been demonstrated. The range of potential vertebrate host for *Ehrlichia* species is not completely defined owing to a lack of clinical signs in many reservoirs hosts, including deer and small mammals. Some mammalian hosts, such as the white-tailed deer, some ruminants, and dogs maintain infectivity for long intervals (months or years) in the absence of clinical signs, whereas other mammals, such as some dog breeds and humans, develop sterile immunity after clinically apparent primary infection. Thus, natural maintenance of *Ehrlichia* is dependent on horizontal transmission involving either acute or persistently infected mammals and ticks.

Target Cells

The target cells depend upon the *Ehrlichia* species involved. *E. chaffeensis*, *E. canis*, and *E. muris* infect monocytes in humans, deer, dogs, and mice, respectively, whereas *E. ewingii* infects neutrophils in canine or human hosts. *E. ruminantium* infects endothelial cells and neutrophils, mainly in cattle. *Ehrlichia* species access host cells by adherence to surface proteins that are usually glycosylated. The bacteria are then internalized within early endosomes. For *E. chaffeensis*, the endosomes selectively accumulate transferrin receptors effectively sequestering the infected vacuole into a receptor salvage pathway that precludes lysosomal fusion (15).

THE GENUS *WOLBACHIA* (1936)
Taxonomy and Phylogeny

The genus *Wolbachia* includes a group of intracellular bacteria found in arthropods (insects, spiders, mites, ticks, and crustacea) and in filarial nematodes (63–65). *W. pipientis* is currently regarded as the sole species of the genus *Wolbachia* (2). Older descriptions of the genus *Wolbachia* included two other species, *W. persica* and *W. Melophagi*, that have characteristics distinguishing them from *W. pipientis*. *W. persica* belongs to the gamma-proteobacteria and has been reclassified as *Francisella persica*. The exact taxonomic position of *W. melophagi* has yet to be determined but a number of its characteristics are not in accordance with the family Anaplasmataceae and in fact are more like the gamma proteobacteria (66). Despite the existence of a single valid *Wolbachia* species, this agent encompasses a wide range of molecular diversity which renders difficult attempts to construct a phylogeny of the genus. To date, at least 105 sequences of the *rrs* gene longer than 1000 bp have been deposited in GenBank®. The phylogeny of the genus has been clarified by polyphasic gene analysis of the *rrs*, *ftsZ*, *dnaA*, and *wsp* genes, and has identified six main lineages of *Wolbachia* provisionally named supergroups A–F (67,68). Interestingly, supergroups A, B, and E include most of the *Wolbachia* thus far detected in arthropods, while supergroups C and D include most of those found in filarial nematodes (67). The remaining supergroup F includes those found in termites and in the filarial nematode *Mansonella ozzardi* (69). It is generally recognized that the level of divergence of the *rrs* gene sequence should be of at least 3% between bacterial species (70). The level of divergence between the six main supergroup is around 3% which suggests that each of these may represent a single species, each with different variants or strains (69). However, there is a general consensus among the *Wolbachia* community to conservatively maintain the single species name *W. pipientis* until new data are generated (69).

Morphology

The bacteria of the genus *Wolbachia* appear as small rods and coccoid forms of 0.5 to 1.3 μm and as the other members of the Anaplasmataceae family are strict intracellular bacteria growing in the vacuoles of the host cell. These bacteria are associated with arthropods and filarial nematodes. Interestingly, they are responsible for reproductive alterations in arthropods. Their role in human disease has recently been demonstrated by the fact that these bacteria are required for persistence of nematode infection in human filariasis. *W. pipientis* is not stained at all with gram stain although its cell wall structure is that of gram-negative bacteria. As with other *Anaplasmataceae*, Romanowsky stains render the agent purple or dark-blue. A peptidoglycan has not yet been observed. A bacteriophage-like element has recently been reported (71). *W. pipientis* multiplies by binary fission in the vacuoles of host cells and is surrounded by a membrane of host origin. In arthropods, the bacteria are present mostly in the cytoplasm of cells of the reproductive organs, but they can also be observed in other tissues, including nervous tissues and hemocytes. In filarial nematodes, *Wolbachia* is present in the lateral cords and in the female reproductive apparatus. In both arthropods and nematodes, *Wolbachia* is transovarially transmitted to the offspring (63). A strain of *W. pipientis* has been established in an *Aedes albopictus*-derived cell line and has been deposited at the ATCC under No. VR-1529.

Host–Parasite Interaction

In arthropods, *Wolbachia* infection is usually associated with alterations in host reproduction, which include killing of male embryos, induction of parthenogenesis, feminization of genetic males, and cytoplasmic incompatibility (CI) (72). It must be noted that females transmit *Wolbachia* to the offspring, whereas males are usually not involved in transmission. All the reproductive alterations effected by *Wolbachia* in arthropods are interpreted as having the overall effect of increasing the transmission rate of *Wolbachia* (72). Parthenogenesis and feminization cause a *Wolbachia*-infected female to generate more female offspring, which will in turn transmit the bacterium. In CI, embryonic death is observed after mating between males that are infected by certain strain of *Wolbachia* and females that are either uninfected or infected with an incompatible *Wolbachia* strain. Males infected by *Wolbachia* do not transmit it, but they sterilize those females that do not carry *Wolbachia* or those that carry a different compatibility type of *Wolbachia*. This reduction of the fitness of uninfected females implies an increase of the fitness of infected ones, thereby favoring the spread of the CI-inducing *Wolbachia* in the host population.

In nematodes, the presence of *Wolbachia* seems restricted to the subfamilies Onchocercinae and Dirofilariinae (69). Within Onchocercinae and Dirofilariinae, there are species that are infected and others that appear refractory; when a species is known to be infected, almost all individuals within that species are infected. Experimental work using antibiotics have provided direct evidence for the existence of a symbiotic relationship. Antibiotics, in reducing the number of *Wolbachia*, reduced the microfilaremia. Clinical trials have shown the efficiency of antibiotics, particularly tetracycline, in the treatment of onchocerciasis (73). Doxycycline administered for six weeks at 200 mg/day resulted in a reduction of more than 95% of *Wolbachia* levels leading to a chronic decline in microfilarial load (74). Filarial nematodes and their *Wolbachia* endosymbionts appear to be reciprocally dependent.

Immune Response

Antibody responses to a number of *Wolbachia* antigens have been observed in both human and animal filariasis, including the major surface protein (WSP), HSP60, HtrA-type serine protease, and aspartate aminotransferase (69). In patients diagnosed with pulmonary dirofilariasis, IgG responses to WSP are elevated compared to healthy individuals and blood donors from nonendemic areas suggesting a possible serodiagnostic test for pulmonary dirofilariasis (75). Studies on WSP serology in human filariasis show an association with the presentation and the duration of chronic disease in lymphatic filariasis. A transient elevation in WSP reactivity seems associated with onset of lymphoedema suggesting that the immune response evoked by *Wolbachia* may trigger the development of disease (76).

GENERAL ORGANIZATION OF THE DIFFERENT GENERA IN THE FAMILY ANAPLASMATACEAE

To summarize the phylogenetic position of the family Anaplasmataceae including most recent published data, we constructed a concatenated phylogenetic tree with available sequences of the *rrs*, *gltA*, and *groEL* genes. Representative species which belong to Anaplasmataceae and of which *rrs*, *gltA*, and *groEL* sequences were available were used to construct the phylogenetic tree. The GenBank® accession numbers of *rrs*, *gltA*, and *groEL* gene sequences used to construct the phylogenetic tree were as follows: *A. centrale*—AF414869, AF304141, and AF414866; *A. marginale*—AF309867, AF304140, and AF414865; *A. platys*—AF303467, AB058782, and AY044161; *A. phagocytophilum*—CP000235, CP000235, and CP000235; *E. canis*—CP000107, CP000107, and U96731; *E. chaffeensis*—CP000236, CP000236, and CP000236; *E. ewingii*—U96436, DQ365879, and AF195273; *E. muris*—U15527, AF304144, and AF210459; *E. ruminantium*—CR925677, CR925677, and CR925677; *N. helminthoeca*—U12457, AF304149, and AY050315; *N. risticii*—AF206300, AF304147, and U24396; *N. sennetsu*—CP000237, CP000237, and CP000237; *Rickettsia conorii*—NC_003103, NC_003103, and NC_003103; and *R. prowazekii*—NC_000963, NC_000963, and NC_000963. For each species that was included, gene sequences (*rrs*, 1389–1402 bp; *gltA*, 1004–1058 bp; *groEL*, 1106–1115 bp; and totally 3504–3566 bp) were concatenated and then alignment was performed using the ClustalW (DDBJ, http://www.ddbj.nig.ac.jp/search/clustalw-e.html). Phylogenies were inferred from aligned sequences using MEGA 3.1 (http://www.megasoftware.net/) using the neighbor-joining algorithm with 1000 bootstrap replicates; 50% consensus trees were selected and are presented in Figure 1. In addition, in order to offer a better overview of the phylogeny of

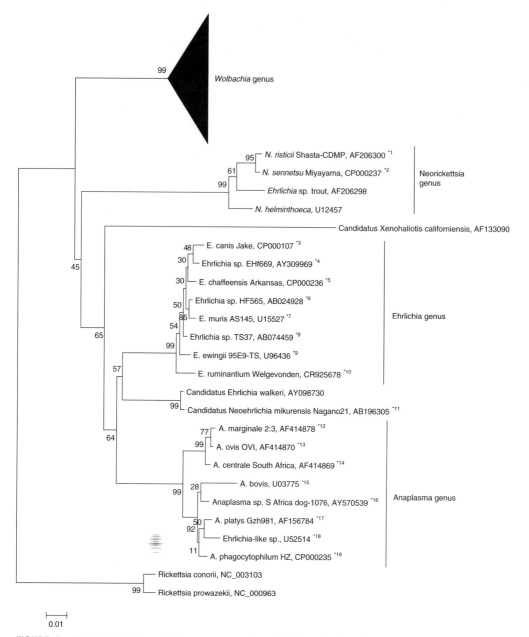

FIGURE 3 Neighbor-Joining method *rrs* sequence-based phylogenic tree of Anaplasmataceae species. Only microorganisms sharing more than 98% of *rrs* sequence similarities are shown. Remaining organisms are shown in Table 2.

the Anaplasmataceae, we constructed a phylogenetic tree based on the *rrs* gene of all Anaplasmataceae members that were available in GenBank®. We decided to include in the analysis only agents which have been recognized as established species, or share the same clade as others which exhibit less than 2% sequence differences with the type strain (70). Other agents were designated as isolates of the same species and included in the table.

rrs gene sequences from Anaplasmataceae species that are greater than 1000 bp were collected from GenBank®, and the phylogenetic tree was constructed as described above (Fig. 3). To avoid confusion in the tree, all microorganisms for which the *rrs* gene is more than

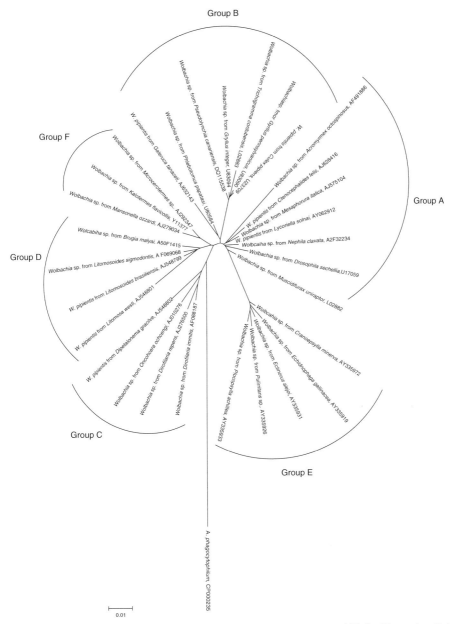

FIGURE 4 Neighbor-Joining method *rrs* sequence-based phylogenic tree of Wolbachia species. Only microorganisms sharing more than 97% of *rrs* sequence similarities are shown. Remaining organisms are shown in Table 3.

98% similar to that of representative bacterium (type strain or establish species) are separately shown in Table 2. *Wolbachia* clade is separately shown in Figure 4. Similarly, all *Wolbachia* microorganisms for which the *rrs* gene is more than 97% similar to that of representative bacterium (type strain or establish species) are separately shown in Table 3. The GenBank® accession numbers used to construct the phylogenetic tree are shown in the figures.

CONCLUSION

Knowledge on the bacteriology and phylogeny of Anaplasmataceae has rapidly improved within recent years due to advances in genomics and analytic techniques. Much more will

TABLE 3 List of all Microorganisms Closely Related to *Wolbachia* Based up on Comparison of the *rrs* Gene Sequence and Listed in GenBank® at July 2006 with Accession Number

Wolbachia supergroup	Bacteria name	GenBank® Accession No.
Group C	*W. pipientis* from *Dipetalonema gracile*	AJ548802
	W. pipientis from *Mansonella* sp.	AJ628417
	Wolbachia sp. from *Dirofilaria immitis*[a]	AF088187
	Wolbachia sp. from *Dirofilaria immitis*	AF487892
	Wolbachia sp. from *Dirofilaria immitis*	Z49261
	Wolbachia sp. from *Dirofilaria. repens*	AJ276500
	Wolbachia sp. from Okinawa2 canine blood	AF537217
	Wolbachia sp. from *Onchocerca gibsoni*	AJ276499
	Wolbachia sp. from *Onchocerca gutturosa*	AJ276498
	Wolbachia sp. from *Onchocerca ochengi*	AJ010276
	Wolbachia sp. from *Rhipicephalus sanguineus*[b]	AF304445
Group D	*W. pipientis* from *Litomosa westi*	AJ548801
	W. pipientis from *Litomosoides brasiliensis*	AJ548799
	W. pipientis from *Litomosa galizai*	AJ548800
	W. pipientis from *Litomosa hamletti*	AJ548798
	Wolbachia sp. from *Brugia malayi*	AF051145
	Wolbachia sp. from *Brugia malayi*	AJ010275
	Wolbachia sp. from *Brugia pahangi*	AJ012646
	Wolbachia sp. from *Litomosoides sigmodontis*	AF069068
	Wolbachia sp. from *Wuchereria bancrofti*	AF093510
Group F	*Wolbachia* sp. from *Cameronieta strandmanni*	DQ288985
	Wolbachia sp. from *Kalotermes flavicollis*	Y11377
	Wolbachia sp. from *Mansoneella ozzardi*	AJ279034
	Wolbachia sp. from *Mansoneella perstans*	AY278355
	Wolbachia sp. from *Microcerotermes* sp.	AJ292347
Group B	Symbiont of *Nasonia vitripennis*	M84686
	W. pipientis from *Culex pipiens*	X61768
	W. pipientis from *Galeruca tanaceti*	AJ619995
	W. pipientis from *Galeruca tanaceti*	AJ632144
	W. pipientis from *Galeruca tanaceti*	AJ632145
	Wolbachia pipientis from *Culex pipiens*	U23709
	Wolbachia pipientis from *Galeruca tanaceti*	AJ632143
	Wolbachia sp. brouquii genotype	DQ402520
	Wolbachia sp. from *Callosobruchus chinensis*	AB025965
	Wolbachia sp. from *Diaphorina citri*	AB038370
	Wolbachia sp. from *Drosophila mauritiana*	U17060
	Wolbachia sp. from *Gryllus tanaceti*	AM180551
	Wolbachia sp. from *Gryllus assimilis*	U83091
	Wolbachia sp. from *Gryllus integer*	U83094
	Wolbachia sp. from *Gryllus integer*	U83095
	Wolbachia sp. from *Gryllus integer*	U83096
	Wolbachia sp. from *Gryllus integer*	U83097
	Wolbachia sp. from *Gryllus ovisopis*	U83093
	Wolbachia sp. from *Gryllus pennsylvanicus*	U83090
	Wolbachia sp. from *Gryllus rubens*	U83092
	Wolbachia sp. from *Metaseiulus occidentalis*	AY754820
	Wolbachia sp. from *Phlebotomus papatasi*	U80584
	Wolbachia sp. from *Phlebotomus. perniciosus*	DQ402518
	Wolbachia sp. from *Pseudolynchia canariensis*	DQ115538
	Wolbachia sp. from *Sitophilus oryzae*	AF035160
	Wolbachia sp. from *Tetranychus urticae*	AY753174
	Wolbachia sp. from *Trichogramma cordubensis*	L02883
	Wolbachia sp. from *Trichogramma deion*	L02884
	Wolbachia sp. from *Trichogramma deion*	L02886
	Wolbachia sp. from *Trichogramma deion*	L02887
	Wolbachia sp. from *Trichogramma deion*	L02888
	Wolbachia sp. from *Trichogramma pretiosum*	L02885
Group A	*W. pipientis* from *Ctenocephalides felis*	AJ628416
	W. pipientis from *Drosophila simulans*	AY833061

(Continued)

TABLE 3 List of all Microorganisms Closely Related to *Wolbachia* Based up on Comparison of the *rrs* Gene Sequence and Listed in GenBank® at July 2006 with Accession Number (*Continued*)

Wolbachia supergroup	Bacteria name	GenBank® Accession No.
	W. pipientis from *Folsomia candida*	AF179630
	W. pipientis from *Folsomia candida*	AY549179
	W. pipientis from *Folsomia candida*	AY549180
	W. pipientis from *Galeruca tanaceti*	AJ632146
	W. pipientis from *Lycoriella solani*	AY026912
	Wolbachia pipientis from *Galeruca tanaceti*	AJ632147
	Wolbachia pipientis from Lycoriella solani	AY026913
	Wolbachia sp. from *Acalymma blandulum*	AY007548
	Wolbachia sp. from *Acalymma vittatum*	AY007549
	Wolbachia sp. from Acromyrmex octospinosus	AF491885
	Wolbachia sp. from *Acromyrmex octospinosus*	AF491886
	Wolbachia sp. from *Acromyrmex octospinosus*	AF491887
	Wolbachia sp. from *Acromyrmex octospinosus*	AF491888
	Wolbachia sp. from *Agelastica alni*	AM180550
	Wolbachia sp. from *Diabrotica cristata*	AY007550
	Wolbachia sp. from *Diabrotica lemniscata*	AY007547
	Wolbachia sp. from *Diabrotica virgifera*	AY007551
	Wolbachia sp. from *Diabrotica virgifera*	U83098
	Wolbachia sp. from *Diabrotica innubila*	AY876253
	Wolbachia sp. from *Diabrotica melanogaster*	AE017196
	Wolbachia sp. from Diabrotica sechellia	U17059
	Wolbachia sp. from Mesaphorura italica	AJ575104
	Wolbachia sp. from *Mesaphorura macrochaeta*	AJ422184
	Wolbachia sp. from Nephila clavata	AF232234
	Wolbachia sp. from *Paratullbergia callipygos*	AJ509026
	Wolbachia sp. from *Thecodiplosis japonensis*	AF220604
Group E	*Wolbachia* sp. from *Adoratopsylla intermedia*	AY335929
	Wolbachia sp. from Craneopsylla minerva	AY335927
	Wolbachia sp. from *Craneopsylla felis*	AY335923
	Wolbachia sp. from Echidnophaga gallinacea	AY335919
	Wolbachia sp. from Ectinorus alejoi	AY335931
	Wolbachia sp. from *Geusibia ashcrafti*	AY335921
	Wolbachia sp. from *Jellisonia* sp.	AY335917
	Wolbachia sp. from *Myodopsylla gentilis*	AY335918
	Wolbachia sp. from *Orchopeas leucopus*	AY335924
	Wolbachia sp. from *Oropsylla hirsuta*	AY335925
	Wolbachia sp. from *Peromyscopsylla selensis*	AY335928
	Wolbachia sp. from *Phtiropsylla agenoris*	AY335932
	Wolbachia sp. from Plocopsylla achillea	AY335933
	Wolbachia sp. from *Polygenis pradoi*	AY335930
	Wolbachia sp. from Pulirritans sp.	AY335926
	Wolbachia sp. from *Pulsimulans* sp.	AY335934
	Wolbachia sp. from *Sphinctopsylla area*	AY335920
	Wolbachia sp. from *Xenopsylla cheopis*	AY335935
	Wolbachia sp. from *Xenopsylla cheopis*	AY335936

Highlighted in bold are microorganisms that do not share more than 97% sequence homology and might reach the species definition. Others should be stains or isolates.
[a]Dog may be infected with *Dirofilaria immitis*.
[b]*Rhipicephalus sanguineus*, brown dog tick, may feed on dog infected with *Dirofilaria immitis*.

undoubtedly be reported in the near future. However, the amount of new data generated, particularly the detection and identification of new gene sequences that may represent new bacteria, may confuse the systematics of this family. Although the taxonomic position of *Ehrlichia* and *Neorickettsia* seems to be clarified and is likely to remain so, the relationship between the erythrocytic *Anaplasma* and the granulocytic *Anaplasma* requires further definition. *Wolbachia* is the larger genus with respect to the number of potentially distinct taxa, although for now *Wolbachia* experts prefer to maintain a single species name, *W. pipientis*. Given the great genetic diversity that is apparent, it is critical that polyphasic studies (cell biology, experimental infection, serological) be done to clarify the taxonomic relevance of such diversity.

ACKNOWLEDGMENT

The authors thank S.R. Telford III for English review of the manuscript and judicious comments that allow us to improve our review.

REFERENCES

1. Dumler JS, Rikihisa Y, Dash G. *Anaplasma*. In: Brenner DJ, Krieg NR, Staley JT, Garrity GM, eds. The Proteobacteria, Part C, Bergey's Manual of Systematic Bacteriology. New York: Springer, 2005: 117–125.
2. Dumler JS, Barbet AF, Bekker CP, et al. Reorganization of genera in the families Rickettsiaceae and Anaplasmataceae in the order Rickettsiales: unification of some species of *Ehrlichia* with *Anaplasma*, *Cowdria* with *Ehrlichia*, and *Ehrlichia* with *Neorickettsia*, descriptions of six new species combinations and designation of *Ehrlichia*, *equi* and 'HGE agent' as subjective synonyms of *Ehrlichia phagocytophila*. Int J Syst Evol Microbiol 2001; 51:2145–2165.
3. Sumner JW, Nicholson WL, Massung RF. PCR amplification and comparison of nucleotide sequences from the *groESL* heat shock operon of *Ehrlichia* species. J Clin Microbiol 1997; 35:2087–2092.
4. Sumner JW, Storch GA, Buller RS, et al. PCR amplification and phylogenetic analysis of *groESL* operon sequences from *Ehrlichia ewingii* and *Ehrlichia muris*. J Clin Microbiol 2000; 38:2746–2749.
5. Dunning Hotopp JC, Lin M, et al. Comparative genomics of emerging human ehrlichiosis agents. PLoS Genet 2006; 2:E21.
6. Misao T, Kobayashi Y. Studies on infectious mononucleosis (glandular fever): isolation of etiologic agent from blood, bone marrow, and lymph node of a patient with infectious monocleosis by using mice. Kyushu J Med Sci 1955; 6:145–152.
7. Barlough JE, Reubel GH, Madigan JE, Vredevoe LK, Miller PE, Rikihisa Y. Detection of *Ehrlichia risticii*, the agent of potomac horse fever, in freshwater stream snails (Pleuroceridae: *Juga* spp.) from northern California. Appl Environ Microbiol 1998; 64:2888–2893.
8. Reubel GH, Barlough JE, Madigan JE. Production and characterization of *Ehrlichia risticii*, the agent of potomac horse fever, from snails (Pleuroceridae: *Juga* spp.) in aquarium culture and genetic comparison to equine strains. J Clin Microbiol 1998; 36:1501–1511.
9. Wen BH, Rikihisa Y, Yamamoto S, Kawabata N, Fuerst PA. Characterization of the SF agent, an *Ehrlichia* sp. isolated from the fluke *Stellantchasmus falcatus*, by 16S rRNA base sequence, serological, and morphological analyses. Int J Syst Bacteriol 1996; 46:149–154.
10. Inokuma H, Brouqui P, Drancourt M, Raoult D. Citrate synthase gene sequence: a new tool for phylogenetic analysis and identification of *Ehrlichia*. J Clin Microbiol 2001; 39:3031–3039.
11. Taillardat-Bisch AV, Raoult D, Drancourt M. RNA polymerase beta-subunit-based phylogeny of *Ehrlichia* spp., *Anaplasma* spp., *Neorickettsia* spp., and *Wolbachia pipientis*. Int J Syst Evol Microbiol 2003; 53:455–458.
12. Rikihisa Y, Stills H, Zimmerman G. Isolation and continuous culture of *Neorickettsia helminthoeca* in a macrophage cell line. J Clin Microbiol 1991; 29:1928–1933.
13. Rikihisa Y. The tribe *Ehrlichieae* and ehrlichial diseases. Clin Microbiol Rev 1991; 4:286–308.
14. Rikihisa Y, Perry BD, Cordes DO. Ultrastructural study of ehrlichial organisms in the large colons of ponies infected with potomac horse fever. Infect Immun 1985; 49:505–512.
15. Barnewall RE, Ohashi N, Rikihisa Y. *Ehrlichia chaffeensis* and *E. sennetsu*, but not the human granulocytic ehrlichiosis agent, colocalize with transferrin receptor and up-regulate transferrin receptor mRNA by activating iron-responsive protein 1. Infect Immun 1999; 67:2258–2265.
16. Brouqui P, Dumler JS, Raoult D, Walker DH. Antigenic characterization of ehrlichiae: protein immunoblotting of *Ehrlichia canis*, *Ehrlichia sennetsu*, and *Ehrlichia risticii*. J Clin Microbiol 1992; 30:1062–1066.
17. Rikihisa Y. Cross-reacting antigens between *Neorickettsia helminthoeca* and *Ehrlichia* species, shown by immunofluorescence and Western immunoblotting. J Clin Microbiol 1991; 29:2024–2029.
18. Zhang Y, Ohashi N, Lee EH, Tamura A, Rikihisa Y. *Ehrlichia sennetsu groE* operon and antigenic properties of the *groEL* homolog. FEMS Immunol Med Microbiol 1997; 18:39–46.
19. Vemulapalli R, Biswas B, Dutta SK. Cloning and molecular analysis of genes encoding two immunodominant antigens of *Ehrlichia risticii*. Microb Pathog 1998; 24:361–372.
20. Weiss E, Dasch GA, Kang YH, Westfall HN. Substrate utilization by *Ehrlichia sennetsu* and *Ehrlichia risticii* separated from host constituents by renografin gradient centrifugation. J Bacteriol 1988; 170:5012–5017.
21. Weiss E, Williams JC, Dasch GA, Kang YH. Energy metabolism of monocytic *Ehrlichia*. Proc Natl Acad Sci USA 1989; 86:1674–1678.

22. Andersson SG, Zomorodipour A, Andersson JO, et al. The genome sequence of *Rickettsia prowazekii* and the origin of mitochondria. Nature 1998; 396:133–140.
23. Nyberg PA, Knapp SE, Millemann RE. "Salmon Poisoning" disease. IV. Transmission of the disease to dogs by *Nanophyetus salmincola* eggs. J Parasitol 1967; 53:694–699.
24. Wells MY, Rikihisa Y. Lack of lysosomal fusion with phagosomes containing *Ehrlichia risticii* in P388D1 cells: abrogation of inhibition with oxytetracycline. Infect Immun 1988; 56:3209–3215.
25. Rikihisa Y, Zhang Y, Park J. Role of Ca^{2+} and calmodulin in ehrlichial infection in macrophages. Infect Immun 1995; 63:2310–2316.
26. Brouqui P, Birg ML, Raoult D. Cytopathic effect, plaque formation, and lysis of *Ehrlichia chaffeensis* grown on continuous cell lines. Infect Immun 1994; 62:405–411.
27. Rikihisa Y, Wada R, Reed SM, Yamamoto S. Development of neutralizing antibody in horses infected with *Ehrlichia risticii*. Vet Microbiol 1993; 36:139–147.
28. Messick JB, Rikihisa Y. Inhibition of binding, entry, or intracellular proliferation of *Ehrlichia risticii* in P388D1 cells by anti-*E. risticii* serum, immunoglobulin G, or Fab fragment. Infect Immun 1994; 62:3156–3161.
29. Rioche M. Bovine rickettsiosis in Senegal. Rev Elev Med Vet Pays Trop 1966; 19:485–494.
30. Gordon WS, Brownlee A, Wilson DR, Macleod J. Tick-borne fever (a hitherto undescribed disease of sheep). J Comp Pathol 1932; 45:301–312.
31. Gribble DH. Equine ehrlichiosis. J Am Vet Med Assoc 1969; 155:462–469.
32. Bakken JS, Dumler JS, Chen SM, Eckman MR, Van Etta LL, Walker DH. Human granulocytic ehrlichiosis in the Upper Midwest United States. J Am Med Assoc 1994; 272:212–218.
33. Parola P. Tick-borne rickettsial diseases: emerging risks in Europe. Comp Immunol Microbiol Infect Dis 2004; 27:297–304.
34. Telford SR III, Dawson JE, Katavolos P, Warner CK, Kolbert CP, Persing DH. Perpetuation of the agent of human granulocytic ehrlichiosis in a deer tick-rodent cycle. Proc Natl Acad Sci USA 1996; 93:6209–6214.
35. Lew AE, Gale KR, Minchin CM, Shkap V, De Waal DT. Phylogenetic analysis of the erythrocytic *Anaplasma* species based on 16S rDNA and *GroEL* (Hsp60) sequences of *A. marginale*, *A. centrale*, and *A. ovis* and the specific detection of *A. centrale* vaccine strain. Vet Microbiol 2003; 92:145–160.
36. Inokuma H, Fujii K, Okuda M, et al. Determination of the nucleotide sequences of heat shock operon *GroESL* and the citrate synthase gene (*Glta*) of *Anaplasma* (*Ehrlichia*) *platys* for phylogenetic and diagnostic studies. Clin Diagn Lab Immunol 2002; 9:1132–1136.
37. Goodfellow M, Manfio GP, Chun J. Towards a practical species concept for cultivable bacteria. In: Clarridge MF, Dawah HA, eds. Species: The Units of Biodiversity. London: Chapman & Hall, 1997:25–29.
38. Stackebrandt E, Frederiksen W, Garrity GM, et al. Report of the ad hoc committee for the re-evaluation of the species definition in bacteriology. Int J Syst Evol Microbiol 2002; 52:1043–1047.
39. Webster P, Ijdo JW, Chicoine LM, Fikrig E. The agent of human granulocytic ehrlichiosis resides in an endosomal compartment. J Clin Invest 1998; 101:1932–1941.
40. Popov VL, Han VC, Chen SM, et al. Ultrastructural differentiation of the genogroups in the genus *Ehrlichia*. J Med Microbiol 1998; 47:235–251.
41. Lin M, Rikihisa Y. *Ehrlichia chaffeensis* and *Anaplasma phagocytophilum* lack genes for lipid a biosynthesis and incorporate cholesterol for their survival. Infect Immun 2003; 71:5324–5331.
42. Barbet AF. Recent developments in the molecular biology of anaplasmosis. Vet Parasitol 1995; 57:43–49.
43. Viseshakul N, Kamper S, Bowie MV, Barbet AF. Sequence and expression analysis of a surface antigen gene family of the Rickettsia *Anaplasma marginale*. Gene 2000; 253:45–53.
44. Asanovich KM, Bakken JS, Madigan JE, Aguero-Rosenfeld M, Wormser GP, Dumler JS. Antigenic diversity of granulocytic *Ehrlichia* isolates from humans in Wisconsin and New York and a horse in California. J Infect Dis 1997; 176:1029–1034.
45. Palmer GH, Eid G, Barbet AF, Mcguire TC, Mcelwain TF. The immunoprotective *Anaplasma marginale* major surface protein 2 is encoded by a polymorphic multigene family. Infect Immun 1994; 62:3808–3816.
46. Palmer GH, Brown WC, Rurangirwa FR. Antigenic variation in the persistence and transmission of the *Ehrlichia anaplasma marginale*. Microbes Infect 2000; 2:167–176.
47. Caspersen K, Park JH, Patil S, Dumler JS. Genetic variability and stability of *Anaplasma phagocytophila* MSP2 (P44). Infect Immun 2002; 70:1230–1234.
48. Park J, Choi KS, Dumler JS. Major surface protein 2 (MSP2) of *Anaplasma phagocytophilum* facilitates adherence to granulocytes. Infect Immun 2003; 71:4018–4025.
49. Scorpio DG, Caspersen K, Ogata H, Park J, Dumler JS. Restricted changes in major surface protein-2 (MSP2) transcription after prolonged in vitro passage of *Anaplasma phagocytophilum*. BMC Microbiol 2004; 4:1.
50. Carlyon JA, Fikrig E. Invasion and survival strategies of *Anaplasma phagocytophilum*. Cell Microbiol 2003; 5:743–754.

51. Herron MJ, Nelson CM, Larson J, Snapp KR, Kansas GS, Goodman JL. Intracellular parasitism by the human granulocytic ehrlichiosis bacterium through the P-selectin ligand, PSGL-1. Science 2000; 288:1653–1656.
52. Gokce HI, Ross G, Woldehiwet Z. Inhibition of phagosome–lysosome fusion in ovine polymorphonuclear leucocytes by *Ehrlichia* (Cytoecetes) *phagocytophila*. J Comp Pathol 1999; 120:369–381.
53. Carlyon JA, Fikrig E. Mechanisms of evasion of neutrophil killing by *Anaplasma phagocytophilum*. Curr Opin Hematol 2006; 13:28–33.
54. Perez M, Bodor M, Zhang C, Xiong Q, Rikihisa Y. Human infection with Ehrlichia canis accompanied by clinical signs in Venezuela. Ann NY Acad Sci 2006; 1078:110–117.
55. Dumler JS. *Anaplasma* and *Ehrlichia* infection. Ann NY Acad Sci 2005; 1063:361–373.
56. Buller RS, Arens M, Hmiel SP, et al. *Ehrlichia ewingii*, a newly recognized agent of human ehrlichiosis. N Engl J Med 1999; 341:148–155.
57. Parola P, Jourdan J, Raoult D. Tick-borne infection caused by *Rickettsia africae* in the West Indies. N Engl J Med 1998; 338:1391.
58. Allsopp MT, Louw M, Meyer EC. *Ehrlichia ruminantium*: an emerging human pathogen? Ann NY Acad Sci 2005; 1063:358–360.
59. Paddock CD, Childs JE. *Ehrlichia chaffeensis*: a prototypical emerging pathogen. Clin Microbiol Rev 2003; 16:37–64.
60. Ohashi N, Rikihisa Y, Unver A. Analysis of transcriptionally active gene clusters of major outer membrane protein multigene family in *Ehrlichia canis* and *E. chaffeensis*. Infect Immun 2001; 69:2083–2091.
61. Yu X, Mcbride JW, Zhang X, Walker DH. Characterization of the complete transcriptionally active *Ehrlichia chaffeensis* 28 kDa outer membrane protein multigene family. Gene 2000; 248:59–68.
62. Reddy GR, Sulsona CR, Barbet AF, Mahan SM, Burridge MJ, Alleman AR. Molecular characterization of a 28 kDa surface antigen gene family of the tribe *Ehrlichiae*. Biochem Biophys Res Commun 1998; 247:636–643.
63. Bandi C, Trees AJ, Brattig NW. *Wolbachia* in filarial nematodes: evolutionary aspects and implications for the pathogenesis and treatment of filarial diseases. Vet Parasitol 2001; 98:215–238.
64. Taylor MJ, Hoerauf A. *Wolbachia* bacteria of filarial nematodes. Parasitol Today 1999; 15:437–442.
65. Werren JH. Biology of *Wolbachia*. Annu Rev Entomol 1997; 42:587–609.
66. La Scola B, Bandi C, Raoult D. *Wolbachia*. In: Brenner DJ, Krieg NR, Staley JT, Garrity GM, eds. The Proteobacteria, Part C, Bergey's Manual of Systematic Bacteriology. New York: Springer, 2005:138–143.
67. Casiraghi M, Bordenstein SR, Baldo L, et al. Phylogeny of *Wolbachia pipientis* based on *Glta, Groel*, and *Ftsz* gene sequences: clustering of arthropod and nematode symbionts in the F supergroup, and evidence for further diversity in the *Wolbachia* tree. Microbiology 2005; 151:4015–4022.
68. Lo N, Casiraghi M, Salati E, Bazzocchi C, Bandi C. How many *Wolbachia* supergroups exist? Mol Biol Evol 2002; 19:341–346.
69. Taylor MJ, Bandi C, Hoerauf A. *Wolbachia* bacterial endosymbionts of filarial nematodes. Adv Parasitol 2005; 60:245–284.
70. Stackebrandt E, Goebel BM. Taxonomic note: a place for DNA–DNA reassociation and 16S rRNA sequence analysis in the present species definition in bacteriology. Int J Syst Bacteriol 1994; 44:846–849.
71. Masui S, Kamoda S, Sasaki T, Ishikawa H. Distribution and evolution of bacteriophage Wo in *Wolbachia*, the endosymbiont causing sexual alterations in arthropods. J Mol Evol 2000; 51:491–497.
72. Werren JH, Hurst GD, Zhang W, Breeuwer JA, Stouthamer R, Majerus ME. Rickettsial relative associated with male killing in the ladybird beetle (*Adalia bipunctata*). J Bacteriol 1994; 176:388–394.
73. Hoerauf A, Mand S, Adjei O, Fleischer B, Buttner DW. Depletion of *Wolbachia* endobacteria in *Onchocerca volvulus* by doxycycline and microfilaridermia after ivermectin treatment. Lancet 2001; 357:1415–1416.
74. Hoerauf A, Mand S, Volkmann L, et al. Doxycycline in the treatment of human onchocerciasis: kinetics of *Wolbachia* endobacteria reduction and of inhibition of embryogenesis in female onchocerca worms. Microbes Infect 2003; 5:261–273.
75. Simon F, Prieto G, Morchon R, Bazzocchi C, Bandi C, Genchi C. Immunoglobulin G antibodies against the endosymbionts of filarial nematodes (*Wolbachia*) in patients with pulmonary dirofilariasis. Clin Diagn Lab Immunol 2003; 10:180–181.
76. Punkosdy GA, Addiss DG, Lammie PJ. Characterization of antibody responses to *Wolbachia* surface protein in humans with lymphatic filariasis. Infect Immun 2003; 71:5104–5114.

14 | Vectors and Reservoir Hosts of Anaplasmataceae

Hisashi Inokuma
Department of Clinical Veterinary Science, Obihiro University of Agriculture and Veterinary Medicine, Obihiro, Japan

INTRODUCTION

Infections with Anaplasmataceae pathogens were previously known only as diseases important to veterinary medicine. However, over the past two decades, several new species or strains have been isolated and characterized as the causative organisms of emerging or reemerging infectious diseases. Anaplasmataceae are now known to be major vector-borne pathogens of both humans and animals. Two major Anaplasmataceae that infect humans are *Anaplasma phagocytophilum* and *Ehrlichia chaffeensis*. Both of these are known to be tick-borne pathogens. *A. phagocytophilum* is transmitted by *Ixodes persulcatus* complex ticks, including *I. scapularis*, *I. pacificas*, and *I. ricinus*, whereas *E. chaffeensis* is transmitted by *Amblyomma americanum*. *I. persulcatus* complex ticks have a worldwide distribution, but *A. americanum* has a strong geographic specificity. This may explain why *E. chaffeensis* has been found only in the United States. As ticks are seasonally active, tick-borne anaplasmosis and ehrlichiosis occur seasonally. For example, *A. phagocytophilum* infection transmitted by *I. scapularis* in the United States occurs from April to October.

Wild animals such as deer or rodents are reservoirs of tick-borne anaplasmosis and ehrlichiosis. Animals which have recovered from clinical disease may harbor the organisms for long periods. A common feature of the tick-associated *Anaplasma* and *Ehrlichia* species is the inefficient transmission from one generation of ticks to the next. This ineffective transovarial transmission implies a reliance on horizontal transmission that further suggests the probable role of persistent infection, probably via persistent bacteremia in reservoir host animals.

An appreciation of the role of animals, animal habitats, and ectoparasites or helminths is needed to understand the infection of Anaplasmataceae in both animals and humans. Knowledge of vectors and reservoirs is also important for an accurate diagnosis and control of specific infectious diseases. With the recent development of molecular biology, specific and sensitive methods to detect pathogens from vectors, reservoirs, and hosts are now widely available. The findings on vectors and reservoirs are still increasing. Thus, vectors and reservoir hosts for Anaplasmataceae with medical and veterinary importance are summarized in this chapter.

VECTORS AND RESERVOIR HOSTS OF HUMAN ANAPLASMOSIS AND EHRLICHIOSIS

A. phagocytophilum: Human Granulocytic Ehrlichiosis

A. phagocytophilum is an agent which causes human granulocytic ehrlichiosis. The disease is characterized by fever, headache, myalgia, leucopenia, anemia, and thrombocytopenia. The agent also causes granulocytic ehrlichiosis in horses. The clinical findings include fever, depression, anorexia, limb edema, icterus, ataxia, and reluctance to move (1); however, the disease is not fatal. In ruminants, it causes disease known as tick-borne fever or Pasture fever. The agent primarily infects neutrophils and other granulocytes of sheep, goat, cattle, and deer. Fever, moderately disturbed general condition, and reduced milk production and growth rate are reported as the main clinical findings (2). Respiratory signs such as nasal discharge and cough may also be present. Mortality is generally low, but secondary infection may cause death to the patients.

The *I. persulcatus* group of ticks is widely distributed around the world, and includes important vectors of human infection with *A. phagocytophilum*. The transmission of *A. phagocytophilum* as a pathogen of tick-borne fever of sheep by *I. ricinus* has been known since 1936 (3). Recently, the pathogens of the human granulocytic ehrlichiosis were isolated or specific DNA fragments of the agents were molecularly detected from various ticks in worldwide. *I. scapularis* is a vector tick in the eastern United States (4–6), and *I. pacificus* in the western United States (7–10). *I. ricinus* is a vector in Europe and western Asia (11–19), and *I. persulcatus* in Asia (20–23). Additionally, *I. dentatus* was recently demonstrated to be a vector of *A. phagocytophilum* in the United States (24).

The best evidence for an animal reservoir is found in small mammals, such as mice and voles, (25,26) and cervids (27–30), which are frequently infected, sustain prolonged bacteremia, and develop no clinical signs (31,32). Woodland rodents, bank voles (*Clethriomys glareous*), and wood mice (*Apodemus syvaticus*) can maintain *A. phagocytophilum* in Great Britain in the absence of other reservoir hosts, and it has been suggested that *I. trianguliceps* is a competent vector for this pathogen (33). Recently, raccoons and gray squirrels were also demonstrated to be reservoir-competent for *A. phagocytophilum* (34). They become naturally infected, and are capable of transmitting the infection to feeding ticks. Because the deer population is expanding rapidly worldwide, tick populations that infest deer are also expanding. That is why Anaplasmosis in humans is now an emerging disease.

Serological and molecular evidence has been accumulated to support the notion that white-tailed deer (*Odocoileus virginanus*) is a major reservoir of *A. phagocytophilum* in the United States (28,32). The results of experimental infection of white-tailed deer with *A. phagocytophilum* confirmed that this animal is susceptible to infection with a human isolate of *A. phagocytophilum* and verify that white-tailed deer produce detectable antibodies upon exposure to the organism. Because adults are the predominant life stage of *I. scapularis* found on deer and because adult *I. scapularis* ticks do not transmit *A. phagocytophilum* transovarially, it is unlikely that white-tailed deer are a significant source of *A. phagocytophilum* for immature ticks even though deer have a high probability of natural infection. However, the susceptibility and immunologic response of white-tailed deer to *A. phagocytophilum* render them suitable candidates as natural sentinels for this zoonotic tick-borne organism (35). Recent findings, however, suggest that white-tailed deer harbor a variant strain not associated with human infection, but contrary to published reports, white-tailed deer are not a reservoir for strains that cause human disease (36). More epidemiological evidence will be required to draw a definitive conclusion about the role of white-tailed deer as a reservoir of *A. phagocytophilum*.

The vector ticks characteristically feed on several hosts, with each life stage having a range of preferred hosts. *A. phagocytophilum* is also well known to be a zoonotic agent that can infect and cause disease in several domestic animals, including dogs, horses, and ruminants. Other animals, including cats, macaques, and baboons, are also infected with the agents experimentally; however, the symptoms are generally mild (37). Thus, a variety of animals are potential reservoirs for *A. phagocytophilum*. Small mammals such as the white-footed mouse (*Peromyscus leucopus*) in the eastern and midwestern United States, the dusky foot woodrat (*Neotoma fuscipes*) in the western United States, and the wood mouse (*A. sylvaticus*), yellow-necked mouse (*A. flavicollis*), bank vole (*Clethrionomys glareolus*), and common shrew (*Sorex araneus*) in Europe are candidate animals for the reservoirs (18,25). Various cervids other than white-tailed deer are also thought to be reservoirs of *A. phagocytophilum*; the candidates include roe deer (*Capreolus capreolus*) and red deer (*Cervus elaphus*) (25). Furthermore, ruminants (goats, sheep, and cattle), rabbits, and coyotes can be reservoirs of the agents (24,38).

Specific gene sequences of *A. phagocytophilum* were detected from ticks that were imported into Sweden by migrant birds. The sequences were identical to those of *A. phagocytophilum* found in domestic animals and humans in Sweden. This finding suggests that birds may play a role in dispersing the pathogen (39).

E. chaffeensis: Human Monocytic Ehrlichiosis

The major tick vector of *E. chaffeensis*, the causative agent of human monocytotropic ehrlichiosis (HME), is *A. americanum*, the lone star tick (40,41). There have been several reports of detection of *E. chaffeensis*-specific DNA from *A. americanum* (42–46). The specific distribution of HME results from association with the distribution pattern of the tick vector, *A. americanum* (47). *A. americanum* is distributed from west-central Texas north to Iowa and eastward in a broad belt spanning the southeastern United States (48). Along the Atlantic coast, the range of this tick extends north through coastal areas of New England (48). The vector tick *A. americanum* transmits the agent in a transstadial manner to mammals, but not in transovarial manner (48a). Thus, nymphs and adults should be important sources of infection. Although DNA fragments of *E. chaffeensis* were also detected from other tick species, including *Dermacentor variablilis* (40,43,49) and *I. pacificus* (42) in the United States, *I. ricinus* in Russia (22), *A. testudinarium* and *Haemaphysalis yeni* in China (20), and *H. longicornis* in Korea (50), further studies will be required to confirm the ability of these ticks to act as definitive vectors of *E. chaffeensis*.

A. americanum is an aggressive host-seeking tick that will feed on many different hosts, including man. All three life stages of *A. americanum* can feed on white-tailed deer, the major reservoir animal of *E. chaffeensis* (41,51). Many cases of detection of *E. chaffeensis* from white-tailed deer have been reported (46,52). Serological evidence also supports the idea that white-tailed deer are a major reservoir of the agent (52). The specific distribution of HME also results from association with the distribution of white-tailed deer (47). The rapid expansion of white-tailed deer populations and geographic range, and the high seroprevalence of infection and evidence of present *E. chaffeensis* bacteremia in the absence of any clinical signs make these animals the most significant reservoir hosts (41). Experimental infection of white-tailed deer with *E. chaffeensis* revealed that primary infection of deer with the agent does not protect against subsequent exposure and confirmed that deer can be simultaneously coinfected with at least two different strains of *E. chaffeensis* (53).

The promiscuous feeding behavior of *A. americanum* ensures that many other species may become infected. Dogs must be important reservoir animals, as dogs can become persistently and subclinically infected and are known vehicles for the transport of infected ticks into the domestic environment (54–56). Although goats are also naturally infected with *E. chaffeensis*, recent studies revealed that this animal may not be susceptible to experimental infection (56a). Coyotes are also thought to be important reservoir animals in the United States, which is especially critical because the numbers and distribution of coyotes are increasing. This animal has been proven to be naturally infected with the agent and the infection rate was reported to be 71% (57). Raccoons (*Procyonis lotor*) are also thought to be an important reservoir. Antibodies against *E. chaffeensis* have been detected from blood samples of raccoon in several studies (58–59,59a). Antibodies reactive with *E. chaffeensis* were also detected in the serum of red foxes (*Vulpes vulpes*), gray foxes (*Urocyon cinereoargenteus*), opossums (*Didelphis virginianus*), and white-footed mice (*Permyscus leucopus*) (60–62,59a). However, more studies, including pathogen isolation, molecular biological examinations, and experimental inoculation will be required to confirm the role of these animals as reservoirs of *E. chaffeensis*. Recently, *E. chaffeensis* DNA was detected in up to 55% of replete nymphs that fed on mice experimentally infected with *E. chaffeensis* (63).

E. chaffeensis DNA fragments were detected by polymerase chain reaction (PCR) from *I. ricinus* ticks recovered from migratory birds in Russia (22). The potential role of avian species that may serve as hosts for immature *A. americanum* stages needs more study.

E. ewingii

Historically, *E. ewingii* was first described as a new strain of *E. canis* that was found in granulocytes and produced a mild form of canine ehrlichiosis (64,65). Evidence of *E. ewingii* infection in a human patient has been reported in the United States (66). *E. chaffeensis*, which occurs most frequently in the southeastern and south-central United States, and *E. ewingii*, a human and canine pathogen that also occurs in the midwestern United States, have been shown to occur in the tick vector *A. americanum* (67). The epidemiological and ecological conditions for *E. ewingii* infection are nearly identical to those for *E. chaffeensis* owing to the shared tick vector, *A. americanum* (47,68).

In infected dogs, nonspecific clinical signs such as fever, lethargy, anorexia, vomiting, diarrhea, anemia, thrombocytopenia, leukocytosis, lymphadenopathy, and polyarthritis were recorded (64,69,70). Dogs exposed to *A. americanum* developed serologic or clinical evidence of infection of *E. ewingii* (71,72). The finding of *E. ewingii* in asymptomatic dogs suggests that dogs could be a reservoir for *E. ewingii* (73).

A few studies have documented the presence of *E. ewingii* DNA in 5% to 20% of white-tailed deer in the midwestern and southeastern United States (68,74). These data suggest that white-tailed deer may be an important reservoir for *E. ewingii*.

VECTORS AND RESERVOIR HOSTS OF ANAPLASMATACEAE THAT ARE OF VETERINARY IMPORTANCE
Genus *Anaplasma*
A. marginale and Closely Related Species: Anaplasmosis of Ruminants

Anaplasmosis of ruminants is an infectious and transmissible disease of cattle, sheep, goats, and other domestic ruminants, characterized by progressive anemia associated with the presence of intraerythrocytic inclusion bodies designated as anaplasma (75). There are three known species: *A. marginale*, *A. centrale*, and *A. ovis*. *A. marginale* is the representative species of this group, and its susceptible host is cattle. *A. centrale* also causes bovine anaplasmosis, and *A. ovis* is the cause of ovine and caprine anaplasmosis. They are not thought to be zoonotic diseases at this time. Once an agent of anaplasmosis is transmitted to a host animal, it invades the mature erythrocytes. Sequential replication, release and new invasion (acute phase) result in the rapid onset of clinical signs that are attributable to severe hemolytic anemia in *A. marginale* infection (75). They include depression, weakness, fever, labored breathing, inappetence, dehydration, constipation, jaundice, abortion, and death. The pathogenic roles of *A. centrale* and *A. ovis* are comparatively weaker than that of *A. marginale*. Thus, little is known about the vectors and reservoirs of *A. centrale* and *A. ovis*.

Although *A. marginale* can be transmitted among cattle mechanically by blood-contaminated mouthparts of biting flies and mosquitoes, it is transmitted biologically by ticks (76). On the basis of experimental and epidemiological data, several insects, including horse flies (Diptera: Tabanidae), stable flies (*Stomoxys*), deer flies (*Chrysops*), horn flies (*Siphona*), and mosquitoes (genus *Psorophora*) have been incriminated as potential vectors (75). About 20 tick species have been shown to transmit anaplasmosis, although field evidence indicating the tick as the principal disease vector is lacking (76,77). *D. andersoni*, *D. occidentalis*, and *D. variabilis* are vector ticks in the United States (78). The ultrastructure and development of the pathogenic agent in *D. andersoni* and *D. variabilis* have been well documented by the series of studies by Kocan. The tropical cattle tick, *Boophilus microplus*, has also been demonstrated to be vector of *A. marginale* (79,80).

Carrier cattle are the main reservoirs of infection. Early serological studies suggested that wild cervids, including white-tailed deer and mule deer (*O. hemionus*), might be reservoirs of *A. marginale* (81–83). Elk (*C. elaphus*) were experimentally infected with *A. marginale*. The pathogen was detected in the blood of these elk and caused disease in splenectomized domestic bovine calves after subinoculation of blood from the elk (84). Experimental infection of *A. marginale* was also demonstrated in splenectomized mule deer (85). Recently, molecular biological techniques were used to detect the agent from reservoir animals, including Iberian red deer (*C. elaphus hispanicus*) (86).

A. bovis is phylogenetically more closely related to *A. phagocytophilum* than to *A. marginale* or *A. centrale*. Morulae are found in monocytes of infected cattle (87). *A. bovis* infection in cattle is seldom reported and is usually associated with subclinical infection (87). Thus, little is known about the epidemiology of this agent. *Hyalomma* spp., *Rhipicephalus appendiculatus*, and *A. variegatum* have been proven to be vectors of *A. bovis* (88–90).

A. platys

A. platys is a platelet-specific rickettsia of dogs that causes canine infectious cyclic thrombocytopenia (91). The pathogenesis of *A. platys* is generally not severe, although a few clinical abnormalities such as fever, anorexia, petechial hemorrhage, and uveitis have been reported (92,93). The agent is found worldwide. Analysis of *R. sanguineus* experimentally infected with *A. platys* revealed that the agent was not detected by light or transmission electron microscopy in the midgut or salivary glands of exposed adult ticks (94); however, this tick species is

TABLE 1 Natural Hosts, Vectors, and Reservoirs of Genus *Anaplasma*

Species	Natural host	Vectors	Reservoirs
A. phagocytophilum	Human Dogs Cattle Sheep Goats Horses	*I. persulcatus* complex *I. scapularis* *I. pacificus* *I. ricinus* *I. persulcatus* *I. dentatus* *I. trianguliceps*	Rodents White-footed mouse Dusty-footed mouse Wood-mouse Yellow-necked mouse Bank vole Common shrew Cervids White-tailed deer Roe deer Red deer Canids Coyotes Racoon Gray Squirrels Others Rabbit Birds
A. marginale	Ruminants Cattle Sheep Goats	Ticks (biological vector) *Dermacentor* spp. *D. andersoni* *D. occidentalis* *D. variabilis* *Boophilus* spp. *B. microplus* Insects (mechanical vector) Biting flies Mosquitoes	Cervids White-tailed deer Mule deer Elk Red deer
A. bovis	Cattle	*Hyalomma* spp. *Rh. appendiculatus* *A. variegatum*	Unknown
A. platys	Dogs	*Rh. sanguineus*	Dogs

thought to be a major vector of *A. platys* based on epidemiological data (93). Although the transmission of the pathogen from ticks to canine hosts has not yet been proven, specific DNA fragments of *A. platys* have been detected from *R. sanguineus* ticks using molecular techniques (95). These data support the notion that this tick species might be a vector of *A. platys*.

Little information is available about the reservoir hosts of *A. platys*. As the suspected tick vector is the same as that for *E. canis*, wild canids are considered to be candidate reservoir animals. More epidemiological studies will be required to prove this.

Genus *Ehrlichia*
E. canis: Canine Monocytic Ehrlichiosis

E. canis infection is known as canine monocytic ehrlichiosis, a potentially fatal tick-borne disease of dogs. The agent causes either an acute, subclinical, or chronic disease in dogs (96). Since the first case report of this disease in 1935, it has been reported worldwide in accord with the broad distribution of its main vector, *Rh. sanguineus*. The development of *E. canis* in the hemocytes, midgut, and salivary glands of female *Rh. sanguineus* was demonstrated by immunofluorescence and electron microscopy (97). The ability of female *Rh. sanguineus* ticks to transmit the pathogen has also been experimentally proven (98,99). Recently, it was reported that male *Rh. sanguineus* can take multiple feedings, and that they can both acquire and transmit *E. canis* in the absence of female ticks (100). However, experimental transmission of *E. canis* by *D. variabilis* to canine hosts was also demonstrated (101).

Canine ehrlichiosis and hepatozoonosis appear to be endemic in the wild red fox populations in Israel, and foxes may serve as a reservoir for infection of other wild canine species and domestic dogs (102). The fact that golden jackals can be infected with *E. canis* suggests that they may serve as a reservoir for the transmission of certain diseases to domestic dogs in Israel (103). *E. canis* was found in eight of 15 free-living jackals (*Canis mesomelas*) and 14 of 31 domestic dogs in rural communities in the same areas of Kenya (104). Red and gray foxes can be reservoir hosts of *E. canis* in the United States (105).

E. ruminantium

E. (*Cowdria*) *ruminantium* infects endothelial cells and neutrophils of ruminants and causes a disease—the so-called "heartwater (Cowdriosis)"—in Africa and the Caribbean. The disease is characterized by high fever, depression, salivation, and neurological signs (106). Peracute or acute disease is usually fatal within a week of the onset of symptoms; however, the clinical symptoms vary according to the strain of *E. ruminantium* (107).

Amblyomma ticks are the only known natural vectors of *E. ruminantium*. The African species include *A. variegatum*, *A. hebraeum*, *A. pomposum*, *A. gemma*, *A. lepidum*, *A. tholloni*, *A. sparsum*, *A. astrion*, *A. cohaerens*, and *A. marmoreum* (108–112). *A. variegatum* and *A. hebraeum* ticks are the two major vectors that transmit *E. ruminantium* to ruminants (113). The American species are *A. maculatum*, *A. cajennense*, and *A. dissimile*. The other American Amblyomma, *A. americanum*, was investigated for its ability to mediate transmission; however, it failed to transmit infection, confirming that low susceptibility to *E. ruminantium* correlates with the poor vector status of these species (114).

Because of the wide susceptibility of ruminants to this agent, African wild ruminants have been considered to be the reservoirs and natural hosts of *E. ruminantium*. Blood and bone marrow samples from healthy, free-ranging Zimbabwean ungulates were taken during translocation from areas harboring *Amblyomma* ticks and tested for the presence of *E. ruminantium* by PCR. Positive reactions were obtained in tsessebe (*Damaliscus lunatus*), waterbuck (*Kobus ellipsiprymnus*), and impala (*Aepyceros melampus*) (115). Similar findings were obtained by experimental inoculation of the agent for sable (*Hippotragus equinus*) (116). *E. ruminantium* can survive for at least two weeks in the back-striped mouse (*Rhabdomys pumilio*), and the multimammate mouse (*Mastomys coucha*) can also be infected (117). Other animals, including tortoises, guinea fowls, scrub hares, and reptiles, can also be subclinical carriers of *E. ruminantium*, and infective to vector ticks (109,118). However, the roles of these wild animals are still unclear.

E. muris and Ehrlichia Species Detected from I. ovatus

Recently, a number of new Anaplasmataceae species have been isolated. *E. muris* was isolated from the spleen of a wild mouse in Japan in 1983 (119). It induces splenomegaly and lymphadenopathy in laboratory mice; however, whether *E. muris* is pathogenic in other animals or humans is still unknown. It is transmitted by *H. flava* and widely distributed in Japan (120). A new *Ehrlichia* species was also isolated from *I. ovatus* ticks in Japan and found to be closely related to *E. chaffeensis* through analysis of the 16S rRNA sequence (121). The *Ehrlichia* detected from *I. ovatus* is more pathogenic and causes mortality in experimentally infected mice, 8 to 10 days postinfection (121). Neither *E. muris* nor the *Ehrlichia* from *I. ovatus* is known to cause disease in humans and other animals, but their suspected tick vectors, *H. flava* and *I. ovatus*, respectively, are widespread throughout mainland Japan. Little is known about the reservoirs and other vector ticks for these two *Ehrlichia* species. Both pathogens are thought to be excellent experimental models of human ehrlichiosis.

Genus Neorickettsia

Pathogens belonging to the genus *Neorickettsia* are known to be transmitted by helminths. Vectors for *Neorickettsia* include trematodes and the intermediate hosts (i.e., fish, snails, and insects) involved in the trematode life cycle. Actually trematodes, such as metacercaria of flukes, are vectors of these species. Fish or snails are reservoirs of these species, and consequently *Neorickettsia* agents are able to infect mammals.

Neorickettsia risticii

This ehrlichia causes equine monocytic ehrlichiosis or Potomac horse fever in horses. The consistent clinical features of Potomac horse fever are fever, depression, anorexia, and diarrhea (122,123). The fever is usually biphasic, whereby an initial increase in rectal temperature of

TABLE 2 Natural Hosts, Vectors, and Reservoirs of Genus *Ehrlichia*

Species	Natural host	Vectors	Reservoirs
E. chaffeensis	Human Dogs	*Amblyomma* ticks *A. americanum* Other ticks (?) *I. pacificus* *I. ricinus* *D. variabilis* *A. testudinarium* *H. yeni* *H. longicornis*	Cervids White-tailed deer Canids Dogs Coyotes Red fox Gray fox Racoons Rodents White-footed mouse Others Goats (?) Birds
E. ewingii	Human Dogs	*A. americanum*	Cervids White-tailed deer Canids Dogs
E. canis	Dogs	*R. sanguineus* *D. variabilis* (experimentally)	Canids Dogs Red fox Gray fox Golden jackal
E. ruminantium	Cattle	*Amblyomma* ticks *A. variegatum* *A. hebraeum* *A. maculatum* *A. cajennense* *A. dissimile* Other species	Ruminants Cattle Impala Waterbuck Tsessebe Sable Rodents Back-striped mouse Multimammate mouse Others Tortoises, guinea fowls Scrub hares, reptiles

limited duration (12–18 hours) may occur several days prior to the onset of depression and anorexia. The clinical course of the disease then progresses to include the following signs: subcutaneous edema of the lower limbs and ventral abdomen, colic, mild to profuse diarrhea, laminitis, and abortion (123).

Since the earliest reports of Potomac horse fever, an association of cases with riverine and other aquatic habitats has been noted. Barlough et al. (124) identified DNA of *N. risticii* by nested PCR in operculate snails (Pleuroceridae: *Juga* spp.) collected from stream water in northern California. *N. risticii* DNA was also found to be associated with virgulate cercariae in snail secretions (125). After that, *N. risticii* DNA was also molecularly detected in xiphidiocercariae from freshwater snails of the *Elimia* (Goniobasis) species (126,127). Because the xiphidiocercariae come from digenetic trematodes that use insects as their second intermediate host, insects should also be the second intermediate hosts of *N. risticii*-infected trematodes. Aquatic insects, including mayflies, caddis flies, stoneflies, damselflies, and dragonflies, carrying metacercariae showed a positive reaction for *N. risticii* by PCR (127,128). Insectivores, such as bats and birds, may serve as the definitive host of the trematode vector. Two potential helminth vectors, *Acanthatrium* sp. and *Lecithodendrium* sp., both infected with *N. risticii*, were found in the gastrointestinal tract of two *Myotis yumanensis* bats in California by PCR analysis (129). Bats and swallows not only act as a host for trematodes, but also as a possible natural reservoir for *N. risticii*. More recently, gravid trematodes (*Acanthatrium oregonense*) recovered from the intestines of *Eptesicus fuscus* (big brown bats) and *M. lucifugus* (little brown bats) from various sites in Pennsylvania were proven to be a natural reservoir and probably a vector of *N. risticii* (130).

Dogs and cats are also susceptible to experimental inoculation with *E. risticii* (131,132). *E. risticii* was isolated from patients with canine ehrlichiosis (133). However, the role of these domestic animals as reservoirs is unclear.

N. helmintoeca and Other Species

N. helminthoeca causes a disease named "salmon poisoning" in dogs and wild Canidae. This name was given because the disease is acquired by eating salmon parasitized with *Neorickettsia*-infected flukes. Clinical findings of "salmon poisoning" are fever, anorexia, depression, dehydration, vomiting, and watery to bloody diarrhea. The fatality rate in untreated infected dogs approaches 90% (134,135). *Nanopyetus salmonicola* is a vector trematode of *N. helmintoeca* that is known to be a pathogen of "salmon poisoning" of fish-eating Canidae (136). Intestinal hemorrhage and inflammation are the main damage in patients. Thus, salmon is thought to be an important reservoir of this agent. The Elokomin fluke fever agent is often classified as *N. elokominica*, but likely is another strain of *N. helmintoeca* (137).

N. sennetsu infection is a human disease characterized by fever, malaise, anorexia, constipation, backache, and lymphadenopathy (138). Although mice are highly susceptible to *N. sennetsu* (139), whether this organism infects domestic animals is unknown. Some epidemiological data regarding *N. sennetsu* infection of humans suggested an association with the consumption of red mullet fish, although it has not yet been proven.

The SF agent was first isolated in Japan in 1962 from *Stellantchasmus falcatus* metacercaria parasitic on gray mullet fish (139). Experimental infection of dogs with the stellantchasmus falcatus (SF) agent causes mild clinical signs including fever, and the SF agent can be reisolated from the dogs (140). However, the pathogenesis in animals in nature is unknown. Thus, the natural host of this agent is still unclear.

FUTURE STUDIES

Recently, a number of new Anaplasmataceae species were isolated. "*Candidatus* Neoehrlichia mikurensis," a novel bacterium that infects laboratory rats was also isolated from wild *Rattus norvegicus* rats in Japan (141). The habitat and pathogenesis of this new species should be intensively surveyed. With the recent development of molecular biology, specific and sensitive methods such as PCR and sequencing methodology are now being used to detect specific pathogens from various samples. Thus, many new uncultured Anaplasmataceae species have

TABLE 3 Natural Hosts, Vectors, and Reservoirs of Genus *Neorickettsia*

Species	Natural host	Vectors	Reservoirs
N. risticii	Horses	Trematode	Snails (first intermediate host of trematodes)
	Acanthatrium sp. *Lecithdendrium* sp. *Elimia* spp.	*Juga* spp.	
			Insects (second intermediate host of trematodes)
			Mayflies
			Caddisflies
			Stoneflies
			Damselflies
			Dragonflies
			Bats (insectovores)
			Myotis spp.
			Eptesicus spp.
			Dogs and cats (?)
N. helminthoeca	Dogs Wild canids	Trematode *Nanophyetus salminoda*	Salmon
N. sennetsu	Human	Trematode	Red mullet fish
SF agents	? *S. falcatus*	Trematode Gray mullet fish	

Abbreviation: SF, stellantchasmus falcatus.

been detected from environmental vertebrates and nonvertebrates throughout the world using these techniques. Many new sequences have been registered in GenBank. The complete information about the habitats of these new Anaplasmataceae species, including vectors, reservoirs, and hosts, and the pathogenesis of the agents are of great interest and should be clarified in future studies.

REFERENCES

1. Madigan JE. Equine ehrlichiosis. In: Woldehiwet Z, Ristic M, eds. Rickettsial and Chlamydial Diseases of Domestic Animals. Oxford: Pergamon Press, 1993:209–214.
2. Woldeiwet Z, Scott GR. Tick-borne (pasture) fever. In: Woldehiwet Z, Ristic M, eds. Rickettsial and Chlamydial Diseases of Domestic Animals. Oxford: Pergamon Press, 1993:233–254.
3. MacLeod F. Studies in tick borne fever of sheep. I. Experiments on transmission and distribution of the disease. Parasitology 1936; 28:320–329.
4. Pancholi P, Kolbert CP, Mitchell PD, et al. *Ixodes dammini* as a potential vector of human granulocytic ehrlichiosis. J Infect Dis 1995; 172:1007–1012.
5. Varde S, Beckley J, Schwartz I. Prevalence of tick-borne pathogens in *Ixodes scapularis* in a rural New Jersey county. Emerg Infect Dis 1998; 4:97–99.
6. Adelson ME, Rao RV, Tilton RC, et al. Prevalence of *Borrelia burgdorferi, Bartonella* spp., *Babesia microti*, and *Anaplasma phagocytophila* in *Ixodes scapularis* ticks collected in Northern New Jersey. J Clin Microbiol 2004; 42:2799–2801.
7. Barlough JE, Madigan JE, DeRock E, et al. Nested polymerase chain reaction for detection of *Ehrlichia equi* genomic DNA in horses and ticks (*Ixodes pacificus*). Vet Parasitol 1996; 63:319–329.
8. Barlough JE, Madigan JE, Kramer VL, et al. *Ehrlichia phagocytophila* genogroup rickettsiae in Ixodid ticks from California collected in 1995 and 1996. J Clin Microbiol 1997; 35:2018–2021.
9. Lane RS, Steinlein DB, Mun J. Human behaviors elevating exposure to *Ixodes pacificus* (Acari: Ixodidae) nymphs and their associated bacterial zoonotic agents in a hardwood forest. J Med Entomol 2004; 41:239–248.
10. Fritz CL, Bronson LR, Smith CR, et al. Clinical, epidemiologic, and environmental surveillance for ehrlichiosis and anaplasmosis in an endemic area of northern California. J Vector Ecol 2005; 30:4–10.
11. Cinco M, Padovan D, Murgia R, et al. Coexistence of *Ehrlichia phagocytophila* and *Borrelia burgdorferi* sensu lato in *Ixodes ricinus* ticks from Italy as determined by 16S rRNA gene sequencing. J Clin Microbiol 1997; 35:3365–3366.
12. Alberdi MP, Walker AR, Paxton EA, et al. Natural prevalence of infection with *Ehrlichia phagocytophila* of *Ixodes ricinus* ticks in Scotland. Vet Parasitol 1998; 78:203–213.
13. Parola P, Beati L, Cambon M, et al. Ehrlichial DNA amplified from *Ixodes ricinus* (Acari: Ixodidae) in France. J Med Entomol 1998; 35:180–183.
14. Ogden NH, Bown K, Horrock BK, et al. Granulocytic *Ehrlichia* infection in Ixodid ticks and mammals in woodlands and uplands of the UK. Med Vet Entomol 1998; 12:423–429.
15. Baumgarten BU, Rollinghoff M, Bogdan C. Prevalence of *Borrelia burgdorferi* and granulocytic and monocytic ehrlichiae in *Ixodes ricinus* ticks from southern Germany. J Clin Microbiol 1999; 37:3348–3451.
16. Pusterla N, Huder JB, Lutz H, et al. Detection of *Ehrlichia phagocytophila* DNA in *Ixodes ricinus* ticks from areas in Switzerland where tick-borne fever is endemic. J Clin Microbiol 1998; 36:2735–2736.
17. Schouls LM, Van de Polo I, Rijpkema SGT, et al. Detection and identification of *Ehrlichia, Borrelia burgdorferi* sensu lato, and *Bartonella* species in Dutch *Ixodes ricinus* ticks. J Clin Microbiol 1999; 37:2215–2222.
18. Liz JS, Anderson L, Sumner JW, et al. PCR detection of granulocytic Ehrlichiae in *Ixodes ricinus* ticks and wild mammals in western Switzerland. J Clin Microbiol 2000; 38:1002–1007.
19. Stanczak J, Gabre RM, Kruminis-Lozowska W, et al. *Ixodes ricinus* as a vector of *Borrelia burgdorferi* sensu lato, *Anaplasma phagocytophilum* and *Babesia microti* in urban and suburban forests. Ann Agric Environ Med 2004; 11:109–114.
20. Cao WC, Zhao QM, Zhang PH, et al. Granulocytic ehrlichiae in *Ixodes persulcatus* ticks from an area in China where Lyme disease is endemic. J Clin Microbiol 2000; 38:4208–4210.
21. Cao WC, Zhao QM, Zhang PH, et al. Prevalence of *Anaplasma phagocytophila* and *Borrelia burgdorferi* in *Ixodes persulcatus* ticks from northeastern China. Am J Trop Med Hyg 2003; 68:547–550.
22. Alekseev A, Dubinina HV, Van de Pol I, et al. Identification of *Ehrlichia* spp. and *Borrelia burgdorferi* in *Ixodes* ticks in the Baltic region of Russia. J Clin Microbiol 2001; 39:2237–2242.
23. Kim CM, Kim MS, Park MS, et al. Identification of *Ehrlichia chaffeensis, Anaplasma phagocytophilum*, and *A. bovis* in *Haemaphysalis longicornis* and *Ixodes persulcatus* ticks from Korea. Vector Borne Zoonotic Dis 2003; 3:17–26.
24. Goethert HK, Telford SR III. Enzootic transmission of the agent of human granulocytic ehrlichiosis among cottontail rabbits. Am J Trop Med Hyg 2003; 68:633–637.

25. Stafford KC III, Massung RF, Magnarelli LA, et al. Infection with agents of human granulocytic ehrlichiosis, Lyme disease, and babesiosis in wild white-footed mice (*Peromyscus leucopus*) in Connecticut. J Clin Microbiol 1999; 37:2887–2892.
26. De Vignes F, Fish D. Transmission of the agent of human granulocytic ehrlichiosis by host-seeking *Ixodes scapularis* (Acari: Ixodidae) in southern New York state. J Med Entomol 1997; 34:379–382.
27. Petrovec M, Bidovec A, Sumner JW, et al. Infection with *Anaplasma phagocytophila* in cervids from Slovenia: evidence of two genotypic lineages. Wien Klin Wochenschr 2002; 114:641–647.
28. Belongia EA, Reed KD, Mitchell PD, et al. Prevalence of granulocytic *Ehrlichia* infection among white-tailed deer in Wisconsin. J Clin Microbiol 1997; 35:1465–1468.
29. Alberdi MP, Walker AR, Urquhart KA. Field evidence that roe deer (*Capreolus capreolus*) are a natural host for *Ehrlichia phagocytophila*. Epidemiol Infect 2000; 124:315–323.
30. Foley JE, Barlough JE, Kimsey RB, et al. *Ehrlichia* spp. in cervids from California. J Wildl Dis 1998; 34:731–737.
31. Stuen S, Handeland K, Frammarsvik T, et al. Experimental *Ehrlichia phagocytophila* infection in red deer (*Cervus elaphus*). Vet Rec 2001; 149:390–392.
32. Magnarelli LA, Ijdo JW, Stafford KC III, et al. Infections of granulocytic ehrlichiae and *Borrelia burgdorferi* in white-tailed deer in Connecticut. J Wildl Dis 1999; 35:266–274.
33. Bown KJ, Begon M, Bennett M, et al. Seasonal dynamics of *Anaplasma phagocytophila* in a rodent-tick (*Ixodes trianguliceps*) system, United Kingdom. Emerg Infect Dis 2003; 9:63–70.
34. Levin ML, Nicholson WL, Massung RF, et al. Comparison of the reservoir competence of medium-sized mammals and *Peromyscus leucopus* for *Anaplasma phagocytophilum* in Connecticut. Vector Borne Zoonotic Dis 2002; 2:125–136.
35. Tate CM, Mead DG, Luttrell MP, et al. Experimental infection of white-tailed deer with *Anaplasma phagocytophilum*, etiologic agent of human granulocytic anaplasmosis. J Clin Microbiol 2005; 43:3595–3601.
36. Massung RF, Courtney JW, Hiratzka SL, et al. *Anaplasma phagocytophilum* in white-tailed deer. Emerg Infect Dis 2005; 11:1604–1606.
37. Lewis GE, Huxell DL, Ristic M, et al. Experimentally induced infection of dogs, cats, and nonhuman primates with *Ehrlichia equi*, etiological agent of equine ehrlichiosis. Am J Vet Res 1975; 36:85–88.
38. Foley JE, Queen EV, Sacks B, et al. GIS-facilitated spatial epidemiology of tick-borne diseases in coyotes (*Canis latrans*) in northern and coastal California. Comp Immunol Microbiol Infect Dis 2005; 28:197–212.
39. Bjoersdorff A, Bergstrom S, Massung RF, et al. *Ehrlichia*-infected ticks on migrant birds. Emerg Infect Dis 2001; 7:877–879.
40. Anderson BE, Sims KG, Olson JG, et al. *Amblyomma americanum*: a potential vector of human ehrlichiosis. Am J Trop Med Hyg 1993; 49:239–244.
41. Ewing SA, Dawson JE, Kocan AA, et al. Experimental transmission of *Ehrlichia chaffeensis* (Rickettsiales: Ehrlichiae) among white-tailed deer by *Amblyomma americanum* (Acari: Ixodidae). J Med Entomol 1995; 32:368–374.
42. Burket CT, Vann CN, Pinger RR, et al. Minimum infection rate of *Amblyomma americanum* (Acari: Ixodidae) by *Ehrlichia chaffeensis* (Rickettsiales: Ehrlichieae) in southern Indiana. J Med Entomol 1998; 35:653–659.
43. Kramer VL, Randolph MP, Hui LT, et al. Detection of the agents of human ehrlichioses in *Ixodid* ticks from California. Am J Trop Med Hyg 1999; 60:62–65.
44. Whitlock JE, Fang QQ, Durden LA, et al. Prevalence of *Ehrlichia chaffeensis* (Rickettsiales: Rickettsiaceae) in *Amblyomma americanum* (Acari: Ixodidae) from the Georgia coast and Barrier Islands. J Med Entomol 2000; 37:276–280.
45. Ijdo JW, Wu C, Magnarelli LA, et al. Detection of *Ehrlichia chaffeensis* DNA in *Amblyomma americanum* ticks in Connecticut and Rhode Island. J Clin Microbiol 2000; 38:4655–4656.
46. Varela AS, Moore VA, Little SE. Disease agents in *Amblyomma americanum* from northeastern Georgia. J Med Entomol 2004; 41:753–759.
47. Childs JE, Paddock CD. The ascendancy of *Amblyomma americanum* as a vector of pathogens affecting humans in the United States. Annu Rev Entomol 2003; 48:307–337.
48. Paddock CD, Childs JE. *Ehrlichia chaffeensis*: a prototypical emerging pathogen. Clin Microbiol Rev 2003; 16:37–64.
48a. Long SW, Zhang X, Zhang J, et al. Evaluation of transovarial transmission and transmissibility of *Ehrlichia chaffeensis* (Rickettsiales: Anaplasmataceae) in *Amblyomma americanum* (Acari: Ixodidae). J Med Entomol 2003; 40:1000–1004.
49. Roland WE, Everett ED, Cyr TL, et al. *Ehrlichia chaffeensis* in Missouri ticks. Am J Trop Med Hyg 1998; 59:641–643.
50. Lee SO, Na DK, Kim CM, et al. Identification and prevalence of *Ehrlichia chaffeensis* infection in *Haemaphysalis longicornis* ticks from Korea by PCR, sequencing and phylogenetic analysis based on 16S rRNA gene. J Vet Sci 2005; 6:151–155.
51. Dawson JE, Stallknecht DE, Howerth EW, et al. Susceptibility of white-tailed deer (*Odocoileus virginianus*) to infection with *Ehrlichia chaffeensis*, the etiologic agent of human ehrlichiosis. J Clin Microbiol 1994; 32:2725–2728.

52. Yabsley MJ, Dugan VG, Stallknecht DE, et al. Evaluation of a prototype *Ehrlichia chaffeensis* surveillance system using white-tailed deer (*Odocoileus virginianus*) as natural sentinels. Vector Borne Zoonotic Dis 2003; 3:195–207.
53. Varela AS, Stallknecht DE, Yabsley MJ, et al. Primary and secondary infection with *Ehrlichia chaffeensis* in white-tailed deer (*Odocoileus virginianus*). Vector Borne Zoonotic Dis 2005; 5:48–57.
54. Dawson JE, Ewing SA. Susceptibility of dogs to infection with *Ehrlichia chaffeensis*, causative agent of human ehrlichiosis. Am J Vet Res 1992; 53:1322–1327.
55. Dawson JE, Biggie KL, Warner CK, et al. Polymerase chain reaction evidence of *Ehrlichia chaffeensis*, an etiological agent of human ehrlichiosis, in dogs from southeast Virginia. Am J Vet Res 1996; 57:1175–1179.
56. Ewing SA, Dawson JE, Panciera RJ, et al. Dogs infected with a human granulocytic *Ehrlichia* spp. J Med Entomol 1997; 34:710–718.
56a. Dugan VG, Varela AS, Stallknecht DE, et al. Attempted experimental infection of domestic goats with *Ehrlichia chaffeensis*. Vector Borne Zoonotic Dis 2004; 4:131–136.
57. Kocan AA, Levesque GC, Whitworth LC, et al. Naturally occurring *Ehrlichia chaffeensis* infection in coyotes from Oklahoma. Emerg Infect Dis 2000; 6:477–480.
58. Dugan VG, Gaydos JK, Stallknecht DE, et al. Detection of *Ehrlichia* spp. in raccoons (*Procyon lotor*) from Georgia. Vector Borne Zoonotic Dis 2005; 5:162–171.
59. Comer JA, Nicholson WL, Olson JG. Detection of antibodies reactive with *Ehrlichia chaffeensis* in the raccoon. J Wildl Dis 2000; 36:705–712.
59a. Lockhart JM, Davidson WR, Stallknecht DE. Natural history of *Ehrlichia chaffeensis* (Rickettsiae: Ehrlichieae) in the piedmont physiographic province of Georgia. J Parasitol 2000; 83:887–894.
60. Lockhart JM, Davidson WR, Stallknecht DE, et al. Lack of seroreactivity to *Ehrlichia chaffeensis* among rodent populations. J Wildl Dis 1998; 34:392–396.
61. Davidson WR, Lockhart JM, Stallknecht DE, et al. Susceptibility for red and gray foxes to infection by *Ehrlichia chaffeensis*. J Wildl Dis 1999; 35:696–702.
62. Magnarelli LA, Anderson JF, Stafford KC, et al. Antibodies to multiple tick-borne pathogens of babesiosis, ehrlichiosis, and Lyme borreliosis in white-footed mice. J Wildl Dis 1997; 33:466–473.
63. Loftis AD, Nicholson WL, Levin ML. Evaluation of immunocompetent and immuno-compromised mice (*Mus musculus*) for infection with *Ehrlichia chaffeensis* and transmission to *Amblyomma americanum* ticks. Vector Borne Zoonotic Dis 2004; 4:323–333.
64. Ewing SA, Roberson WR, Buckner RG, et al. A new strain of *Ehrlichia canis*. J Am Vet Med Assoc 1971; 159:1771–1774.
65. Anderson BE, Greene CE, Jones DC, et al. *Ehrlichia ewingii* sp. nov., the etiological agent of canine granulocytic ehrlichiosis. Int J Syst Bacteriol 1992; 42:299–302.
66. Buller RS, Arens M, Hmiel SP, et al. *Ehrlichia ewingii*, a newly recognized agent of human ehrlichiosis. N Engl J Med 1999; 341:148–155.
67. Lockhart JM, Davidson WR, Stallknecht DE, et al. Site-specific geographic association between *Amblyomma americanum* (Acari: Ixodidae) infestations and *Ehrlichia chaffeensis*-reactive (Rickettsiales: Ehrlichieae) antibodies in white-tailed deer. J Med Entomol 1996; 33:153–158.
68. Yabsley MJ, Varela AS, Tate CM, et al. *Ehrlichia ewingii* infection in white-tailed deer (*Odocoileus virginianus*). Emerg Infect Dis 2002; 8:668–671.
69. Carrillo JM, Green RA. A case report of canine ehrlichiosis: neutrophilic strain. J Am Anim Hosp Assoc 1978; 14:100–104.
70. Goldman EE, Breitschwerdt EB, Grindem CB, et al. Granulocytic ehrlichiosis in dogs from North Carolina and Virginia. J Vet Intern Med 1998; 12:61–70.
71. Anziani AS, Ewing SA, Barker RW. Experimental transmission of a granulocytic form of the tribe Ehrlichiae by *Dermacentor variabilis* and *Amblyomma americanum* to dogs. Am J Vet Res 1990; 51:929–931.
72. Goodman RA, Hawkins EC, Olby NJ, et al. Molecular identification of *Ehrlichia ewingii* infection in dogs 15 cases (1997–2001). J Am Vet Med Assoc 2003; 222:1102–1107.
73. Liddell AM, Stockham SL, Scott MA, et al. Predominance of *Ehrlichia ewingii* in Missouri dogs. J Clin Microbiol 2003; 41:4617–4622.
74. Steiert JG, Gilfoy F. Infection rates of *Amblyomma americanum* and *Dermacentor variabilis* by *Ehrlichia chaffeensis* and *Ehrlichia ewingii* in southwest Missouri. Vector Borne Zoonotic Dis 2002; 2:53–60.
75. Wanduragala L, Rictic M. Anaplasmosis. In: Woldehiwet Z, Ristic M, eds. Rickettsial and Chlamydial Diseases of Domestic Animals. Oxford: Pergamon Press, 1993:65–87.
76. Ewing SA. Transmission of *Anaplasma marginale* by arthropods. In: Hidalgo RJ, Jones EW, eds. Proceedings 7th National Anaplasmosis Conference. State College: Mississippi State University Press, 1981:395–423.
77. Dikmans G. The transmission of anaplasmosis. Am J Vet Res 1950; 38:5–16.
78. Ristic M. Anaplasmosis. In: Weinman D, Ristic M, eds. Infectious Blood Diseases of Man and Animals. New York: Academic Press, 1968:478–542.
79. Aguirre DH, Gaido AB, Vinabal AE, et al. Transmission of *Anaplasma marginale* with adult *Boophilus microplus* ticks fed as nymphs on calves with different levels of rickettsaemia. Parasite 1994; 1:405–407.

80. Leatch G. Preliminary studies on the transmission of *Anaplasma marginale* by *Boophilus microplus*. Aust Vet J 1973; 49:16–19.
81. Chomel BB, Carniciu ML, Kasten RW, et al. Antibody prevalence of eight ruminant infectious diseases in California mule and black-tailed deer (*Odocoileus heminus*). J Wildl Dis 1994; 30:51–59.
82. Aguirre AA, McLean RG, Cook RS, et al. Serologic survey from selected arboviruses and other potential pathogens in wildlife from Mexico. J Wildl Dis 1992; 28:435–442.
83. Morley RS, Hugh-Jones ME. Seroepidemiology of *Anaplasma marginale* in white-tailed deer (*Odocoileus virginanus*) from Louisiana. J Wildl Dis 1989; 25:342–346.
84. Zaugg JL, Goff WL, Foreyt W, et al. Susceptibility of elk (*Cervus elaphus*) to experimental infection with *Anaplasma marginale* and *A. ovis*. J Wildl Dis 1996; 32:62–66.
85. Zaugg JL. Experimental anaplasmosis in mule deer: persistence of infection of *Anaplasma marginale* and susceptibility to *A. ovis*. J Wildl Dis 1988; 24:120–126.
86. De La Fuente J, Vincente J, Hofle U. *Anaplasma* infection in free-ranging Iberian red deer in the region of Castilla-La Mancha, Spain. Vet Microbiol 2004; 100:163–173.
87. Stewart CG. Bovine ehrlichiosis. In: Fivaz B, Petrey T, Horak I, eds. Ticks Vector Biology—Medical and Veterinary Aspects. Berlin: Springer, 1992:101–107.
88. Donatien A, Lestoquard F. *Rickettsia bovis*, nouvelle espece pathogene pour le boeuf. Bull Soc Pathol Exot 1936; 29:1057–1061.
89. Matson BA. Theileriosis in Rhodesia (Zimbabwe): a study of diagnostic specimens over two seasons. J S Afr Vet Med Assoc 1967; 38:93–97.
90. Rioche M. Lesion microscopique de la rickettsiose generale bovine *Rickettsia (Ehrlichia) bovis* (Donatient et Lestoquard 1936). Rev Elev Med Vet Pays Trop 1967; 20:415–427.
91. Harvey JW, Simpson CF, Gaskin JM. Cyclic thrombocytopenia induced by a Rickettsia-like agent in dogs. J Infect Dis 1978; 137:182–188.
92. Bradfield JF, Vore SJ, Pryor WH Jr. *Ehrlichia platys* infection in dogs. Lab Anim Sci 1996; 46:565–568.
93. Hoskins JD. Ehrlichial diseases of dogs: diagnosis and treatment. Canine Pract 1991; 16:13–21.
94. Simpson RM, Gaunt SD, Hair JA, et al. Evaluation of *Rhipicephalus sanguineus* as a potential biologic vector of *Ehrlichia platys*. Am J Vet Res 1991; 52:1537–1541.
95. Inokuma H, Raoult D, Brouqui P. Detection of *Ehrlichia platys* DNA in brown dog ticks (*Rhipicephalus sanguineus*) in Okinawa Island, Japan. J Clin Microbiol 2000; 38:4219–4221.
96. Harrus S, Waner T, Bark H. Canine monocytic ehrlichiosis—an update. Compend Contin Educ Prac Vet 1997; 19:431–444.
97. Smith RD, Sells DM, Stephenson EH, et al. Development of *Ehrlichia canis*, causative agent of canine ehrlichiosis, in the tick *Rhipicephalus sanguineus* and its differentiation from a symbiotic *Rickettsia*. Am J Vet Res 1976; 37:119–126.
98. Groves MG, Dennis GL, Amyx HL, et al. Transmission of *Ehrlichia canis* to dogs by ticks (*Rhipicephalus sanguineus*). Am J Vet Res 1975; 36:937–940.
99. Lewis GE, Ristic M, Smith RD, et al. The brown dog tick *Rhipicephalus sanguineus* and the dog as experimental hosts of *Ehrlichia canis*. Am J Vet Res 1975; 38:1953–1955.
100. Bremer WG, Schaefer JJ, Wagner ER, et al. Transstadial and intrastadial experimental transmission of *Ehrlichia canis* by male *Rhipicephalus sanguineus*. Vet Parasitol 2005; 131:95–105.
101. Johnson EM, Ewing SA, Barker RW, et al. Experimental transmission of *Ehrlichia canis* by *Dermacentor variabilis*. Vet Parasitol 1998; 74:277–288.
102. Fishman Z, Gonen L, Harrus S, et al. Serosurvey of *Hepatozoon canis* and *Ehrlichia canis* antibodies in wild red foxes (*Vulpes vulpes*) from Israel. Vet Parasitol 2004; 119:21–26.
103. Shamir M, Yakobson B, Baneth G, et al. Antibodies to selected canine pathogens and infestation with intestinal helminths in golden jackals (*Canis aureus*) in Israel. Vet J 2001; 162:66–72.
104. Price JE, Karstad LH. Free-living jackals (*Canis mesomelas*)—potential reservoir hosts for *Ehrlichia canis* in Kenya. J Wildl Dis 1980; 16:469–473.
105. Amyx HL, Huxsoll DL. Red and gray foxes—potential reservoir hosts for *Ehrlichia canis*. J Wildl Dis 1973; 9:47–50.
106. Uilenberg G, Camus E. Heartwater (Cowdriosis). In: Woldehiwet Z, Ristic M, eds. Rickettsial and Chlamydial Diseases of Domestic Animals. Oxford: Pergamon Press, 1993:293–332.
107. Van De Pypekamp HE, Prozesky L. Heartwater: an overview of the clinical signs, susceptibility and differential diagnoses of the disease in domestic ruminants. Onderstepoort J Vet Res 1987; 54:263–268.
108. Bezuidenhout JD. Natural transmission of heartwater. Onderstepoort J Vet Res 1987; 54:349–351.
109. Jongejan F. Experimental transmission of *Cowdria ruminantium* (Rickettsiales) by the American reptile tick *Amblyomma dissimile* Koch, 1844. Exp Appl Acarol 1992; 15:117–121.
110. Peter TF, Burridge MJ, Mahan SM. Competence of the African tortoise tick, *Amblyomma marmoreum* (Acari: Ixodidae), as a vector of the agent of heartwater (*Cowdria ruminantium*). J Parasitol 2000; 86:438–441.
111. Peter TF, Barbet AF, Alleman AR, et al. Detection of the agent of heartwater, *Cowdria ruminantium*, in *Amblyomma* ticks by PCR: validation and application of the assay to field ticks. J Clin Microbiol 2000; 38:1539–1544.

112. Bryson NR, Horak IG, Venter EH, et al. The prevalence of *Cowdria ruminantium* in free-living adult *Amblyomma hebraeum* collected at a communal grazing area and in 2 wildlife reserves in South Africa. J S Afr Vet Assoc 2002; 73:131–132.
113. Peter TF, Bryson NR, Perry BD, et al. *Cowdria ruminantium* infection in ticks in the Kruger National Park. Vet Rec 1999; 145:304–307.
114. Mahan SM, Peter TF, Simbi BH, et al. Comparison of efficacy of American and African *Amblyomma* ticks as vectors of heartwater (*Cowdria ruminantium*) infection by molecular analyses and transmission trials. J Parasitol 2000; 86:44–49.
115. Kock ND, van Vliet AH, Charlton K, et al. Detection of *Cowdria ruminantium* in blood and bone marrow samples from clinically normal, free-ranging Zimbabwean wild ungulates. J Clin Microbiol 1995; 33:2501–2504.
116. Peter TF, Anderson EC, Burridge MJ, et al. Susceptibility and carrier status of impala, sable, and tsessebe for *Cowdria ruminantium* infection (heartwater). J Parasitol 1999; 85:468–472.
117. Mackenzie PKI, McHardy N. The culture of *Cowdria ruminantium* in mice: significance in respect of the epidemiology and control of heartwater. Prev Vet Med 1984; 2:227–237.
118. Bezuidenhout JD. Recent research finding on cowdriosis. In: Williams JC, Kakoma I, eds. A Vector-Borne Disease of Animals and Humans. Boston: Kluwer Academic Publishers, 1990:125–135.
119. Kawahara M, Suto C, Rikihisa Y, et al. Characterization of ehrlichial organisms isolated from a wild mouse. J Clin Microbiol 1993; 31:89–96.
120. Kawahara M, Ito T, Suto C, et al. Comparison of *Ehrlichia muris* strains isolated from wild mice and ticks and serologic survey of humans and animals with *E. muris* as antigen. J Clin Microbiol 1999; 37:1123–1129.
121. Shibata SI, Kawahara M, Rikihisa Y, et al. New *Ehrlichia* species closely related to *E. chaffeensis* isolated from *Ixodes ovatus* ticks in Japan. J Clin Microbiol 2000; 38:1331–1338.
122. Mulville P. Equine monocytic ehrlichiosis (Potomac horse fever): a review. Equine Vet J 1991; 23:400–404.
123. Holland CJ, Ristic M. Equine monocytic ehrlichiosis (Syn., Potomac horse fever). In: Woldehiwet Z, Ristic M, eds. Rickettsial and Chlamydial Diseases of Domestic Animals. Oxford: Pergamon Press, 1993:215–232.
124. Barlough JE, Reubel GH, Madiogan JE, et al. Detection of *Ehrlichia risticii*, the agent of Potomac horse fever, in freshwater stream snails (Pleuroceridae: *Juga* spp.) from Northern California. Appl Environ Microbiol 1998; 64:2888–2893.
125. Reubel GH, Barlough JE, Madiogan JE. Production and characterization of *Ehrlichia risticii*, the agent of Potomac horse fever, from snails (Pleuroceridae: *Juga* spp.) in aquarium culture and genetic comparison to equine strains. J Clin Microbiol 1998; 36:1501–1511.
126. Kanter M, Mott J, Ohashi N, et al. Analysis of 16S rRNA and 51-kilodalton antigen gene and transmission in mice of *Ehrlichia risticii* in virgulate trematodes from *Elimia livescens* snails in Ohio. J Clin Microbiol 2000; 38:3349–3358.
127. Mott J, Muramatsu Y, Seaton E, et al. Molecular analysis of *Neorickettsia risticii* in adult aquatic insects in Pennsylvania, in horses infected by ingestion of insects, and isolated in cell culture. J Clin Microbiol 2002; 40:690–693.
128. Chae JS, Pusterla N, Johnson E, et al. Infection of aquatic insects with trematode metacercariae carrying *Ehrlichia risticii*, the cause of Potomac horse fever. J Med Entomol 2000; 37:619–625.
129. Pusterla N, Johnson EM, Chae JS, et al. Digenetic trematodes, *Acanthatrium* sp. and *Lecithodendrium* sp., as vectors of *Neorickettsia risticii*, the agent of Potomac horse fever. J Helminthol 2003; 77:335–339.
130. Gibson KE, Rikihisa Y, Zhang C, et al. *Neorickettsia risticii* is vertically transmitted in the trematode *Acanthatrium oregonense* and horizontally transmitted to bats. Environ Microbiol 2005; 7:203–212.
131. Dawson JE, Abeygunawardena I, Holland CJ, et al. Susceptibility of cats to infection with *Ehrlichia risticii*, causative agent of equine monocytic ehrlichiosis. Am J Vet Res 1988; 49:2096–2100.
132. Ristic M, Dawson J, Holland CJ, et al. Susceptibility of dogs to infection with *Ehrlichia risticii*, causative agent of equine monocytic ehrlichiosis (Potomac horse fever). Am J Vet Res 1988; 49:1497–1500.
133. Kacoma I, Hansen RD, Anderson BE, et al. Culture, molecular, and immunological characterization of the etiological agent for atypical canine ehrlichiosis. J Clin Microbiol 1994; 32:170–175.
134. Cordy DR, Gorham JR. The pathology and etiology of salmon poisoning disease in dogs and fox. Am J Pathol 1950; 26:617–637.
135. Philip CB, Hadlow WJ, Hughes LE. Studies on salmon poisoning disease in canines. I. The rickettsial relationships and pathogenicity of *Neorickettsia helminthoeca*. Exp Parasitol 1954; 3:336–350.
136. Gorham JR, Foreyt WJ. Salmon poisoning disease. In: Woldehiwet Z, Ristic M, eds. Rickettsial and Chlamydial Diseases of Domestic Animals. Oxford: Pergamon Press, 1993:281–292.
137. Frank DW, McGuire TC, Gorman JR, et al. Lymphoreticular lesions of canine rickettsiosis. J Infect Dis 1974; 129:163–171.

138. Misao T, Kobayashi Y. Studies on infectious mononucleosis (glandular fever). I. Isolation of etiologic agent from blood, bone marrow and lymph node of a patient with infectious mononucleosis by using mice. Kyushu J Med Sci 1955; 6:145–152.
139. Fukuda T, Sasahara T, Kitao T. Studies on the causative agent of "Hyuganetsu disease". XI. Characterization of rickettsia-like organism isolated from metacercaria of *Stellantchasmus falcatus* parasitic in gray mullet. J Jpn Assoc Infect Dis 1973; 47:474–482.
140. Fukuda T, Yamamoto S. Neorickettsia-like organism isolated from metacercaria of a fluke, *Stellantchasmus falcatus*. Jpn J Med Sci Biol 1981; 34:103–107.
141. Kawahara M, Rikihisa Y, Isogai E, et al. Ultrastructure and phylogenetic analysis of '*Candidatus* Neoehrlichia mikurensis' in the family Anaplasmataceae, isolated from wild rats and found in *Ixodes ovatus* ticks. Int J Syst Evol Microbiol 2004; 54:1837–1843.

15 | Human Ehrlichioses

Juan P. Olano
Department of Pathology, University of Texas Medical Branch, Galveston, Texas, U.S.A.

INTRODUCTION

On the basis of the taxonomic reorganization of the family Anaplasmataceae proposed in 2000 (1), ehrlichial pathogens affecting humans include *Ehrlichia chaffeensis*, *E. ewingii*, and sporadic reports (Olano and McBride, Unpublished data) of *E. canis* infections in humans (2). This chapter will discuss in detail human monocytotropic ehrlichiosis (HME), caused by *E. chaffeensis*, and ehrlichiosis ewingii, a form of granulocytotropic ehrlichiosis, caused by *E. ewingii*. Before the taxonomic reorganization of the Anaplasmataceae family occurred, a pathogen formerly known as the HGE agent or *E. equi/E. phagocytophila* was identified as the cause of human granulocytotropic ehrlichiosis. Such pathogen is now in the genus *Anaplasma* and is known as *Anaplasma phagocytophilum*. The disease it causes is now known as human granulocytotropic anaplasmosis, described in another chapter.

DEFINITION

Ehrlichia are obligate intracellular bacteria that belong to the alpha subdivision of the proteobacteria and survive in phagosomal vacuoles within the host cell. By electron microscopy, they show two different forms known as dense-cored cells and reticulate cells, both of which are capable of binary fission (3,4). Phagosomes can contain tens of ehrlichial organisms that can be seen in the cytoplasm of their target cell as mulberry-like structures known as morulae on peripheral blood smears stained with Romanowsky-derived dyes. Typically, *Ehrlichia* spp. infect cells of leukocytic lineage (monocytes and polymorphonuclear leukocytes) in humans and other mammals, in contrast to *Anaplasma* spp., which infect bone-marrow-derived cells of all lineages (erythrocytes, platelets, and leukocytes).

EPIDEMIOLOGY

These infections are transmitted via a tick bite and are all zoonoses maintained in nature in a cycle that involves a mammal and an arthropod. In arthropods, ehrlichial organisms are transmitted transstadially (molting from larvae to nymphs and nymphs to adults), but not transovarially (5). Therefore, an infected mammalian host is needed for maintenance of the life cycle in nature.

Human Monocytotropic Ehrlichiosis

Its agent, *E. chaffeensis*, was proposed as an agent of human disease in 1991 after gene sequence analysis of a human isolate revealed enough genetic divergence from *E. canis* for it to be considered a novel bacterium (6,7). The first human case of agent for human monocytotropic ehrlichiosis (HME) occurred in 1986 (8). More than 1300 cases of HME were reported by the Centers for Disease Control and Prevention between 1999 and 2004 (9–11). Passive surveillance obtained from a large commercial reference laboratory diagnosed a total of 722 cases between 1992 and 1995 (12). Over 480 cases were reported from another commercial laboratory between 1997 and 1998 (13). Furthermore, a prospective study in Cape Girardeau, Missouri, conducted between 1996 and 1999 revealed an incidence between 2 and 4.7 per 100,000 population which represents an order of magnitude that is nearly higher than the incidence obtained by passive surveillance (14). Most cases of HME occur in the south-central and southeastern regions of the United States. However, cases also occur in the mid-Atlantic states (15). Cases have also been described in California, a state in which *Amblyomma americanum* (the main vector for HME) is not found. Therefore, alternate vectors (*Ixodes pacificus*) are thought to be involved (15). Reports from other parts of the world (16–19) including Latin America, Europe, Africa, and Asia also exist although the diagnosis is based on serological studies, so the possibility of a closely related organism as the cause of HME cannot be completely ruled out. However, *E. chaffeensis* DNA has been amplified from blood samples of patients in Cameroon (McBride, Personal communication). Polymerase chain reaction (PCR) detection of *E. chaffeensis* gene fragments has been reported from ticks trapped in continental China and Korea (19). In the United States, the main arthropod vector is *A. americanum* or the Lone Star tick, found in the regions where the disease has been described (20,21). *E. chaffeensis* DNA has also been detected by PCR from *Dermacentor variabilis* ticks in areas of the Midwest (22). The main mammal reservoir in nature for *E. chaffeensis* is the white-tailed deer (*Odocoileus virginianus*) (23–25). Domestic dogs are also implicated as natural reservoirs (26). Minor reservoirs also described include oppossums, foxes, wolves, raccoons, voles, coyotes, and goats (15).

Ehrlichiosis Ewingii

The disease was first described in 1999 in Missouri by demonstration of *E. ewingii* DNA sequences in the blood of four patients, three of whom were immunosuppressed (27). Two years later, four additional cases were described associated with HIV/AIDS (28). The clinical picture is similar to that of HME although based on a small number of human cases; it appears that *E. ewingii* is less virulent than *E. chaffeensis*. In fact, none of the cases with HIV and *E. ewingii* coinfection died as opposed to an increased mortality rate and severity in cases of HIV and *E. chaffeensis* coinfection (28). *E. ewingii* was first described as a canine pathogen in 1992 and is responsible for the disease known as canine granulocytotropic ehrlichiosis (29). Its main vector is also *A. americanum* although *E. ewingii* has also been detected in *D. variabilis* ticks (22,30). White-tailed deer are also reservoirs for this pathogen and therefore the geographic distribution of the disease is similar to HME (31). In humans, as in dogs, the target cell is the polymorphonuclear neutrophil. Human cases have been described so far in Missouri, Oklahoma, and Tennessee (28).

PATHOGENESIS AND PATHOLOGY

Ehrlichial organisms enter the body via a tick bite (nymph or adult). Attachment must extend for 24 to 48 hours in order for disease to appear. The mean incubation time is around 10 days. The elucidation of the pathogenesis and pathology of *E. chaffeensis* is a work in progress and has been studied extensively in vitro using monocyte-derived cell lines, and in vivo using murine animal models available for both chronic and acute ehrlichial infections (32–34). In addition, complete genome sequences have already been completed for *E. chaffeensis* and *E. canis*, therefore facilitating the study of pathogenesis of these organisms (35,36). *Ehrlichia* attach to a host cell receptor (E- and L-selectin) through surface-exposed glycoproteins (most likely the 120-kDa protein) (37). Internalization occurs through receptor-mediated endocytosis and requires phosphorylation of phospholipase C gamma 2 isoform that leads to production of inositide triphosphate, which in turn releases calcium from the endoplasmic reticulum and allows entry of calcium from the extracellular fluid via voltage-gated channels on the cellular membrane (37). It has also been shown that cholesterol-containing lipid rafts are involved in the internalization process and glycosylphosphatidylinositol (GPI) anchored proteins are also needed (38). Once internalized, ehrlichia reside in early endosomal compartments and inhibit fusion of endosomes with lysosomes (39,40). This inhibitory process is mediated by proteins such as RAB5A, SNAP23, and STX16. Accumulation of transferring receptors in the endosomal membrane has been demonstrated and is necessary for iron acquisition and ehrlichial survival within the endosome (39). In fact, ehrlichiae have conserved ferric-binding proteins, one of which is a 37-kDa protein known as ferric-binding protein (41). Inclusions containing replicative ehrlichiae are maintained in the caveolar trafficking system and interact with the endosomal pathway. Once inside the cell, ehrlichial organisms have evolved means to subvert the host cell response in order to favor their survival. Mechanisms of subversion of the host cell response include inhibition of phosphorylation of Janus kinases and signal transducer and activators of transcription (Jaks/Stat pathways) induced by IFN-γ (42). Additional modulation of host cell genes includes reduced activities of mitogen activated protein (MAP) kinases (MAPKs), NF-κB activation, upregulation of apoptotic inhibitors, and differential regulation of cell cyclins to improve cell survival (43). Recent experimental work indicates that ehrlichial glycoproteins are translocated to the nucleus and might influence transcription (McBride, Personal communication).

Histopathologic studies are mostly based on murine animal models available to study both acutely fatal and chronic infections (32–34). Systematic evaluation of human histopathology is not available due to the scarcity of tissues available for such studies. However, based on animal models and the few studies published on human pathology, it seems likely that the pathologic lesions seen in the different organs are in most part due to the immune response from the host leading to perivascular lymphohistiocytic aggregates present in liver, spleen, lungs, and bone marrow (12,44,45). Additional lesions include poorly formed granulomas in the bone marrow and liver and interstitial pneumonitis (46). If severe enough, the latter can lead to diffuse alveolar damage. In the central nervous system (CNS), *E. chaffeensis* induces a meningoencephalitis with the presence of perivascular lesions in both the meninges and brain parenchyma. The cellular infiltrates seen in affected organs, including the perivascular lesions, are, for the most part, due to induction of chemokines in the target cell by ehrlichial glycoproteins. In addition, cytokine responses have also been demonstrated both in vitro and in vivo and include elevated levels of IL-1β, IL-6, IL-8, TNF-α, and IFN-γ (47–51). In fact, in the animal model of fatal ehrlichiosis, markedly elevated levels of TNF-α produced by CD8 T-cells were demonstrated in the serum of fatally infected animals (34).

CLINICAL FEATURES

Clinical manifestations of HME range from a mild febrile illness to multisystem organ failure (13,14,52,53). Reports of asymptomatic seroconversion in humans with documented tick bites have been published, although the actual antigenic stimulus in those cases has never been fully characterized, suggesting the possibility of inoculation with a nonpathogenic ehrlichial organism (54). The most common presentation is that of fever (almost always >38°C), headache, myalgias, and arthralgias. Other symptoms and signs include nausea, vomiting, abdominal pain, respiratory, and CNS-related manifestations (Table 1) (13,14,52,53,55–58). A skin rash that involves the trunk and extremities, and less commonly the face, occurs in 12% to 36% of patients but it is present at the time of consultation in less than 10% of patients. The rash is far more common in children in whom it can appear in up to 67% of cases (59–61). The initial symptoms and signs appear after an average of 11 days after tick exposure but the incubation period may be as high as 34 days. Tick bite or tick exposure can be documented in up to 90% of cases. The disease is seasonal, with most cases occurring between April and September, time at which ticks are most actively looking for blood meals. HME is more frequent in males (3:2) and can affect people of all ages, including children and the elderly. The most important risk factor identified for development of severe disease besides immunosuppression due to AIDS or any other immunocompromising condition is age. The rate of life-threatening complications or death is higher in patients over 60 years old. The overall case-fatality rate is 2% to 3%.

Routine, nonspecific laboratory tests may aid in the diagnostic process of HME. Approximately two-thirds of the patients with HME show leucopenia and thrombocytopenia (13,14,53). Leucopenia usually appears by the third day of illness and peaks around day 6, after which gradually increases over a period of two weeks. The decline is more pronounced on the lymphocyte counts which can be decreased by up to 50% to 60% of normal values. During the second week of illness, a "rebound" lymphocytosis is present in almost all patients (62–64). The significance of this finding is unknown but immunophenotyping reveals that the lymphocytosis is due to a marked increased in $\gamma\delta$ T-lymphocytes which in some cases is so severe that false-positive results for the diagnosis of T-cell lymphomas can occur when T-cell receptor

TABLE 1 Main Signs and Symptoms Reported in Different Published Series of Human Monocytotropic Ehrlichiosis

Clinical feature	Eng et al. (52)	Fishbein et al. (58)	Everett et al. (56)	Schutze et al. (60)[a]	Olano et al. (13)	Olano et al. (14)
Fever	100	97	100	100	95[b]	100
Malaise/weakness	61	84	30	NR	NR	38
Chills/rigor	65	61	73	NR	NR	45
Cephalea	77	81	63	25	NR	72
Myalgia	53	68	43	58	NR	69
Arhtralgia	28	41	33	NR	NR	69
Anorexia	50	66	27	NR	NR	NR
Nausea	54	48	50	NR	NR	38
Vomiting	49	37	27	25	NR	38
Diarrhea	38	24	10	25	NR	10
Diaphoresis	21	53	NR	17	NR	NR
Abdominal pain	23	21	10	17	27	7
Cough	39	26	<10	17	NR	24
Pharyngitis	33	25	NR	17	NR	21
Rash	47	36	20	67	17	21
Confusion	29	20	20	8[c]	22	21
Photophobia	11	NR	13	NR	27	NR
Stupor	NR	NR	NR	NR	7	NR
Coma	NR	NR	NR	NR	2	NR
Seizures	NR	NR	NR	NR	2	NR
Lymphadenopathy	26	25	NR	NR	29	NR
Jaundice	15	NR	NR	NR	NR	NR
Dyspnea	23	NR	<10	NR	NR	NR
Hepatomegaly	15	NR	<10	25	2	NR
Splenomegaly	15	NR	NR	25	2	NR

All values expressed as % of total number of cases.
[a]This series includes pediatric cases only ($n = 12$). Other reported signs and symptoms included puffy eyes, murmur, and dehydration.
[b]Malaise and headache usually accompanied fever in this series.
[c]Described as irritable or combative instead of confusion.

rearrangements are analyzed by molecular techniques. $\gamma\delta$ T-cell lymphocytosis disappears in two to four weeks. Platelets also start decreasing from days 1 to 3 of illness and reach the lowest values around day 6, after which a gradual recovery is seen over the next two to three weeks. Another useful but nonspecific finding is the presence of mildly to moderately elevated liver enzymes which can reach values of up to 400 to 500 IU/L ("transaminitis"). Both aspartate amino transferase (AST) and alanine amino transferase (ALT) levels are elevated and parallel each other. However, ALT levels are usually higher than AST levels (Table 2).

LABORATORY DIAGNOSIS

There are four categories of testing available for diagnosis of HME, namely direct visualization of the ehrlichial organisms on peripheral blood smears or other tissues, molecular detection of ehrlichial DNA or RNA by nucleic acid amplification techniques, detection of antibodies in serum by immunofluorescence antibody (IFA) or Western immunoblotting, and cultivation of *E. chaffeensis* in cell monolayers.

Ethylenediamine tetraacetic acid (EDTA)-anticoagulated blood and serum are the most important specimens that should be obtained for diagnosis of HME during the acute phase of the disease. If the patient has prominent neurologic signs and symptoms, a CSF specimen is usually obtained and reveals mild pleocytosis with lymphocytosis. Occasionally, visualization of typical ehrlichial morulae in CSF monocytes has been described. Visualization of morulae in peripheral blood monocytes is rather insensitive as a diagnostic tool for HME but a careful search should be performed on peripheral blood smears stained with Romanowsky-derived stains when suspicion of HME is high. An excellent alternative is the examination of buffy coat smears which increase the number of cells available for analysis by an order of magnitude.

TABLE 2 Summary of Laboratory Values Reported in Different Published Series of Patients with Human Monocytotropic Ehrlichiosis

Test result	Eng et al. (52)	Fishbein et al. (53)	Everett et al. (56)	Schutze et al. (60)[a]	Olano et al. (13)	Olano et al. (14)
Leucopenia	74	50	57	58	54	60
Thrombocytopenia	72	88	70	92	70	57
Anemia	50	63	NR	42	59	NR
Increased AST	88	NR	85	91	86	52
Increased ALT	78	88	74	67	83	NR
Increased BUN	31	NR	4	17	NR	NR
Increased creatinine	24	NR	4	17	NR	NR
Increased bilirubin	39	13	24	NR	NR	NR

All values expressed as % of total number of cases.
[a]This series includes pediatric cases only ($n = 12$).
Abbreviations: ALT, alanine amino transferase; AST, aspartate amino transferase; BUN; blood urea nitrogen.

Under ideal conditions, the sensitivity of this method is up to 30% in culture-proven cases (7,66,67). The number of cells with morulae is higher in immunocompromised patients. Immunocytologic/immunohistologic methods using mostly polyclonal antibodies against *E. chaffeensis* have been developed in selected research laboratories but are not available commercially (44,68). Tissues used for this purpose include lungs, spleen, bone marrow, and liver and are usually available when a postmortem diagnosis is needed. For premortem diagnosis, the most frequently obtained tissue is the bone marrow for evaluation of blood cytopenias, although it is obtained infrequently.

Detection of ehrlichial DNA/RNA from samples of peripheral blood is probably the best method to diagnose HME during the acute phase. EDTA-anticoagulated samples are also used for this purpose, and extraction of DNA can be performed from whole blood or buffy coats. The most extensively evaluated set of primers is the one designed for amplification of the 16S rRNA gene (HE1/HE3 primers) (14,56,69,70). The product is a 389-bp fragment that can be detected by nucleic acid staining after gel electrophoresis or by Southern blotting using an internal probe. The latter increases the analytical sensitivity of the assay. A clinical evaluation of the HE1/HE3 primers using gel electrophoresis and visualization of the specific band with ethidium bromide showed a sensitivity of 79% to 100% when using seroconversion during convalescence as the gold standard. It is worth noting that isolated reports of lack of seroconversion in culture-proven cases has been reported and appears to be related to administration of specific therapy early in the course of the disease (67). Nested-PCR techniques have also been described in order to increase the analytical sensitivity of the test but the risk of DNA-amplicon contamination increases with "open-nested" techniques.

Other PCR targets that are not as extensively evaluated include the *groESL* operon, a variable-length PCR target (which codes for a 40 to 50 kDa glycoprotein with variable tandem-repeat units), the 120-kDa antigen gene which codes for a surface-exposed glycoprotein with tandem-repeat units, the *nadA* gene, and the p28 multigene family (14,28,67,71). In a prospective study, the 120-kDa protein gene, the *nadA* gene, and the 16S rRNA gene all had similar sensitivity and specificity when using ethidium bromide for visualization of specific products. In this particular study, the overall sensitivity was 56% and the specificity was 100% (14). However, many samples were obtained from patients during the late convalescent phase (based on high antibody titers by IFA and clinical history) when ehrlichial organisms circulating in blood are already at low concentrations. When sensitivity was calculated based on seroconversion rates as gold standard, it rose to 84%.

Recently, a real-time multicolor PCR and real-time multiplex reverse transcriptase PCR assays were developed and both have extremely high analytical sensitivities and specificities. The analytical sensitivity is as low as 50 ehrlichial organisms and the main advantages include speed, low risk of contamination, cost, and the possibility of detecting multiple ehrlichial pathogens in a single amplification run (72,73).

Serological methods are the most widely used method for confirmation of ehrlichial infections. However, the diagnosis is usually made on a retrospective basis since the percentage of patients with ehrlichial antibodies at the time of the first visit during the acute phase is less than 30% (74,75). IFA is the most widely used technique and it is available in research and commercial reference laboratories (15,76–78). IFA standardization is lacking, and each laboratory is responsible for validating the IFA technique using either home-made antigen glass slides or commercially available slides. Samples are usually screened at 1:64 or 1:80 dilutions and titrated if reactivity is detected. IFA testing is performed using anti-Ig conjugates (detect all IgG, IgA, and IgM antibodies), anti-IgM alone, or anti-IgG alone conjugates. Careful evaluation of all conjugates is not available although a single report suggests that detection of IgM antibodies in the acute phase might be slightly more sensitive than detection of the other antibodies (75). This finding underscores the difficulty in interpreting IgM antibody titers when performing ehrlichial serology. IgM titers are considered elevated when titers are 1:32 or greater.

Immunoblotting procedures are available in research laboratories and theoretically have increased specificity when compared to IFA. Differentiation between HME and human granulocytic anaplasmosis, which can sometimes induce formation of cross-reactive antibodies, is possible by immunoblotting. Antibodies reactive with one or more of the 22, 28, 29, 46, 54, 120, or 200 kDa proteins confirm the presence of HME (79–82). A recombinant 120-kDa protein used in a dot-blot format proved to be both sensitive and specific as a confirmation tool (83).

Cultivation of *E. chaffeensis* is possible in only selected research laboratories around the world. Isolation of *E. chaffeensis* has been reported in approximately 30 patients around the country (7,66,67). The most widely used cell type for isolation is the canine hystiocytic cell line DH82 but successful isolation has also been reported using THP-1 (a human monocytic leukemia cell line), HEL-22 cells (fibroblast-like cells), Vero cells, and a human promyelocytic leukemia cell line (HL-60). The latter has to undergo treatment with retinoic acid to induce differentiation through the monocytic pathway (84). Monolayers are inoculated either with whole blood or ideally with buffy coats obtained by lysis of red blood cells or density gradient centrifugation with Ficoll-Paque. The generation time of *E. chaffeensis* has been calculated at 19 hours. Therefore, cell monolayers or suspensions must be maintained at a low growth rate to avoid overgrowth of ehrlichial organisms by rapidly proliferating host cells. Cultures are maintained for four to six weeks and examined every five to seven days by scraping monolayers or cytocentrifugation (cytospins) followed by immunofluorescent staining or Romanowsky stains to detect intracytoplasmic morulae. The main confounding factor is the presence of apoptotic cell fragments being phagocytosed by neighboring cells. Confirmation is done with IFA and PCR (Table 3).

The laboratory diagnosis of ehrlichiosis ewingii rests on the detection of *E. ewingii* DNA in peripheral blood of infected patients by standard PCR techniques. As mentioned above, a newly developed real-time PCR assay is capable of detecting and differentiating *E. ewingii* DNA in a multiplex format. Serological assays are not specific due to the extensive cross-reactivity between *E. chaffeensis* and *E. ewingii*. Cultivation of *E. ewingii* has been elusive.

DIFFERENTIAL DIAGNOSIS

Due to the nonspecific nature of the signs and symptoms, the differential diagnosis of the human ehrlichioses is very broad (13,77,85). Cases in which the only manifestations are

TABLE 3 Case Definitions for Human Monocytotropic Ehrlichiosis (2000)

Confirmed case of HME
A clinically compatible illness (febrile patient with history of tick bite or tick exposure), and demonstration of a fourfold change in antibody titer to *Ehrlichia chaffeensis* by IFA in paired serum samples, or Positive PCR assay and confirmation of *E. chaffeensis* DNA, or Identification of morulae in peripheral monocytes and a positive IFA titer to *E. chaffeensis*, or Immunostaining of biopsy or autopsy material, or Culture of *E. chaffeensis* from clinical specimen

Probable case of HME
A clinically compatible illness (febrile patient with a history of tick bite or tick exposure), and Presence of a single positive IFA titer or stationary titer in paired samples (if titer >fourfold above cut-off value) or visualization of morulae in leukocytes or positive PCR assay without sequencing confirmation

Abbreviations: HME, human monocytotropic ehrlichiosis; IFA, immunofluorescence antibody, PCR, polymerase chain reaction.
Source: From Ref. 90.

constitutional signs and symptoms such as fever, headache, malaise, myalgias, and arthralgias, HME must be differentiated from other acute febrile illnesses including viruses leading to "flu-like" clinical pictures. In cases where the predominant manifestations are related to the CNS, the differential diagnosis comprises bacterial and viral meningoencephalitis, including vector-borne agents. Cases with pulmonary or GI manifestations must be differentiated from acute viral and bacterial illnesses affecting those organs. Severe cases presenting as multiorgan failure must be differentiated from other entities such as bacterial sepsis, toxic sock syndrome, endocarditis, meningococcemia, and typhoid fever. In cases where the rash is present, the differential diagnosis will include Rocky Mountain spotted fever, relapsing fever, murine typhus, vasculitis, thrombotic thrombocytopenic purpura, and collagen vascular diseases, among others. The diagnosis of ehrlichiosis should be considered in any patient presenting with fever, generalized aching, leucopenia, thrombocytopenia, and abnormal liver function tests.

TREATMENT AND PROGNOSIS

Antibiotic regimens for human ehrlichioses have not been evaluated in controlled, prospective, double-blind randomized trials. On the basis of retrospective empirical clinical data and in vitro susceptibility testing, doxycycline is the drug of choice (86–89). Because of concerns with fetal welfare in pregnant women, doxycycline should be substituted with rifampin which has shown some success. Duration of treatment has not been evaluated but the consensus is treatment for three to five days after complete defervescence which equates to at least 10 days of therapy.

The prognosis is very favorable when therapy is administered early in the disease process. In cases that present or progress to multiorgan failure, the prognosis worsens. The overall case-fatality ratio for HME is around 2% to 3%.

Even though acute signs and symptoms respond quickly to treatment in noncomplicated cases, asthenia persists for weeks or months. The basis for this phenomenon is completely unknown but evidence of chronic infections in humans due to *E. chaffeensis* or *E. ewingii* is lacking. Antibody titers might be high for weeks or months after successful treatment, and treatment should not be restarted because of high antibody titers in the presence of fatigability.

In summary, the field of human ehrlichioses continues to evolve rapidly as more efforts are devoted to their study around the world. Major advances have been made in the field in the last 15 years from the time in which HME was first described, especially in the areas of pathogenesis, genetics, and epidemiology. However, these diseases still remain grossly underdiagnosed. Powerful diagnostic techniques are available, although standardization and widespread availability are lacking.

REFERENCES

1. Dumler JS, Barbet AF, Bekker CP, et al. Reorganization of genera in the families Rickettsiaceae and Anaplasmataceae in the order Rickettsiales: unification of some species of *Ehrlichia* with *Anaplasma*, *Cowdria* with *Ehrlichia* and *Ehrlichia* with *Neorickettsia*, descriptions of six new species combinations and designation of *Ehrlichia equi* and "HGE agent" as subjective synonyms of *Ehrlichia phagocytophila*. Int J Syst Evol Microbiol 2001; 51:2145–2165.
2. Perez M, Rikihisa Y, Wen B. *Ehrlichia canis*-like agent isolated from a man in Venezuela: antigenic and genetic characterization. J Clin Microbiol 1996; 34:2133–2139.
3. Popov VL, Han VC, Chen SM, et al. Ultrastructural differentiation of the genogroups in the genus *Ehrlichia*. J Med Microbiol 1998; 47:235–251.
4. Popov VL, Chen SM, Feng HM, Walker DH. Ultrastructural variation of cultured *Ehrlichia chaffeensis*. J Med Microbiol 1995; 43:411–421.
5. Long SW, Zhang X, Zhang J, Ruble RP, Teel P, Yu XJ. Evaluation of transovarial transmission and transmissibility of *Ehrlichia chaffeensis* (Rickettsiales: Anaplasmataceae) in *Amblyomma americanum* (Acari: Ixodidae). J Med Entomol 2003; 40:1000–1004.
6. Anderson BE, Dawson JE, Jones DC, Wilson KH. *Ehrlichia chaffeensis*, a new species associated with human ehrlichiosis. J Clin Microbiol 1991; 29:2838–2842.
7. Dawson JE, Anderson BE, Fishbein DB, et al. Isolation and characterization of an *Ehrlichia* sp. from a patient diagnosed with human ehrlichiosis. J Clin Microbiol 1991; 29:2741–2745.
8. Maeda K, Markowitz N, Hawley RC, Ristic M, Cox D, McDade JE. Human infection with *Ehrlichia canis*, a leukocytic rickettsia. N Engl J Med 1987; 316:853–856.

9. Prevention CDCa. Summary of provisional cases of selected notifiable diseases, United States 2004. Morb Mortal Wkly Rep 2005; 53:1213.
10. Prevention CDCa. Summary of notifiable diseases, United States, 2003. Morb Mortal Wkly Rep 2005; 55:16, 20, 27, 72.
11. Gardner SI, Holman RC, Krebs JW, Berkelman R, Childs JE. National surveillance for the human ehrlichioses in the United States, 1997–2001, and proposed methods of data quality. Ann NY Acad Sci 2003; 990:80–89.
12. Walker DH, Dumler JS. Emergence of the ehrlichioses as human health problems. Emerg Infect Dis 1996; 2:18–29.
13. Olano JP, Hogrefe W, Seaton B, Walker DH. Clinical manifestations, epidemiology, and laboratory diagnosis of human monocytotropic ehrlichiosis in a commercial laboratory setting. Clin Diagn Lab Immunol 2003; 10:891–896.
14. Olano JP, Masters E, Hogrefe W, Walker DH. Human monocytotropic ehrlichiosis, Missouri. Emerg Infect Dis 2003; 9:1579–1586.
15. Paddock CD, Childs JE. *Ehrlichia chaffeensis*: a prototypical emerging pathogen. Clin Microbiol Rev 2003; 16:37–64.
16. Brouqui P, Le Cam C, Kelly PJ, et al. Serologic evidence for human ehrlichiosis in Africa. Eur J Epidemiol 1994; 10:695–698.
17. Cinco M, Barbone F, Grazia Ciufolini M, et al. Seroprevalence of tick-borne infections in forestry rangers from northeastern Italy. Clin Microbiol Infect 2004; 10:1056–1061.
18. Gongora-Biachi RA, Zavala-Velazquez J, Castro-Sansores CJ, Gonzalez-Martinez P. First case of human ehrlichiosis in Mexico. Emerg Infect Dis 1999; 5:481.
19. Ripoll CM, Remondegui CE, Ordonez G, et al. Evidence of rickettsial spotted fever and ehrlichial infections in a subtropical territory of Jujuy, Argentina. Am J Trop Med Hyg 1999; 61:350–354.
20. Lockhart JM, Davidson WR, Dawson JE, Stallknecht DE. Temporal association of *Amblyomma americanum* with the presence of *Ehrlichia chaffeensis* reactive antibodies in white-tailed deer. J Wildl Dis 1995; 31:119–124.
21. Lockhart JM, Davidson WR, Stallknecht DE, Dawson JE. Site-specific geographic association between *Amblyomma americanum* (Acari: Ixodidae) infestations and *Ehrlichia chaffeensis*-reactive (Rickettsiales: Ehrlichiae) antibodies in white-tailed deer. J Med Entomol 1996; 33:153–158.
22. Steiert JG, Gilfoy F. Infection rates of *Amblyomma americanum* and *Dermacentor variabilis* by *Ehrlichia chaffeensis* and *Ehrlichia ewingii* in southwest Missouri. Vector Borne Zoonotic Dis 2002; 2:53–60.
23. Lockhart JM, Davidson WR, Stallknecht DE, Dawson JE, Howerth EW. Isolation of *Ehrlichia chaffeensis* from wild white-tailed deer (*Odocoileus virginianus*) confirms their role as natural reservoir hosts. J Clin Microbiol 1997; 35:1681–1686.
24. Dawson JE, Stallknecht DE, Howerth EW, et al. Susceptibility of white-tailed deer (*Odocoileus virginianus*) to infection with *Ehrlichia chaffeensis*, the etiologic agent of human ehrlichiosis. J Clin Microbiol 1994; 32:2725–2728.
25. Dawson JE, Childs JE, Biggie KL, et al. White-tailed deer as a potential reservoir of *Ehrlichia* spp. J Wildl Dis 1994; 30:162–168.
26. Dawson JE, Ewing SA. Susceptibility of dogs to infection with *Ehrlichia chaffeensis*, causative agent of human ehrlichiosis. Am J Vet Res 1992; 53:1322–1327.
27. Buller RS, Arens M, Hmiel SP, et al. *Ehrlichia ewingii*, a newly recognized agent of human ehrlichiosis [see comment]. N Engl J Med 1999; 341:148–155.
28. Paddock CD, Folk SM, Shore GM, et al. Infections with *Ehrlichia chaffeensis* and *Ehrlichia ewingii* in persons coinfected with human immunodeficiency virus. Clin Infect Dis 2001; 33:1586–1594.
29. Anderson BE, Greene CE, Jones DC, Dawson JE. *Ehrlichia ewingii* sp. nov., the etiologic agent of canine granulocytic ehrlichiosis. Int J Syst Bacteriol 1992; 42:299–302.
30. Wolf L, McPherson T, Harrison B, Engber B, Anderson A, Whitt P. Prevalence of *Ehrlichia ewingii* in *Amblyomma americanum* in North Carolina. J Clin Microbiol 2000; 38:2795.
31. Arens MQ, Liddell AM, Buening G, et al. Detection of *Ehrlichia* spp. in the blood of wild white-tailed deer in Missouri by PCR assay and serologic analysis. J Clin Microbiol 2003; 41:1263–1265.
32. Sotomayor EA, Popov VL, Feng HM, Walker DH, Olano JP. Animal model of fatal human monocytotropic ehrlichiosis. Am J Pathol 2001; 158:757–769.
33. Olano JP, Wen G, Feng HM, McBride JW, Walker DH. Histologic, serologic, and molecular analysis of persistent ehrlichiosis in a murine model. Am J Pathol 2004; 165:997–1006.
34. Ismail N, Soong L, McBride JW, et al. Overproduction of TNF-alpha by CD8 + type 1 cells and down-regulation of IFN-gamma production by CD4 + Th1 cells contribute to toxic shock-like syndrome in an animal model of fatal monocytotropic ehrlichiosis. J Immunol 2004; 172:1786–1800.
35. Mavromatis K, Doyle CK, Lykidi A, et al. The genome of the obligately intracellular bacterium *Ehrlichia caviis* reveals themes of complex membrance structure and immune evasion strategies. J Bacteriology 2006; 188:4015–4023.
36. Hotopp JC, Lin M, Madupu R, et al. Comparative genomics of energing human ehrlichios agents. PLoS Genetics 2006; 2(2):e21.

37. Zhang JZ, McBride JW, Yu XJ. L-selectin and E-selectin expressed on monocytes mediating *Ehrlichia chaffeensis* attachment onto host cells. FEMS Microbiol Lett 2003; 227:303–309.
38. Lin M, Rikihisa Y. Obligatory intracellular parasitism by *Ehrlichia chaffeensis* and *Anaplasma phagocytophilum* involves caveolae and glycosylphosphatidylinositol-anchored proteins. Cell Microbiol 2003; 5:809–820.
39. Barnewall RE, Rikihisa Y, Lee EH. *Ehrlichia chaffeensis* inclusions are early endosomes which selectively accumulate transferrin receptor. Infect Immun 1997; 65:1455–1461.
40. Rikihisa Y. Mechanisms to create a safe haven by members of the family *Anaplasmataceae*. Ann NY Acad Sci 2003; 990:548–555.
41. McBride JW, Ndip LM, Popov VL, Walker DH. Identification and functional analysis of an immunoreactive DsbA-like thio-disulfide oxidoreductase of *Ehrlichia* spp. Infect Immun 2002; 70:2700–2703.
42. Lee EH, Rikihisa Y. Protein kinase A-mediated inhibition of gamma interferon-induced tyrosine phosphorylation of Janus kinases and latent cytoplasmic transcription factors in human monocytes by *Ehrlichia chaffeensis*. Infect Immun 1998; 66:2514–2520.
43. Lin M, Rikihisa Y. *Ehrlichia chaffeensis* downregulates surface Toll-like receptors 2/4, CD14 and transcription factors PU.1 and inhibits lipopolysaccharide activation of NF-kappa B, ERK 1/2 and p38 MAPK in host monocytes. Cell Microbiol 2004; 6:175–186.
44. Dumler JS, Dawson JE, Walker DH. Human ehrlichiosis: hematopathology and immunohistologic detection of *Ehrlichia chaffeensis*. Hum Pathol 1993; 24:391–396.
45. Sehdev AE, Dumler JS. Hepatic pathology in human monocytic ehrlichiosis: *Ehrlichia chaffeensis* infection. Am J Clin Pathol 2003; 119:859–865.
46. Walker DH, Dumler JS. Human monocytic and granulocytic ehrlichioses: discovery and diagnosis of emerging tick-borne infections and the critical role of the pathologist. Arch Pathol Lab Med 1997; 121:785–791.
47. Feng HM, Walker DH. Mechanisms of immunity to *Ehrlichia muris*: a model of monocytotropic ehrlichiosis. Infect Immun 2004; 72:966–971.
48. Kim HY, Rikihisa Y. Expression of interleukin-1beta, tumor necrosis factor alpha, and interleukin-6 in human peripheral blood leukocytes exposed to human granulocytic ehrlichiosis agent or recombinant major surface protein P44. Infect Immun 2000; 68:3394–3402.
49. Tuo W, Palmer GH, McGuire TC, Zhu D, Brown WC. Interleukin-12 as an adjuvant promotes immunoglobulin G and type 1 cytokine recall responses to major surface protein 2 of the ehrlichial pathogen *Anaplasma marginale*. Infect Immun 2000; 68:270–280.
50. Lee EH, Rikihisa Y. Anti-*Ehrlichia chaffeensis* antibody complexed with *E. chaffeensis* induces potent proinflammatory cytokine mRNA expression in human monocytes through sustained reduction of IkappaB-alpha and activation of NF-kappaB. Infect Immun 1997; 65:2890–2897.
51. Lee EH, Rikihisa Y. Absence of tumor necrosis factor alpha, interleukin-6 (IL-6), and granulocyte-macrophage colony-stimulating factor expression but presence of IL-1beta, IL-8, and IL-10 expression in human monocytes exposed to viable or killed *Ehrlichia chaffeensis*. Infect Immun 1996; 64:4211–4219.
52. Eng TR, Harkess JR, Fishbein DB, et al. Epidemiologic, clinical, and laboratory findings of human ehrlichiosis in the United States, 1988. J Am Med Assoc 1990; 264:2251–2258.
53. Fishbein DB, Kemp A, Dawson JE, Greene NR, Redus MA, Fields DH. Human ehrlichiosis: prospective active surveillance in febrile hospitalized patients. J Infect Dis 1989; 160:803–809.
54. Yevich SJ, Sanchez JL, DeFraites RF, et al. Seroepidemiology of infections due to spotted fever group rickettsiae and *Ehrlichia* species in military personnel exposed to areas of the United States where such infections are endemic. J Infect Dis 1995; 171:1266–1273.
55. Eng TR, Fishbein DB, Dawson JE, Greene CR, Redus M. Surveillance of human ehrlichiosis in the United States: 1988. Ann NY Acad Sci 1990; 590:306–307.
56. Everett ED, Evans KA, Henry RB, McDonald G. Human ehrlichiosis in adults after tick exposure: diagnosis using polymerase chain reaction. Ann Intern Med 1994; 120:730–735.
57. Ratnasamy N, Everett ED, Roland WE, McDonald G, Caldwell CW. Central nervous system manifestations of human ehrlichiosis. Clin Infect Dis 1996; 23:314–319.
58. Fishbein DB, Dawson JE, Robinson LE. Human ehrlichiosis in the United States. Ann Intern Med 1994; 120:736–743.
59. Marshall GS, Jacobs RF, Schutze GE, et al. *Ehrlichia chaffeensis* seroprevalence among children in the southeast and south-central regions of the United States. Arch Pediatr Adolesc Med 2002; 156:166–170.
60. Schutze GE, Jacobs RF. Human monocytic ehrlichiosis in children. Pediatrics 1997; 100:E10.
61. Jacobs RF, Schutze GE. Ehrlichiosis in children. J Pediatr 1997; 131:184–192.
62. Caldwell CW, Everett ED, McDonald G, Yesus YW, Roland WE. Lymphocytosis of gamma/delta T cells in human ehrlichiosis. Am J Clin Pathol 1995; 104:761–766.
63. Heeb HL, Wilkerson MJ, Chun R, Ganta RR. Large granular lymphocytosis, lymphocyte subset inversion, thrombocytopenia, dysproteinemia, and positive *Ehrlichia* serology in a dog. J Am Anim Hosp Assoc 2003; 39:379–384.

64. Caldwell CW, Everett ED, McDonald G, Yesus YW, Roland WE, Huang HM. Apoptosis of gamma/delta T cells in human ehrlichiosis. Am J Clin Pathol 1996; 105:640–646.
65. Aguero-Rosenfeld M, Olano JP. *Ehrlichia*, *Anaplasma* and related intracellular bacteria. In: ASM Manual for Clinical Microbiology. 9th Ed. In press
66. Paddock CD, Sumner JW, Shore GM, et al. Isolation and characterization of *Ehrlichia chaffeensis* strains from patients with fatal ehrlichiosis. J Clin Microbiol 1997; 35:2496–2502.
67. Standaert SM, Yu T, Scott MA, et al. Primary isolation of *Ehrlichia chaffeensis* from patients with febrile illnesses: clinical and molecular characteristics. J Infect Dis 2000; 181:1082–1088.
68. Yu X, Brouqui P, Dumler JS, Raoult D. Detection of *Ehrlichia chaffeensis* in human tissue by using a species-specific monoclonal antibody. J Clin Microbiol 1993; 31:3284–3288.
69. Anderson BE, Sumner JW, Dawson JE, et al. Detection of the etiologic agent of human ehrlichiosis by polymerase chain reaction. J Clin Microbiol 1992; 30:775–780.
70. Standaert SM, Dawson JE, Schaffner W, et al. Ehrlichiosis in a golf-oriented retirement community [see comment]. N Engl J Med 1995; 333:420–425.
71. Sumner JW, Sims KG, Jones DC, Anderson BE. *Ehrlichia chaffeensis* expresses an immunoreactive protein homologous to the *Escherichia coli* GroEL protein. Infect Immun 1993; 61:3536–3539.
72. Sirigireddy KR, Ganta RR. Multiplex detection of *Ehrlichia* and *Anaplasma* species pathogens in peripheral blood by real-time reverse transcriptase-polymerase chain reaction. J Mol Diagn 2005; 7:308–316.
73. Doyle CK, Labruna MB, Breitschwerdt EB, et al. Detection of medically important *Ehrlichia* by quantitative multicolor TaqMan real-time polymerase chain reaction of the *dsb* gene. J Mol Diagn 2005; 7:504–510.
74. Comer JA, Nicholson WL, Sumner JW, Olson JG, Childs JE. Diagnosis of human ehrlichiosis by PCR assay of acute-phase serum. J Clin Microbiol 1999; 37:31–34.
75. Childs JE, Sumner JW, Nicholson WL, Massung RF, Standaert SM, Paddock CD. Outcome of diagnostic tests using samples from patients with culture-proven human monocytic ehrlichiosis: implications for surveillance. J Clin Microbiol 1999; 37:2997–3000.
76. Walker DH. Diagnosing human ehrlichiosis. ASM News 2000; 66:287–290.
77. Olano JP, Walker DH. Human ehrlichioses. Med Clin North Am 2002; 86:375–392.
78. Olano JP, Walker DH. Current recommendations for diagnosis and treatment of the human ehrlichioses. Infect Med 2002; 318–325.
79. Brouqui P, Dumler JS, Raoult D, Walker DH. Antigenic characterization of ehrlichiae: protein immunoblotting of *Ehrlichia canis*, *Ehrlichia sennetsu*, and *Ehrlichia risticii*. J Clin Microbiol 1992; 30:1062–1066.
80. Chen SM, Dumler JS, Feng HM, Walker DH. Identification of the antigenic constituents of *Ehrlichia chaffeensis*. Am J Trop Med Hyg 1994; 50:52–58.
81. Chen SM, Cullman LC, Walker DH. Western immunoblotting analysis of the antibody responses of patients with human monocytotropic ehrlichiosis to different strains of *Ehrlichia chaffeensis* and *Ehrlichia canis*. Clin Diagn Lab Immunol 1997; 4:731–735.
82. Wong SJ, Brady GS, Dumler JS. Serological responses to *Ehrlichia equi*, *Ehrlichia chaffeensis*, and *Borrelia burgdorferi* in patients from New York State. J Clin Microbiol 1997; 35:2198–2205.
83. Yu XJ, Crocquet-Valdes P, Cullman LC, Walker DH. The recombinant 120-kilodalton protein of *Ehrlichia chaffeensis*, a potential diagnostic tool. J Clin Microbiol 1996; 34:2853–2855.
84. Heimer R, Tisdale D, Dawson JE. A single tissue culture system for the propagation of the agents of the human ehrlichioses [see comment]. Am J Trop Med Hyg 1998; 58:812–815.
85. Stone JH, Dierberg K, Aram G, Dumler JS. Human monocytic ehrlichiosis. J Am Med Assoc 2004; 292:2263–2270.
86. Branger S, Rolain JM, Raoult D. Evaluation of antibiotic susceptibilities of *Ehrlichia canis*, *Ehrlichia chaffeensis*, and *Anaplasma phagocytophilum* by real-time PCR. Antimicrob Agents Chemother 2004; 48:4822–4828.
87. Maurin M, Abergel C, Raoult D. DNA gyrase-mediated natural resistance to fluoroquinolones in *Ehrlichia* spp. Antimicrob Agents Chemother 2001; 45:2098–2105.
88. Rolain JM, Maurin M, Bryskier A, Raoult D. In vitro activities of telithromycin (HMR 3647) against *Rickettsia rickettsii*, *Rickettsia conorii*, *Rickettsia africae*, *Rickettsia typhi*, *Rickettsia prowazekii*, *Coxiella burnetii*, *Bartonella henselae*, *Bartonella quintana*, *Bartonella bacilliformis*, and *Ehrlichia chaffeensis*. Antimicrob Agents Chemother 2000; 44:1391–1393.
89. Brouqui P, Raoult D. In vitro antibiotic susceptibility of the newly recognized agent of ehrlichiosis in humans, *Ehrlichia chaffeensis*. Antimicrob Agents Chemother 1992; 36:2799–2803.
90. http://www.cdc.gov.epo/dphsi/print/ehrlichiosis_current.htm.

16 Anaplasmosis in Humans

Anna Grzeszczuk
Department of Infectious Diseases, Medical University of Bialystok, Bialystok, Poland

Nicole C. Barat
Division of Medical Microbiology, Department of Pathology, The Johns Hopkins University School of Medicine, Baltimore, Maryland, U.S.A.

Johan S. Bakken
Department of Family Medicine, School of Medicine, University of Minnesota at Duluth and St. Luke's Infectious Disease Associates, St. Luke's Hospital, Duluth, Minnesota, U.S.A.

J. Stephen Dumler
Division of Medical Microbiology, Department of Pathology, The Johns Hopkins University School of Medicine, Baltimore, Maryland, U.S.A.

INTRODUCTION

Changes in ecology wrought by human behavior have had a substantial effect on the environment (1). One such effect, evident to those interested in infectious diseases has been the increase in zoonoses, particularly vector-transmitted infections (2,3). Unanticipated changes occurring with human environmental modifications have led to the concurrence of several important events: increases in the abundance of some wild animal populations owing to the loss of natural predators or adaptation to peridomestic environments, a consequent increase and spread of ectoparasites, such as ticks, associated with these wild animal populations, and the human desire to live, work, or recreate in natural, wild, or otherwise "pristine" habitats for which humans are nonnatural inhabitants. Such is the case with the emergence and reemergence of important tick-transmitted infections such as Lyme disease, but also the more deadly rickettsial pathogens, including one not previously recognized in humans now assigned to the genus *Anaplasma*. The purpose of this chapter is to describe various features of the clinical and pathologic aspects of human disease, and important related components of ecology and epidemiology, recognized to occur with infection by *Anaplasma phagocytophilum*, the sole member of the genus known to infect and cause disease in humans.

MICROBIOLOGY, PATHOLOGY, AND PATHOGENESIS
Taxonomy and Nomenclature

Human granulocytic anaplasmosis (HGA) is a tick-borne zoonotic infection that is caused by *A. phagocytophilum* (4). HGA has become increasingly recognized in the United States and in several European countries. The increased desire of humans to pursue outdoor recreational activities during the summer months has also amplified their potential exposure to pathogenic bacteria, for which a portion of the lifecycle occurs in nonvertebrate bloodsucking enzootic hosts. Just like *Borrelia burgdorferi*, the agent of Lyme borreliosis, *A. phagocytophilum* cycles within hard-bodied ticks that are members of the *Ixodes persulcatus* complex.

Although agents now recognized as *A. phagocytophilum* have been known as veterinary pathogens since 1932 (5), Bakken et al. (6) were the first to describe the infection, now called HGA, found among older men in the upper midwestern states in 1994. This human outbreak allowed an intensive molecular and serologic study among infected humans, California horses infected with *Ehrlichia equi*, and some European ruminants infected with *E. phagocytophilum* (7). Because of substantial serological and molecular data, these agents have now been reclassified in the genus *Anaplasma*. In fact, this and similar analyses prompted an extensive reorganization of the families Rickettsiaceae and Anaplasmataceae such that many species in the genera *Ehrlichia*, *Anaplasma*, and *Neorickettsia* were reassigned, and at least one genus, *Cowdria*, was eliminated (4).

The genus *Anaplasma* now encompasses the ruminant species *A. marginale*, *A. centrale*, *A. phagocytophilum*, *A. platys*, and *A. bovis*, all of which have the capacity for persistence in ruminants and possibly other hosts in the absence of significant clinical signs of infection. All members of this genus are tick-transmitted to various degrees, but each has a predilection for infection of a different host's bone marrow-derived cell. *A. phagocytophilum* chiefly infects granulocytes, mostly peripheral blood neutrophils, while limited data suggest the potential for a broader host cell range (8).

Microbiology and Pathogenesis

The ability to survive within neutrophils is a highly unique adaptation, and the mechanism by which *A. phagocytophilum* has achieved this niche is a matter of intense investigation (9,10). It is known that *A. phagocytophilum* substantially alters host neutrophil function, by in part promoting inflammation and recruitment of additional inflammatory cells that could serve as new hosts (11–13), while preventing substantial margination and tissue distribution to facilitate maximal bacteremia for transmission to biting ticks (14–16). In natural hosts, this interaction seems to have minimal disease impact, and the bacteremia persists for long intervals, an obvious survival adaptation for the bacterium (17,18). However, when introduced into inadvertent hosts for which adaptation is poorly tolerated, it is apparent that the proinflammatory changes induced in neutrophils can cause substantial tissue injury, disease, and immune suppression (10,19,20). In concert with these observations is that inflammatory histopathology in the mouse model and disease manifestations in the horse model are mediated not only by the bacterium itself, but also by the inflammatory response initiated by the bacterium (13,21). This is shown with elimination of the key cytokine that mediates control of obligate intracellular bacteria, interferon-γ, or by downregulation of inflammatory and immune response by pharmacological manipulation with dexamethasone (22,23). In both cases, the average bacteremia substantially increases, whereas tissue inflammatory lesions are inhibited in IFN-γ deficient mice, and fever and other clinical signs are reversed in experimentally infected horses.

It is not entirely clear that these events also occur in humans, although identical histopathologic lesions and substantial elevations in serum IFNγ are observed during the active phase of HGA (24). Initially, *A. phagocytophilum* is introduced into the dermis of a patient via the infected salivary secretions of *Ixodes* spp. ticks. The bacterium presumably infects neutrophils migrating to the tick-bite wound and is disseminated as the cell migrates further; alternately, the bacterium replicates locally to spread by infecting other host cells such as macrophages or endothelial cells, or drains through the local lymph nodes to eventually reach the blood where widespread dissemination occurs. Mature neutrophils and even myeloid precursors in the bone marrow are susceptible to infection by *A. phagocytophilum* (25,26), which inactivates antibacterial machinery by a combination of direct (superoxide dismutase) (27,28) and indirect (downregulation of antimicrobial genes such as *CYBB* and *RAC2*) effects (29,30). Inhibition of apoptosis via stabilization of *bcl2* family gene transcription prolongs neutrophil life and ensures enough time for the bacterium to replicate at least through several generations (average generation time for *A. phagocytophilum* is 26 hours) (31–33). Degranulation of metalloproteases, induction of innate immune responses via toll-like receptor-2 and MyD88, and upregulated expression of chemokines promote inflammation that facilitates recruitment of new host cells to expand infection (12,13,31,34,35). The histopathologic consequences are the production of small inflammatory lesions in the liver associated with elevated serum transaminase activities, and the activation of macrophages exposed to such signals as IFN-γ. Although not clearly demonstrated, some features of human and animal infections suggest a macrophage activation or hemophagocytic syndrome that could lead to destruction or sequestration of a variety of blood cells, explaining the occurrence of neutropenia, lymphopenia, thrombocytopenia, and to some degree, anemia (36). It is currently not possible to account for the significant reductions in these cell concentrations during infection by direct bacterial-mediated loss, and there is very little evidence of bone marrow suppression, although considerable study is still needed.

Severe consequences of HGA include pulmonary and peripheral nerve involvement, both presumably related to the induction of local inflammation (10,36,37). There is some evidence that adult respiratory distress syndrome may infrequently occur after HGA (38,39), and one hypothesis is that this could be related to a poorly regulated production of proinflammatory cytokines (24). An interesting observation with HGA is the extreme rarity of central nervous system (CNS) infection. The precise reasons for this are unclear; however, that infected neutrophils shed selectin adhesins needed for the first stage of margination prior to transmigration of endothelial cell barriers, such as the blood–brain barrier, could provide an explanation (14,40). Rarely, hemorrhage occurs as a complication of HGA (6,41). The underlying mechanism of this manifestation is also unknown, although various conjectures include: consumptive coagulopathy with disseminated intravascular coagulation, for which very little evidence exists; platelet dysfunction, for which little data also exist; and thrombocytopenia, a clear occurrence in HGA. The rarity of hemorrhage in human disease and in experimentally infected horses that develop profound thrombocytopenia indicates that much more study of this phenomenon is needed (36,42).

ECOLOGY AND EPIDEMIOLOGY
Ecology

Ticks in the *Ixodes* genus are known vectors for *A. phagocytophilum*, and are also vectors of *B. burgdorferi* (Lyme borreliosis) and *Babesia microti* (human babesiosis) (37,43,44). The most important tick vector of *A. phagocytophilum* in North America is *I. scapularis* that is distributed broadly across the east to the midwestern region of the United States (45,46); a smaller region on the Pacific coast of northern California, Oregon, and Washington is endemic for *I. pacificus* that are also competent vectors (47). Transmission in Europe is largely by the bites of *I. ricinus* ticks, and a role for *I. persulcatus* in Eastern Europe and Asia is also supported by increasing data (48,49). Although *A. phagocytophilum* is occasionally identified within other tick genera, no evidence exists to show that non-*Ixodes* spp. ticks are competent vectors (50). *A. phagocytophilum* is very inefficiently transmitted by transovarian passage from adult female ticks to eggs and larvae, but transstadial transmission does occur (5,46). The lack of vertical transmission indicates that a tick–mammal–tick cycle is most critical for survival, further suggesting that persistent high levels of bacteremia would be important survival mechanisms. The reservoir hosts for *A. phagocytophilum* have not been completely established, but likely include cervids, some ruminants, rodents, and perhaps other small and intermediate-size mammals (45,46,51–54). The relatively high prevalence of *A. phagocytophilum* in some nidiculous *Ixodes* spp. ticks that do not frequently bite humans suggests that important natural cycles exist into which promiscuous tick species are occasionally introduced (55–58). The importance of this concept is that the ecology of *A. phagocytophilum* is likely to be extremely complex and highly flexible, perhaps even refractory to attempts to control disease by ecological interventions.

Epidemiology

HGA has only recently become a reportable disease in humans, but at least some surveillance and case reporting data are available through the Centers for Disease Control and Prevention (CDC) and its reports dating to the first identification in humans (59,60). Reported cases have steadily increased since the first case was identified in 1990 and reported in 1994; a total of 2963 cases of HGA have been recorded in the U.S. since 1994, and for 2005, a tentative total of 700 cases was identified—more than ever before—comprising a 30% increase from 2004 and a 272% increase from 2000 (Fig. 1) (61). Among several prospective European studies that examined febrile patients with a tick-bite history, the prevailing tick-borne diseases identified were tick-borne encephalitis in Slovenia and Poland (62–64) and Lyme borreliosis in Sweden and Switzerland (65,66). However, about 3% were confirmed HGA, and when probable HGA cases

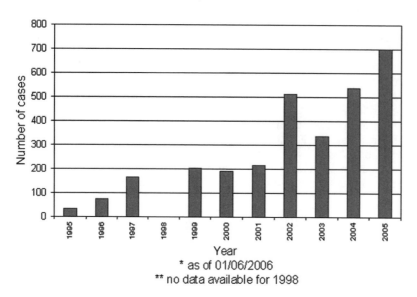

FIGURE 1 Cases of HGA reported to the U.S. CDC since 1994. *Abbreviations*: HGA, human granulocytic anaplasmosis; CDC, Centers for Disease Control and Prevention.

were considered, the rate was at least doubled. HGA is also reported from Austria, Italy, Latvia, The Netherlands, Norway, Poland, Spain, France, and Sweden. Blanco and Oteo (67), and later Strle (68), compared the features of HGA in European patients to those reported in the United States, comprising up to only 60 individuals so far. However, seroepidemiologic studies clearly show that *A. phagocytophilum* infection in humans is highly prevalent in both the United States and in Europe (Table 1) (69–72). Given that median seroprevalence rates of 4% to 9% exceed recognized maximal incidence rates of approximately 0.05% to 0.06% by a factor of 100, it is anticipated that most infections are mild or even asymptomatic, although significant underdiagnosis owing to lack of physician awareness and availability of laboratory diagnostics confound these data (69,70,73,74). Most symptomatic patients recover without any sequelae in one to two weeks even without specific antibiotic therapy (75). Unlike the situation for *A. phagocytophilum* in reservoir hosts, infection in humans and other animals that develop clinical signs, persistent or chronic infection has not been detected. Although the case-fatality rate for HGA is 0.5%, approximately 50% of symptomatic patients will require hospitalization, and 7% of patients will need admission to an intensive care unit (37,41). Persons with underlying diseases such as diabetes mellitus or immune compromise, and those for whom diagnosis and/or treatment are delayed are at increased risk for severe disease. As a result, prompt antimicrobial therapy is needed for all patients with a diagnosis of HGA (37).

Because of the shared tick vector, HGA may occasionally occur concurrently with Lyme disease or babesiosis (76–79). Among 12 published studies that examined Lyme disease patients for serologic evidence of coinfection, the median proportion was 10.1%, with a maximum of 35.6% and a minimum of 3.8% (70,75,80–89).

CLINICAL FEATURES AND DIAGNOSIS
Clinical Presentation

HGA appears most commonly as an undifferentiated febrile illness, resembling an influenza-like infection (41,67,90,91). The majority of patients recall tick bite or tick exposure 7 to 14 days prior to onset of the disease (37,92). However, other routes of transmission, such as exposure to deer blood (93), blood transfusion (94) or perinatal infection have been reported (95).

TABLE 1 Meta-analysis of Reported Human Seroprevalence Rates (%) for *A. phagocytophilum* Infection Among Various Populations at Different Degrees of Acquisition Risk

		Mean	Median	Maximum	Minimum	Number studies (number sera)
Overall[a]						
	Asia	8.9	8.9	8.9	8.9	1 (271)
	Europe	7.2	6.2	21.0	0.0	35 (8344)
	North America	4.5	5.1	35.6	0.3	11 (4126)
Cross-sectional[b]						
	Asia					0 (4038)
	Europe	8.2	5.6	15.4	0.0	19 (2939)
	North America	3.7	3.0	14.9	0.3	6
At risk[c]						
	Asia	8.9	8.9	8.9	8.9	1 (271)
	Europe	6.3	9.1	21.0	0.1	15 (4288)
	North America	6.4	5.3	35.6	0.4	5 (1184)
Lyme borreliosis[d]						
	Asia					0
	Europe	11.4	10.8	21.0	3.8	8 (1362)
	North America	20.9	5.5	35.6	5.3	3 (230)

[a]Overall—combination of all seroprevalence results regardless of study population risk status.
[b]Cross-sectional—seroprevalence determined among populations reflecting no increased risk for geographic region studied.
[c]At-risk populations deemed to have increased risk for tick bites or exposures, including forestry and farm workers, persons with tick bites or exposure, persons with fever, and populations with evidence of Lyme borreliosis.
[d]Lyme disease—populations with evidence of Lyme borreliosis.

After an incubation period of 7 to 10 days (37), high-grade fever (>39°C) develops, most often accompanied by malaise, weakness, headache, myalgia, and/or arthralgia (41,44,67,90,96–98). Myalgia can be severe, described by many patients as being "beaten" or "run over by a truck (6,37)." Other symptoms are observed in less than half of North American patients and can include anorexia, nausea, vomiting, abdominal pain, diarrhea, cough, or confusion (41,90). Several cases presenting as atypical pneumonitis have been described, and *A. phagocytophilum* infection associated with dermatologic manifestations of Sweet syndrome are also reported (39,99–101). Clinical features reported from Europe are similar to those reported from the United States (Table 2) although disease appears to be generally milder (67,68,99,103–105). However, the frequency of symptoms among European patients is difficult to estimate because more than 30% occur concurrently with other tick-borne infections, such as Lyme borreliosis (64,104,106) or tick-borne encephalitis (64,107). Moreover, given the infrequency of its recognition in Europe, the complete clinical spectrum of HGA is still a matter for investigation.

Results of physical examinations are generally unremarkable; however, conjunctivitis, cervical lymphadenopathy, slight hepatomegaly, and splenomegaly have been reported (99,102) in European patients, whereas these features are not often documented in patients from North America. Skin rash is rare with HGA, and usually results from the recognition of erythema migrans with concurrent Lyme borreliosis (10,108). Similarly, manifestations attributable to CNS involvement are observed in approximately 20% of patients, although objective findings that implicate CNS infection are exceedingly rare (59,109). Laboratory findings frequently identified in patients with corroborated HGA include thrombocytopenia, leucopenia, a left shift during the first week, a mild to moderate increase in serum transaminase activities, and an increased C-reactive protein level. Occasionally, reactive lymphocytosis is observed. Normalization of leukocyte counts and thrombocytopenia occurs during the second week, even without treatment (41,90,110,111).

Disease Course

In the vast majority of cases, the course of the disease is mild and favorable, with reported clinical improvement within 24 to 48 hours after doxycycline therapy and complete recovery

TABLE 2 Meta-analysis of Clinical Manifestations and Laboratory Abnormalities in Patients with HGA (36,64,102)

Symptom or sign	All		North America		Europe	
	Mean %	n	Mean %	n	Mean %	n
Fever	93	521	92	448	99	73
Myalgia	77	516	79	448	66	68
Headache	76	385	71	316	95	69
Malaise	94	288	96	271	53	17
Nausea	38	258	36	207	47	51
Vomiting	26	90	34	41	19	49
Diarrhea	16	95	22	41	11	54
Cough	19	260	22	207	10	53
Arthralgias	46	504	47	448	41	56
Rash	6	357	6	289	5	68
Stiff neck	21	24	22	18	17	6
Confusion	17	211	17	207	0	4
Laboratory abnormality						
Leucopenia	49	336	50	282	46	54
Thrombocytopenia	71	336	72	282	63	54
Anemia	37	59	37	59	n.d.	n.d.
Elevated serum AST or ALT	71	177	79	123	53	54
Elevated serum creatinine	43	72	49	59	15	13

Abbreviations: ALT, alanine transaminase; AST, asperate transaminase; HGA, human granulocytic anaplasmosis; n.d., not determined.

within two months, even without appropriate antibiotic treatment (67,69,111). Elderly patients are more prone to severe infections and death as are individuals with underlying medical conditions (e.g., immunosuppressive treatment, malignancies) or with delayed specific antibiotic treatment (60,92,106,112). A severe course of HGA can present as a septic or toxic-shock-like syndrome, myositis, rhabdomyolysis, myocarditis, or neurological involvement, such as brachial plexopathy or demyelinating polyneuropathy (38,41,109,113–116). Life-threatening complications were described in 7% (30 of 457) of patients in 2001–2002 (59), including acute respiratory distress syndrome (three patients), disseminated intravascular coagulation (one patient), renal failure (three patients), and others. The long-term outcome for HGA is usually favorable, showing no differences in physical functioning, general health, and vitality in one case-controlled study; however, HGA patients showed lower scores for "pain and health" relative to one year earlier (117).

No convincing clinical data support increased severity of Lyme disease with HGA (37,44,97,117), and there is no evidence for chronic or persistent HGA in humans (41,111). In contrast, experimental coinfection with *A. phagocytophilum* and *B. burgdorferi* in mice results in increased *B. burgdorferi* burden and severity of Lyme arthritis (118–120), and antibody response to *A. phagocytophilum* but not to *B. burgdorferi* is decreased in coinfected C3H/HeN mice (119). Moreover, coinfection in vitro facilitates migration of *B. burgdorferi* through endothelial cell barriers, including models of the blood–brain barrier (121). Much more study of how these interactions mechanistically explain the biological alterations is required.

The case-fatality rate is estimated at 0.7% based on U.S. surveillance data (59). So far, only one fatal case has been reported in Europe (122). In most unfavorable outcomes, opportunistic infections superimposed on HGA are observed. These included disseminated candidiasis, invasive pulmonary aspergillosis, necrotizing herpes esophagitis, and cryptococcosis, among others (41,114,123–125).

Not all *A. phagocytophilum* infections result in disease. Asymptomatic *A. phagocytophilum* seroconversion (68,74,111,126) and high seroprevalence rates in North America, Europe, and Asia suggest that most infections are subclinical or asymptomatic (69–71,74,127,128). Whether the serologic reactions represent true *A. phagocytophilum* infection that is cleared, infections by "nonpathogenic" strains, or simply false-positive serologic tests is not known (70,129,130).

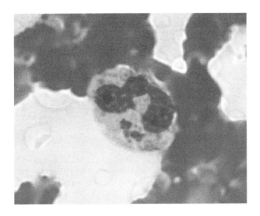

FIGURE 2 A. phagocytophilum appears as a cluster of small, dark-stained stipples in the cytoplasm of peripheral blood neutrophils and immature granulocytes, as shown here [Romanowsky (Hema-3) stain; original magnification: ×1060].

Diagnosis

The diagnosis can be confirmed by detection of a typical cluster of bacteria, called a morula, within a cytoplasmic vacuole of granulocytes on peripheral blood or buffy coat smears stained by Romanowsky methods. Morulae (Fig. 2) are seen in 20% to 80% of North American patients, but are rarely identified in the blood of European patients (41,66,67,90,102,104,111,131–133). A. phagocytophilum infection can be confirmed by polymerase chain reaction (PCR) detection of bacterial DNA in acute-phase blood (6,37,41,69,90,111,134). Isolation of A. phagocytophilum is performed by cell culture (Fig. 3), which requires an experienced laboratory and can take from several days to two or more weeks, thus limiting the utility of this method (37,135). The vast majority of patients produce specific antibodies, which can be detected by the indirect fluorescent antibody test, preferably performed on matched acute and convalescent serum samples separated by several weeks and that demonstrate seroconversion or a fourfold change in titer (41,75,90,105,111,136–138). IgM antibodies are detectable only during first 45 to 50 days after inoculation and the sensitivity is not higher than detection of IgG antibodies in the same time interval (139).

Case definitions for HGA have been proposed by the CDC in the United States (140) and also by the European Society of Clinical Microbiology and Infectious Disease (ESCMID) study group (Table 3) (105). The ESCMID definition is more restrictive than that of the CDC in that sequence determination is required for confirmation of PCR amplicons. The differential diagnosis includes viral infections, Q fever, *Mycoplasma* pneumonia, human monocytic ehrlichiosis, sepsis, endocarditis, tularemia, leptospirosis, relapsing fever, Kawasaki disease, collagen-vascular disease, and leukemia. When gastrointestinal symptoms are presented, different

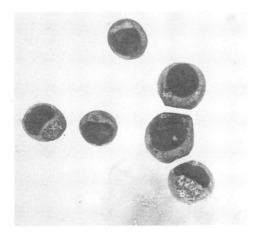

FIGURE 3 A. phagocytophilum appears similar in HL-60 cell culture, except that multiple morulae may be observed in single cells, and a high proportion of infected cells can be observed [Romanowsky (Hema-3) stain; original magnification: ×260].

TABLE 3 Human Granulocytic Anaplasmosis Case Definitions

Confirmed human anaplasmosis
Febrile illness with a history of a tick bite or tick exposure and
Demonstration of *A. phagocytophilum* infection by seroconversion or ≥ 4-fold
Change in antibody titer (IFA)
Or
Positive PCR result with subsequent sequencing of the amplicons demonstrating *Anaplasma*-specific DNA in blood
Or
Isolation of *A. phagocytophilum* in blood culture
Probable human anaplasmosis
Febrile illness with a history of a tick bite or tick exposure
And
Presence of stable titer of *A. phagocytophilum* antibodies in acute and convalescent sera if Titer >4-fold above the cut-off value (IFA)
Or
Positive PCR result without sequencing confirmation
Or
Presence of intracytoplasmic morulae in a blood smear

Abbreviations: IFA, immunofluorescence antibody; PCR, polymerase chain reaction.
Source: From Refs. 105, 140.

enteric infections should be considered including hepatitis. History of tick-bite is suggestive for tick-borne encephalitis, Lyme borreliosis, Colorado tick fever, Rocky Mountain spotted fever, and other rickettsioses and babesiosis (105,111).

TREATMENT

Tetracyclines appear to be very effective in treating HGA, and doxycycline is currently a first-line antibiotic (41,91,111). When the antibiotic susceptibilities of North American strains were tested in vitro, doxycycline and rifampin were most effective (141–143). Studies based on a quantitative real-time PCR assay confirmed that doxycycline and rifampin are highly active against *A. phagocytophilum* with variable susceptibility to fluoroquinolones (32,144). β-Lactam compounds, cotrimoxazole, macrolide compounds, and telithromycin showed no activity against *A. phagocytophilum* (32,144,145).

The recommended therapy for adults is doxycycline 100 mg given orally at 12-hour intervals (Table 4) (37,108,111). Children older than eight years should also be treated with doxycycline given in divided doses adjusted to the patient's weight (4.4 mg/kg/24 hours, maximum 100 mg per dose administered) (145,146). Doxycycline is the drug of choice for children who are seriously ill regardless of age (146). For children less than eight years who are not seriously ill, limited data support the use of rifampin (141,147). Patients treated with doxycycline usually defervesce within 24 to 48 hours (37,41,75,111,148). Thus, patients who fail to respond to treatment within this time frame should be reevaluated for alternative diagnoses and treatment.

The optimal duration of the therapy has yet to be determined. It is recommended that tetracycline treatment be continued for 7 to 10 days, or at least three to five days after defervescence (37,75,91,95,108,111,149). Myocarditis attributed to HGA was successfully treated with

TABLE 4 Recommended Adult and Pediatric Antibiotic Treatment for HGA

Antibiotic	Doxycycline hyclate	Tetracycline hydrochloride
Dose (adults)	100 mg iv[a] or po[b] Q 12 hr	500 mg PO Q 6 hrs or
Dose (children)	2.2 mg/kg po Q 12 hr[c]	25–50 mg/kg/day po in 4 divided doses[c]
Therapy duration (days)	5–14[d]	5–14[d]

[a]Intravenous administration.
[b]Oral administration.
[c]Until fever has resolved and for three additional days.
[d]Fourteen days recommended if coincubating *B. burgdorferi* infection is suspected.
Abbreviation: HGA, human granulocytic anaplasmosis.
Source: Refs. 37, 90, 108, 145, 146.

doxycycline for 30 days, to be certain that any coinfecting *B. burgdorferi* were also eradicated (150). Relapse or chronic infection has never been reported, even for those patients who were never treated with an active antibiotic. Reinfection, albeit rare, may occur, and was recently demonstrated in the case of a 60-year-old woman from Westchester County in New York State (151). Adult patients who are considered at risk for coinfection with *B. burgdorferi* should continue doxycycline therapy for a full 14 days. A shorter course of doxycycline (five to seven days) has been advocated for pediatric age-group patients because of the potential risk for adverse effects (dental staining) seen occasionally in young children (145,146,152). A small number of pediatric patients and pregnant women who had HGA were treated successfully with rifampin (147,153,154). Thus, patients who have HGA and who are unsuited for tetracycline treatment due to a history of drug allergy or pregnancy, and children younger than eight years of age who are not seriously ill should be considered for rifampin therapy.

REFERENCES

1. Patz JA, Daszak P, Tabor GM, et al. Unhealthy landscapes: policy recommendations on land use change and infectious disease emergence. Environ Health Perspect 2004; 112:1092–1098.
2. Taylor LH, Latham SM, Woolhouse ME. Risk factors for human disease emergence. Philos Trans R Soc Lond B Biol Sci 2001; 356:983–989.
3. Gubler DJ, Reiter P, Ebi KL, et al. Climate variability and change in the United States: potential impacts on vector- and rodent-borne diseases. Environ Health Perspect 2001; 109(suppl 2):223–233.
4. Dumler JS, Barbet AF, Bekker CP, et al. Reorganization of genera in the families *Rickettsiaceae* and *Anaplasmataceae* in the order *Rickettsiales*: unification of some species of *Ehrlichia* with *Anaplasma*, *Cowdria* with *Ehrlichia* and *Ehrlichia* with *Neorickettsia*, descriptions of six new species combinations and designation of *Ehrlichia equi* and 'HGE agent' as subjective synonyms of *Ehrlichia phagocytophila*. Int J Syst Evol Microbiol 2001; 51:2145–2165.
5. MacLeod GW Jr. Studies in tick-borne fever of sheep. I. Transmission by the tick, *Ixodes ricinus*, with a description of the disease produced. Parasitology 1933; 25:273–285.
6. Bakken JS, Dumler JS, Chen SM, et al. Human granulocytic ehrlichiosis in the upper Midwest United States: a new species emerging? J Am Med Assoc 1994; 272:212–218.
7. Dumler JS, Asanovich KM, Bakken JS, et al. Serologic cross-reactions among *Ehrlichia equi*, *Ehrlichia phagocytophila*, and human granulocytic *Ehrlichia*. J Clin Microbiol 1995; 33:1098–1103.
8. Munderloh UG, Lynch MJ, Herron MJ, et al. Infection of endothelial cells with *Anaplasma marginale* and *A. phagocytophilum*. Vet Microbiol 2004; 101:53–64.
9. Carlyon JA, Fikrig E. Mechanisms of evasion of neutrophil killing by *Anaplasma phagocytophilum*. Curr Opin Hematol 2006; 13:28–33.
10. Dumler JS, Choi KS, Garcia-Garcia JC, et al. Human granulocytic anaplasmosis and *Anaplasma phagocytophilum*. Emerg Infect Dis 2005; 11:1828–1834.
11. Akkoyunlu M, Malawista SE, Anguita J, et al. Exploitation of interleukin-8-induced neutrophil chemotaxis by the agent of human granulocytic ehrlichiosis. Infect Immun 2001; 69:5577–5588.
12. Choi KS, Grab DJ, Dumler JS. *Anaplasma phagocytophilum* infection induces protracted neutrophil degranulation. Infect Immun 2004; 72:3680–3683.
13. Scorpio DG, Von Loewenich FD, Bogdan C, et al. Innate immune tissue injury and murine HGA: tissue injury in the murine model of granulocytic anaplasmosis relates to host innate immune response and not pathogen load. Ann NY Acad Sci 2005; 1063:425–428.
14. Choi KS, Garyu J, Park J, et al. Diminished adhesion of *Anaplasma phagocytophilum*-infected neutrophils to endothelial cells is associated with reduced expression of leukocyte surface selectin. Infect Immun 2003; 71:4586–4594.
15. Park J, Choi KS, Dumler JS. Major surface protein 2 of *Anaplasma phagocytophilum* facilitates adherence to granulocytes. Infect Immun 2003; 71:4018–4025.
16. Scorpio DG, Akkoyunlu M, Fikrig E, et al. CXCR2 blockade influences *Anaplasma phagocytophilum* propagation but not histopathology in the mouse model of human granulocytic anaplasmosis. Clin Diagn Lab Immunol 2004; 11:963–968.
17. Levin ML, Nicholson WL, Massung RF, et al. Comparison of the reservoir competence of medium-sized mammals and *Peromyscus leucopus* for *Anaplasma phagocytophilum* in Connecticut. Vector Borne Zoonotic Dis 2002; 2:125–136.
18. Foley JE, Foley P, Brown RN, et al. Ecology of *Anaplasma phagocytophilum* and *Borrelia burgdorferi* in the western United States. J Vector Ecol 2004; 29:41–50.
19. Greig B, Asanovich KM, Armstrong PJ, et al. Geographic, clinical, serologic, and molecular evidence of granulocytic ehrlichiosis, a likely zoonotic disease, in Minnesota and Wisconsin dogs. J Clin Microbiol 1996; 34:44–48.

20. Engvall EO, Egenvall A. Granulocytic ehrlichiosis in Swedish dogs and horses. Int J Med Microbiol 2002; 291(suppl 33):100–103.
21. Martin ME, Bunnell JE, Dumler JS. Pathology, immunohistology, and cytokine responses in early phases of human granulocytic ehrlichiosis in a murine model. J Infect Dis 2000; 181:374–378.
22. Martin ME, Caspersen K, Dumler JS. Immunopathology and ehrlichial propagation are regulated by interferon-gamma and interleukin-10 in a murine model of human granulocytic ehrlichiosis. Am J Pathol 2001; 158:1881–1888.
23. Madigan JE. 2006. Personal communication.
24. Dumler JS, Trigiani ER, Bakken JS, et al. Serum cytokine responses during acute human granulocytic ehrlichiosis. Clin Diagn Lab Immunol 2000; 7:6–8.
25. Klein MB, Miller JS, Nelson CM, et al. Primary bone marrow progenitors of both granulocytic and monocytic lineages are susceptible to infection with the agent of human granulocytic ehrlichiosis. J Infect Dis 1997; 176:1405–1409.
26. Bunnell JE, Trigiani ER, Srinivas SR, et al. Development and distribution of pathologic lesions are related to immune status and tissue deposition of human granulocytic ehrlichiosis agent-infected cells in a murine model system. J Infect Dis 1999; 180:546–550.
27. Carlyon JA, Abdel-Latif D, Pypaert M, et al. *Anaplasma phagocytophilum* utilizes multiple host evasion mechanisms to thwart NADPH oxidase-mediated killing during neutrophil infection. Infect Immun 2004; 72:4772–4783.
28. Ijdo JW, Mueller AC. Neutrophil NADPH oxidase is reduced at the *Anaplasma phagocytophilum* phagosome. Infect Immun 2004; 72:5392–5401.
29. Banerjee R, Anguita J, Roos D, et al. Cutting edge: infection by the agent of human granulocytic ehrlichiosis prevents the respiratory burst by down-regulating gp91phox. J Immunol 2000; 164:3946–3949.
30. Carlyon JA, Chan WT, Galan J, et al. Repression of *rac2* mRNA expression by *Anaplasma phagocytophila* is essential to the inhibition of superoxide production and bacterial proliferation. J Immunol 2002; 169:7009–7018.
31. Choi KS, Park JT, Dumler JS. *Anaplasma phagocytophilum* delay of neutrophil apoptosis through the p38 mitogen-activated protein kinase signal pathway. Infect Immun 2005; 73:8209–8218.
32. Branger S, Rolain JM, Raoult D. Evaluation of antibiotic susceptibilities of *Ehrlichia canis*, *Ehrlichia chaffeensis*, and *Anaplasma phagocytophilum* by real-time PCR. Antimicrob Agents Chemother 2004; 48:4822–4828.
33. Ge Y, Yoshiie K, Kuribayashi F, et al. *Anaplasma phagocytophilum* inhibits human neutrophil apoptosis via upregulation of bfl-1, maintenance of mitochondrial membrane potential and prevention of caspase 3 activation. Cell Microbiol 2005; 7:29–38.
34. Choi KS, Scorpio DG, Dumler JS. *Anaplasma phagocytophilum* ligation to toll-like receptor (TLR) 2, but not to TLR4, activates macrophages for nuclear factor-kappa B nuclear translocation. J Infect Dis 2004; 189:1921–1925.
35. Klein MB, Hu S, Chao CC, et al. The agent of human granulocytic ehrlichiosis induces the production of myelosuppressing chemokines without induction of proinflammatory cytokines. J Infect Dis 2000; 182:200–205.
36. Dumler JS. *Anaplasma* and *Ehrlichia* infection. Ann NY Acad Sci 2005; 1063:361–373.
37. Bakken JS, Dumler JS. Human granulocytic ehrlichiosis. Clin Infect Dis 2000; 31:554–560.
38. Wong S, Grady LJ. *Ehrlichia* infection as a cause of severe respiratory distress. N Engl J Med 1996; 334:273.
39. Remy V, Hansmann Y, De Martino S, et al. Human anaplasmosis presenting as atypical pneumonitis in France. Clin Infect Dis 2003; 37:846–848.
40. Park J, Choi KS, Grab DJ, et al. Divergent interactions of *Ehrlichia chaffeensis*- and *Anaplasma phagocytophilum*-infected leukocytes with endothelial cell barriers. Infect Immun 2003; 71:6728–6733.
41. Bakken JS, Krueth J, Wilson-Nordskog C, et al. Clinical and laboratory characteristics of human granulocytic ehrlichiosis. J Am Med Assoc 1996; 275:199–205.
42. Madigan JE, Gribble D. Equine ehrlichiosis in northern California: 49 cases (1968–1981). J Am Vet Med Assoc 1987; 190:445–448.
43. Anderson JF. The natural history of ticks. Med Clin North Am 2002; 86:205–218.
44. Krause PJ, McKay K, Thompson CA, et al. Disease-specific diagnosis of coinfecting tickborne zoonoses: babesiosis, human granulocytic ehrlichiosis, and Lyme disease. Clin Infect Dis 2002; 34:1184–1191.
45. Levin ML, des Vignes F, Fish D. Disparity in the natural cycles of *Borrelia burgdorferi* and the agent of human granulocytic ehrlichiosis. Emerg Infect Dis 1999; 5:204–208.
46. Telford SR III, Dawson JE, Katavolos P, et al. Perpetuation of the agent of human granulocytic ehrlichiosis in a deer tick-rodent cycle. Proc Natl Acad Sci USA 1996; 93:6209–6214.
47. Richter PJ Jr, Kimsey RB, Madigan JE, et al. *Ixodes pacificus* (Acari: Ixodidae) as a vector of *Ehrlichia equi* (Rickettsiales: Ehrlichieae). J Med Entomol 1996; 33:1–5.
48. Oteo JA, Gil H, Barral M, et al. Presence of granulocytic ehrlichia in ticks and serological evidence of human infection in La Rioja, Spain. Epidemiol Infect 2001; 127:353–358.

49. Cao WC, Zhao QM, Zhang PH, et al. Prevalence of *Anaplasma phagocytophila* and *Borrelia burgdorferi* in *Ixodes persulcatus* ticks from northeastern China. Am J Trop Med Hyg 2003; 68:547–550.
50. Des Vignes F, Levin ML, Fish D. Comparative vector competence of *Dermacentor variabilis* and *Ixodes scapularis* (Acari: Ixodidae) for the agent of human granulocytic ehrlichiosis. J Med Entomol 1999; 36:182–185.
51. Ogden NH, Bown K, Horrocks BK, et al. Granulocytic *Ehrlichia* infection in *Ixodid* ticks and mammals in woodlands and uplands of the U.K. Med Vet Entomol 1998; 12:423–429.
52. Walls JJ, Greig B, Neitzel DF, et al. Natural infection of small mammal species in Minnesota with the agent of human granulocytic ehrlichiosis. J Clin Microbiol 1997; 35:853–855.
53. Castro MB, Nicholson WL, Kramer VL, et al. Persistent infection in *Neotoma fuscipes* (Muridae: Sigmodontinae) with *Ehrlichia phagocytophila* sensu lato. Am J Trop Med Hyg 2001; 65:261–267.
54. Grzeszczuk A, Ziarko S, Radziwon PM, Prokopowicz D. Evidence of *Anaplasma phagocytophilum* infection of European bisons in the Bialowieza Primeval Forest. Med Weter 2004; 60:600–601.
55. Zeidner NS, Burkot TR, Massung R, et al. Transmission of the agent of human granulocytic ehrlichiosis by *Ixodes spinipalpis* ticks: evidence of an enzootic cycle of dual infection with *Borrelia burgdorferi* in Northern Colorado. J Infect Dis 2000; 182:616–619.
56. Goethert HK, Telford SR III. Enzootic transmission of the agent of human granulocytic ehrlichiosis among cottontail rabbits. Am J Trop Med Hyg 2003; 68:633–637.
57. Bown KJ, Begon M, Bennett M, et al. Seasonal dynamics of *Anaplasma phagocytophila* in a rodent-tick (*Ixodes trianguliceps*) system, United Kingdom. Emerg Infect Dis 2003; 9:63–70.
58. Santos AS, Santos-Silva MM, Almeida VC, et al. Detection of *Anaplasma phagocytophilum* DNA in *Ixodes* ticks (Acari: Ixodidae) from Madeira Island and Setubal District, mainland Portugal. Emerg Infect Dis 2004; 10:1643–1648.
59. Demma LJ, Holman RC, McQuiston JH, et al. Epidemiology of human ehrlichiosis and anaplasmosis in the United States, 2001–2002. Am J Trop Med Hyg 2005; 73:400–409.
60. McQuiston JH, Paddock CD, Holman RC, et al. The human ehrlichioses in the United States. Emerg Infect Dis 1999; 5:635–642.
61. Prevention CfDCa. Notifiable diseases/deaths in selected cities weekly information. Morb Mortal Wkly Rep 2006; 54:1320–1330.
62. Arnez M, Luznik-Bufon T, Avsic-Zupanc T, et al. Etiology of tick-borne febrile illnesses in Slovenian children. Ann NY Acad Sci 2003; 990:353–354.
63. Lotric-Furlan S, Petrovec M, Avsic-Zupanc T, et al. Prospective assessment of the etiology of acute febrile illness after a tick bite in Slovenia. Clin Infect Dis 2001; 33:503–510.
64. Grzeszczuk AZS, Kovalchuk O, et al. Etiology of tick-borne febrile illnesses in adult residents of northeastern Poland: report from a prospective clinical study. Int J Med Microbiol 2006; 296(40):242–249.
65. Bjoersdorff A, Bagert B, Massung RF, et al. Isolation and characterization of two European strains of *Ehrlichia phagocytophila* of equine origin. Clin Diagn Lab Immunol 2002; 9:341–343.
66. Baumann D, Pusterla N, Peter O, et al. Fever after a tick bite: clinical manifestations and diagnosis of acute tick bite-associated infections in northeastern Switzerland. Dtsch Med Wochenschr 2003; 128:1042–1047.
67. Blanco JR, Oteo JA. Human granulocytic ehrlichiosis in Europe. Clin Microbiol Infect 2002; 8:763–772.
68. Strle F. Human granulocytic ehrlichiosis in Europe. Int J Med Microbiol 2004; 293(suppl 37):27–35.
69. Bakken JS, Goellner P, Van Etten M, et al. Seroprevalence of human granulocytic ehrlichiosis among permanent residents of northwestern Wisconsin. Clin Infect Dis 1998; 27:1491–1496.
70. Aguero-Rosenfeld ME, Donnarumma L, Zentmaier L, et al. Seroprevalence of antibodies that react with *Anaplasma phagocytophila*, the agent of human granulocytic ehrlichiosis, in different populations in Westchester County, New York. J Clin Microbiol 2002; 40:2612–2615.
71. Cizman M, Avsic-Zupanc T, Petrovec M, et al. Seroprevalence of ehrlichiosis, Lyme borreliosis and tick-borne encephalitis infections in children and young adults in Slovenia. Wien Klin Wochenschr 2000; 112:842–845.
72. Dumler JS, Dotevall L, Gustafson R, et al. A population-based seroepidemiologic study of human granulocytic ehrlichiosis and Lyme borreliosis on the west coast of Sweden. J Infect Dis 1997; 175:720–722.
73. Hilton E, DeVoti J, Benach JL, et al. Seroprevalence and seroconversion for tick-borne diseases in a high-risk population in the northeast United States. Am J Med 1999; 106:404–409.
74. Woessner R, Gaertner BC, Grauer MT, et al. Incidence and prevalence of infection with human granulocytic ehrlichiosis agent in Germany: a prospective study in young healthy subjects. Infection 2001; 29:271–273.
75. Bakken JS, Haller I, Riddell D, et al. The serological response of patients infected with the agent of human granulocytic ehrlichiosis. Clin Infect Dis 2002; 34:22–27.
76. De Martino SJ, Carlyon JA, Fikrig E. Coinfection with *Borrelia burgdorferi* and the agent of human granulocytic ehrlichiosis. N Engl J Med 2001; 345:150–151.
77. Belongia EA, Reed KD, Mitchell PD, et al. Tickborne infections as a cause of nonspecific febrile illness in Wisconsin. Clin Infect Dis 2001; 32:1434–1439.

78. Moss WJ, Dumler JS. Simultaneous infection with *Borrelia burgdorferi* and human granulocytic ehrlichiosis. Pediatr Infect Dis J 2003; 22:91–92.
79. Thompson C, Spielman A, Krause PJ. Coinfecting deer-associated zoonoses: Lyme disease, babesiosis, and ehrlichiosis. Clin Infect Dis 2001; 33:676–685.
80. Santino I, Grillo R, Nicoletti M, et al. Prevalence of IgG antibodies against *Borrelia burgdorferi* s.l. and *Ehrlichia phagocytophila* in sera of patients presenting symptoms of Lyme disease in a central region of Italy. Int J Immunopathol Pharmacol 2002; 15:245–248.
81. Grzeszczuk A, Stanczak J, Kubica-Biernat B, et al. Human anaplasmosis in north-eastern Poland: seroprevalence in humans and prevalence in *Ixodes ricinus* ticks. Ann Agric Environ Med 2004; 11:99–103.
82. Guillaume B, Heyman P, Lafontaine S, et al. Seroprevalence of human granulocytic ehrlichiosis infection in Belgium. Eur J Clin Microbiol Infect Dis 2002; 21:397–400.
83. Hunfeld KP, Brade V. Prevalence of antibodies against the human granulocytic ehrlichiosis agent in Lyme borreliosis patients from Germany. Eur J Clin Microbiol Infect Dis 1999; 18:221–224.
84. Lebech AM, Hansen K, Pancholi P, et al. Immunoserologic evidence of human granulocytic ehrlichiosis in Danish patients with Lyme neuroborreliosis. Scand J Infect Dis 1998; 30:173–176.
85. Fingerle V, Goodman JL, Johnson RC, et al. Human granulocytic ehrlichiosis in southern Germany: increased seroprevalence in high-risk groups. J Clin Microbiol 1997; 35:3244–3247.
86. Bakken JS, Krueth J, Tilden RL, et al. Serological evidence of human granulocytic ehrlichiosis in Norway. Eur J Clin Microbiol Infect Dis 1996; 15:829–832.
87. Mitchell PD, Reed KD, Hofkes JM. Immunoserologic evidence of coinfection with *Borrelia burgdorferi*, *Babesia microti*, and human granulocytic *Ehrlichia* species in residents of Wisconsin and Minnesota. J Clin Microbiol 1996; 34:724–727.
88. Skarphedinsson S, Sogaard P, Pedersen C. Seroprevalence of human granulocytic ehrlichiosis in high-risk groups in Denmark. Scand J Infect Dis 2001; 33:206–210.
89. Magnarelli LA, Dumler JS, Anderson JF, et al. Coexistence of antibodies to tick-borne pathogens of babesiosis, ehrlichiosis, and Lyme borreliosis in human sera. J Clin Microbiol 1995; 33:3054–3057.
90. Aguero-Rosenfeld ME, Horowitz HW, Wormser GP, et al. Human granulocytic ehrlichiosis: a case series from a medical center in New York State. Ann Intern Med 1996; 125:904–908.
91. Olano JP, Walker DH. Human ehrlichioses. Med Clin North Am 2002; 86:375–392.
92. Bakken JS. The discovery of human granulocytotropic ehrlichiosis. J Lab Clin Med 1998; 132:175–180.
93. Bakken JS, Krueth JK, Lund T, et al. Exposure to deer blood may be a cause of human granulocytic ehrlichiosis. Clin Infect Dis 1996; 23:198.
94. Eastlund T, Persing D, Mathiesen D, et al. Human granulocytic ehrlichiosis after red cell transfusion. Transfusion 1999; 39:117S.
95. Horowitz HW, Kilchevsky E, Haber S, et al. Perinatal transmission of the agent of human granulocytic ehrlichiosis. N Engl J Med 1998; 339:375–378.
96. Wallace BJ, Brady G, Ackman DM, et al. Human granulocytic ehrlichiosis in New York. Arch Intern Med 1998; 158:769–773.
97. Belongia EA, Reed KD, Mitchell PD, et al. Clinical and epidemiological features of early Lyme disease and human granulocytic ehrlichiosis in Wisconsin. Clin Infect Dis 1999; 29:1472–1477.
98. Horowitz HW, Aguero-Rosenfeld ME, McKenna DF, et al. Clinical and laboratory spectrum of culture-proven human granulocytic ehrlichiosis: comparison with culture-negative cases. Clin Infect Dis 1998; 27:1314–1317.
99. Lotric-Furlan S, Petrovec M, Avsic-Zupanc T, et al. Human granulocytic ehrlichiosis in Slovenia. Ann NY Acad Sci 2003; 990:279–284.
100. Karlsson U, Bjoersdorff A, Massung RF, et al. Human granulocytic ehrlichiosis—a clinical case in Scandinavia. Scand J Infect Dis 2001; 33:73–74.
101. Halasz CL, Niedt GW, Kurtz CP, et al. A case of Sweet syndrome associated with human granulocytic anaplasmosis. Arch Dermatol 2005; 141:887–889.
102. Walder G, Fuchs D, Sarcletti M, et al. Human granulocytic anaplasmosis in Austria: epidemiological, clinical and laboratory findings in five consecutive patients from Tyrol, Austria. Int J Med Microbiol 2006; 296(40):287–301.
103. Arnez M, Petrovec M, Lotric-Furlan S, et al. First European pediatric case of human granulocytic ehrlichiosis. J Clin Microbiol 2001; 39:4591–4592.
104. Bjoersdorff A, Wittesjo B, Berglun J, et al. Human granulocytic ehrlichiosis as a common cause of tick-associated fever in Southeast Sweden: report from a prospective clinical study. Scand J Infect Dis 2002; 34:187–191.
105. Brouqui P, Bacellar F, Baranton G, et al. Guidelines for the diagnosis of tick-borne bacterial diseases in Europe. Clin Microbiol Infect 2004; 10:1108–1132.
106. Hulinska D, Votypka J, Plch J, et al. Molecular and microscopical evidence of *Ehrlichia* spp. and *Borrelia burgdorferi* sensu lato in patients, animals and ticks in the Czech Republic. New Microbiol 2002; 25:437–448.
107. Lotric-Furlan S, Petrovec M, Avsic-Zupanc T, et al. Concomitant tickborne encephalitis and human granulocytic ehrlichiosis. Emerg Infect Dis 2005; 11:485–488.

108. Bakken JS, Dumler JS. Clinical diagnosis and treatment of human granulocytotropic anaplasmosis. Ann NY Acad Sci 2006; 1075:284–297.
109. Lee FS, Chu FK, Tackley M, et al. Human granulocytic ehrlichiosis presenting as facial diplegia in a 42-year-old woman. Clin Infect Dis 2000; 31:1288–1291.
110. Bakken JS, Aguero-Rosenfeld ME, Tilden RL, et al. Serial measurements of hematologic counts during the active phase of human granulocytic ehrlichiosis. Clin Infect Dis 2001; 32:862–870.
111. Dumler JS, Walker DH. Tick-borne ehrlichioses. Lancet Inf Dis 2001; 0:21–28.
112. Bjoersdorff A, Berglund J, Kristiansen BE, et al. Varying clinical picture and course of human granulocytic ehrlichiosis: twelve Scandinavian cases of the new tick-borne zoonosis are presented. Lakartidningen 1999; 96:4200–4204.
113. Shea KW, Calio AJ, Klein NC, et al. *Ehrlichia equi* infection associated with rhabdomyolysis. Clin Infect Dis 1996; 22:605.
114. Jahangir A, Kolbert C, Edwards W, et al. Fatal pancarditis associated with human granulocytic ehrlichiosis in a 44-year-old man. Clin Infect Dis 1998; 27:1424–1427.
115. Horowitz HW, Marks SJ, Weintraub M, et al. Brachial plexopathy associated with human granulocytic ehrlichiosis. Neurology 1996; 46:1026–1029.
116. Heller HM, Telford SR III, Branda JA. Case records of the Massachusetts General Hospital. Case 10-2005. A 73-year-old man with weakness and pain in the legs. N Engl J Med 2005; 352:1358–1364.
117. Ramsey AH, Belongia EA, Gale CM, et al. Outcomes of treated human granulocytic ehrlichiosis cases. Emerg Infect Dis 2002; 8:398–401.
118. Holden K, Hodzic E, Feng S, et al. Coinfection with *Anaplasma phagocytophilum* alters *Borrelia burgdorferi* population distribution in C3H/HeN mice. Infect Immun 2005; 73:3440–3444.
119. Thomas V, Anguita J, Barthold SW, et al. Coinfection with *Borrelia burgdorferi* and the agent of human granulocytic ehrlichiosis alters murine immune responses, pathogen burden, and severity of Lyme arthritis. Infect Immun 2001; 69:3359–3371.
120. Zeidner NS, Dolan MC, Massung R, et al. Coinfection with *Borrelia burgdorferi* and the agent of human granulocytic ehrlichiosis suppresses IL-2 and IFN gamma production and promotes an IL-4 response in C3H/HeJ mice. Parasite Immunol 2000; 22:581–588.
121. Nyarko EGD, Dumler JS. *Anaplasma phagocytophilum*-infected neutrophils enhance transmigration of *Borrelia burgdorferi* across the human blood–brain barrier in vitro. Int J Paracitol 2006; 34:601–605.
122. Hulinska D, Kurzova D, Drevova H, et al. First detection of Ehrlichiosis detected serologically and with the polymerase chain reaction in patients with borreliosis in the Czech Republic. Cas Lek Cesk 2001; 140:181–184.
123. Chen SM, Dumler JS, Bakken JS, et al. Identification of a granulocytotropic *Ehrlichia* species as the etiologic agent of human disease. J Clin Microbiol 1994; 32:589–595.
124. Lepidi H, Bunnell JE, Martin ME, et al. Comparative pathology, and immunohistology associated with clinical illness after *Ehrlichia phagocytophila*-group infections. Am J Trop Med Hyg 2000; 62:29–37.
125. Hardalo CJ, Quagliarello V, Dumler JS. Human granulocytic ehrlichiosis in Connecticut: report of a fatal case. Clin Infect Dis 1995; 21:910–914.
126. Grzeszczuk A, Puzanowska B, Miegoc H, et al. Incidence and prevalence of infection with *Anaplasma phagocytophilum*: prospective study in healthy individuals exposed to ticks. Ann Agric Environ Med 2004; 11:155–157.
127. Zeman P, Pazdiora P, Rebl K, et al. Antibodies to granulocytic ehrlichiae in the population of the western and central part of the Czech Republic. Epidemiol Mikrobiol Imunol 2002; 51:13–18.
128. Park JH, Heo EJ, Choi KS, et al. Detection of antibodies to *Anaplasma phagocytophilum* and *Ehrlichia chaffeensis* antigens in sera of Korean patients by western immunoblotting and indirect immunofluorescence assays. Clin Diagn Lab Immunol 2003; 10:1059–1064.
129. Wormser GP, Horowitz HW, Nowakowski J, et al. Positive Lyme disease serology in patients with clinical and laboratory evidence of human granulocytic ehrlichiosis. Am J Clin Pathol 1997; 107:142–147.
130. Wong SJ, Thomas JA. Cytoplasmic, nuclear, and platelet autoantibodies in human granulocytic ehrlichiosis patients. J Clin Microbiol 1998; 36:1959–1963.
131. Arnez M, Luznik-Bufon T, Avsic-Zupanc T, et al. Causes of febrile illnesses after a tick bite in Slovenian children. Pediatr Infect Dis J 2003; 22:1078–1083.
132. Prukk T, Ainsalu K, Laja E, et al. Human granulocytic ehrlichiosis in Estonia. Emerg Infect Dis 2003; 9:1499–1500.
133. Walder G, Falkensammer B, Aigner J, et al. First documented case of human granulocytic ehrlichiosis in Austria. Wien Klin Wochenschr 2003; 115:263–266.
134. Courtney JW, Massung RF. Multiplex Taqman PCR assay for rapid detection of *Anaplasma phagocytophila* and *Borrelia burgdorferi*. Ann NY Acad Sci 2003; 990:369–370.
135. Aguero-Rosenfeld ME, Kalantarpour F, Baluch M, et al. Serology of culture-confirmed cases of human granulocytic ehrlichiosis. J Clin Microbiol 2000; 38:635–638.
136. Lotric-Furlan S, Petrovec M, Zupanc TA, et al. Human granulocytic ehrlichiosis in Europe: clinical and laboratory findings for four patients from Slovenia. Clin Infect Dis 1998; 27:424–428.

137. Aguero-Rosenfeld ME. Diagnosis of human granulocytic ehrlichiosis: state of the art. Vector Borne Zoonotic Dis 2002; 2:233–239.
138. Belongia EA, Gale CM, Reed KD, et al. Population-based incidence of human granulocytic ehrlichiosis in northwestern Wisconsin, 1997–1999. J Infect Dis 2001; 184:1470–1474.
139. Walls JJ, Aguero-Rosenfeld M, Bakken JS, et al. Inter- and intralaboratory comparison of *Ehrlichia equi* and human granulocytic ehrlichiosis (HGE) agent strains for serodiagnosis of HGE by the immunofluorescent-antibody test. J Clin Microbiol 1999; 37:2968–2973.
140. http://www.cdc.gov/epo/dphsi/casedef/case_definitions.htm (March 2, 2006).
141. Klein MB, Nelson CM, Goodman JL. Antibiotic susceptibility of the newly cultivated agent of human granulocytic ehrlichiosis: promising activity of quinolones and rifamycins. Antimicrob Agents Chemother 1997; 41:76–79.
142. Maurin M, Bakken JS, Dumler JS. Antibiotic susceptibilities of *Anaplasma* (*Ehrlichia*) *phagocytophilum* strains from various geographic areas in the United States. Antimicrob Agents Chemother 2003; 47:413–415.
143. Horowitz HW, Hsieh TC, Aguero-Rosenfeld ME, et al. Antimicrobial susceptibility of *Ehrlichia phagocytophila*. Antimicrob Agents Chemother 2001; 45:786–788.
144. Hunfeld KP, Bittner T, Rodel R, et al. New real-time PCR-based method for in vitro susceptibility testing of *Anaplasma phagocytophilum* against antimicrobial agents. Int J Antimicrob Agents 2004; 23:563–571.
145. Bakken JS, Dumler JS. *Ehrlichia* and *Anaplasma* Species: Antimicrobial Therapy and Vaccines. 2nd ed. New York: Apple Trees Productions, 2002:875–882.
146. Anonymous. *Ehrlichia* infections (human ehrlichioses). Red Book: 2003 Report of the Committee of Infectious Diseases. Elk Grove Village, IL: American Academy of Pediatrics, 2003:266–269.
147. Krause PJ, Corrow CL, Bakken JS. Successful treatment of human granulocytic ehrlichiosis in children using rifampin. Pediatrics 2003; 112:e252–e253.
148. Fishbein DB, Dawson JE, Robinson LE. Human ehrlichiosis in the United States, 1985 to 1990. Ann Intern Med 1994; 120:736–743.
149. Asanovich KM, Bakken JS, Madigan JE, et al. Antigenic diversity of granulocytic *Ehrlichia* isolates from humans in Wisconsin and New York and a horse in California. J Infect Dis 1997; 176:1029–1034.
150. Malik A, Jameel MN, Ali SS, et al. Human granulocytic anaplasmosis affecting the myocardium. J Gen Intern Med 2005; 20:C8–C10.
151. Horowitz HW, Aguero-Rosenfeld M, Dumler JS, et al. Reinfection with the agent of human granulocytic ehrlichiosis. Ann Intern Med 1998; 129:461–463.
152. Anonymous. Tetracyclines. AHFS Drug Information. Bethesda, MD: American Society of Health-System Pharmacists, 2004:433–457.
153. Buitrago MI, Ijdo JW, Rinaudo P, et al. Human granulocytic ehrlichiosis during pregnancy treated successfully with rifampin. Clin Infect Dis 1998; 27:213–215.
154. Elston DM. Perinatal transmission of human granulocytic ehrlichiosis. N Engl J Med 1998; 339:1941–1942.

Section IV: *ORIENTIA TSUTSUGAMUSHI* AND SCRUB TYPHUS

17 | *Orientia tsutsugamushi* and Scrub Typhus

George Watt
Family Health International, Asia-Pacific Regional Office, Bangkok, Thailand

Pacharee Kantipong
Department of Internal Medicine, Chiangrai Regional Hospital, Chiangrai, Thailand

INTRODUCTION

Scrub typhus is a chigger-borne zoonosis that is of greatest public health importance in tropical rural Asia. Humans are accidental hosts who acquire the disease by intruding into often sharply localized foci colonized by infected larval trombiculid mites, popularly known as chiggers. *Orientia tsutsugamushi*, the causative agent, is an obligate intracellular bacterium that was recently reclassified from the genus *Rickettsia* into a separate genus because it differs from rickettsiae in genetic composition, cell wall structure, and multiplication cycle (1).

Scrub typhus occurs only in Asia. For a short time, during World War II, Westerners feared the disease because of its ferocity when untreated and because of the estimated 18,000 cases acquired by Allied troops deployed to the Asian theater. Some 1255 cases were reported in just four months on two small islands off the north coast of Irian Jaya, then Dutch New Guinea (2). Since that time, scrub typhus has returned to obscurity in the western world. There have been no large military outbreaks and the disease is not a major threat to travelers to endemic areas. Scientific enthusiasm has also been suppressed by the dramatic discovery shortly after World War II that chloramphenicol and later the safer tetracyclines could both cure and prevent *O. tsutsugamushi* infection (3–7). Lyme disease, first described in Connecticut and a far less common arthropod-transmitted disease than scrub typhus, was the subject of 68 National Institute of Allergy and Infectious Disease grants in 1997, *O. tsutsugamushi* infection of none (8). Yet it is estimated that more than a million cases of scrub typhus are transmitted annually in Asia and more than a billion people are at risk (8), making it the most medically important rickettsial disease.

Scrub typhus was a dreaded disease in the preantibiotic era. Noad and Haymaker (9) wrote in 1953 that "scrub typhus has been robbed of its terror by the introduction of chloromycetin (chloramphenicol)." The chief architect of the discovery that antibiotics were remarkably effective against *O. tsutsugamushi* was Joseph Smadel. Smadel et al. (3–7,10–12) delineated much of what we know today about scrub typhus in a series of landmark papers beginning with a publication in Science in 1947. The extraordinary scope of their work ranged from basic immunology and pathogenesis, to some of the first trials of antibiotic efficacy and pharmacokinetics, to the development and efficacy testing of scrub typhus vaccines.

The most common clinical presentation in mild cases is fever and cough, Adult respiratory distress syndrome (ARDS) is the principal cause of death in severe disease. The response of mild scrub typhus to treatment with doxycycline or chloramphenicol is typically so rapid that resolution of fever is used as a diagnostic test; if the temperature has not returned to normal within 48 hours after beginning doxycycline treatment, infection is not due to *O. tsutsugamushi* (13). Recently, however, strains of *O. tsutsugamushi* from Chiangrai, northern Thailand, have shown reduced susceptibility to traditional antirickettsial antibiotics in the first demonstration of naturally occurring antibiotic resistance in rickettsiae (8,13,14). Another recent finding was that HIV-1viremia falls in some AIDS patients who acquire *O. tsutsugamushi* infection, possibly due to cross-reacting antibodies (15,16). Although the clinical characteristics of scrub typhus disease and the morphology of the mite vector were first described in a

Chinese clinical manual that appeared in the year 313 A.D., the continued public health importance of *O. tsutsugamushi* infection and the regular appearance of unexplained and unexpected new findings underscore the wisdom in the statement that "a disease first documented by the Chinese nearly 2000 years ago cannot be described as emerging, but it is to be hoped that our appreciation of it is" (8).

THE ORGANISM

Nagayo et al. (17) demonstrated the causative organism inside human and animal macrophages in 1924 and were able to passage *O. tsutsugamushi* six years later in Descemet's membrane. Intraperitoneal infection of mice was shown to be a useful method of isolating *O. tsutsugamushi* in 1932 and remains the method of choice today (18). The organisms are rods approximately 0.5 μm in width and from 1.2 to 3.0 μm in length, slightly larger than typhus and spotted fever group rickettsiae. *O. tsutsugamushi* is an obligate intracellular parasite that invades host cells by induced phagocytosis and escapes from the phagosome to the cytosol. Once free in the host cytoplasm, the bacteria replicate by transverse binary fission in the perinuclear area. Organisms are released from the cell by pushing out the host cytoplasmic membrane from inside, and budding organisms accumulate at a high density on the host cell surface. New cells can be infected either by free bacteria or by contact with budding projections from infected cells (18). The organism enters the cytosol of the new cell by lysing intervening host cell membranes. Organisms stain deep purple by Giemsa and characteristically are grouped in perinuclear clusters (Fig. 1). *O. tsutsugamushi* is less stable than other rickettsiae in an extracellular environment and multiplies slowly in culture—approximately three times per 24 hours.

Taxonomy

In 1995, the causative agent of scrub typhus was moved from the genus *Rickettsia* to a separate genus, *Orientia* (1). The cell wall of *O. tsutsugamushi* differs strikingly from that of other *Rickettsia* when seen by electron microscopy, contains unique proteins, and lacks peptidoglycan and lipopolysaccharide (1,19–21). The budding process that figures so prominently in the multiplication cycle of *O. tsutsugamushi* is uncharacteristic of *Rickettsia* species (1). Analyses of 16S ribosomal RNA gene sequences indicate 98.5% to 99.9% homology between scrub typhus organisms but only 90.2% to 90.6% homology with organisms of the genus *Rickettsia* (22).

Intracellular Survival Strategies

O. tsutsugamushi has evolved a variety of mechanisms to remain viable in its intracellular habitat. The organism can enter and replicate inside macrophages, which normally provide an environment hostile to the survival of microorganisms (23). *O. tsutsugamushi* suppresses the

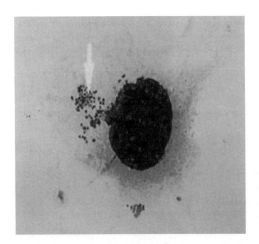

FIGURE 1 The organism. Perinuclear clusters of Giemsa-stained *O. tsutsugamushi*. *Source*: Photo courtesy of Dr. Kriangkrai Lerdthusnee, Department of Entomology, AFRIMS.

production of the inflammatory cytokines tumor necrosis factor (TNF)-alpha and interleukin-6 in murine macrophages (24); TNF-alpha production appears to be inhibited by the induction of interleukin-10 (25). Apoptosis of host cells would deprive this obligate intracellular pathogen of its intracellular hideout. Scrub typhus bacteria are able to inhibit apoptosis of macrophages by retarding intracellular calcium release (26).

Antigens of *O. tsutsugamushi*

O. tsutsugamushi exhibits great antigenic variation and this heterogeneity among strains is greater than that encountered in other groups of rickettsiae. Three classical strains (Karp, Gilliam, and Kato) and new antigenic types from Thailand have been used as prototype strains in many studies. The major surface protein antigen of *O. tsutsugamushi* is the variable 56-kDa protein, which accounts for 10% to 15% of its total protein (27). This protein is an immunodominant antigen, is reactive with group- and strain-specific monoclonal antibodies, and is recognized by sera from most scrub typhus patients. There is 59% to 82% overall amino acid homology among the various strains (28). The four other major surface proteins are at 110, 47, and 25 kDa, respectively, and also display considerable antigenic variability (27,29). The strain heterogeneity among scrub typhus rickettsiae appears to be a result of multiple components that exhibit variability in a background of strong homology.

EPIDEMIOLOGY

Scrub typhus transmission occurs within a triangular-shaped area of more than 5 million square miles bounded to the north by Siberia and the Kamchatka Peninsula, to the south by Queensland, Australia, and to the west by Afghanistan (Fig. 2). The public health impact of *O. tsutsugamushi* infection is greatest in agricultural laborers in the rural Asian tropics (30).

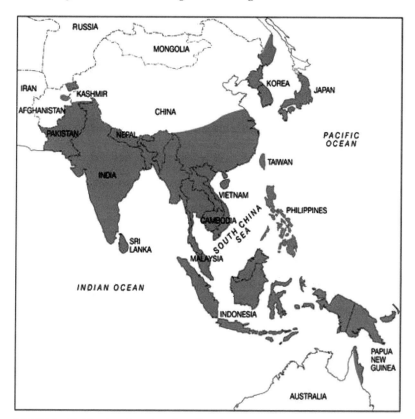

FIGURE 2 Distribution of scrub typhus. Note that the disease is only endemic in Asia. *Source*: Photo courtesy of D.A. Warrell, editor, Oxford Textbook of Medicine.

Disease transmission has been reported in suburban areas (31), but residents of city centers are not at risk. Travelers to endemic areas can become infected (32), particularly those who engage in eco-tourism (30) or visit rural areas to engage in activities such as trekking, rafting, or camping (33,34). However, scrub typhus is an uncommon cause of fever in the returning traveler; only about 20 cases of travel-associated *O. tsutsugamushi* infection have been reported since 1986 (34). In contrast, there were 1402 reported cases of malaria in travelers returning to the U.S.A. alone during the year 2000 (35).

The majority of scrub typhus cases go undiagnosed because commercial diagnostic tests are generally unavailable in the rural tropics where most infections occur and symptoms and signs are often nonspecific. However, longitudinal studies have shown that scrub typhus is an exceedingly common infection. Twenty-three percent of all febrile illnesses at one Malaysian hospital were scrub typhus (36), and *O. tsutsugamushi* was documented to be the most common cause of acute, undifferentiated fever in both rural Malaysia and northern Thailand (13,37). More than 75% of adults have serological evidence of exposure to scrub typhus in some rural Thai villages (38) as do more than 80% of rural Malaysian adults (39). During the Second World War, there were an estimated 18,000 cases of *O. tsutsugamushi* infection in Allied soldiers, 35,000 cases in Japanese troops, and "eighteen percent of a single battalion ... got scrub typhus in two months, and in that time 5% of the total strength had died of it" (40).

Habitat and Ecology

O. tsutsugamushi is transmitted in the tropics, in temperate zones, and even in the high Himalayas (41). Thai physicians have long observed that the majority of their scrub typhus patients are rice farmers, but the importance of active rice fields as a niche of transmission has not been reflected in the literature. Although infected chiggers and rodents can be found in rice fields year-round, cases occur with human contact and their numbers peak during rice-planting and rice-harvesting seasons (Fig. 3). Agricultural exposure on oil palm and rubber plantations

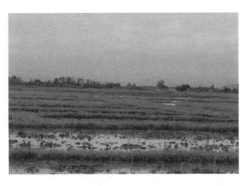
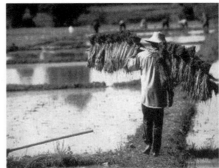
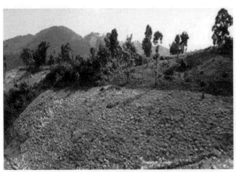
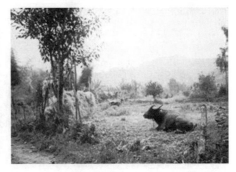

FIGURE 3 (*See color insert.*) Scrub typhus habitats. Transmission occurs in active rice fields (*top left*). Farmers intrude on the chigger-rodent cycle taking place on walkways between flooded fields (*top right*). Typical "scrub" or secondary vegetation in Thailand (*bottom panels*). *Source*: Top left photo courtesy of Dr. Kriangkrai Lerdthusnee, Department of Entomology, AFRIMS.

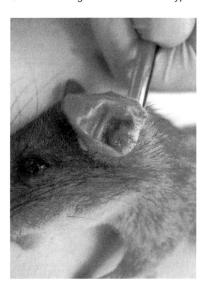

FIGURE 4 Chiggers and rats. Numerous larval trombiculid mites (chiggers) attached to the earlobe of a rodent (*Rattus rattus*). *Source*: Photo courtesy of Dr. Kriangkrai Lerdthusnee, Department of Entomology, AFRIMS.

and forestry also poses a major risk (30). Transmission often occurs in zones where primary forest has been cleared and replaced by secondary, or scrub, vegetation, hence the name scrub typhus (Fig. 3). However, infected mites have been collected in areas as ecologically diverse as semideserts, sandy beaches, and alpine meadows (41).

Humans are accidental hosts, acquiring *O. tsutsugamushi* during feeding of a larval trombiculid mite of the genus *Leptotrombidium*. These chiggers only feed on mammalian tissue fluid once in their lifetime (41), and constitute the reservoir of infection through transovarial transmission. Mites are normally maintained in nature by feeding on a variety of wild rodents (Fig. 4). Rodents are the key to the population density of chiggers but are not a reservoir of *O. tsutsugamushi*. Only a low proportion of chiggers acquire *O. tsutsugamushi* from infected rats, and chiggers infected by feeding neither develop a generalized infection nor transmit the organisms transovarially to their offspring (42). Humans become infected when they accidentally encroach on a zone where the rodent–chigger cycle is taking place. Transmission depends on the seasonal activities of both chiggers and humans. Chigger activity is determined by temperature and humidity, both of which are relatively stable in the tropics. In much of southeast Asia where climatic conditions are favorable throughout the year, populations of mites and maintaining rodent hosts may be high and endemic areas extensive. However, in more temperate zones, seasonal variations in climatic conditions are influential and endemic areas are scattered. *Leptotrombidium deliense* is the most important vector species in Southeast Asia and southern China, whereas *L. akamushi*, *L. scutellare*, and *L. pallidum* are the main vectors in Korea and Japan (30,41). *L. chiangraiensis* is a newly described vector found in cultivated rice fields in Thailand (Fig. 5) (43).

PATHOLOGY, PATHOGENESIS, AND IMMUNITY

Much remains to be learned about the pathogenesis of scrub typhus, and most pathology studies were done before modern histopathological techniques were available. *O. tsutsugamushi* infection appears to be a vasculitis, but clinical findings correlate poorly with pathology. Marked geographical variations in severity of illness were reported in the preantibiotic era, but determinants of severity remain uncharacterized. Evaluation of the results of both experimental animal infections and studies in cell culture is confounded by the unclear relevance of the target cells in these models. In mice, the route of inoculation determines the distribution of rickettsiae. The host cell in human scrub typhus is not known with certainty, and studies examining chemokine and cytokine production in patients with naturally acquired scrub typhus are lacking.

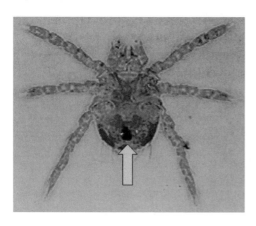

FIGURE 5 Mite vector of scrub typhus. *L. chiangraiensis*, a mite associated with disease transmission in Thailand. Note the posterior oil droplet (*arrow*), thought to be an adaptation to life in open fields. *Source*: Photo courtesy of Dr. Kriangkrai Lerdthusnee, Department of Entomology, AFRIMS.

Pathology

In fatal cases, the histopathology is chiefly disseminated focal vasculitis and perivasculitis, particularly in vessels of the skin, lungs, heart, and brain. Endovasculitis and focal hemorrhage may be present but are less prominent than in Rocky Mountain spotted fever and epidemic typhus (44). Pathologic abnormalities often correlate poorly with the clinical picture. Several series report consistent vasculitic lesions in the kidney and heart (44), but neither primary myocarditis nor renal failure are often seen clinically. The basic histopathological lesions, disseminated perivasculitis, and focal interstitial mononuclear infiltrations associated with edema suggest that macrophages are a more important target cell than the endothelium (45). Thrombotic lesions are rare, and little histologically evident vascular damage was seen in the most important histopathologic study of *O. tsutsugamushi* infection (46). The most important lesions are interstitial pneumonia with alveolar edema, hemorrhage, occasionally hyaline membranes, interlobular septal edema, and meningoencephalitis (44–46).

Pathogenesis

In humans, it is not known with precision whether organisms deposited in the skin spread to internal organs via the bloodstream, the lymphatics, or by another mechanism. However, a standard method for isolating *O. tsutsugamushi* is to inoculate patient's peripheral blood into mice, implying that organisms are present in the circulation. Human volunteers fed upon by infected chiggers developed a febrile illness with an eschar and regional lymphadenopathy after an 8- to 10-day incubation period during which organisms were apparently inoculated from the salivary glands of the chiggers into the dermis and subsequently spread to the regional lymph nodes and bloodstream (47). Bacteremia was detected one to three days before onset of fever. Mononuclear white blood cells from three of seven patients with naturally acquired acute scrub typhus stained positively for *O. tsutsugamushi* before and for two days after treatment (Fig. 6) (48). Specific staining subsequently identified the infected cells as monocytes; organisms were not found within lymphocytes.

Heparan sulfate proteoglycans contribute to the attachment of *O. tsutsugamushi* to cells (49), but a specific cellular receptor has not been identified. Scrub typhus bacteria have been demonstrated in a variety of cells in humans, including monocytes (Fig. 6), macrophages, Kupffer cells, cardiac myocytes, hepatocytes, and endothelial cells (44,46,48,50,51). A recently characterized monoclonal antibody that reacts exclusively against intracellular scrub typhus organisms could be used to stain viable intracellular *O. tsutsugamushi* and provide a valuable resource for increasing our understanding of the pathogenesis of this infection (52). Endothelial cell activation leads to the recruitment of macrophages, and subsets of chemokine genes are produced in macrophages and endothelial cells infected with *O. tsutsugamushi* (53,54). Activation of transcription factor activator protein 1 is involved in the induction of the gene encoding macrophage chemoattractant protein 1 by scrub typhus in endothelial cells (55).

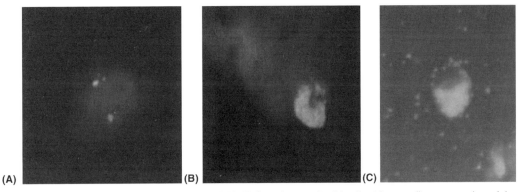

FIGURE 6 Specific staining for *O. tsutsugamushi*. (**A, B**) Organisms stained by direct immunofluorescence in peripheral blood smears of a patient with acute scrub typhus. *Source*: Photos courtesy of Dr. Douglas S. Walsh. (**C**) Organisms cultured in Vero cells. *Source*: Photo courtesy of Dr. Stuart Blacksell, Faculty of Tropical Medicine, Mahidol University, Bangkok, Thailand.

Marked variations in virulence of prototype strains of *O. tsutsugamushi* for mice is documented and there is evidence that mouse virulence correlates with severity of human disease (56). In human disease, widespread variations in scrub typhus virulence have been reported, particularly during the preantibiotic era. Case-fatality rates were higher in the elderly (57) and there was marked geographic variation in morbidity and mortality. Among Allied troops during World War II, case-fatality rates ranged from less than 1% in some camps to more than 30% in others (5). In Niigata Prefecture, Japan, 35% of more than 2000 cases reported between 1917 and 1952 were fatal, but there were no deaths among 780 cases on the Izo-Shichito Islands (58). The reasons underlying these differences in disease severity have never been adequately explained. A relationship between a particular strain of *O. tsutsugamushi*, the geographic origin of the rodent host, the mite vector, and disease severity has been demonstrated in Japan, but not in either Thailand or in West Pakistan (59).

Immunity

Infection with *O. tsutsugamushi* usually results in an acute, self-limiting febrile illness. The critical role played by the host immune response in controlling scrub typhus has been clearly documented (60). Experimental evidence from laboratory infections of mice (61) and circumstantial evidence from natural infections of humans (5,62) suggested that reduction of the relapse rate after withdrawal of chloramphenicol therapy was related to the development of a protective immune response. Mice receiving chloramphenicol therapy two days before being experimentally infected with scrub typhus died after withdrawal of drug but mice treated one week after infection survived (60). The production of antibody and the development of cellular immunity were more rapid in those animals in which rickettsial proliferation was allowed to proceed for seven days before initiation of chemotherapy (60).

However, the process by which scrub typhus rickettsiae are eliminated is not completely understood. Antibodies enhance clearance of *O. tsutsugamushi* from the blood, and B-lymphocyte depletion increases the susceptibility of mice to a moderately pathogenic strain (63). A T-cell-mediated cytotoxic immune mechanism exists that may play an important role (64). The potential importance of macrophages is suggested by the conversion of infection with a sublethal dose to a fatal infection when macrophage function is impaired by treatment with silica (65). *O. tsutsugamushi* has been shown to upregulate the β-chemokine regulated on activation normal T expressed and secreted (RANTES) in a cell culture model (54), and *O. tsutsugamushi* is a potent inducer of chemokines and cytokines in experimentally inoculated mice (66). To date, however, no studies examining chemokine and cytokine production in patients with naturally acquired sequence typing have been published.

Immunity to *O. tsutsugamushi* is incomplete, with frequent reinfections. Studies of humans have indicated that protective heterologous immunity lasts for only one to three months, whereas homologous immunity lasts for approximately one to three years (12). Reinfection with a heterologous strain produces a milder disease (67) and first infections are more often symptomatic than are subsequent infections (68).

CLINICAL FEATURES
Symptoms and Signs

The chigger bite can occur on any part of the body, is painless, and is not usually remembered by the patient (69). An eschar forms at the bite site in about half of primary infections and in a lesser proportion of secondary infections. However, eschars are often located in hard-to-examine areas such as the genital region or under the axilla and are often missed. The eschar develops during the 6- to 20-day (average 10 days) incubation period and is usually well developed by the time fever appears. It begins as a small papule, enlarges, undergoes central necrosis, and acquires a blackened crust to form a lesion resembling a cigarette burn (Fig. 7). A typical eschar is pathognomonic when viewed by a clinician experienced in scrub typhus diagnosis. Regional lymph nodes are enlarged and sometimes tender, and generalized lymphadenopathy and splenomegaly are not uncommon.

Fever and headache begin abruptly and are frequently accompanied by myalgias and malaise. Muscle tenderness is either absent or mild. A transient macular rash may appear at the end of the first week of illness. The rash appears on the trunk, becomes maculopapular, and spreads peripherally (Fig. 8). However, it is often difficult to detect on dark-skinned persons. The rash does not become hemorrhagic. Conjunctival suffusion is a helpful but nonspecific physical finding (Fig. 9). Hearing loss concurrent with the onset of fever occurs in about one-third of cases and is a very useful diagnostic clue (70). However, true hearing loss must be distinguished from tinnitus, which sometimes coexists with hearing loss, and from transient hearing loss due to nasal congestion, also a common feature of scrub typhus (69). Sensorineural hearing loss was documented by audiometry in Thai patients during acute *O. tsutsugamushi* infection and resolved after treatment. Acoustic nerve damage caused by scrub typhus has been well documented pathologically (9).

Cough, sometimes accompanied by infiltrates on the chest radiograph, is one of the most common presentations of scrub typhus infection (71). In severe cases, tachypnea progresses to dyspnea, the patient becomes cyanotic, and full-blown ARDS may develop. ARDS is associated with older age and preceding infiltrates on chest radiographs (72). Respiratory failure is the most common cause of death in severe scrub typhus infection, but survivors recover without sequelae.

Myocardial involvement during scrub typhus has been reported but is rare (73), and electrocardiographs are generally normal or have only minor nonspecific changes (74). Relative bradycardia, an unexpectedly low heart rate response for a given temperature increase, has been reported as a feature of a number of infectious diseases, particularly those caused by intracellular Gram-negative organisms. Relative bradycardia is mentioned in reports of scrub typhus case series from the preantibiotic era (69) and was recently quantified and found to occur in more than 50% of patients with mild *O. tsutsugamushi* infection (75). Confusion, apathy, and other mild personality changes can occur and sporadic cases of meningoencephalitis have been reported, but coma is rare (76,77). Hepatomegaly and mild jaundice are occasionally seen, but severe liver involvement is exceptional (78,79).

Scrub Typhus in Children

Scrub typhus is an underrecognized cause of febrile illness in childhood. In two Thai studies, one from the north (80) and one from the south (81), older male children were most often affected. Signs and symptoms were similar to those described in adults, except that vomiting was more common. Respiratory findings were prominent.

Scrub Typhus in Pregnancy

There is little information about the prevalence and effects of scrub typhus during pregnancy. According to the few studies published, clinical findings are no more severe in the pregnant

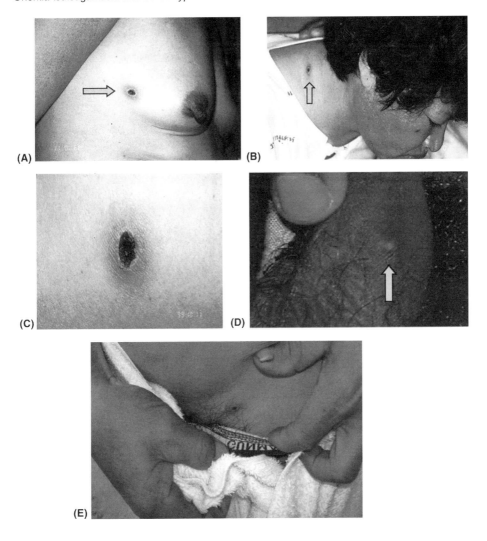

FIGURE 7 (*See color insert.*) Two eschars (*gray arrows*) in exposed areas (**A, B**). Eschars (**C**) may be atypical and lose their crust in moist locations such as the scrotum (**D**). Typical eschars may be missed because they are located in difficult to examine areas (**E**). *Source*: Photos courtesy of Dr. Kriangkrai Lerdthushee.

mother, and response to antibiotic treatment is prompt (82–86). However, fetal distress, premature delivery, stillbirth, abortion, and low birth-weight appear to occur in a high proportion of cases (82–84,87). In some cases, the adverse effects on pregnancy may have been caused by antibiotic therapy rather than by the disease itself (84). Neonatal scrub typhus has been reported (87), as has a case of vertical transmission from an infected mother (86).

Laboratory Findings

There is no amalgam of laboratory results that suggest the diagnosis of scrub typhus. Basic hematology and biochemistry results are often more useful for suggesting other diagnoses rather than hinting at *O. tsutsugamushi* infection. Complete blood count findings may be normal, although moderate elevations in the white blood cell count are common. Slight rises in serum hepatic transaminase levels occur often.

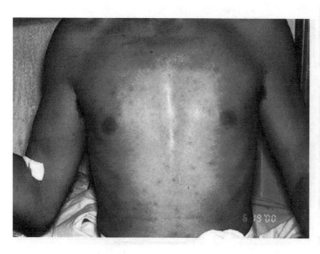
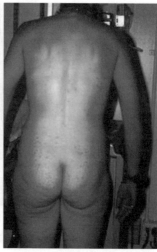

FIGURE 8 (*See color insert.*) Scrub typhus rash. The subtle rash seen in *O. tsutsugamushi* infection is fleeting and predominates on the trunk.

DIAGNOSIS

The clinical and laboratory features of scrub typhus are notoriously nonspecific. The eschar is the single most useful diagnostic clue, and is pathognomonic for *O. tsutsugamushi* when seen by a physician experienced in diagnosing this infection (Fig. 7). The importance of a careful search for an eschar in suspected cases of scrub typhus cannot be overstated.

Positive Diagnosis

The diagnosis can be simple in a patient who has visited or lives in an endemic area and presents with a fever, eschar, acute hearing loss, and lymphadenopathy. Unfortunately, this setting is rarely the case. Scrub typhus is an often overlooked cause of both acute undifferentiated fever and of pneumonitis of undetermined etiology (36,71). The single most useful diagnostic clue is the eschar, but even a typical eschar can be overlooked (33), eschars without crusts are often misdiagnosed, and eschars appear in only a minority of *O. tsutsugamushi* infections.

Laboratory Confirmation
Serodiagnosis

Clinical suspicion generally requires laboratory confirmation. Current diagnosis relies on the demonstration of specific antibody. For many years, the serodiagnosis of scrub typhus depended on the Weil–Felix test, which detects antibodies produced during *O. tsutsugamushi* infection that

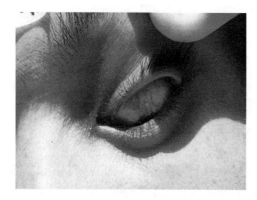

FIGURE 9 Conjunctival hyperemia in scrub typhus. This sign may be difficult to find, as shown here.

cross-react by agglutination with the OX-K antigen of an unrelated bacteria, *Proteus mirabilis*. The Weil–Felix test is grossly insensitive, with sensitivity rates consistently measured at less than 50% (30,88), yet it remains commercially available in much of Asia. Indeed, it is the only commercially available diagnostic test for scrub typhus in most areas endemic for the disease. The gold standard confirmatory tests are the indirect immunoperoxidase test and the immunofluorescent assay (IFA), which use yolk-sac-propagated or cell-culture-derived *O. tsutsugamushi* antigens (89,90). However, the complexity of these tests limits their use to a small number of reference centers. A rapid dot blot immunoassay (Fig. 10), which does not require a microscope, has been found to be as sensitive and specific as the more complex confirmatory assays (91,92). In a prospective field trial, more than 90% of scrub typhus cases could be diagnosed in about one hour by testing a single, admission blood specimen with this assay (91). However, the accuracy of these rapid tests should be validated against gold standard methods before they are deployed into a region where their sensitivity and specificity have not been previously established. An even more rapid lateral flow assay for the detection of IgG and IgM antibodies has been developed (93), but has not been prospectively field tested and is not commercially available. Recombinant scrub typhus proteins could provide a more standardized, easily stored, inexpensive, and plentiful source of antigens for use in test kits, and avoid the potential hazards of cultivating living rickettsiae (94). Initial evaluations indicate that recombinant-based assays are effective (92,94,95), but further appraisals, including prospective field testing, are necessary.

Demonstration of the Causative Organism

O. tsutsugamushi can be isolated from blood or tissues. Whole blood from patients with acute scrub typhus is injected intraperitoneally into white mice, which are then observed for signs of illness or death. Organisms can be demonstrated in Giemsa-stained impression smears taken from the surface of the spleen or peritoneum. Reported isolation rates vary widely, but remain less than 50% even when performed under the most favorable conditions by experienced workers. The causative organism can also be demonstrated by standard and by nested polymerase chain reaction (PCR) (96,97). Recently, detection of *O. tsutsugamushi* by quantitative real-time PCR has been reported (98,99). The qPCR assay was more sensitive than was mouse inoculation at demonstrating rickettsiae (99). However, the use of PCR is constrained by expense and technical requirements and at present its use is limited to the research setting. The use of PCR for routine diagnosis is probably not necessary because excellent, less expensive, rapid antibody-based serological tests have been developed (92). Rapid tests are positive in more than 90% of patients with scrub typhus infection during the first week of fever (91), and thus far the sensitivity of PCR is considerably lower (96–99). A relapse of scrub typhus cannot be distinguished from other causes of fever by serology, and PCR could help in this setting.

Differential Diagnosis

Tularemia, spotted fever rickettsiosis, and anthrax can cause eschars but have a different epidemiology, and the lesions differ from those seen in *O. tsutsugamushi* infection. Eschars frequently

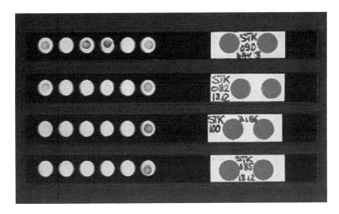

FIGURE 10 Dot blot immunoassay for the diagnosis of scrub typhus. Dots within the four leftmost circles indicate *O. tsutsugamushi* infection. The top strip clearly demonstrates a positive result, while the bottom strip is negative.

occur in the genital region where they often lose their crust (Fig. 7B). Thus they can be confused with the ulcers of lymphogranuloma venereum, chancroid, or syphilis.

The differential diagnosis depends on the diseases prevalent in the area in which the illness originated. Findings from a Malaysian study are fairly typical of the major causes of acute undifferentiated fever in areas endemic for scrub typhus (37). Scrub typhus was the most frequent diagnosis (19.3%), followed in frequency by typhoid (7.4%), flavivirus infection (7.0%), leptospirosis (6.8%), and malaria (6.2%). Murine typhus often coexists with *O. tsutsugamushi* infection in Asian populations (31,100–102). Unlike the other entities, however, malaria can be easily diagnosed by demonstrating plasmodia in blood films and so will not be considered further in this discussion.

Typhoid fever, scrub typhus, murine typhus, dengue virus infection, and leptospirosis all present as acute undifferentiated fever and also coexist in the same areas. Their signs and symptoms may be nonspecific, and confirmatory diagnostic tests are often not available in areas where these diseases are common. A correct initial diagnosis would avoid harm caused by performing inappropriate treatments, permit the prompt initiation of correct therapy, and contribute to accurate epidemiologic records. Attempts to develop a diagnostic kit capable of identifying one of several tropical infections simultaneously on a single assay have not yet yielded success. One such test, a multitest strip dot blot immunoassay for the diagnosis of typhoid fever, scrub typhus, murine typhus, dengue virus infection, and leptospirosis, was evaluated in Thai adults presenting to hospital with acute, undifferentiated fever (103). Unfortunately, the kit gave multiple positive test results in 92% of patients with verified, single infections and was therefore not a useful admission diagnostic tool. Antigen or genetic detection may eventually provide a solution to the problem of trying to simultaneously diagnose one of several possible infections with a single test.

Scrub Typhus, Typhoid Fever, and Murine Typhus

Typhoid fever is uncommon in the better developed countries of the Asian-Pacific region such as Thailand, Japan, Malaysia, Singapore, Taiwan, Korea, and Hong Kong (104). *Salmonella typhi* infection rarely causes generalized lymphadenopathy or conjunctival suffusion, while sustained fever is unusual in scrub typhus (104). Murine typhus is generally a more mild illness than is *O. tsutsugamushi* infection and is less often associated with serious pneumonitis (100). Febrile patients from urban areas are more likely to have murine typhus than scrub typhus, although transmission of *O. tsutsugamushi* occurs in suburban areas of Bangkok (31).

Scrub Typhus and Dengue Fever

A rash that is hemorrhagic, particularly if associated with leucopenia and thrombocytopenia, suggests infection with dengue virus rather than *O. tsutsugamushi*. In a study of adults with acute, undifferentiated fever in northern Thailand, dengue virus infection was associated with hemorrhagic manifestations, particularly bleeding from the gums, which was reported by 27% of the dengue patients, but by none of the scrub typhus patients (105). The white blood cell count is useful in differentiating the two diseases; a low platelet count ($<140,000\,\text{mm}^{-3}$) and low white blood cell count ($<5000\,\text{mm}^{-3}$) were strongly associated with dengue infections (odds ratio 26.3 for platelets and 8.2 for leukocytes) (105). Although mild elevations of serum transaminase concentrations occur in scrub typhus patients, marked rises in liver enzymes are more characteristic of dengue virus infection, where fulminant hepatic failure can occur (106).

Scrub Typhus and Leptospirosis

Differentiating leptospirosis from *O. tsutsugamushi* infection is a frequently encountered and important clinical problem. Both infections are common in agricultural workers, occur in travelers returning from endemic areas, and have been associated with ecotourism (30,107). A history of contact with water, marked myalgia, liver involvement, and renal dysfunction suggest leptospirosis rather than scrub typhus. Patients with leptospirosis tend to have higher white blood cell counts, a higher percentage of neutrophils, and higher levels of serum bilirubin and serum creatinine than do patients with scrub typhus infection. Although patients with both diseases often complain of myalgia, the response to palpation of the affected muscles can differ and provide diagnostic help. In leptospirosis, even the pressure of the bed sheets can be painful, and muscles are exquisitely painful to the touch. Patients with *O. tsutsugamushi* infection, however, sometimes report that myalgia is lessened by rubbing the muscles involved. Conjunctival suffusion occurs in both infections but a combination of suffusion, bleeding, and jaundice sometimes give a characteristic orange discoloration of the sclera in leptospirosis which is uncommon in scrub typhus infection. Renal compromise is unusual in scrub typhus, but is the hallmark of Weil's disease, the severe form of leptospirosis. Lethal pulmonary complications occur in both infections, but unlike the ARDS-like syndrome that is the most common cause of death in *O. tsutsugamushi* infection, pulmonary hemorrhage is the predominant severe respiratory problem in leptospirosis (108).

Dual Infections

The problem of differentiating *O. tsutsugamushi* infection from other causes of acute undifferentiated fever in the tropics is made more complex by the possibility that scrub typhus may coexist with another infection (109). Dual infections should be considered in patients at risk of both who have atypical clinical features of either disease alone and in patients responding poorly to treatment. Rice farmers in north-eastern Thailand, and possibly much of southeast Asia, are commonly infected with both leptospirosis and scrub typhus (109). Mud and water in flooded rice fields provide a fertile environment for leptospirosis while the rodent–chigger cycle takes place on the drier walkways between the flooded paddies (Fig. 3). Specific signs of scrub typhus such as hearing loss or an eschar in a patient with a clinical picture typical for leptospirosis suggest the presence of a double infection. It can be critical to identify mixed leptospirosis–scrub typhus infections. *O. tsutsugamushi* is not susceptible to penicillin, the standard treatment for severe leptospirosis. Similarly, intravenous chloramphenicol is often used to treat severe scrub typhus infections in the tropics, but will not cure leptospirosis. Patients with acute scrub typhus coinfected with dengue fever or malaria are seen with some regularity in regions where these infections are endemic.

TREATMENT

Scrub typhus is said to respond even more promptly to antibiotics than do other rickettsial diseases, with patients generally becoming afebrile within 24 to 36 hours after beginning antibiotic therapy. Indeed, *O. tsutsugamushi* infection is usually so responsive to treatment with doxycycline or chloramphenicol that if fever has not abated within 48 hours, the diagnosis of scrub typhus is considered unlikely (13). Early antibiotic treatment shortens the disease course, reduces mortality, and accelerates convalescence. Treatment must often be presumptive, but the benefits of avoiding severe scrub typhus by early antibiotic administration generally outweigh the risks of a one-week course of doxycycline—the treatment of choice. Either oral tetracycline 500 mg four times daily or oral doxycycline 100 mg twice daily for seven days is recommended. Shorter treatment courses are often curative, but may result in relapse (79). A one-week course of chloramphenicol 50 to 75 mg/kg/day is also effective although less so than tetracyclines. Parenteral therapy should be given to patients who are vomiting or have severe disease. Intravenous chloramphenicol is a useful alternative in areas where parenteral formulations of tetracyclines are unavailable or unaffordable. Scrub typhus was a dreaded disease in the preantibiotic era. Prompt antibiotic therapy generally prevents death, but good supportive care and early detection of complications are important in severe cases if a good outcome is to be obtained.

Treatment of Pregnant Women and Children

The antimicrobial treatment of pregnant women and children poses several problems. The tetracyclines are contraindicated in pregnancy because of their teratogenic potential, and repeated long courses administered to young children cause staining of the permanent teeth. Chloramphenicol is best avoided during pregnancy and cannot be given to neonates. Macrolide antibiotics would be safer alternatives for the treatment of *O. tsutsugamushi* infection during pregnancy and early childhood. Roxithromycin, one such macrolide, was as effective as doxycycline and chloramphenicol in a trial of 39 Korean children (110). Three Japanese patients were treated successfully with clarithromycin (111), as were 47 Korean patients with azithromycin (112).

Drug-Resistant Scrub Typhus

The antibiotic susceptibility of different *O. tsutsugamushi* strains can be determined in mice, in cell culture, by flow cytometry and by application of a monoclonal antibody specific for intracellular *O. tsutsugamushi* to the IFA test (113–115). The occurrence of chloramphenicol- and doxycycline-resistant strains of *O. tsutsugamushi* in Chiangrai, northern Thailand, has been documented by mouse antibiotic susceptibility testing and in tissue culture (13,116). Median fever clearance times after doxycycline treatment were longer in patients infected in northern Thailand than in a control group of patients infected with scrub typhus in the western part of the country (13). Even though the treatment response was slowed, all patients were cured. Whether resistant strains occur elsewhere is unknown and the mechanism of resistance has not yet been elucidated. How resistant strains could be transmitted from a human to another host is unclear since chiggers are the reservoir of infection and neither human-to-human nor human-to-chigger transmission of *O. tsutsugamushi* has been reported (8).

Rifampin and rifabutin were the only antibiotics identified as more active than doxycycline against resistant strains of scrub typhus and were equally effective against drug-sensitive strains in mouse antibiotic susceptibility testing. Rifampin alone controlled fever more rapidly than did doxycycline in a controlled, blinded treatment trial of mild scrub typhus acquired in Chiangrai Province in northern Thailand (14). Treatment failures were seen with the combination of doxycycline plus rifampicin. The reduced susceptibility to doxycycline manifests itself as prolonged fever clearance time, but not complete therapeutic failure. All patients were eventually cured. However, the use of an antibiotic to which the organism is fully susceptible could be life-saving in severe disease. Neither the efficacy of rifampin for severe disease nor the optimal therapeutic regimen for drug-resistant scrub typhus has been determined. The widespread use of single-dose rifampin could potentially contribute to the problem of drug-resistant tuberculosis in areas where both *O. tsutsugamushi* and *Mycobacterium tuberculosis* infection are highly prevalent.

When tested in an in vitro assay system, azithromycin was more effective than doxycycline against doxycycline-susceptible and -resistant strains of *O. tsutsugamushi* (116). However, in susceptibility testing in mice, azithromycin was no more effective than was doxycycline against drug-resistant strains and was less effective than both rifampin and rifabutin. Symptoms, signs, and fever abated rapidly in two azithromycin-treated pregnant women who acquired scrub typhus in northern Thailand, where drug-resistant strains occur (82). Limited data suggest that ciprofloxacin is not efficacious in *O. tsutsugamushi* infection (114,117). There is an critical need for prospective, randomized trials to improve antibiotic treatment of severe and resistant scrub typhus, and of *O. tsutsugamushi* infection in pregnancy and childhood. Newer technologies can perhaps accelerate the process of improving scrub typhus therapy. Flow cytometry and application of a monoclonal antibody specific for intracellular *O. tsutsugamushi* to the IFA test could help identify potentially useful new antimicrobials, and quantitative PCR could serve as an objective marker of treatment response in clinical trials of agents found effective in preclinical testing (99,113,115).

PREVENTION
Chemoprophylaxis

Chemoprophylaxis should be considered for persons with anticipated intense but transient exposure to *O. tsutsugamushi*. Soldiers and road construction crews are typical examples, but chemoprophylaxis should also be considered in high-risk travelers such as trekkers or eco-tourists. Weekly doses of 200 mg of doxycycline can prevent *O. tsutsugamushi* infection (118,119). However, several questions about doxycycline chemoprophylaxis remain unanswered. It is not known whether doxycycline chemoprophylaxis would be protective against northern Thai strains of *O. tsutsugamushi* with reduced susceptibility to this antimicrobial agent. It is also not known whether the daily doxycycline prophylaxis regimen recommended for the chemoprophylaxis of malaria would protect against scrub typhus, and there are theoretical reasons for suspecting that it might not. Intermittent prophylaxis would allow an immune response to develop against organisms acquired between two doses of antibiotic, whereas no such response would be allowed by daily drug administration (60). Indeed, weekly chloramphenicol was shown to prevent scrub typhus, but daily chloramphenicol did not (5).

Reduction of Chigger Contact

Contact with chiggers can be reduced by applying repellent to the tops of boots, socks, and trouser legs and by not sitting or lying directly on the ground. Unfortunately, these measures are frequently too impractical to be used by those exposed occupationally.

Scrub Typhus Vaccine

Vaccines offer the potential of long-term prevention from morbidity and mortality caused by scrub typhus. They also obviate the difficulties posed by drug resistance, vector control, and preventive chemoprophylaxis. Currently, there is no vaccine in use. During the 1940s, attempts to protect people against scrub typhus by immunization with killed rickettsial vaccines gave uniformly discouraging results under the conditions of field exposure, although animal trials had been successful (120,121). The failure of these vaccines in humans was most likely due to the inability of the killed organisms used to stimulate long-lasting heterologous protection. Other vaccine strategies have included using gamma-irradiated organisms that were metabolically active but incapable of growth, and combined infection and antibiotic prophylaxis (10,122). A DNA vaccine relying on the immunodominant 56-kDa outer membrane protein provided some protection in mice (123). A recombinant 56-kDa protein vaccine stimulated both T- and B-lymphocyte responses in mice and in two monkeys (124,125). These results provide some encouragement, and several groups in the United States and Asia are currently working on the development of a scrub typhus vaccine. However, the existence of countless disparate heterologous strains and multiple previous unsuccessful attempts suggest that a broadly effective vaccine may not be imminent.

SCRUB TYPHUS AND HIV-1
Effects of HIV on *O. tsutsugamushi* Infection

O. tsutsugamushi can be detected in the organs of mice, rats, and guinea pigs for months after the acute manifestations of disease have disappeared, and also persists in tissues of patients recovered from scrub typhus for appreciable lengths of time (11). This raises the possibility that dormant organisms could become active as immunity wanes. One setting where this eventuality might manifest would be northern Thailand, an area at the epicenter of the AIDS epidemic where *O. tsutsugamushi* infection is also common. However, no upsurge of scrub typhus cases was seen as the AIDS epidemic ravaged northern Thailand. Indeed, *O. tsutsugamushi* infection was no more common in HIV-infected subjects than in those who were not infected with HIV.

AIDS patients coinfected with some intracellular organisms have been found to have more severe disease and more frequent and prolonged bacteremia. Varicella-zoster virus produces more severe clinical manifestations in HIV-infected patients than in individuals that are not infected, whereas Salmonella species cause bacteremia more often in patients with AIDS than in non-HIV-infected patients. However, the opposite appears to be the case with the intracellular bacterium *O. tsutsugamushi*. *O. tsutsugamushi* blood culture positivity rates were significantly higher in HIV-uninfected subjects (48.6%) than in HIV-infected individuals (14.3%) and there are no differences in scrub typhus disease severity between HIV-infected and non-HIV-infected patients (126).

Effects of Scrub Typhus on HIV-1

Among HIV-1-seropositive individuals, acute infection with other organisms usually results in a transient rise in plasma viral load (127). In contrast, coinfection with *O. tsutsugamushi* was found to be associated with a substantial decrease in HIV-1 RNA levels in about 40% of patients in northern Thailand (15,16,127). Scrub typhus appears to shift the viral population from CXCR4-using (X4) to CCR5-utilizing (R5) strains of HIV-1, but the exact mechanism of this shift and of suppression is unclear. Preliminary data suggest that some soluble inhibitory factors, such as cross-reactive antibodies, play an important role while others, such as HIV-inhibitory chemokines, do not. *O. tsutsugamushi* antibody appears to colocalize with HIV-envelope proteins.

REFERENCES

1. Tamura A, Ohashi N, Urakami H, et al. Classification of *Rickettsia tsutsugamushi* in a new genus, *Orientia* gen. nov. as *Orientia tsutsugamushi* comb. nov. Int J Syst Bacteriol 1995; 45(3):589–591.
2. Irons EN, Armstrong HE. Scrub typhus in Dutch New Guinea. Ann Intern Med 1947; 26:201–220.
3. Smadel JE, Jackson EB. Chloromycetin, an antibiotic with chemotherapeutic activity in experimental rickettsial and viral infections. Science 1947; 106:418–419.
4. Smadel JE, Woodward TE, Ley HT, et al. Chloromycetin in the treatment of scrub typhus. Science 1948; 108(2798):160–161.
5. Smadel JE, Traub R, Ley HL, et al. Chloramphenicol (chloromycetin) in the chemoprophylaxis of scrub typhus (tsutsugamushi disease). II. Results with volunteers exposed in hyperendemic areas of scrub typhus. Am J Hyg 1949; 50(1):75–91.
6. Smadel JE, Jackson EB, Ley HL. Terramycin as a rickettsiostatic agent and its usefulness in patients with scrub typhus. Ann NY Acad Sci 1950; 53(2):375–384.
7. Smadel JE, Traub R, Frick LP, et al. Chloramphenicol (chloromycetin) in the chemoprophylaxis of scrub typhus (tsutsugamushi disease). III. Suppression of overt disease by prophylactic regimens of four-week duration. Am J Hyg 1950; 51(2):216–228.
8. Rosenberg R. Drug-resistant scrub typhus: paradigm and paradox. Parasitol Today 1997; 13(4):131–132.
9. Noad KB, Haymaker W. The neurological features of tsutsugamushi fever, with special reference to deafness. Brain 1953; 76(1):113–131.
10. Smadel JE, Ley HL, Diercks FH, et al. Immunization against scrub typhus. I. Combined living vaccine and chemoprophylaxis in volunteers. Am J Hyg 1951; 53(3):317–325.
11. Smadel JE, Ley HL, Diercks FH, et al. Persistence of *Rickettsia tsutsugamushi* in tissues of patients recovered from scrub typhus. Am J Hyg 1952; 56(3):294–302.
12. Smadel JE, Ley HL Jr, Diercks FH, et al. Immunization against scrub typhus: duration of immunity in volunteers following combined living vaccine and chemoprophylaxis. Am J Trop Med Hyg 1952; 1(1):87–99.
13. Watt G, Chouriyagune C, Ruangweerayud R, et al. Scrub typhus infections poorly responsive to antibiotics in Northern Thailand. Lancet 1996; 348(9020):86–89.
14. Watt G, Kantipong P, Jongsakul K, et al. Doxycycline and rifampicin for mild scrub-typhus infections in northern Thailand: a randomized trial. Lancet 2000; 356(9235):1057–1061.
15. Watt G, Kantipong P, de Souza M, et al. HIV-1 suppression during acute scrub typhus infection. Lancet 2003; 356(9228):475–479.
16. Watt G, Kantipong P, Jongsakul K, et al. Passive transfer of scrub typhus plasma to patients with AIDS: a descriptive clinical study. Q J Med 2001; 94(11):599–607.
17. Nagayo M, Tamiya T, Mitamura T, et al. On the virus of tsutsugamushi disease and its demonstration by a new method. Jpn J Exp Med 1930; 8:309–318.
18. Kawamura A Jr, Tanaka H, Tamura A. Tsutsugamushi Disease. Tokyo: University of Tokyo Press, 1995.
19. Silverman DJ, Wisseman CL Jr. Comparative ultrastructural study on the cell envelopes of *Rickettsia prowazekii*, *Rickettsia rickettsii*, and *Rickettsia tsutsugamushi*. Infect Immun 1978; 21(3):1020–1023.
20. Tamura A, Ohashi N, Urakami H, et al. Analysis of polypeptide composition and antigenic components of *Rickettsia tsutsugamushi* by polyacrylamide gel electrophoresis and immunoblotting. Infect Immun 1985; 48(3):671–675.
21. Amano K, Tamura A, Ohashi N, et al. Deficiency of peptidoglycan and lipopolysaccharide components in *Rickettsia tsutsugamushi*. Infect Immun 1987; 55(9):2290–2292.
22. Ohashi N, Fukuhara M, Shimada M, et al. Phylogenetic position of *Rickettsia tsutsugamushi* and the relationship among its antigenic variants by analyses of 16S rRNA gene sequences. FEMS Microbiol Lett 1995; 125(2–3):299–304.
23. Seong S-Y, Choi M-S, Kim I-S. *Orientia tsutsugamushi* infection: overview and immune responses. Microbes Infect 2001; 3(1):11–21.
24. Kim M-K, Kang JS. *Orientia tsutsugamushi* suppresses the production of inflammatory cytokines induced by its own heat-stable component in murine macrophages. Microb Pathog 2001; 31(3):145–150.
25. Kim MJ, Kim MK, Kang JS. *Orientia tsutsugamushi* inhibits tumor necrosis factor alpha production by inducing interleukin 10 secretion in murine macrophages. Microb Pathog 2006; 40(1):1–7.
26. Kim M-K, Seong S-Y, Seoh J-Y, et al. *Orientia tsutsugamushi* inhibits apoptosis of macrophages by retarding intracellular calcium release. Infect Immun 2002; 70(8):4692–4696.
27. Hanson B. Identification and partial characterization of *Rickettsia tsutsugamushi* major protein immunogens. Infect Immun 1985; 50(3):603–609.
28. Ohashi N, Nashimoto H, Ikeda H, et al. Diversity of immunodominant 56-kDa type-specific antigen (TSA) of *Rickettsia tsutsugamushi*: sequence and comparative analyses of the genes encoding TSA homologues from four antigenic variants. J Biol Chem 1992; 267(18):12728–12735.
29. Oaks EV, Rice RM, Kelly DJ, et al. Antigenic and genetic relatedness of eight *Rickettsia tsutsugamushi* antigens. Infect Immun 1989; 57(10):3116–3122.

30. Silpapojakul S. Scrub typhus in the western Pacific region. Ann Acad Med Singapore 1997; 26:794–800.
31. Strickman D, Tanskul P, Eamsila C, et al. Prevalence of antibodies to rickettsiae in the human population of suburban Bangkok. Am J Trop Med Hyg 1994; 51(2):149–153.
32. Thiebaut MM, Bricaire F, Raoult D. Scrub typhus after a trip to Vietnam. N Engl J Med 1997; 336(22):1613–1614.
33. Watt G, Strickman D. Life-threatening scrub typhus in a traveler returning from Thailand. Clin Infect Dis 1994; 18(4):624–626.
34. Jensenius M, Fournier P-E, Raoult D. Rickettsioses and the international traveller. Clin Infect Dis 2004; 39(10):1493–1499.
35. Anon. Malaria surveillance—United States, 2000. Morb Mortal Wkly Rep 2002; 51(SS-5):9–23.
36. Brown GW, Robinson DM, Huxsoll DL, et al. Scrub typhus: a common cause of illness in indigenous populations. Trans R Soc Trop Med Hyg 1977; 70(5–6):444–448.
37. Brown GW, Shirai A, Jegathesan M, et al. Febrile illness in Malaysia—an analysis of 1,629 hospitalized patients. Am J Trop Med Hyg 1984; 33(2):311–315.
38. Johnson DE, Crum JW, Hanchalay S, et al. Sero-epidemiological survey of *Rickettsia tsutsugamushi* infection in a rural Thai village. Trans R Soc Trop Med Hyg 1982; 76(1):1–3.
39. Brown GW, Robinson DM, Huxsoll DL. Serologic evidence for a high incidence of transmission of *Rickettsia tsutsugamushi* in two Orang Asli settlements in peninsular Malaysia. Am J Trop Med Hyg 1978; 27(1):121–123.
40. Philip CB. Tsutsugamushi disease (scrub typhus) in World War II. J Parasitol 1948; 34(3):169–191.
41. Traub R, Wisseman CL Jr. The ecology of chigger-borne rickettsiosis (scrub typhus). J Med Entomol 1974; 11(3):237–303.
42. Burgdorfer W. Ecological and epidemiological considerations of Rocky Mountain spotted fever and scrub typhus. In: Walker DH, ed. Biology of Rickettsial Diseases. Boca Raton, FL: CRC Press, 1988:33.
43. Lerdthusnee K, Khuntirat B, Leepitakrat WL, et al. Scrub typhus: vector competence of *Leptotrombidium chiangraiensis* chiggers and transmission efficacy and isolation of *Orientia tsutsugamushi*. Ann NY Acad Sci 2003; 990:25–35.
44. Settle EB, Pinkerton H, Corbett AJ. A pathologic study of tsutsugamushi disease (scrub typhus) with notes on clinicopathologic correlation. J Lab Clin Med 1945; 30:639–661.
45. Park JH, Hart MS. The pathology of scrub typhus. Am J Clin Pathol 1946; 16:139–149.
46. Allen AC, Spitz S. A comparative study of the pathology of scrub typhus (tsutsugamushi disease) and other rickettsial diseases. Am J Pathol 1945; 21:603–681.
47. Shirai A, Saunders JP, Dohany AL, et al. Transmission of scrub typhus to human volunteers by laboratory-reared chiggers. Jpn J Med Sci Biol 1982; 35(1):9–16.
48. Walsh DS, Myint KS, Kantipong P, et al. *Orientia tsutsugamushi* in peripheral white blood cells of patients with acute scrub typhus. Am J Trop Med Hyg 2001; 65(6):899–901.48.
49. Ihn K-S, Han S-H, Kim M-S, et al. Cellular invasion of *Orientia tsutsugamushi* requires initial interaction with cell surface heparin sulfate. Microb Pathog 2000; 28(4):227–233.
50. Pongponratn E, Maneerat Y, Chaisri U, et al. Electron-microscopic examination of *Rickettsia tsutsugamushi*-infected human liver. Trop Med Int Health 1998; 3(3):242–248.
51. Moron CG, Popov VL, Feng HM, et al. Identification of the target cells of *Orientia tsutsugamushi* in human cases of scrub typhus. Mod Pathol 2001; 14(8):752–759.
52. Kim MK, Odgerel Z, Chung MH, et al. Characterization of monoclonal antibody reacting exclusively against intracellular *Orientia tsutsugamushi*. Microbiol Immunol 2002; 46(11):733–740.
53. Cho N-H, Seong S-Y, Huh M-S, et al. Expression of chemokine genes in murine macrophages infected with *Orientia tsutsugamushi*. Infect Immun 2000; 68(2):594–602.
54. Cho N-H, Seong MS, Choi MS, et al. Expression of chemokine genes in human dermal microvascular endothelial cell lines infected with *Orientia tsutsugamushi*. Infect Immun 2001; 69(3):1265–1272.
55. Cho N-H, Seong S-Y, Huh M-S, et al. Induction of the gene encoding macrophage chemoattractant protein 1 by *Orientia tsutsugamushi* in human endothelial cells involves activation of transcription factor activator protein 1. Infect Immun 2002; 70(9):4841–4850.
56. Jackson EB, Smadel JE. Immunization against scrub typhus. II. Preparation of lyophilized living vaccine. Am J Hyg 1950; 53(3):326–331.
57. Blake FG, Maxcy KF, Sadusk JF Jr, et al. Studies on tsutsugamushi disease (scrub typhus, mite-borne typhus) in New Guinea and adjacent islands: epidemiology, clinical observations and etiology in the Dobadura area. Am J Hyg 1945; 41:243–373.
58. Maxcy KF. Scrub typhus (tsutsugamushi disease) in the U.S. Army during World War II. In: Moulton FR, ed. Rickettsial Diseases of Man. Boston, MA: Thomas, Adams & Davis, 1946:36.
59. Philip RN. Scrub typhus. In: Stoenner H, Kaplan W, Torten M, eds. CRC Handbook Series in Zoonoses. Section A: Bacterial, Rickettsial, and Mycotic Diseases. Vol. II. Boca Raton, FL: CRC Presss, 1980:303–315.
60. Shirai A, Catanzaro PJ, Eisenberg GH, et al. Host defenses in experimental scrub typhus: effect of chloramphenicol. Infect Immun 1977; 18(2):324–329.
61. Smadel JE, Jackson EB, Cruise AB. Chloromycetin in experimental rickettsial infections. J Immunol 1949; 62:49–65.

62. Sheehy TW, Hazlett D, Turk RE. Scrub typhus: a comparison of chloramphenicol and tetracycline in its treatment. Arch Intern Med 1973; 132(1):77–80.
63. Jerrells TR, Li H, Walker DH. In vivo and in vitro role of gamma interferon in immune clearance of Rickettsia species. Adv Exp Med Biol 1988; 239:193–200.
64. Rollwagen FM, Dasch GA, Jerrells TR. Mechanisms of immunity to rickettsial infection: characterization of a cytotoxic effector cell. J Immunol 1986; 136(4):1418–1421.
65. Jerrells TR, Osterman JV. Role of macrophages in innate and acquired host resistance to experimental scrub typhus infection of inbred mice. Infect Immun 1982; 37(3):1066–1073.
66. Koh YS, Yun JH, Seong SY, et al. Chemokine and cytokine production during *Orientia tsutsugamushi* infection in mice. Microb Pathog 2004; 36(1):51–57.
67. Smadel JE, Ley HL Jr, Diercks FH, et al. Immunity in scrub typhus: resistance to induced reinfection. Arch Pathol 1950; 50(6):847–861.
68. Olson JG, Bourgeois AL. *Rickettsia tsutsugamushi* infection and scrub typhus incidence among Chinese military personnel in the Pescadores Islands. Am J Epidemiol 1977; 106(2):172–175.
69. Sayen JJ, Pond HS, Forrester JS, et al. Scrub typhus in Assam and Burma. Medicine (Baltimore) 1946; 25:155–214.
70. Premaratna R, Chandrasena TGAN, Dassayake AS, et al. Acute hearing loss due to scrub typhus: a forgotten complication of a reemerging disease. Clin Infect Dis 2006; 42(1):e6–e8.
71. Chaykul P, Panich V, Silpapojakul K. Scrub typhus pneumonitis: an entity which is frequently missed. Q J Med 1988; 68(256):595–602.
72. Tsay RW, Chang FY. Acute respiratory distress syndrome in scrub typhus [Letter]. Q J Med 2002; 95(2):126–128.
73. Shah SS, McGowan JP. Ricketsial, ehrlichial and bartonella infections of the myocardium and pericardium. Front Biosci 2003; 8:E197–E201.
74. Watt G, Kantipong P, Jirajarus K. Acute scrub typhus in northern Thailand: EKG changes. Southeast Asian J Trop Med Public Health 2002; 33(2):312–313.
75. Aronoff DM, Watt G. Prevalence of relative bradycardia in *Orientia tsutsugamushi* infection. Am J Trop Med Hyg 2003; 68(4):477–479.
76. Kim DE, Lee SH, Park KI, et al. Scrub typhus encephalomyelitis with prominent focal neurologic signs. Arch Neurol 2000; 57(12):1770–1772.
77. Silpapojakul K, Ukkachoke C, Krisman S, et al. Rickettsial meningitis and encephalitis. Arch Intern Med 1991; 151(9):1753–1757.
78. Machella TE, Forrester JS. Mite or scrub typhus: a clinical and laboratory study of 64 cases. Am J Med Sci 1945; 38:38–61.
79. Berman SJ, Kundin WD. Scrub typhus in South Vietnam. Ann Int Med 1973; 79(1):26–30.
80. Sirisanthana V, Poneprasert B. Scrub typhus in children at Chiang Mai University hospital. J Infect Dis Antimicrob Agents 1989; 6(1):22–27.
81. Silpapojakul K, Varachit B, Silpapojakul K. Paediatric scrub typhus in Thailand: a study of 73 confirmed cases. Trans Roy Soc Trop Med Hyg 2004; 98(6):354–359.
82. Watt G, Kantipong P, Jongsakul K, et al. Azithromycin activities against *Orientia tsutsugamushi* strains isolated in cases of scrub typhus in northern Thailand. Antimicrob Agents Chemother 1999; 43(11): 2817–2818.
83. Phupong V, Srettakraikul K. Scrub typhus during pregnancy: a case report and review of the literature. Southeast Asian J Trop Med Public Health 2004; 35(2):358–360.
84. Mathai E, Rolain JM, Verghese L, et al. Case reports: scrub typhus during pregnancy in India. Trans R Soc Trop Med Hyg 2003; 97:570–572.
85. Tsui M-S, Fang RCY, Su Y-M, et al. Scrub typhus and pregnancy: a case report and literature review. Chin Med J 1992; 49:61–63.
86. Suntharasaj T, Janjindamai W, Krisanapan S. Pregnancy with scrub typhus and vertical transmission: a case report. J Obstet Gynaecol Res 1997; 23(1):75–78.
87. Wang C-L, Yang KD, Cheng S-N, et al. Neonatal scrub typhus: a case report. Pediatrics 1992; 89(5, Pt 1):965–968.
88. Pradutkanchana J, Silpapojakul K, Paxton H, et al. Comparative evaluation of four serodiagnostic tests for scrub typhus in Thailand. Trans R Soc Trop Med Hyg 1997; 91(4):425–428.
89. Brown GW, Shirai A, Rogers C, et al. Diagnostic criteria for scrub typhus: probability values for immunofluorescent antibody and *Proteus* OXK agglutinin titers. Am J Trop Med Hyg 1983; 32(5): 1101–1107.
90. Yamamoto S, Minamishima Y. Serodiagnosis of tsutsugamushi fever (scrub typhus) by the indirect immunoperoxidase technique. J Clin Microbiol 1982; 15(6):1128–1132.
91. Watt G, Strickman D, Kantipong P, et al. Performance of a dot blot immunoassay for the rapid diagnosis of scrub typhus in a longitudinal case series. J Infect Dis 1998; 177(3):800–802.
92. Coleman RE, Sangkasuwan V, Suwanabun N, et al. Comparative evaluation of selected diagnostic assays for the detection of IgG and IgM antibody to *Orientia tsutsugamushi* in Thailand. Am J Trop Med Hyg 2002; 67(5):497–503.
93. Wilkinson R, Rowland D, Ching WM. Development of an improved rapid lateral flow assay for the detection of *Orientia tsutsugamushi*-specific IgG/IgM antibodies. Ann NY Acad Sci 2003; 990:386–390.

94. Kim IS, Seong SY, Woo SG, et al. High level expression of a 56-kilodalton protein gene (*bor* 56) of *Rickettsia tsutsugamushi* Boryong and its application to enzyme-linked immunosorbent assays. J Clin Microbiol 1993; 31(3):598–605.
95. Jiang J, Marienau KJ, May LA, et al. Laboratory diagnosis of two scrub typhus outbreaks at Camp Fuji, Japan in 2000 and 2001 by enzyme-linked immunosorbent assay, rapid flow assay, and Western blot assay using outer membrane 56 kDa recombinant proteins. Am J Trop Med Hyg 2003; 69(1):60–66.
96. Furuya Y, Yoshida Y, Katayama T, et al. Serotype-specific amplification of *Rickettsia tsutsugamushi* DNA by nested polymerase chain reaction. J Clin Microbiol 1993; 31(6):1637–1640.
97. Murai K, Tachibana N, Okayama A, et al. Sensitivity of polymerase chain reaction assay for *Rickettsia tsutsugamushi* in patients' blood samples. Microbiol Immunol 1992; 36(11):1145–1153.
98. Jiang J, Chan T-C, Temenak JJ, et al. Development of a quantitative real-time polymerase chain reaction assay specific for *Orientia tsutsugamushi*. Am J Trop Med Hyg 2004; 70(4):351–356.
99. Singhsilarak T, Leowattana W, Looareesuwan S, et al. Short report: detection of *Orientia tsutsugamushi* in clinical samples by quantitative real-time polymerase chain reaction. Am J Trop Med Hyg 2005; 72(5):640–641.
100. Lee HC, Ko WC, Lee HL, et al. Clinical manifestations and complications of rickettsiosis in southern Taiwan. J Formos Med Assoc 2002; 101(6):385–392.
101. Duffy PE, Le Guillouzic H, Gass RF, et al. Murine typhus identified as a major cause of febrile illness in a camp for displaced Khmers in Thailand. Am J Trop Med Hyg 1990; 43(5):520–526.
102. Wilde H, Pornsilapatip J, Sokly T, et al. Murine and scrub typhus at Thai–Kampuchean border displaced persons camps. Trop Geogr Med 1991; 43(4):363–369.
103. Watt G, Jongsakul K, Ruangvirayuth R, et al. Short report: prospective evaluation of a multi-test strip for the diagnoses of scrub and murine typhus, leptospirosis, dengue fever, and *Salmonella typhi* infection. Am J Trop Med Hyg 2005; 72(1):10–12.
104. Wang JL, Kao JH, Tseng SP, et al. Typhoid fever and typhoid hepatitis in Taiwan. Epidemiol Infect 2005; 133(6):1073–1079.
105. Watt G, Jongsakul K, Chouriyagune C, et al. Differentiating dengue virus infection from scrub typhus in Thai adults with fever. Am J Trop Med Hyg 2003; 68(5):536–538.
106. Lawn SD, Tilley R, Lloyd G, et al. Dengue hemorrhagic fever with fulminant hepatic failure in an immigrant returning to Bangladesh. Clin Infect Dis 2003; 37:e1–e4.
107. Stone SC, McNutt E. Update: outbreak of acute febrile illness among athletes participating in Eco-Challenge-Sabah 2000, Borneo, Malaysia. Ann Emerg Med 2000; 38(1):83–84.
108. McBride AJ, Athanazio DA, Reis MG, et al. Leptospirosis. Curr Opin Infect Dis 2005; 18(5):36–386.
109. Watt G, Jongsakul K, Suttinont C. Possible scrub typhus coinfections in Thai agricultural workers hospitalized with leptospirosis. Am J Trop Med Hyg 2003; 68(1):89–91.
110. Lee K-Y, Lee H-S, Hong J-H, et al. Roxithromycin treatment of scrub typhus (tsutsugamushi disease) in children. Pediatr Infect Dis J 2003; 22(2):130–133.
111. Miura N, Kudoh Y, Osabe M, et al. Three cases of tsutsugamushi disease successfully treated with clarithromycin. Acta Med Nagasaki 1995; 40:44–47.
112. Kim Y-S, Yun H-J, Shim SK, et al. A comparative trial of a single dose of azithromycin versus doxycycline for the treatment of mild scrub typhus. Clin Infect Dis 2004; 39:1329–1335.
113. Kelly DJ, Salata KF, Strickman D, et al. *Rickettsia tsutsugamushi* infection in cell culture: antibiotic susceptibility determined by flow cytometry. Am J Trop Med Hyg 1995; 53(6):602–606.
114. McClain JB, Joshi B, Rice R. Chloramphenicol, gentamicin, and ciprofloxacin against murine scrub typhus. Antimicrob Agents Chemother 1988; 32(2):285–286.
115. Kim M-K, Odgerel Z, Kim M-J, et al. Application of monoclonal, specific for intracellular *Orientia tsutsugamushi*, to immunofluorescent antibody test for determining antibiotic susceptibility. Microbiol Immunol 2004; 48(9):655–660.
116. Strickman D, Sheer T, Salata K, et al. In vitro effectiveness of azithromycin against doxycycline-resistant and -susceptible strains of *Rickettsia tsutsugamushi*, etiologic agent of scrub typhus. Antimicrob Agents Chemother 1995; 39(11):2406–2410.
117. Mathai E, Rolain JM, Verghese GM, et al. Outbreak of scrub typhus in southern India during the cooler months. Ann NY Acad Sci 2003; 990:359–364.
118. Olson JG, Bourgeois AL, Fang RCY, et al. Prevention of scrub typhus: prophylactic administration of doxycycline in a randomized double blind trial. Am J Trop Med Hyg 1980; 29(5):989–997.
119. Twartz JC, Shirai A, Selvaraju G, et al. Doxycycline prophylaxis for human scrub typhus. J Infect Dis 1982; 146(6):811–818.
120. Berge TO, Gauld RL, Kitaoka M. A field trial of a vaccine prepared from the Volner strain of *Rickettsia tsutsugamushi*. Am J Hyg 1949; 50(3):337–342.
121. Card WI, Walker JM. Scrub typhus vaccine: field trial in South-East Asia. Lancet 1945; 1:481–483.
122. Eisenberg GHG Jr, Osterman JV. Gamma-irradiated scrub typhus immunogens: broad-spectrum immunity with combinations of rickettsial strains. Infect Immun 1979; 26(1):131–136.
123. Ni Y-S, Chan T-C, Chao C-C, et al. Protection against scrub typhus by a plasmid vaccine encoding the 56-kDa outer membrane protein antigen gene. Am J Trop Med Hyg 2005; 73(5):936–941.

124. Seong SY, Huh MS, Jang WJ, et al. Induction of homologous immune response to *Rickettsia tsutsugamushi* Boryong with a partial 56-kilodalton recombinant antigen fused with the maltose-binding protein MBP-BOR56. Infect Immun 1997; 65(4):1541–1545.
125. Chattopadhyay S, Jiang J, Chan T-C, et al. Scrub typhus vaccine candidate Kp r56 induces humoral and cellular immune responses in cynomolgus monkeys. Infect Immun 2005; 73(8):5039–5047.
126. Kantipong P, Watt G, Jongsakul K, et al. HIV infection does not influence the clinical severity of scrub typhus. Clin Infect Dis 1996; 23:1168–1170.
127. Kannangara S, DeSimone JA, Pomerantz RJ. Attenuation of HIV-1 infection by other microbial agents. J Infect Dis 2005; 192(15): 1003–1009.

Section V: *COXIELLA BURNETII* AND Q FEVER

18 | Bacteriology of *Coxiella*

Katja Mertens and James E. Samuel
Department of Microbial and Molecular Pathogenesis, Texas A&M University System Health Science Center, College Station, Texas, U.S.A.

INTRODUCTION

Coxiella burnetii, a gram-negative, pleomorphic coccobacillus, is characterized by its obligate intracellular localization and close association with arthropod and mammalian hosts. An infection with this organism causes Q (query) fever in humans and animals, first described by Derrick (1) in 1937 during an outbreak of a febrile illness among abattoir workers in Australia. Q fever, a zoonosis with a worldwide distribution, normally appears in humans as an acute, flu-like, and self-limiting illness, with fever and severe headaches. The less common chronic form can be life-threatening and manifests primarily as endocarditis or hepatitis (2). Impressive is the extremely broad host range of *C. burnetii*, including domestic animals, such as sheep, goats, and cattle, but also wild animals (3). This wide spectrum of reservoirs and the unique resistance of *C. burnetii* to environmental factors make tracing the source of infection difficult. Furthermore, the low infective dose, aerosolic transmission, and the capacity to disable a large group of humans led to the classification of *C. burnetii* as potential biological weapon in 1942 (4) and recently as a category B Select Agent by the Centers for Disease Control and Prevention. This renewed concern has led to new efforts to investigate the epidemiology, pathogenesis, and genomic aspects of this organism and to develop new vaccine and treatment strategies.

Among intracellular bacteria, *C. burnetii* occupies a unique position, in that it shares the absolute requirement for intracellular parasitism with members of the genera *Rickettsia*, but unlike cytoplasmic *Rickettsia*, it resides within a parasitophorous vacuole (PV) (5,6). *C. burnetii* and the phylogenetic-related pathogen *Legionella pneumophila* are both transmitted primarily by aerosols and survive in the environment, but *L. pneumophila* inhibits the phagosome–lysosome fusion to survive in an alkaline environment, whereas *C. burnetii* remains in an acidified phagolysosomal compartment (7). This unique biological niche is a hostile environment for most bacteria, because of hydrolytic enzymes, bactericidal factors, oxygen, and nitrogen radicals, as well as acidic pH ($\approx$4.8) (8,9). The latter condition is known as an absolute requirement for metabolic activation and replication initiation of *C. burnetii* (10–13). A developmental life cycle and phase transition as part of an adaptive lifestyle are subject to continuing studies (14,15).

The progress in understanding genetic events in *C. burnetii* is slow, because standard techniques for genetic manipulations are unavailable. The obligate intracellular lifestyle, cellular localization, slow growth rate, and the tendency for host cell persistence rather than lysis have hampered the development of new transformation techniques. Initial approaches to studying gene function and regulation in *C. burnetii* used cloning into heterologous systems such as *Escherichia coli* of several genes encoding housekeeping functions, surface proteins, and stress response for characterization (16–21). The identification of an autonomous replication sequence (*ars*), which is likely to be the chromosomal origin and mediates plasmid replication in *E. coli*, provided new possibilities for the development of genetic manipulation (22,23). The recently published genome sequence of *C. burnetii* Nine Mile provides new opportunities to understand the biology and pathogenesis of this organism and may lead to new genetic tools (24). This review focuses on the recent discoveries and advances in phylogenetical classification, microbiological attributes, and genetic aspects in context of the intracellular lifestyle of *C. burnetii*.

TAXONOMY

The characteristically obligate intracellular lifestyle and close association to arthropods was the reason for the historical classification of *C. burnetii* within the α-1 subdivision of the

Proteobacteria to the Rickettsiaceae family and *Rickettsiae* tribe, together with the genera *Rickettsia* and *Rochalimaea* (now reclassified as *Bartonella*) (25). Genome comparison and 16S rRNA gene sequence analysis showed that *C. burnetii* is phylogenetically distant from *Rickettsia* and resulted in reclassification to the order of *Legionellales* in the γ subdivision of the *Proteobacteria*, with the more closely related genera *Legionella*, *Francisella*, and *Rickettsiella* (24,26,27). Furthermore, these data indicated a high degree of genetic homogeneity and supports the assumption that the genus *Coxiella* consists of a single species (26,28).

Originally, *C. burnetii* isolates were described by their source of isolation, geographic origin, and clinical manifestation. Several attempts were made to discriminate between these organisms based on phenotypic and genomic characteristics including lipopolysaccharide (LPS) banding pattern comparison and plasmid-type determination (29,30). Currently, five different plasmid types are known, designated as QpH1, QpRS, QpDG, QpDV, and one nondesignated plasmid from a Chinese isolate (31,32). The first described plasmid was QpH1 (36 kb), isolated from *C. burnetii* Nine Mile strain RSA493. This plasmid has been sequenced, and several loci were identified and characterized (*qsopAB*, *roa307*, *cbhE'*) (33–37). Plasmid QpRS (39 kb), originally isolated from *C. burnetii* Priscilla Q177, a strain obtained from a goat abortion, contains highly conserved and unique sequences compared to QpH1 (38,39). QpDG (51 kb) was isolated from the *C. burnetii* isolate Dugway 5J108-111, obtained from a rodent. This strain was shown to be avirulent in guinea pigs (40). Plasmid QpDV (33.5 kb) was isolated from two different sources: *C. burnetii* Q321 and Q1140, Russian isolates from human pneumonia and cow's milk, respectively. QpDV showed both unique and QpH1 homologous sequence regions (41). Cross-hybridization experiments indicated that all of these four plasmids, as well as the plasmidless isolate *C. burnetii* Scurry Q217, harbor the same 16-kb fragment, designated as the "core fragment" (33,34,42,43). It was suggested that these genes are essential for *C. burnetii*, but no functional data have been reported to support this idea.

Restriction fragment length polymorphism (RFLP) analysis of genomic DNA from *C. burnetii* isolates demonstrates a considerable heterogenic banding pattern for the classification of genomic groups. In initial studies, 36 *C. burnetii* isolates of different origins were analyzed by RFLP with three restriction enzymes (*Bam*HI, *Eco*RI, *Hind*III). Six distinct genomic groups (I–VI) were identified, which have been confirmed in subsequent studies (44,45). This grouping, as shown in Table 1, can be correlated with specific plasmid types and clinical manifestations (30). Group I, II, and III isolates were mainly associated with an acute infection and harbor the QpH1 plasmid, whereas QpRS is present in group IV isolates that were associated with a chronic disease. Genomic variation of *C. burnetii* has also been demonstrated by RFLP pattern analysis in other studies and single loci sequence analysis (47–51).

In a recent study, 173 *Coxiella* isolates from Europe, Canada, the United States, and Japan were phylogenetically analyzed by multispacer sequence typing (MST) (52). This new method compared the nucleotide sequences of internal regions between different genes, which are considered to be highly variable because of a lower selection pressure compared to the adjacent genes. For each region, a difference in a determined sequence represents an allele and these, as a whole, define the allelic profile of an organism. On the basis of sequence type (ST) distribution and frequency of 10 chromosomal spacers and one spacer for each plasmid QpH1, QpRS, and QpDV, three monophylogenetic groups with several subgroups were calculated. A correlation between the geographical and ST distribution, as well as phylogenetic relatedness of worldwide distributed strains, could be shown. The latter may indicate the spreading of a single ancestral strain. Concordant results were obtained by MST in comparison with plasmid type and genotype analysis. Interestingly, these data demonstrate a correlation between genotype, plasmid type, and disease outcome. QpRS was found in association with chronic infections and QpDV with acute and chronic infections. Another promising tool to analyze and correlate genetic diversity with phylogenetic aspects, pathogenic, and virulence potential of bacteria is the comparative genome hybridization (CGH). Genetic polymorphism, defined as negative hybridization of single or multiple open reading frames (ORFs) relative to the reference strain, were detected by probe sets on a custom Affimetrix microarray chip, representing all *C. burnetii* Nine Mile RSA493 ORFs (46). RFLP grouping of 20 previously typed *Coxiella* isolates was confirmed by CGH, and two new genomic groups, VII and VIII, were classified. In correlation with Glazunova et al., the worldwide distribution of group I isolates and the surprisingly low genetic

TABLE 1 *C. burnetii* Genomic Groups

Group[a]	Plasmid type[b]	Isolate	Phase[c]	Origin	Disease
I	QpH1	**Nine Mile RSA493**	I	**Montana, tick, 1935**	—
		Nine Mile RSA439	II	Montana, tick, 1935	—
		Nine Mile RSA514	I/II	Montana, tick, 1935	—
		Dyer RSA345	II	U.S.A., human blood, 1938	Acute
		Australia QD RSA425	II	Australia, human blood, ~1939	Acute
		Turkey RSA333	II	Turkey, human blood, 1948	Acute
		African RSA334	I	**Central Africa, human blood, 1949**	**Acute**
		El Tayeb RSA342	I	Egypt, tick, 1967	—
		California 33 RSA329	I	California, cow's milk, 1947	Persistent
II	QpH1	M44 RSA459	II	Italo-Greek, 'Grita', ~1945	Acute
		Henzerling RSA331	II	**Italy, human blood, 1945**	**Acute**
III	QpH1	Idaho goat Q195	I	Idaho, goat, 1981	Abortion
		Koka	I	Ethiopia, tick, 1963	—
IV	QpRS	**MSU Goat Q177**	I	**Montana, goat cotyledon, 1980**	**Abortion**
		K Q154	I	**Oregon, human heart valve, 1976**	**Endocarditis**
		P Q173	I	California, human heart valve, 1979	Endocarditis
V	NP	L Q216	I	Nova Scotia, human heart valve, 1981	Endocarditis
		G Q212	I	**Nova Scotia, human heart valve, 1981**	**Endocarditis**
		S Q217	I	Montana, human liver biopsy, 1981	Hepatitis
VI	QpDG	**Dugway 5J106-111**	I	**Utah, rodents, 1958**	—
VII	QpDV	Q321	ND	Russia, cow's milk	—
VIII	ND	Le Brunges	ND	France, unknown source	—

Isolates of TIGR and NIAID genome sequencing project are highlighted.
[a]Described by Hendrix et al. (44), except groups VII and VIII determined by Baere et al. (46).
[b]Described by Samuel et al. (30).
[c]Defined by Rocky Mountain Laboratories, Hamilton, MT, U.S.A.
Abbreviations: ND, not determined; NIAID, National Institute of Allergy and Infectious Disease; —, no disease associated; NP, no plasmid; TIGR, The Institute for Genome Research.

polymorphism within this group support the assumption of an common ancestral strain, which has undergone a limited evolution since its first isolation. Data also indicate that group I isolates represent the ancestor for the other genomic groups, which are clustered together in two phylogenetic clades: groups I, II, III, and VI, as well as groups IV, VII, and VIII.

MICROBIOLOGY

C. burnetii is an obligate intracellular, nonmotile, pleomorphic coccobacillus (0.3–1.0 μM), which replicates to high numbers within a PV of eukaryotic host cells, with an estimated doubling time of 20 to 45 hours (3,53). Although *C. burnetii* posses a membrane similar to other gram-negative bacteria, with outer membrane proteins, LPS, and peptidoglycan, it shows a nonreliable Gram-staining behavior, and the Giminez staining method is widely used for detection (54).

C. burnetii, naturally transmitted by aerosol, is primarily internalized by alveolar macrophages and monocytes through parasite-directed endocytosis. These endocytic vesicles mature normally to secondary phagolysosomes, where microorganisms are killed and degraded. Many invasive bacteria display the ability to escape from the endocytic pathway, either by lysis of the phagocytic vesicle (*Rickettsia*, *Shigella*), maturation arrest of the phagosome (*Mycobacterium*) or inhibition of phagosome–lysosome fusion (*Legionella*, *Chlamydia*) (55). After internalization, *Coxiella* containing vacuoles show a high fusogenity to form a large spacious PV, which can occupy nearly the whole cytoplasm of the host cell without affecting the viability (56–58). This PV shows specific markers of a secondary phagolysosome, such as acid phosphatase, cathepsin D, Rab7, and the lysosomal glycoproteins LAMP-1 and LAMP-2 (6,59–61). Maturation of the phagosome can selectively be modified by invasive bacteria to allow growth within a specific intracellular environment. For instance, the phylogenetic-related pathogen *L. pneumophilia* alters the phagocytic pathway and evades the endocytic traffic. Remodeling of the *Legionella* containing vacuole by the rough endoplasmic reticulum is controlled through the type IV secretion system released effector molecules (*icm/dot* genes) (7).

C. burnetii contains nearly all of the icm/dot genes and may alter the phagosome–lysosome fusion in a novel way (62). The observation of a delayed fusogenity of the PV containing metabolic active compared to dead bacteria and the demonstration of autophagosomal markers support the idea of a C. burnetii-specific altered PV maturation (57,60,63).

Acidophilic Lifestyle

Within the PV, C. burnetii becomes highly activated by the low pH and metabolic processes including nutrient transport and substrate metabolism are induced (11–13). To allow active transport across the membrane, a neutral cytoplasmic pH is maintained by active and passive mechanisms. Several sodiumion/proton exchangers are annotated as well as the characteristically high content of proteins with basic p*I* values that may contribute to maintaining a stable intracellular pH homeostasis (15,24). The pH difference between the bacterial cytoplasm and phagolysosome milieu likely energizes nutrient transport, enabled and driven by proton motive force (PMF) (64,65). The highly adapted lifestyle becomes more apparent by the cyclic generation of adenosine triphosphate (ATP). Under acidic conditions, high cellular levels of ATP are generated in the presence of glutamate (oxidative phosphorylation), a preferred substrate of C. burnetii. This ATP pool is stable at pH 7.0 and allows sustained minimal metabolic activity outside the host until reentry (10,66). Furthermore, expression of chaperones such as CbMip (peptidylprolyl isomerase) and Com-1 (disulfide oxidoreductase/isomerase), might be necessary to facilitate an appropriate folding of proteins in this reductive environment (67,68). Several studies demonstrated a reversible effect of C. burnetii replication and PV maturation in interferon-γ (IFN-γ) and tumor necrosis factor-α (TNF-α) and TNF α-treated host cells. This induced upregulation of nitrogen radical production together with the presence of oxygen radicals has a synergistic effect and contributes to the control of C. burnetii replication in the PV (53,69,70). C. burnetii posses several enzymes involved in protection and modulation of the oxidative burst. Detoxification of superoxide anions is mediated by two superoxide dismutase (SOD) enzymes, a cytoplasmically localized *Sod*A and secreted *Sod*C, distinguishable from the host enzyme. In a subsequent step, a catalase converts hydrogen peroxide to water and oxygen (71,72). Catalase activity was demonstrated for C. burnetii, but sequence analysis revealed an ORF encoding a defective enzyme. Genome annotation indicates several alkylhydroxy peroxidase genes, which may provide this catalase function. The observation that macrophage and neutrophils infected with C. burnetii fail to trigger a significant oxidative burst, lead to the identification of a C. burnetiih specific and phosphatase (ACP). As shown for the facultative intracellular microorganisms L. micdadei and Leishmania promastigotes, a reduced amount of host specific second messengers, responsible for inhibition of the oxidative burst results from the activity of parasitic expressed ACPs. The activity level of the C. burnetii ACP is significant higher as described for other microorganisms and imply a similar function for protection against the primarily host defense (73,74).

Metabolic Pathways

C. burnetii demonstrate an unusually broad spectrum of biosynthetic capabilities and can utilize sugar via the Entner–Doudoroff (glycolysis), the Embden–Meyerhof–Parnas (gluconeogenesis), the pentose-phosphate pathway, and the tricarboxylic acid cycle (TCA). Genes for the glyoxylate bypass of the TCA are absent and might explain the dependency of C. burnetii on exogenously acquired amino acids. Furthermore, several complete amino acid biosynthetic pathways or key enzymes, including lysine and tryptophan synthesis, are absent. The latter may be generated from host intermediates. Energy from ATP is generated through oxidative phosphorylation and the electron transport chain reaction. Pathways for purine and pyrimidine nucleotide metabolism, fatty acid, phospholipid, and cofactor synthesis are intact, based on sequence annotation. Isoprenoid or isopentyl diphosphate, precursor for the lipid carrier undecaprenol, involved in cell wall biosynthesis as well as menaquinones and ubiquinones involved in electron transport are synthesized via the mevalonate pathway (24).

Transport

Genome reduction, including metabolic capabilities, is a common phenomenon among obligate intracellular bacteria and reflects their increasing dependency on host factors. Development of transport mechanisms to facilitate nutrient and precursor uptake are essential under these conditions. C. burnetii possesses two proton-driven transport systems for glucose and xylose, 15 amino acid transporters, and three peptide transporters (24). Despite intact synthetic pathways for purines and pyrimidines, active uptake and incorporation of purine nucleosides were demonstrated, whereas pyrimidine uptake was passive and may rely on diffusion (75). C. burnetii maintains a cytoplasmic pH homeostasis, similar to other acidophilic bacteria for cellular processes depending on a physiological neutral pH. Three mechanosensitive ion channels, three transporters for osmoprotectants, and four sodium ion/proton exchangers are annotated, likely to provide resistance against osmotic shock and maintenance of a pH homeostasis (24). A significant portion of the cellular transporter genes are drug-efflux systems, which probably mediate resistance against host-produced defensin or antibiotics. C. burnetii lacks an ATP/adenosine diphosphate (ADP) exchanger to scavenge ATP from the host, typical for several other obligate intracellular bacteria. ATP is rarely present within the phagolysosome, and acquisition of a ATP/ADP exchanger may not be relevant for C. burnetii in this specific environment (24,75).

Developmental Life Cycle

The unusually high resistance against chemical and physical factors is one of the most impressive attributes of C. burnetii. It enables this organism to persist in the environment over extended time and remain infectious. The basis for this stability is the expression of different cell types during an incompletely characterized biphasic life cycle. C. burnetii can be separated into distinct cell forms within the phagolysosomal compartment of eukaryotic host cells and this pleomorphic nature was first described by Davis and Cox in 1938 (76). McCaul and Williams (77) formulated a developmental life cycle, which included differentiation of vegetative cells and sporogenesis. They described two cell forms of C. burnetii and established the terms small cell variant (SCV) and large cell variant (LCV), as different stages of a developmental life cycle (77). These cell types can be separated by density-gradient centrifugation and differentiated upon morphological markers. SCVs are typically 0.2 to 0.5 µm in diameter, rod shaped with electron-dense, condensed chromatin and a close network of intracytoplasmic membranes. This cell form is resistant to heat shock, pressure, sonication, osmotic shock, and oxidative stress. LCVs are larger (length exceeds 1 µm) and more pleomorphic, with a dispersed, filamentous chromatin. They show characteristics of a typical gram-negative bacterium in the exponential phase with a cytoplasmic membrane, periplasmic space, and outer membrane (15,78).

To facilitate the understanding of the developmental life cycle of C. burnetii, several attempts have been made to identify genes involved in regulation of the morphological cell differentiation within the PV. Antigenic differences between SCVs and LCVs have been demonstrated by immunoblotting, surface ionization, and two-dimensional polyacrylamide gel electrophoresis and lead to the identification of a 29-kDa outer membrane protein designated P1 (15,79). It was the first described cell variant specific protein in the literature and is highly expressed in LCVs. P1 functions as an anion-selective porin, which opens in a pH-dependent manner. The porin is predominantly open at a neutral pH of 7.4, reflecting the extracellular state. At a low pH of 4.6, similar to the phagolysosome, the porin activity changes and is mainly closed, but opens frequently. The open stage at this pH is stabilized by glutamate, a preferred carbon source of C. burnetii (80).

Gene expression profile analysis demonstrated that LCV- and SCV-specific genes, CBU0311 (P1), the alternative sigma factor *rpoS*, and *hcbA* are upregulated in an early stage after infection (81). According to previous studies, an essential role for P1 in nutrient acquisition in the acidic phagolysosome was indicated (15). In E. coli, gene regulation in response to transition from the exponential to stationary phase or under certain stress conditions is regulated by RpoS. An upregulation of RpoS in LCV and the absence of C. burnetii in SCV were previously shown and indicate that morphological differentiation may not correspond to exponential and stationary phase, instead they likely represent a specific adaption to the intra- and extracellular environment (82). Another example for differentiated gene expression is the elongation factors EF-Ts (*tsf*) and EF-Tu (*tufB*), identified as translational elements specific for LCVs. They may fulfill multiple function in promoting aminoacyl tRNA ribosome binding, transcription activation, and stress response in C. burnetii (83).

The SCV-specific gene *hcbA* encodes for Hq1, a protein similar to the histone-like protein Hc1 of *Chlamydia* (84). Hq1 is likely to play a role in formation of a condensed nucleoid during the LCV to SCV differentiation, similar to the chlamydial Hc1, which is involved in chromatin condensation during elementary body (EB) formation (85). Function of ScvA, small cell variant protein A (*scvA*), is not well understood. Because of its DNA binding activity in vitro, a structural function in chromosome stabilization or induction of topological DNA changes that alter the gene expression during the LCV to SCV differentiation was proposed (14).

Morphological differentiation of *C. burnetii* demonstrates superficial similarities to the developmental life cycles of *Chlamydia* spp. and *Legionella* spp. Both SCV and the chlamydial EB contain condensed chromatin, are less metabolically active, and are adapted for extracellular survival (86). Compared to *C. burnetii*, *L. pneumophilia* undergoes morphological differentiation within the natural amoebic host. The "cyst-like" or mature intracellular form (MIF) is comparable to the SCV, in that both cell variants appear during intracellular growth and represent a environmentally stable, infectious form (87). The described biphasic life cycle of *C. burnetii* includes two different phases, a replicative, metabolic active LCV and a dormant-like, resistant SCV, which may reflect the highly adaptive nature of these bacteria to different stages of an infection cycle.

Phase Variation
Structure of Phase I and Phase II Lipopolysaccharides

C. burnetii displays antigenic variation in a host-dependent manner. After several passages in embryonated hen eggs or cell culture, the bacterial population shifts from a virulent (phase I) to an avirulent phase (phase II), similar to the smooth to rough variation described for many Enterobacteriaceae (88,89). *C. burnetii* phase I bacteria express a smooth, full-length LPS, they are highly infective, and naturally found in infected animals, humans, and ticks. Phase variation is probably not a single-step process, as intermediate-phase or semi-rough LPS types have been described (90,91). Avirulent phase II bacteria express a truncated, rough LPS molecule and may differ in surface protein composition, surface charge, and cell density (29,92–95).

The O-antigenic polysaccharide chain is composed of a galactosaminuronyl-α-(1,6)-glucosamine disaccharide [GalU-α-(1,6)-GlcN] and the two unusual sugars, β-D-virenose (6-deoxy-3-C-methylgulose) and L-dihydroxystreptose [3-C-(hydroxymethyl)-lyxose]. The exact O-antigenic repeating unit structure is not determined but a terminal position of β-D-virenose and L-dihydroxystreptose has been assumed (96). Intrastrain heterogeneity in LPS structure and antigenicity have been described for phase I bacteria upon LPS banding pattern and, interestingly, pattern distribution correlated with acute or chronic clinical manifestation of Q fever (29). Furthermore, chemical comparison of *C. burnetii* Nine Mile and Priscilla isolate prototypes for acute and chronic disease revealed small differences in the overall composition, but noticeable differences in the O-polysaccharide side chain sugar composition and therefore existence of different *Coxiella* O-serotypes is possible (97). Semirough LPS has a sugar composition identical to phase I bacteria, except for the absence of β-D-virenose, whereas phase II bacteria demonstrate a typically rough LPS phenotype and completely lack the phase I O-polysaccharide side chain (90,91,98,99). Phase II LPS is composed of D-mannose (D-Man), D-*glycero*-D-*manno*-heptose (D,D-Hep), and 3-deoxy-α-D-*manno*-oct-2-ulopyranoside (Kdo), in the molar ratio 2:2:3, comparable to the enterobacterial inner core region. Usually the outer core is composed of a branched oligosaccharide of common pyranosidic hexoses. In *C. burnetii* phase II, a terminal D-Man residue is present at Hep II, which may indicate a mutation in the synthetic pathway for the outer core region (100,101). *C. burnetii* lipid A contains the typical β-(1,6)-linked D-glucosamine (GlcN) disaccharide backbone, phosphorylated in position 1 and 4'. Considerably different from the classical hexaacylated enterobacterial lipid A, *C. burnetii* lipid A is tetraacylated (102,103).

Activation of immune cells by LPS depends on a conserved primary lipid A structure, and variations result in a dramatic reduction of biological activity. The capability to induce cytokine production in human monocytes is significantly lower for *C. burnetii* compared to a typically enterobacterial LPS or lipid A (103). It was demonstrated that toll like receptor 4 (TLR4) plays an important role in phagocytosis, cytokine production, and granuloma formation in vivo, but is not important for *C. burnetii* infection control (104). In fact, TLR2-deficient macrophages were highly susceptible to *C. burnetii* phase II infection, and production of inflammatory cytokines was not induced (105). Additionally, *C. burnetii* lipid A demonstrated an antagonistic effect and interfered with TLR4 activation by enterobacterial LPS, comparable to the biosynthetic precursor lipid IV$_A$ (105,106). Activation and maturation of dendritic cells (DCs) in a TLR4-independent manner was only achieved by phase II infection. Full-length LPS of *C. burnetii* phase I may have a masking effect and protects the bacteria from TLR2 recognition (107). Various pathogen-associated patterns are recognized by the innate immune system, and it is likely that protection depends on a variety of TLR interactions.

Genetic Organization and Lipopolysaccharide Biosynthesis

Genetic coding for the biosynthesis of the O-polysaccharide and core oligosaccharide of the LPS molecule is normally organized in clusters of continuous genes, which can be located in distinct regions or close association on the bacterial chromosome. Lipid A biosynthesis directing genes are highly conserved among the gram-negative bacteria and usually scattered around the genome. For *C. burnetii*, two distinct regions are dedicated as O-antigen and core oligosaccharide gene cluster, at coordinates 612249-642009 and 779513-806124 (24). The O-polysaccharide gene cluster spans a region of approximately 30 kb and contains several genes for the synthesis of nucleotide diphosphate (NDP)-activated sugar precursor, glycosyltransferases, as well as genes for assembly and export of the O-specific polysaccharide. The cluster organization is limited and possible transcriptional units are interrupted by non-O-polysaccharide-associated genes. Chromosomal localization of the O-polysaccharide gene cluster is conserved among the *Enterobacteriaceae* and maps adjacent to the *his* locus. In *C. burnetii*, the *his* locus is not annotated, but interestingly, a *hisB* similar gene (CBU0673) is present within the 5′ end of the gene cluster. This unusual organization may indicate gene acquisition or genomic rearrangement events, potentially associated with two transposases located up- and downstream of the gene cluster (CBU0664 and CBU0715), respectively.

In accordance with the described O-antigen-repeating unit structure, the activated sugar precursor for formation of the GalU-α-(1,6)-GlcN disaccharide is likely provided by the housekeeping metabolite pool. Synthetic pathways for the *C. burnetii*-specific sugar β-D-virenose and L-dihydroxystreptose have not yet been described, but similar sugar residues are present in nature. The O-antigen of *Yersinia enterocolitica* O:8 contains a 6-deoxy-gulose residue, which only differs in the C3 methylation status (108). Following the proposed biosynthesis pathway in *Yersinia*, 6-deoxy-gulose may be synthesized from an NDP-hexose precursor in several steps. NDP-4-keto-6-deoxy-hexose as intermediate can be converted to 6-deoxy-gulose by reduction of the keto group and C3 or C5 epimerization, in dependence of the hexose precursor. C3 methylation may either be mediated by CBU0682, an *S*-adenosyl-L-methionine (*S*-AdoMet)-dependent methyltransferase or CBU0691, an NDP-hexose 3-*C*-methyltransferase. L-Dihydroxystreptose is known as a sugar moiety of streptomycin and synthesized by *Streptomyces griseus* as a product of the secondary metabolism. The biosynthetic pathway is well characterized and enzymes with analogous function may be present in *C. burnetii* (109).

Two genes, downstream of the dedicated O-polysaccharide cluster, CBU0703 and CBU0704, are similar to *wzm* and *wzt*, components of an ABC-(ATP-binding cassette) transporter. Synthesis of the O-polysaccharide in *C. burnetii* might be directed via an ABC-transporter-dependent pathway, typically involved in assembly of unbranched homopolymeric or structurally simple heteropolymeric O-polysaccharides, reviewed in Ref. (110). The O-polysaccharide chain is completely synthesized at the cytoplasmic face of the cytoplasmic membrane, and processive addition of glycosyl residues is catalyzed by highly specific glycosyltransferases. Two glycosyltransferases (CBU0690 and CBU0694) are annotated for *C. burnetii* within the O-polysaccharide gene cluster, and additional transferases may be necessary. Terminal modification of the O-polysaccharide chain is a common phenomenon in the ABC-transporter-dependent pathway and has been speculated to be involved in chain termination (110). Terminal position of β-D-virenose and L-dihydroxystreptose is reported for *C. burnetii* and transfer of either sugar residue may lead to chain termination and initiation of the O-polysaccharide export. Incorporation frequency may be responsible for the described antigenic heterogeneity of *C. burnetii* isolates. As shown for *Vibrio cholerae* O1, the addition of a terminal 2-*O*-methyl residues is associated with seroconversion from Ogawa to Inaba (111,112).

The dedicated region for the core oligosaccharide gene cluster spans a region of approximately 27 kb and contains genes for sugar precursor synthesis and sequential transfer of the hexose residues. Genes necessary for synthesis and transfer of Kdo and D,D-Hep are located outside the dedicated region, more or less scattered.

Phase transition of *C. burnetii* Nine Mile is accompanied with sequential loss of the O-side chain specific sugar β-D-virenose or L-dihydroxystreptose and the GalU-α-(1,6)-GlcN disaccharide. RFLP pattern comparison from *C. burnetii* phase I and phase II isolates initially demonstrated a correlation between loss of the O-antigen and a chromosomal deletion within the O-polysaccharide gene cluster (90,113). However, sequence analyses of several isolates revealed no correlation between deletion and LPS chemotype. *C. burnetii* RSA514 and the Australian strain AUST II display a semirough LPS chemotype, which lacks only the β-D-virenose residue in the O-specific chain. Interestingly, the AUST II strain harbors an intact O-antigen cluster similar to RSA514, which has a deletion of approximately 32 kb in this region. Further on, *C. burnetii* RSA439 and the European vaccine strain M44 express a rough LPS, but only RSA439 has a deletion of approximately 26 kb within the O-antigen cluster (114,115). Phase variation in Gram-negative bacteria is often shown to be a random process, caused by replication errors, which may result in frameshift mutations or early termination. Alternatively, bacterial-sensing systems, such as PmrA/PmrB and PhoP/PhoQ, are involved in alterations of the LPS molecule as response to different environmental conditions to adapt and survive in specific niches within the host (116,117). Chromosomal deletions in *C. burnetii* are not the only mechanism for phase transition, and analysis of the LPS biosynthetic pathway will contribute to understanding of this process.

GENOME

C. burnetii possesses a small circular chromosome of approximately 2 Mbp. Most isolates harbor additionally one of four previously described plasmids of 32 to 51 kb in size, which carry about 2% of the genome information. Strains without a resident plasmid carry instead a 16-kb plasmid-like sequence integrated in the chromosome (118). The genome has a G+C content of 43 mol.% and 2134 coding sequences (CDS) are predicted, of which 719 (33.7%) are hypothetical, with no significant similarity to other genes in the database (24,119). Genome reduction is a common feature for obligate intracellular bacteria and represents an adaptation process to the specific selection pressure in the occupied niche. During this process, irrelevant genes are eliminated. For *C. burnetii*, 83 pseudogenes have been identified. Many of these genes contain single frameshifts, point mutations, or truncations, which imply a recent origin and indicate that genome reduction is a relatively early, ongoing process in *C. burnetii* (24). Unlike some other intracellular bacteria, a variety of mobile genetic elements are present in the genome of *C. burnetii*. Three degenerate transposons and 29 IS elements are identified, with 21 copies of a unique IS110-related isotype IS*1111*, five IS30, and three ISAs1 family elements (24). The IS*1111* element includes an insertion sequence of approximately 1400 bp with a single transposase-like ORF, flanked by 7 bp inverted repeats. Sequence analyses of three IS*1111* elements revealed less than 2% divergence, which may indicate a recent introduction or homogenization by concerted evolution (24,120).

In cooperation with The Institute for Genome Research (TIGR) and the National Institute of Allergy and Infectious Disease (NIAID, Rocky Mountain Laboratories), genome sequencing of serven *C. burnetii* isolates is in progress (Table 1). Comparison of obtained sequence data may reveal strain-specific variations responsible for differences in virulence and pathogenicity.

Autonomous Replication Sequence

A chromosomal origin search carried out by a plasmid rescue technique led to the isolation of an autonomous replication sequence (*ars*) located on a 5.8-kb *Eco*RI fragment. The minimal region required for plasmid replication was narrowed down to a 403-bp fragment. This minimal *ars* lacks significant homology to other well-characterized origins, but resembles a chromosomal origin-like structure. Two of typically four DnaA boxes, three A+T-rich 21mers as well as potential integration host factor and factor of inversion stimulation binding sites are predicted within this region. Adjacent ORFs are similar to a 60-kDa inner membrane protein, *rnpA* and *rpmH* genes, normally located near the *oriC* in other bacteria. Despite these structural similarities and the ability to support plasmid replication in *E. coli*, no experimental evidence for chromosomal replication initiation within the *ars* was demonstrated, and function as an *oriC* in *C. burnetii* remains unclear (22,23). With identification and isolation of the *ars*, the development of stable genetic systems for manipulation of *C. burnetii* becomes possible. In first experiments, the *ars* was used as a *C. burnetii*-specific replicon for construction of a ColE1-type shuttle vector, designated as pSKO(+)1000 encoding for β-lactamase. Genetic analyses of resultant transformants revealed integrated and autonomously replicating states for the vector. Duplication of the ARS in these transformants, harboring an integrated vector, had no influence on replication fitness or viability and indicated the potential for genetic manipulation of *C. burnetii*, based on homologous recombination. The selection process was hampered by spontaneous resistant bacteria, which did not maintain plasmid DNA after long-term treatment with ampicillin (121,122). To overcome these difficulties, a green fluorescent protein expressing shuttle vector, containing the 5.8-kb *ars* fragment as an additional replicon, was generated. This new method allows a visual detection of transformants in cell culture and provides new possibilities to study pathogen–host interactions (123). Improvement of these promising techniques and development of better selection markers will lead to useful and stable genetic systems for *C. burnetii*.

DNA Repair Mechanisms

C. burnetii is likely exposed to a variety of DNA-damaging agents in the acidic environment of the phagolysosome, and maintenance of genomic stability and integrity may be a critical factor for persistence and generation of genetic diversity. DNA repair mechanisms are divided into three major categories: direct repair, excision repair, and the recombinational repair system. Direct repair is the simplest form, and the normal DNA structure is enzymatically restored without breaking the backbone. This includes the photoreactivation system (*phrAB*) and removal of methyl groups by methyltransferases. *C. burnetii* possess one gene, *phrB* of the photolyase system, and at least one methyltransferase, *ogt*, is annotated.

Excision repair involves the active removal and replacement of the damaged base or section of neighboring nucleotides. This includes nucleotide excision (NER), base excision (BER), and mismatch repair (MMR). The NER system (*unrABCD*) is completely annotated for *C. burnetii*. DNA glycosylases and endonucleases involved in BER, a DNA-3-methyladenine glycosidase (*tag*), and uracil-DNA glycosylase (*ung*), are present in *C. burnetii*. The mismatch repair system recognizes improperly paired bases and functions immediately after DNA replication. *C. burnetii* contains an incomplete MMR system: only *mutL* and *mutS* are present and, as shown for other bacteria, lack of *mutH* results in mismatch repair deficiency (124). Oxidative DNA damage, one of the major defense mechanisms of the host cell, results in formation of 7,8-dihydro-8-oxo-deoxyguanosine (8-oxodG or GO) and promotes misincorporation of adenine in the next replication round, producing a G:C→T:A mutation. The GO system prevents and repairs oxidative lesions and involves at least three genes, *mutM*, *mutY*, and *mutT*. *C. burnetii* lacks MutM, which can be complemented by MutS of the MMR system as shown for other bacteria (125).

Two major recombinational DNA repair systems are known, the *recBCD* and *recFOR* pathway, involved in gap or double-strand break repair, respectively. RecA plays a major regulatory role in these systems and in the induction of the SOS response after DNA damage. Within the PV, protection against DNA damage by host-released ROS and NOS may be essential, and surprisingly, essential components of the recombinational (*recBCD*, *recE*, *recT*) and the SOS repair system (*lexA*, *umuCD*) are not annotated for *C. burnetii*. A constitutive expression of the SOS response genes, indicated by the absence of LexA, might have a compensatory effect. Additionally, the *recFOR* pathway can complement for *recBCD*-mediated homologous recombination and this may be sufficient for maintenance of genomic stability (126).

SUMMARY AND PROSPECTS

Since the original description of Q fever by Derrick in 1937, substantial progress has been made in understanding the complex nature of *C. burnetii*. Reclassification to the order of *Legionellales* within the γ *Proteobacteria* accounts for phenotypic and genomic similarities between *C. burnetii* and *L. pneumophilia*. Both pathogens reside within a membrane-bound vacuole and undergo cellular differentiation with appearance of a highly resistant extracellular form. Most intracellular bacteria have the capability to modify specifically their intracellular environment and allow growth within a unique niche. Evidently, the type IV secretion system of *L. pneumophilia* and secreted effector molecules play a major role in alteration of the endocytic pathway. A similar role for *C. burnetii* is likely, and secreted effector molecules may be involved in delay of phagosome maturation, formation of a spacious vacuole, and for inhibition of an oxidative burst (127).

The PV resembles a secondary phagolysosome, a specific compartment of professional phagocytic cells of the innate immune system and contains several enzymes, defensin, oxygen, and nitrogen radicals for inactivation and degradation of invasive bacteria. Survival of *C. burnetii* within this destructive environment requires protective mechanisms and highly adapted physiological attributes. Genome sequencing and characterization of biological and biochemical properties of *C. burnetii* revealed a broad spectrum of metabolic capabilities and transport systems. Generation of an ATP pool to sustain minimal metabolic activity outside the host represents a biochemical stratagem for optimal adaption to the host and infection cycle. Additionally, expression of several enzymes, two SODs, alkylhydroxy peroxidase and ACP, as well as a wide variety of DNA repair systems may be sufficient for protection against host released reactive oxygen and nitrogen radicals in nonactivated phagocytic host cells.

Phase variation of *C burnetii* is accompanied by transition from a smooth to rough LPS chemotype and loss of virulence. The molecular mechanism of phase transition is not well understood and was initially correlated with a chromosomal deletion. Full-length LPS may have a shielding effect and protect phase I bacteria against TLR-dependent recognition. With identification of an autonomous replication sequence, genetic manipulation of *C. burnetii* will become available and facilitate understanding of the pathogenic nature of this organism. The TIGR and NIAID genome sequencing projects include isolates representing various genomic groups with differences in host specificity and disease outcome. Comparative genome analyses of these isolates will provide information about genetic variations and may lead to the identification of virulence specific genes.

REFERENCES

1. Derrick EH. "Q" fever, a new fever entity: clinical features, diagnosis and laboratory investigation. Med J Aust 1937; 2:281–299.
2. Maurin M, Raoult D. Q fever. Clin Microbiol Rev 1999; 12(4):518–553.
3. Baca OG, Paretsky D. Q fever and *Coxiella burnetii*: a model for host–parasite interactions. Microbiol Rev 1983; 47(2):127–149.
4. Madariaga MG, Rezai K, Trenholme GM, et al. Q fever: a biological weapon in your backyard. Lancet Infect Dis 2003; 3(11):709–721.
5. Heinzen RA, Grieshaber SS, Van Kirk LS, et al. Dynamics of actin-based movement by *Rickettsia rickettsii* in Vero cells. Infect Immun 1999; 67(8):4201–4207.
6. Heinzen RA, Scidmore MA, Rockey DD, et al. Differential interaction with endocytic and exocytic pathways distinguish parasitophorous vacuoles of *Coxiella burnetii* and *Chlamydia trachomatis*. Infect Immun 1996; 64(3):796–809.
7. Vogel JP, Isberg RR. Cell biology of *Legionella pneumophila*. Curr Opin Microbiol 1999; 2(1):30–34.
8. Fang FC. Antimicrobial reactive oxygen and nitrogen species: concepts and controversies. Nat Rev Microbiol 2004; 2(10):820–832.
9. Maurin M, Benoliel AM, Bongrand P, et al. Phagolysosomes of *Coxiella burnetii*-infected cell lines maintain an acidic pH during persistent infection. Infect Immun 1992; 60(12):5013–5016.
10. Hackstadt T, Williams JC. Biochemical stratagem for obligate parasitism of eukaryotic cells by *Coxiella burnetii*. Proc Natl Acad Sci USA 1981; 78(5):3240–3244.
11. Hendrix L, Mallavia LP. Active transport of proline by *Coxiella burnetii*. J Gen Microbiol 1984; 130(11):2857–2863.
12. Chen SY, Vodkin M, Thompson HA, et al. Isolated *Coxiella burnetii* synthesizes DNA during acid activation in the absence of host cells. J Gen Microbiol 1990; 136(1):89–96.
13. Zuerner RL, Thompson HA. Protein synthesis by intact *Coxiella burnetii* cells. J Bacteriol 1983; 156(1):186–191.

14. Heinzen RA, Hackstadt T, Samuel JE. Developmental biology of *Coxiella burnetii*. Trends Microbiol 1999; 7(4):149–154.
15. Samuel JE, Kiss K, Varghees S. Molecular pathogenesis of *Coxiella burnetii* in a genomics era. Ann NY Acad Sci 2003; 990:653–663.
16. Heinzen RA, Mallavia LP. Cloning and functional expression of the *Coxiella burnetii* citrate synthase gene in *Escherichia coli*. Infect Immun 1987; 55(4):848–855.
17. Nguyen SV, To H, Yamaguchi T, et al. Characterization of the *Coxiella burnetii* sucB gene encoding an immunogenic dihydrolipoamide succinyltransferase. Microbiol Immunol 1999; 43(8):743–749.
18. Hendrix LR, Mallavia LP, Samuel JE. Cloning and sequencing of *Coxiella burnetii* outer membrane protein gene *com1*. Infect Immun 1993; 61(2):470–477.
19. Zhang G, To H, Russell KE, et al. Identification and characterization of an immunodominant 28-kilodalton *Coxiella burnetii* outer membrane protein specific to isolates associated with acute disease. Infect Immun 2005; 73(3):1561–1567.
20. Vodkin MH, Williams JC. A heat shock operon in *Coxiella burnetii* produces a major antigen homologous to a protein in both mycobacteria and *Escherichia coli*. J Bacteriol 1988; 170(3):1227–1234.
21. Macellaro A, Tujulin E, Hjalmarsson K, et al. Identification of a 71-kilodalton surface-associated Hsp70 homologue in *Coxiella burnetii*. Infect Immun 1998; 66(12):5882–5888.
22. Chen SY, Hoover TA, Thompson HA, et al. Characterization of the origin of DNA replication of the *Coxiella burnetii* chromosome. Ann NY Acad Sci 1990; 590:491–503.
23. Suhan M, Chen SY, Thompson HA, et al. Cloning and characterization of an autonomous replication sequence from *Coxiella burnetii*. J Bacteriol 1994; 176(17):5233–5243.
24. Seshadri R, Paulsen IT, Eisen JA, et al. Complete genome sequence of the Q-fever pathogen *Coxiella burnetii*. Proc Natl Acad Sci USA 2003; 100(9):5455–5460.
25. Weiss E, Moulder JW. Order I *Rickettsiales*. In: Holt JH, ed. Bergey's Manual of Systematic Bacteriology. Vol. 1. Baltimore: The Williams and Wilkins Co., 1984:687–704.
26. Stein A, Saunders NA, Taylor AG, et al. Phylogenic homogeneity of *Coxiella burnetii* strains as determinated by 16S ribosomal RNA sequencing. FEMS Microbiol Lett 1993; 113(3):339–344.
27. Weisburg WG, Dobson ME, Samuel JE, et al. Phylogenetic diversity of the *Rickettsiae*. J Bacteriol 1989; 171(8):4202–4206.
28. Vodkin MH, Williams JC, Stephenson EH. Genetic heterogeneity among isolates of *Coxiella burnetii*. J Gen Microbiol 1986; 132(2):455–463.
29. Hackstadt T. Antigenic variation in the phase I lipopolysaccharide of *Coxiella burnetii* isolates. Infect Immun 1986; 52(1):337–340.
30. Samuel JE, Frazier ME, Mallavia LP. Correlation of plasmid type and disease caused by *Coxiella burnetii*. Infect Immun 1985; 49(3):775–779.
31. Thompson HA, Suhan ML. Genetics of *Coxiella burnetii*. FEMS Microbiol Lett 1996; 145(2):139–146.
32. Ning Z, Yu SR, Quan YG, et al. Molecular characterization of cloned variants of *Coxiella burnetii* isolated in China. Acta Virol 1992; 36(2):173–183.
33. Samuel JE, Frazier ME, Kahn ML, et al. Isolation and characterization of a plasmid from phase I *Coxiella burnetii*. Infect Immun 1983; 41(2):488–493.
34. Thiele D, Willems H, Haas M, et al. Analysis of the entire nucleotide sequence of the cryptic plasmid QpH1 from *Coxiella burnetii*. Eur J Epidemiol 1994; 10(4):413–420.
35. Lin Z, Howe D, Mallavia LP. Roa307, a protein encoded on *Coxiella burnetii* plasmid QpH1, shows homology to proteins encoded in the replication origin region of bacterial chromosomes. Mol Gen Genet 1995; 248(4):487–490.
36. Lin Z, Mallavia LP. Functional analysis of the active partition region of the *Coxiella burnetii* plasmid QpH1. J Bacteriol 1999; 181(6):1947–1952.
37. Minnick MF, Small CL, Frazier ME, et al. Analysis of the *cbhE'* plasmid gene from acute disease-causing isolates of *Coxiella burnetii*. Gene 1991; 103(1):113–118.
38. Minnick MF, Heinzen RA, Douthart R, et al. Analysis of QpRS-specific sequences from *Coxiella burnetii*. Ann NY Acad Sci 1990; 590:514–522.
39. Lautenschlager S, Willems H, Jager C, et al. Sequencing and characterization of the cryptic plasmid QpRS from *Coxiella burnetii*. Plasmid 2000; 44(1):85–88.
40. Mallavia LP, Samuel JE. Genetic diversity of *Coxiella burnetii*. In: Moulder J, ed. Intracellular Parasitism. Vol. 1. Boca Raton, FL: CRC Press, 1989:117–126.
41. Valkova D, Kazar J. A new plasmid (QpDV) common to *Coxiella burnetii* isolates associated with acute and chronic Q fever. FEMS Microbiol Lett 1995; 125(2–3):275–280.
42. Savinelli EA, Mallavia LP. Comparison of *Coxiella burnetii* plasmids to homologous chromosomal sequences present in a plasmidless endocarditis-causing isolate. Ann NY Acad Sci 1990; 590:523–533.
43. Willems H, Ritter M, Jager C, et al. Plasmid-homologous sequences in the chromosome of plasmidless *Coxiella burnetii* Scurry Q217. J Bacteriol 1997; 179(10):3293–3297.
44. Hendrix LR, Samuel JE, Mallavia LP. Differentiation of *Coxiella burnetii* isolates by analysis of restriction-endonuclease-digested DNA separated by SDS–PAGE. J Gen Microbiol 1991; 137(2):269–276.
45. Heinzen R, Stiegler GL, Whiting LL, et al. Use of pulsed field gel electrophoresis to differentiate *Coxiella burnetii* strains. Ann NY Acad Sci 1990; 590:504–513.

46. Baere PA, Samuel JE, Howe D, et al. Genetic diversity of the Q fever agent, *Coxiella burnetii*, assessed by microarray-based whole-genome comparisons. J Bacteriol 2006; 188(6):2309–2324.
47. Thiele D, Willems H, Kopf G, et al. Polymorphism in DNA restriction patterns of *Coxiella burnetii* isolates investigated by pulsed field gel electrophoresis and image analysis. Eur J Epidemiol 1993; 9(4):419–425.
48. Jager C, Willems H, Thiele D, et al. Molecular characterization of *Coxiella burnetii* isolates. Epidemiol Infect 1998; 120(2):157–164.
49. Nguyen SV, Hirai K. Differentiation of *Coxiella burnetii* isolates by sequence determination and PCR-restriction fragment length polymorphism analysis of isocitrate dehydrogenase gene. FEMS Microbiol Lett 1999; 180(2):249–254.
50. Zhang GQ, To H, Yamaguchi T, et al. Differentiation of *Coxiella burnetii* by sequence analysis of the gene (*com1*) encoding a 27-kDa outer membrane protein. Microbiol Immunol 1997; 41(11):871–877.
51. Sekeyova Z, Roux V, Raoult D. Intraspecies diversity of *Coxiella burnetii* as revealed by *com1* and *mucZ* sequence comparison. FEMS Microbiol Lett 1999; 180(1):61–67.
52. Glazunova O, Roux V, Freylikman O, et al. *Coxiella burnetii* genotyping. Emerg Infect Dis 2005; 11(8):1211–1217.
53. Brennan RE, Russell K, Zhang G, et al. Both inducible nitric oxide synthase and NADPH oxidase contribute to the control of virulent phase I *Coxiella burnetii* infections. Infect Immun 2004; 72(11):6666–6675.
54. Gimenez DF. Staining *Rickettsiae* in yolk-sac cultures. Stain Technol 1964; 39:135–140.
55. Meresse S, Steele-Mortimer O, Moreno E, et al. Controlling the maturation of pathogen-containing vacuoles: a matter of life and death. Nat Cell Biol 1999; 1(7):E183–E188.
56. Baca OG, Klassen DA, Aragon AS. Entry of *Coxiella burnetii* into host cells. Acta Virol 1993; 37(2–3):143–155.
57. Howe D, Melnicakova J, Barak I, et al. Fusogenicity of the *Coxiella burnetii* parasitophorous vacuole. Ann NY Acad Sci 2003; 990:556–562.
58. Veras PS, Moulia C, Dauguet C, et al. Entry and survival of *Leishmania amazonensis* amastigotes within phagolysosome-like vacuoles that shelter *Coxiella burnetii* in Chinese hamster ovary cells. Infect Immun 1995; 63(9):3502–3506.
59. Howe D, Mallavia LP. *Coxiella burnetii* exhibits morphological change and delays phagolysosomal fusion after internalization by J774A.1 cells. Infect Immun 2000; 68(7):3815–3821.
60. Beron W, Gutierrez MG, Rabinovitch M, et al. *Coxiella burnetii* localizes in a Rab7-labeled compartment with autophagic characteristics. Infect Immun 2002; 70(10):5816–5821.
61. Sauer JD, Shannon JG, Howe D, et al. Specificity of *Legionella pneumophila* and *Coxiella burnetii* vacuoles and versatility of *Legionella pneumophila* revealed by coinfection. Infect Immun 2005; 73(8):4494–4504.
62. Sexton JA, Vogel JP. Type IVB secretion by intracellular pathogens. Traffic 2002; 3(3):178–185.
63. Howe D, Melnicakova J, Barak I, et al. Maturation of the *Coxiella burnetii* parasitophorous vacuole requires bacterial protein synthesis but not replication. Cell Microbiol 2003; 5(7):469–480.
64. Hackstadt T, Williams JC. pH dependence of the *Coxiella burnetii* glutamate transport system. J Bacteriol 1983; 154(2):598–603.
65. Hackstadt T. Estimation of the cytoplasmic pH of *Coxiella burnetii* and effect of substrate oxidation on proton motive force. J Bacteriol 1983; 154(2):591–597.
66. Hackstadt T, Williams JC. Stability of the adenosine 5'-triphosphate pool in *Coxiella burnetii*: influence of pH and substrate. J Bacteriol 1981; 148(2):419–425.
67. Mo YY, Cianciotto NP, Mallavia LP. Molecular cloning of a *Coxiella burnetii* gene encoding a macrophage infectivity potentiator (Mip) analogue. Microbiology 1995; 141(pt 11):2861–2871.
68. Hendrix LR, Samuel JE, Mallavia LP. Identification and cloning of a 27-kDa *Coxiella burnetii* immunoreactive protein. Ann NY Acad Sci 1990; 590:534–540.
69. Zamboni DS, Rabinovitch M. Nitric oxide partially controls *Coxiella burnetii* phase II infection in mouse primary macrophages. Infect Immun 2003; 71(3):1225–1233.
70. Howe D, Barrows LF, Lindstrom NM, et al. Nitric oxide inhibits *Coxiella burnetii* replication and parasitophorous vacuole maturation. Infect Immun 2002; 70(9):5140–5147.
71. Heinzen RA, Frazier ME, Mallavia LP. *Coxiella burnetii* superoxide dismutase gene: cloning, sequencing, and expression in *Escherichia coli*. Infect Immun 1992; 60(9):3814–3823.
72. Akporiaye ET, Baca OG. Superoxide anion production and superoxide dismutase and catalase activities in *Coxiella burnetii*. J Bacteriol 1983; 154(1):520–523.
73. Baca OG, Roman MJ, Glew RH, et al. Acid phosphatase activity in *Coxiella burnetii*: a possible virulence factor. Infect Immun 1993; 61(10):4232–4239.
74. Baca OG, Li YP, Kumar H. Survival of the Q fever agent *Coxiella burnetii* in the phagolysosome. Trends Microbiol 1994; 2(12):476–480.
75. Miller JD, Thompson HA. Permeability of *Coxiella burnetii* to ribonucleosides. Microbiology 2002; 148(pt 8):2393–2403.
76. Davis GE, Cox HR. A filter-passing infectious agent isolated from ticks. I. Isolation from *Dermacentor andersonii*, reactions in animals, and filtration. Public Health Rep 1938; 53:2259–2282.

77. McCaul TF, Williams JC. Developmental cycle of *Coxiella burnetii*: structure and morphogenesis of vegetative and sporogenic differentiations. J Bacteriol 1981; 147(3):1063–1076.
78. Wiebe ME, Burton PR, Shankel DM. Isolation and characterization of two cell types of *Coxiella burnetii* phase I. J Bacteriol 1972; 110(1):368–377.
79. McCaul TF, Banerjee-Bhatnagar N, Williams JC. Antigenic differences between *Coxiella burnetii* cells revealed by postembedding immunoelectron microscopy and immunoblotting. Infect Immun 1991; 59(9):3243–3253.
80. Varghees S, Kiss K, Frans G, et al. Cloning and porin activity of the major outer membrane protein P1 from *Coxiella burnetii*. Infect Immun 2002; 70(12):6741–6750.
81. Coleman SA, Fischer ER, Howe D, et al. Temporal analysis of *Coxiella burnetii* morphological differentiation. J Bacteriol 2004; 186(21):7344–7352.
82. Seshadri R, Samuel JE. Characterization of a stress-induced alternate sigma factor, RpoS, of *Coxiella burnetii* and its expression during the development cycle. Infect Immun 2001; 69(8):4874–4883.
83. Seshadri R, Hendrix LR, Samuel JE. Differential expression of translational elements by life cycle variants of *Coxiella burnetii*. Infect Immun 1999; 67(11):6026–6033.
84. Heinzen RA, Hackstadt T. A developmental stage-specific histone H1 homolog of *Coxiella burnetii*. J Bacteriol 1996; 178(16):5049–5052.
85. Grieshaber NA, Grieshaber SS, Fischer ER, et al. A small RNA inhibits translation of the histone-like protein Hc1 in *Chlamydia trachomatis*. Mol Microbiol 2006; 59(2):541–550.
86. Abdelrahman YM, Belland RJ. The chlamydial developmental cycle. FEMS Microbiol Rev 2005; 29(5):949–959.
87. Garduno RA, Garduno E, Hiltz M, et al. Intracellular growth of *Legionella pneumophila* gives rise to a differentiated form dissimilar to stationary-phase forms. Infect Immun 2002; 70(11):6273–6283.
88. Ftacek P, Skultety L, Toman R. Phase variation of *Coxiella burnetii* strain Priscilla: influence of this phenomenon on biochemical features of its lipopolysaccharide. J Endotoxin Res 2000; 6(5):369–376.
89. Hotta A, Kawamura M, To H, et al. Phase variation analysis of *Coxiella burnetii* during serial passage in cell culture by use of monoclonal antibodies. Infect Immun 2002; 70(8):4747–4749.
90. Vodkin MH, Williams JC. Overlapping deletion in two spontaneous phase variants of *Coxiella burnetii*. J Gen Microbiol 1986; 132(9):2587–2594.
91. Amano K, Williams JC, Missler SR, et al. Structure and biological relationships of *Coxiella burnetii* lipopolysaccharides. J Biol Chem 1987; 262(10):4740–4747.
92. Hackstadt T, Peacock MG, Hitchcock PJ, et al. Lipopolysaccharide variation in *Coxiella burnetii*: intrastrain heterogeneity in structure and antigenicity. Infect Immun 1985; 48(2):359–365.
93. Moos A, Hackstadt T. Comparative virulence of intra- and interstrain lipopolysaccharide variants of *Coxiella burnetii* in the guinea pig model. Infect Immun 1987; 55(5):1144–1150.
94. Vishwanath S, Hackstadt T. Lipopolysaccharide phase variation determines the complement-mediated serum susceptibility of *Coxiella burnetii*. Infect Immun 1988; 56(1):40–44.
95. Hackstadt T. Steric hindrance of antibody binding to surface proteins of *Coxiella burnetii* by phase I lipopolysaccharide. Infect Immun 1988; 56(4):802–807.
96. Slaba K, Hussein A, Palkovic P, et al. Studies on the immunological role of virenose and dihydrohydroxystreptose present in the *Coxiella burnetii* phase I lipopolysaccharide. Ann NY Acad Sci 2003; 990:505–509.
97. Skultety L, Toman R, Pätoprsty V. A comparative study of lipopolysaccharides from two *Coxiella burnetii* strains considered to be associated with acute and chronic Q fever. Carbohydr Polym 1998; 35:189–194.
98. Amano K, Williams JC. Chemical and immunological characterization of lipopolysaccharides from phase I and phase II *Coxiella burnetii*. J Bacteriol 1984; 160(3):994–1002.
99. Toman R, Skultety L, Ftacek P, et al. NMR study of virenose and dihydrohydroxystreptose isolated from *Coxiella burnetii* phase I lipopolysaccharide. Carbohydr Res 1998; 306(1–2):291–296.
100. Toman R, Skultety L. Analysis of the 3-deoxy-D-manno-2-octulosonic acid region in a lipopolysaccharide isolated from *Coxiella burnetii* strain Nine Mile in phase II. Acta Virol 1994; 38(4):241–243.
101. Toman R, Skultety L. Structural study on a lipopolysaccharide from *Coxiella burnetii* strain Nine Mile in avirulent phase II. Carbohydr Res 1996; 283:175–185.
102. Toman R, Hussein A, Palkovic P, et al. Structural properties of lipopolysaccharides from *Coxiella burnetii* strains Henzerling and S. Ann NY Acad Sci 2003; 990:563–567.
103. Toman R, Garidel P, Andra J, et al. Physicochemical characterization of the endotoxins from *Coxiella burnetii* strain Priscilla in relation to their bioactivities. BMC Biochem 2004; 5:1.
104. Honstettre A, Ghigo E, Moynault A, et al. Lipopolysaccharide from *Coxiella burnetii* is involved in bacterial phagocytosis, filamentous actin reorganization, and inflammatory responses through Toll-like receptor 4. J Immunol 2004; 172(6):3695–3703.
105. Zamboni DS, Campos MA, Torrecilhas AC, et al. Stimulation of toll-like receptor 2 by *Coxiella burnetii* is required for macrophage production of pro-inflammatory cytokines and resistance to infection. J Biol Chem 2004; 279(52):54405–54415.
106. Golenbock DT, Hampton RY, Qureshi N, et al. Lipid A-like molecules that antagonize the effects of endotoxins on human monocytes. J Biol Chem 1991; 266(29):19490–19498.

107. Shannon JG, Howe D, Heinzen RA. Virulent *Coxiella burnetii* does not activate human dendritic cells: role of lipopolysaccharide as a shielding molecule. Proc Natl Acad Sci USA 2005; 102(24):8722–8727.
108. Zhang L, Radziejewska-Lebrecht J, Krajewska-Pietrasik D, et al. Molecular and chemical characterization of the lipopolysaccharide O-antigen and its role in the virulence of *Yersinia enterocolitica* serotype O:8. Mol Microbiol 1997; 23(1):63–76.
109. Pissowotzki K, Mansouri K, Piepersberg W. Genetics of streptomycin production in *Streptomyces griseus*: molecular structure and putative function of genes strELMB2N. Mol Gen Genet 1991; 231(1):113–123.
110. Raetz CR, Whitfield C. Lipopolysaccharide endotoxins. Annu Rev Biochem 2002; 71:635–700.
111. Ito T, Higuchi T, Hirobe M, et al. Identification of a novel sugar, 4-amino-4,6-dideoxy-2-O-methylmannose in the lipopolysaccharide of *Vibrio cholerae* O1 serotype Ogawa. Carbohydr Res 1994; 256(1):113–128.
112. Stroeher UH, Karageorgos LE, Morona R, et al. Serotype conversion in *Vibrio cholerae* O1. Proc Natl Acad Sci USA 1992; 89(7):2566–2570.
113. O'Rourke AT, Peacock M, Samuel JE, et al. Genomic analysis of phase I and II *Coxiella burnetii* with restriction endonucleases. J Gen Microbiol 1985; 131(6):1543–1546.
114. Hoover TA, Culp DW, Vodkin MH, et al. Chromosomal DNA deletions explain phenotypic characteristics of two antigenic variants, phase II and RSA 514 (crazy), of the *Coxiella burnetii* Nine Mile strain. Infect Immun 2002; 70(12):6726–6733.
115. Thompson HA, Hoover TA, Vodkin MH, et al. Do chromosomal deletions in the lipopolysaccharide biosynthetic regions explain all cases of phase variation in *Coxiella burnetii* strains? An update. Ann NY Acad Sci 2003; 990:664–670.
116. Gunn JS, Lim KB, Krueger J, et al. PmrA–PmrB-regulated genes necessary for 4-aminoarabinose lipid A modification and polymyxin resistance. Mol Microbiol 1998; 27(6):1171–1182.
117. Guo L, Lim KB, Gunn JS, et al. Regulation of lipid A modifications by *Salmonella typhimurium* virulence genes phoP–phoQ. Science 1997; 276(5310):250–253.
118. Mallavia LP. Genetics of *Rickettsiae*. Eur J Epidemiol 1991; 7(3):213–221.
119. Tyeryar FJ Jr, Weiss E, Millar DB, et al. DNA base composition of *Rickettsiae*. Science 1973; 180(84):415–417.
120. Hoover TA, Vodkin MH, Williams JC. A *Coxiella burnetii* repeated DNA element resembling a bacterial insertion sequence. J Bacteriol 1992; 174(17):5540–5548.
121. Suhan ML, Chen SY, Thompson HA. Transformation of *Coxiella burnetii* to ampicillin resistance. J Bacteriol 1996; 178(9):2701–2708.
122. Suhan ML, Thompson HA. Expression of beta-lactamase in *Coxiella burnetii* transformants. FEMS Microbiol Lett 2000; 184(2):303–306.
123. Lukacova M, Valkova D, Quevedo Diaz M, et al. Green fluorescent protein as a detection marker for *Coxiella burnetii* transformation. FEMS Microbiol Lett 1999; 175(2):255–260.
124. Lahue RS, Au KG, Modrich P. DNA mismatch correction in a defined system. Science 1989; 245(4914):160–164.
125. Wyrzykowski J, Volkert MR. The *Escherichia coli* methyl-directed mismatch repair system repairs base pairs containing oxidative lesions. J Bacteriol 2003; 185(5):1701–1704.
126. Morimatsu K, Kowalczykowski SC. RecFOR proteins load RecA protein onto gapped DNA to accelerate DNA strand exchange: a universal step of recombinational repair. Mol Cell 2003; 11(5):1337–1347.
127. Vogel JP. Turning a tiger into a house cat: using *Legionella pneumophila* to study *Coxiella burnetii*. Trends Microbiol 2004; 12(3):103–105.

19 | Immune Response to Q Fever

Jean-Louis Mege
Unité des Rickettsies, Université de la Méditerranée, Marseille, France

INTRODUCTION

Q fever is caused by *Coxiella burnetii*, an obligate intracellular bacterium phylogenetically related to *Legionellae* species and *Francisella tularensis* (1). Q fever has a wide spectrum of clinical manifestations (2). Naïve patients usually contract Q fever via aerosol (few bacteria being infective) and develop primary infection. Very few primary infections are diagnosed because more than half of patients will not show any symptoms associated with seroconversion and only 2% will develop significant disease leading to specific blood samplings and/or hospitalization. Among diagnosed and severe cases, most are middle-aged males (between 50 and 60 years). Almost always, acute Q fever resolves without specific antibiotic treatment. However, *C. burnetii* sometimes persists in seemingly cured patients (3). In special hosts, the primary infection (symptomatic or not) may evolve to a chronic infection (4). The latency between acute and chronic infection may last from months to years. Patients with valvular damage or evolutive cancer such as lymphomas and pregnant women are at high risk of evolution to chronic infection (5). The main clinical manifestation of chronic Q fever is the endocarditis (6). Among blood culture-negative infective endocarditis, 48% are associated with *C. burnetii* (7). Q fever endocarditis is characterized by fibrosis, calcification, slight inflammation and vascularization, and small or absent vegetations (8). Patients have a spontaneous evolution to death and exhibit high level of antibodies specific for *C. burnetii* (1). The combination of doxycycline and chloroquine has changed the prognosis of the disease: fewer than 5% of patients experience relapses after 18 months of therapy (9). Circulating concentrations of doxycycline and decreased titers of anti-*C. burnetii* antibodies are correlated (10). Besides the two major clinical presentations of Q fever, two new evolutive forms have been recently reported. The hyperinflammatory syndrome is associated with hepatitis and autoantibodies in middle-aged male patients; corticosteroids improve patient cure (1). Persistent asthenia lasting for months or years has been reported in some patients with acute Q fever (11). Finally, Q fever is deemed a category B biological terrorist agent (12).

IMMUNOLOGICAL OVERVIEW OF Q FEVER

In contrast to humoral response (1,13), cell-mediated immunity is protective in *C. burnetii* infection, as attested by the formation of granulomas in acute Q fever (14). When the immune response does not control infection, as exemplified in chronic Q fever or in mice with severe combined immunodeficiency, *C. burnetii* may persist and, eventually, infection leads to death (15).

Protective Immune Response in Primary Q Fever

The control of the infection in patients with primary Q fever involves systemic cell-mediated immune response and granuloma formation. The granulomatous lesions have a central open space and a fibrin ring, and are referred to as doughnut granulomas. They consist of macrophages with epithelioid morphology and of multinucleated giant cells, and are paucibacillary (16–18). A systemic cell-mediated immune response, manifesting as a marked proliferative response to *C. burnetii* antigen, is observed in patients who have convalesced from acute Q fever and patients with acute Q fever hepatitis (19). The individuals vaccinated with formalin-inactivated *C. burnetii* exhibit specific lymphoproliferation and interferon (IFN)-γ production in response to *C. burnetii* challenge (20,21). The combination of IFN-γ production and granuloma formation suggest a Th1-type polarization of immune response. Nevertheless, immune control of Q fever does not lead to *C. burnetii* eradication as animals exhibit persistent shedding of *C. burnetii* (1), and *C. burnetii* DNA is found in circulating monocytes and bone marrow several months to years after acute Q fever (3).

It is likely that factors, such as the route of infection and the inoculum size, affects the expression of *C. burnetii* infection. Indeed, the respiratory route is associated with pneumonia, and the intraperitoneal route with hepatitis in mice and guinea pigs (22). High inocula are associated with myocarditis in guinea pigs (1). Gender and age also affect the expression of *C. burnetii* infection. Men are symptomatic more often than women, with a man:woman ratio of 2.5, despite comparable exposure and seroprevalence (23,24). The predisposition for infection in men may be explained by differences in sex hormones such as 17β-estradiol. Indeed, female C56BL/6 mice have fewer granulomas and lower bacterial burden than males, and ovarectomized mice have disease rates comparable to males. The administration of 17β-estradiol prevents the effect of ovarectomy on host response and tissue burden (25). Age also appears as a risk factor for Q fever. The prevalence of clinical cases in children significantly increases with age (24). Symptomatic Q fever occurs more frequently in people over 15 years of age than in people under 15 years. We have recently found that bacterial burden and granuloma number were increased in tissues of 14-month-old mice as compared with one-month-old mice (Leone et al., submitted manuscript).

Defective Immune Response in Chronic Q Fever

C. burnetii infection may become chronic in immunocompromised hosts. Nude mice that exhibit major impairment of cell-mediated immunity can develop a chronic infection (26). Corticosteroid treatment or whole body irradiation favors the occurrence of relapses in mice previously challenged by *C. burnetii* (27). The relapses may be associated with endocarditis when mice received cyclophosphamide (28). Pregnant mice infected with *C. burnetii* experience chronic infection associated with miscarriage, premature birth, and endocarditis (29). In humans, previous valvulopathy, pregnancy, and acquired immunodeficiencies may make Q fever chronic (4,5,30,31).

Once established, chronic Q fever is characterized by defective cell-mediated immunity, thus emphasizing the major role of cell-mediated immunity in the protection against *C. burnetii*. Impaired cell-mediated immunity is characterized by a scarcity of granulomas, which are replaced by lymphocyte infiltration and necrosis foci in liver (32). Lymphocytes from patients with Q fever endocarditis do not proliferate in response to *C. burnetii* antigen, in contrast to lymphocytes from patients with acute Q fever (19). The mechanisms of this specific unresponsiveness may include alterations in T-cell subsets, but $CD4^+$ T-cell lymphopenia was observed in patients with Q fever endocarditis and in cured patients who exhibited normal immune response (33). More likely, this specific suppression is mediated by immunoregulatory mediators such as prostaglandins E2 (34) or cytokines. Interleukin (IL)-10, an immunoregulatory cytokine that is overproduced in chronic Q fever (35,36), may be involved in Q-fever-associated immunosuppression perhaps via the induction of regulatory T-cells. Finally, defective imbalance of cytokines and chemokines may result in impaired migration of immunocompetent cells to targets (36a). Indeed, *C. burnetii*-infected monocytes exhibit defective transmigration through endothelium activated by tumor necrosis factor (TNF) (37).

The immune suppression of chronic Q fever is associated with exacerbated inflammatory response. A severe inflammation is found in almost every patient with Q fever endocarditis (1). They exhibit upregulated circulating levels of TNF and IL-6, two inflammatory cytokines, type II TNF receptors (TNF-RII), and IL-1 receptor antagonist (IL-1ra). Although IL-1ra levels are significantly higher in acute Q fever than in chronic Q fever, the levels of soluble CD23, a leukocyte activation marker also known as the low-affinity receptor for immunoglobulins E, are specifically increased in chronic Q fever (38). In addition, monocyte production of TNF and IL-1β is increased in patients with Q fever endocarditis, whereas it remains low in patients with uncomplicated acute Q fever (39,40). TNF production is related to disease activity. First, the production of TNF is higher in patients with Q fever recently diagnosed than in those monitored for more than 12 months and in cured patients. Second, the greatest increase in TNF production is observed in patients with the highest titers of immunoglobulins G directed against *C. burnetii* (39). The production of the chemokines RANTES (Regulated upon Activation, Normal T-cell Expressed and Secreted, CCL5) and MCP-1 (Monocyte Chemoattractant Protein-1, CCL2) is increased in monocytes from patients with Q fever endocarditis (40a). IL-6 production is high in both acute and chronic Q fever (38), which agrees with the overproduction of IL-6 reported in patients with post-Q fever fatigue syndrome (41). Clearly, immunosuppression and exacerbated inflammation are associated with chronic Q fever.

INNATE IMMUNE SYSTEM IN Q FEVER
Macrophages, the Critical Host Cells for *Coxiella burnetii*

C. burnetii is an obligate intracellular microorganism that lives in vivo in cells of the myeloid lineage. Its survival in the hostile environment of macrophages requires subversion of their microbicidal functions, including phagocytosis, intracellular trafficking, and killing activities.

Phagocytosis of Coxiella burnetii

C. burnetii has developed a strategy of phagocytosis subversion not previously observed in other intracellular organisms (42). In human monocytes, *C. burnetii* organisms are poorly internalized but they survive successfully, whereas avirulent variants of *C. burnetii* are efficiently phagocytosed but are rapidly eliminated. The phagocytosis of virulent *C. burnetii* requires the engagement of $\alpha v \beta 3$ integrin and that of avirulent variants of *C. burnetii* is mediated by $\alpha v \beta 3$ integrin and CR3 ($\alpha M \beta 2$ integrin, CD11b/CD18). As the efficiency of CR3-mediated phagocytosis depends on CR3 activation via $\alpha v \beta 3$ integrin, the low phagocytic efficiency observed with virulent *C. burnetii* results from the interference with integrin cross-talk. Indeed, pretreatment of monocytes with virulent organisms prevents CR3-mediated phagocytosis and CR3 activation. The uncoupling of $\alpha v \beta 3$ integrin from CR3 results from inappropriate activation of macrophages and is characterized by reorganization of actin cytoskeleton and activation of protein tyrosine kinase (PTK) pathway. Virulent *C. burnetii* organisms stimulate the formation of pseudopodal extensions and transient reorganization of filamentous actin (F-actin), whereas avirulent variants have no effect (43). F-actin reorganization is due to PTK activation. Indeed, virulent *C. burnetii* induce early PTK activity and tyrosine phosphorylation of three main endogenous substrates including src-related PTK. Tyrosine kinase activity is found in cytoskeleton fraction of stimulated cells and tyrosine phosphoproteins colocalize with F-actin inside the protrusions. Finally, specific inhibitors of src-related kinases prevent *C. burnetii*-stimulated reorganization of cytoskeleton (44). Pseudopodal extensions play an apparently complex role in the internalization of *C. burnetii*. On one hand, they are associated with phagocytosis impairment, as described in pedestal formation in macrophages stimulated by enteropathogenic *Escherichia coli* (45). On the other hand, they are required for *C. burnetii* entry because only virulent organisms are found in close apposition with F-actin protrusions (43). We also showed that CR3 molecules remain outside the peudopodal extensions induced by *C. burnetii* in monocytes, whereas $\alpha v \beta 3$ integrin molecules are present in pseudopods. When CR3 is allowed to localize with $\alpha v \beta 3$ integrin in pseudopodal extensions, for instance, after monocyte stimulation by RANTES, *C. burnetii* phagocytosis is increased in a CR3-dependent manner. Hence, the localization of phagocytosis receptors controls *C. burnetii* uptake and its intracellular fate (46).

Intracellular Traffic of Coxiella burnetii

The adaptation of internalized *C. burnetii* to acidic environment has so far been considered as a prerequisite for its survival and multiplication in contrast to other bacteria, which rather subvert phagosome maturation (47,48). The adaptation of *C. burnetii* to intracellular life is linked with acidic pH of its phagosome. Acidic pH allows the entry of nutrients necessary for *C. burnetii* metabolism (49), and also protects bacteria from antibiotics by altering their activity.

Hence, when lysosomotropic agents such as chloroquine, known to alkalinize the phagosomal compartment, are combined with doxycycline, the microbicidal activity of macrophages toward *C. burnetii* is increased (50). As *C. burnetii* lives in an acidic compartment, it has been supposed that this compartment is a phagolysosome. In murine macrophage cell lines and nonphagocytic cells, *C. burnetii* multiplies within a large vacuole that fuses with lysosomes (51). These vacuoles are able to fuse with other intracellular vacuoles containing yeasts (52) or *Mycobacterium avium* (53). In nonphagocytic cells such as Vero cells or HeLa cells, *C. burnetii*-containing vacuoles fulfill the criteria of mature phagolysosomes, including the sequestration of fluid-phase markers, the expression of proton ATPase, lysosome-associated membrane proteins (LAMP)-1 and -2, and lysosomal enzymes such as cathepsin D and acid phosphatase (54). They also accumulate two molecules of the major histocompatibility complex, HLA-DR and HLA-DM. Their interaction with bacterial vacuoles may delay presentation of antigenic peptides by affecting the efficiency of peptide loading (55). As these studies used avirulent variants of *C. burnetii*, they cannot highlight the survival mechanism of virulent organisms in macrophages, the natural hosts of *C. burnetii*. For example, the replication of virulent *C. burnetii* is limited to a few murine macrophage cell lines such as P388D1 or J774-1 while avirulent variants are able to proliferate in a large number of cells (56). In addition, virulent organisms survive in human macrophages, whereas avirulent variants are eliminated (42).

This finding prompted us to revisit the paradigm of *C. burnetii* survival (57). Both virulent and avirulent organisms are present in acidic phagosomes, confirming the previous reports in nonphagocytic cells. Hence, the survival of *C. burnetii* in human macrophages does not depend on vacuolar pH. We have found that the maturation of phagosomes containing virulent *C. burnetii* is impaired. Virulent organisms are present in phagosomes that express endosomal markers such as mannose-6-phosphate receptor, LAMP-1, and proton ATPase, but they do not acquire a lysosomal marker such as cathepsin D. Avirulent variants, which are eliminated, are present in mature phagosomes that colocalize with cathepsin D, in agreement with findings in nonphagocytic cells. These findings suggest that the survival of *C. burnetii* in human macrophages is based on the control of phagocytosis and the prevention of ultimate phagosome–lysosome (PL) fusion. We next extended these findings to Q fever. Monocytes from patients with chronic Q fever in evolution, who do not control the infection, exhibit defective phagosome maturation and impaired *C. burnetii* killing. In contrast, both responses are stimulated in patients recovering from Q fever, who exhibit Th1 immune response. Defective phagosome maturation is induced by exogenous IL-10 in monocytes from patients with microbicidal competence, and is corrected by IL-10 neutralization in patients with chronic Q fever (58). Hence, phagosome maturation and *C. burnetii* killing are linked in Q fever and are controlled by cytokines.

The analysis of *C. burnetii* genome provides several candidates able to control phagosome maturation in macrophages. Indeed, a type IV secretion system has been identified in both *L. pneumophila* and *C. burnetii* with similar genetic organization. It may be involved in bacterial growth (59,60), as emphasized by host cell cocultures in which *L. pneumophila*-containing vacuoles are associated with *C. burnetii*-containing vacuoles (61). A family of phagosomal transporters has been recently identified in three related pathogens, *L. pneumophila*, *F. tularensis*, and *C. burnetii*. These transporters may be involved in phagosomal nutrient supply (62).

Toll-Like Receptors, Sensors of Coxiella burnetii
Toll-like receptors (TLRs) play a critical role in both innate resistance and initiation of adaptive immunity to infectious pathogens (63). They recognize conserved molecular structures on microbes, and multiple TLRs determine pathogen control (64). The recognition of *C. burnetii* by immune cells requires at least two TLRs, TLR4, and TLR2. The presence of lipopolysaccharide (LPS) on *C. burnetii*, a Gram-negative bacterium, as major virulence factor suggests a role for TLR4, the sensor of LPS, in bacterial recognition. The phagocytosis of *C. burnetii* partly depends on TLR4 and LPS (65). It is likely that the engagement of TLR4 by LPS provides an activating signal for $\alpha v \beta 3$ integrin. The interaction of *C. burnetii* with macrophages results in the reorganization of actin cytoskeleton that largely depends on TLR4. Indeed, *C. burnetii*-stimulated formation of filopods and ruffles is prevented in the absence of TLR4. Once internalized, the fate of *C. burnetii* (phagosome maturation and microbicidal activity) is similar in macrophages from

wild type and TLR4-deficient mice (65), demonstrating that TLR4 is involved in initial macrophage responses to infection. It is noteworthy that in vitro responses of macrophages to avirulent variants of *C. burnetii* were independent of TLR4.

We also studied the role of TLR4 in tissue infection and granuloma formation using TLR4-deficient mice infected with *C. burnetii* (65). The pattern of tissue infection and the clearance of *C. burnetii* are similar in wt- and TLR4-deficient mice. In contrast, the formation of granulomas and the production of cytokines (TNF, IFN-γ) are impaired in TLR4-deficient mice. Hence, TLR4 controls inflammatory response and its organization into granulomas, but not microbicidal competence (65), suggesting that other factors are needed to acquire microbicidal competence.

TLR2, known to recognize peptidoglycan and lipopeptides, is also involved in *C. burnetii* infection. Using cell lines expressing TLR2, macrophages from TLR2-deficient mice, and avirulent variants of *C. burnetii*, Zamboni et al. (66) showed that TLR2 is involved in TNF and IFN-γ production. Macrophages from TLR2-deficient mice are highly permissive for the intracellular growth of avirulent *C. burnetii*. In vivo experiments showed that TLR2 is also involved in granuloma formation as do TLR4 (67). It is likely that other TLR-related receptors are involved in the response to *C. burnetii* as reported for other infectious pathogens.

Dendritic Cells

Dendritic cells (DCs) are central in mediating both the initiation of antimicrobial immunity and the maintenance of tolerance to self. Immature DCs are present in peripheral tissues and exhibit high capacity of bacterial uptake; once activated, they migrate to lymph nodes to differentiate into mature DCs that support adaptive immune response (68). Among DC subsets, monocyte-derived DCs represent the main cell subset supporting antimicrobial immunity against intracellular bacteria (69). It has been recently demonstrated that myeloid DCs can be infected by *C. burnetii*. DCs likely constitute a protective niche for *C. burnetii* as organisms replicate within DCs (70). In addition, *C. burnetii* is unable to stimulate the maturation of DCs, as assessed by expression of costimulation receptors, and is a poor stimulator of IL-12 production. In contrast, avirulent variants of *C. burnetii*, which are eliminated by host immune response, stimulate DC maturation and IL-12 production. Such findings suggest that defective immune response to *C. burnetii* may be due to the ability of *C. burnetii* to block DC1 program and, consequently, Th1 response. Further work would be necessary to demonstrate that immune deficiency of Q fever results from impaired response of myeloid DCs.

CYTOKINE NETWORK AND *COXIELLA BURNETII* DEATH OR REPLICATION

The resolution of infectious diseases requires Th1 immune response that is based on the production of microbicidal cytokines such as IFN-γ. In contrast, the chronic evolution of infectious diseases is based on Th2 immune response or the dampering of Th1 immune response by immunoregulatory cytokines such as IL-10. It is likely that acute Q fever, which is spontaneously resolutive, is controlled by Th1 immune response, whereas chronic Q fever is related to reorientation of immune response toward Th2-type pattern or to its control by IL-10.

Interferon Gamma

IFN-γ is produced in acute Q fever, but its production seems defective in chronic Q fever. IFN-γ is a powerful cytokine able to induce microbicidal competence in macrophages through oxygen-dependent and -independent mechanisms (71). IFN-γ mediates *C. burnetii* killing by monocytes and macrophages (72).

The microbicidal mechanism of IFN-γ directed against *C. burnetii* does not depend on the production of reactive oxygen intermediates (ROIs). Although *C. burnetii* has developed specific strategies to scavenge ROIs (73) and to prevent ROI production (74,75), it is likely that ROIs do not play a protective role against *C. burnetii*. First, *C. burnetii* does not stimulate the release of superoxide anion and hydrogen peroxide by monocytes (72), emphasizing previous results obtained in neutrophils (76). Second, the survival of *C. burnetii* is similar in control monocytes and in monocytes from patients with chronic granulomatous disease, in which

NADPH oxidase complex is not functional (72). The conclusions concerning the role of reactive nitrogen intermediates are less clear. *C. burnetii* induces the production of nitric oxide (NO) by murine alveolar macrophages, but inhibitors of NO production do not modify the infection rate of macrophages (77). IFN-γ controls *C. burnetii* infection despite the absence of NO synthase in one report (78) and less efficiently in another report (79). In THP-1 cells, *C. burnetii* does not induce NO production, even in the presence of IFN-γ, and L-arginine inhibitors have no effect on the survival of *C. burnetii* (72).

IFN-γ stimulates the microbicidal program directed against *C. burnetii* through an oxygen-independent mechanism. IFN-γ restores PL fusion when it is added to monocytes before or after their infection (57). It is likely that this mechanism accounts for the restoration of PL fusion in monocytes from patients with acute Q fever (58). When IFN-γ is added to infected monocytes, it has no effect on phagosomal pH, whereas its addition to monocytes before their infection results in phagosome alkalinization (57). Hence, in a context of Th1-like type of immune response as found in acute Q fever, changing vacuolar pH may have some therapeutical consequences. The antibiotics, even used in combination for prolonged periods, do not have bactericidal activity against *C. burnetii*. The combination of doxycycline and chloroquine, which promotes vacuolar alkalinization, induces in vitro bactericidal activity against *C. burnetii* (1). The ability of IFN-γ to induce killing of *C. burnetii*, by modulating iron metabolism and PL fusion, may complete the action of doxycycline and chloroquine.

The survival of obligate intracellular organisms requires the prevention of the death of host cells (80,81), and additional signals are needed to induce cell apoptosis and bacterial killing. IFN-γ is able to promote the apoptosis of *C. burnetii*-infected macrophages. The apoptotic effect of IFN-γ on *C. burnetii*-infected cells depends on TNF. Indeed, IFN-γ upregulates TNF production and induces the expression of membrane TNF. Neutralizing TNF with specific antibodies prevents both macrophage apoptosis and *C. burnetii* killing (72). Concomitantly, IFN-γ induces homotypic adherence of *C. burnetii*-infected macrophages, which depends on β2 integrins and CD54. When adherence is disrupted by mechanical dissociation or blocking integrin receptors, both cell apoptosis and bacterial killing induced by IFN-γ are inhibited (82). These findings may help to understand the mechanisms of granuloma formation in acute Q fever. A contrario, decreased IFN-γ production may impair the aggregation and the microbicidal activity of monocytes as found in chronic Q fever.

Finally, IFN-γ may control *C. burnetii* infection by mechanisms such as cytokine production and/or regulation of nutrient supply. *C. burnetii*-infected monocytes stimulated by IFN-γ release high amounts of TNF (72). Besides its role in apoptosis, TNF may contribute to microbicidal activity of macrophages. It affects the phagocytosis step but not the later steps of microbicidal process. Indeed, neutralizing anti-TNF antibodies decrease *C. burnetii* internalization by monocytes from patients with Q fever endocarditis but they do not affect the long-term survival of bacteria (40). As described for other intracellular organisms, the prevention of production and/or activity of inflammatory cytokines may be considered as a subversion strategy. Virulent *C. burnetii* organisms are less efficient than avirulent organisms in inducing the synthesis and the release of TNF by human monocytes. This limited efficiency is not the consequence of poor activity of LPS because purified LPS from virulent organisms is more potent than LPS from avirulent organisms at stimulating TNF release (83). In fact, virulent organisms, which poorly bind to monocytes, would present fewer LPS molecules to target cells than would avirulent bacteria, which efficiently bind to monocytes (83). In addition, IFN-γ controls iron metabolism in macrophages through the down-modulation of transferrin receptors, resulting in decreased assimilation of iron (84). *C. burnetii* upregulates the expression of transferrin receptors in murine macrophage cell lines, which results in increased cell iron content and bacterial burden. The intracellular iron chelator, desferoxamine, suppresses the replication of *C. burnetii* (85). It remains to determine whether IFN-γ-mediated killing of *C. burnetii* involves decreased iron content.

Macrophage-Deactivating Cytokines

IL-10 shares with IL-4, IL-13, and transforming growth factor (TGF)-β the ability to down-modulate microbicidal activity of macrophages, and it has been associated with increased susceptibility to intracellular organisms (86,87). It is likely that IL-10 is involved in the chronic evolution of patients with acute Q fever and the inefficient immune response found in patients with chronic Q fever. First, IL-10 is produced by mononuclear cells from patients with Q fever endocarditis and patients with Q fever and valvulopathy who had a risk of chronic evolution (35,36). Second, IL-10, but not IL-4 and TGF-β1, induces *C. burnetii* replication in monocytes. IL-10 acts through the down-modulation of TNF production because TNF restores the microbicidal activity towards *C. burnetii* in IL-10-treated monocytes (88). IL-10 also upregulates TNF-RII release. In chronic Q fever, the expression of TNF-RII on monocytes and their release are increased. It is likely that soluble TNF-RII interferes with TNF-stimulated microbicidal activity of monocytes, thus sustaining bacterial replication. Third, IL-10 is related to microbicidal defect of chronic Q fever. Indeed, *C. burnetii* is eliminated in monocytes from patients with acute Q fever and low IL-10 production, whereas it replicates in monocytes from patients with chronic Q fever and high IL-10 production. Microbicidal activity of monocytes from patients with Q fever endocarditis is restored by neutralizing IL-10 (88). As the fusion of *C. burnetii*-containing phagosomes with lysosomes is a key component of the microbicidal activity of monocytes (57), we have studied the colocalization of *C. burnetii* with cathepsin D, a marker of PL fusion, in monocytes from patients with chronic Q fever. PL fusion is impaired in these patients compared to patients with acute Q fever, and the neutralization of endogenous IL-10 restores PL fusion (58). Fourth, IL-10 seems to be involved in the migration of immune cells to peripheral tissues. Indeed, the transendothelial migration of mononuclear cells is defective in patients with Q fever endocarditis and this defect is corrected by neutralizing IL-10 (36a). Defective transendothelial migration of mononuclear cells partly accounts for defective granuloma formation. Indeed, using mice overexpressing IL-10 in myeloid compartment reveals two major features of chronic Q fever: lack of granulomas and tissue persistence of *C. burnetii* (manuscript in preparation). Finally, it is likely that IL-10 plays a complex role in the interplay between mammalian host and *C. burnetii*. For instance, the CD28 deficiency decreases *C. burnetii* burden in the infected tissues and impairs the production of IL-10 by peritoneal macrophages, suggesting that IL-10 does not exert an univocal role on *C. burnetii* infection (89).

CONCLUSIONS

The pathophysiology of Q fever depends on the ability of *C. burnetii* to survive and replicate in human macrophages. This condition is obtained when deactivating cytokines such as IL-10 are produced. Situations like pregnancy, in which the success of fetal allograft depends on deactivating cytokines, favor disease reactivation or chronic evolution of Q fever. In contrast, resting monocytes create the conditions for *C. burnetii* survival without replication, which depends on limitation of bacterial phagocytosis, impairment of PL fusion, and modulation of inflammatory cytokine production. This strategy for escaping death may account for *C. burnetii* persistence in macrophages but should not interfere with the development of cell-mediated immune response as observed in acute Q fever. The consequence of specific cell-mediated immunity is the production of IFN-γ, which is responsible for the killing of *C. burnetii* through the restoration of PL fusion, the stimulation of TNF production, and the apoptosis of infected cells. When the production of IFN-γ is impaired, the killing step cannot occur, leading to bacterial persistence and/or replication. The role of other immune effectors such as DCs and regulatory T-cells will probably open new perspectives in understanding Q fever pathophysiology.

REFERENCES

1. Maurin M, Raoult D. Q fever. Clin Microbiol Rev 1999; 12(4):518–553.
2. Raoult D, Marrie T, Mege JL. Natural history and pathophysiology of Q fever. Lancet Infect Dis 2005; 5(4):219–226.
3. Harris RJ, Storm PA, Lloyd A, et al. Long-term persistence of *Coxiella burnetii* in the host after primary Q fever. Epidemiol Infect 2000; 124(3):543–549.
4. Raoult D. Host factors in the severity of Q fever. Ann NY Acad Sci 1990; 590:33–38.
5. Fenollar F, Fournier PE, Carrieri MP, et al. Risks factors and prevention of Q fever endocarditis. Clin Infect Dis 2001; 33(3):312–316.
6. Brouqui P, Dupont HT, Drancourt M, et al. Chronic Q fever: ninety-two cases from France, including 27 cases without endocarditis. Arch Intern Med 1993; 153(5):642–648.

7. Houpikian P, Raoult D. Blood culture-negative endocarditis in a reference center: etiologic diagnosis of 348 cases. Medicine (Baltimore) 2005; 84(3):162–173.
8. Lepidi H, Houpikian P, Liang Z, et al. Cardiac valves in patients with Q fever endocarditis: microbiological, molecular, and histologic studies. J Infect Dis 2003; 187(7):1097–1106.
9. Houpikian P, Habib G, Mesana T, et al. Changing clinical presentation of Q fever endocarditis. Clin Infect Dis 2002; 34(5):E28–E31.
10. Rolain JM, Mallet MN, Raoult D. Correlation between serum doxycycline concentrations and serologic evolution in patients with *Coxiella burnetii* endocarditis. J Infect Dis 2003; 188(9):1322–1325.
11. Raoult D, Mege JL, Marrie TJ. Q fever: queries remaining after decades of research. In: Scheld WM, Craig WA, Hughes JM, eds. Emerging Infections. Washington, DC: ASM Press, 2001:29–56.
12. Madariaga MG, Rezai K, Trenholme GM, et al. Q fever: a biological weapon in your backyard. Lancet Infect Dis 2003; 3(11):709–721.
13. Kishimoto RA, Burger GT. Appearance of cellular and humoral immunity in guinea pigs after infection with *Coxiella burnetii* administered in small-particle aerosols. Infect Immun 1977; 16(2):518–521.
14. Ascher MS, Williams JC, Berman MA. Dermal granulomatous hypersensitivity in Q fever: comparative studies of the granulomatous potential of whole cells of *Coxiella burnetii* phase I and subfractions. Infect Immun 1983; 42(3):887–889.
15. Andoh M, Naganawa T, Hotta A, et al. SCID mouse model for lethal Q fever. Infect Immun 2003; 71(8):4717–4723.
16. Pellegrin M, Delsol G, Auvergnat JC, et al. Granulomatous hepatitis in Q fever. Hum Pathol 1980; 11(1):51–57.
17. Srigley JR, Vellend H, Palmer N, et al. Q-fever: the liver and bone marrow pathology. Am J Surg Pathol 1985; 9(10):752–758.
18. Voigt JJ, Delsol G, Fabre J. Liver and bone marrow granulomas in Q fever. Gastroenterology 1983; 84(4):887–888.
19. Koster FT, Williams JC, Goodwin JS. Cellular immunity in Q fever: specific lymphocyte unresponsiveness in Q fever endocarditis. J Infect Dis 1985; 152(6):1283–1289.
20. Izzo AA, Marmion BP, Worswick DA. Markers of cell-mediated immunity after vaccination with an inactivated, whole-cell Q fever vaccine. J Infect Dis 1988; 157(4):781–789.
21. Izzo AA, Marmion BP. Variation in interferon-gamma responses to *Coxiella burnetii* antigens with lymphocytes from vaccinated or naturally infected subjects. Clin Exp Immunol 1993; 94(3):507–515.
22. Marrie TJ, Stein A, Janigan D, et al. Route of infection determines the clinical manifestations of acute Q fever. J Infect Dis 1996; 173(2):484–487.
23. Tissot Dupont H, Raoult D, Brouqui P, et al. Epidemiologic features and clinical presentation of acute Q fever in hospitalized patients: 323 French cases. Am J Med 1992; 93(4):427–434.
24. Maltezou HC, Raoult D. Q fever in children. Lancet Infect Dis 2002; 2(11):686–691.
25. Leone M, Honstettre A, Lepidi H, et al. Effect of sex on *Coxiella burnetii* infection: protective role of 17β-estradiol. J Infect Dis 2004; 189(2):339–345.
26. Kishimoto RA, Rozmiarek H, Larson EW. Experimental Q fever infection in congenitally athymic nude mice. Infect Immun 1978; 22(1):69–71.
27. Sidwell RW, Thorpe BD, Gebhardt LP. Studies of latent Q fever infections. II. Effects of multiple cortisone injections. Am J Hyg 1964; 79:320–327.
28. Atzpodien E, Baumgartner W, Artelt A, et al. Valvular endocarditis occurs as a part of a disseminated *Coxiella burnetii* infection in immunocompromised BALB/cJ (H-2d) mice infected with the Nine Mile isolate of *C. burnetii*. J Infect Dis 1994; 170(1):223–226.
29. Stein A, Lepidi H, Mege JL, et al. Repeated pregnancies in BALB/c mice infected with *Coxiella burnetii* cause disseminated infection, resulting in stillbirth and endocarditis. J Infect Dis 2000; 181(1):188–194.
30. Raoult D, Tissot-Dupont H, Foucault C, et al. Q fever 1985–1998: clinical and epidemiologic features of 1,383 infections. Medicine (Baltimore) 2000; 79(2):109–123.
31. Stein A, Raoult D. Q fever during pregnancy: a public health problem in southern France. Clin Infect Dis 1998; 27(3):592–596.
32. Raoult D, Raza A, Marrie TJ. Q fever endocarditis and other forms of chronic Q fever. In: Marrie TJ, ed. Q Fever: The Disease. Vol. 1. Boca Raton, FL: CRC Press, 1990:3784–3786.
33. Sabatier F, Dignat-George F, Mege JL, et al. CD4+ T-cell lymphopenia in Q fever endocarditis. Clin Diagn Lab Immunol 1997; 4(1):89–92.
34. Koster FT, Williams JC, Goodwin JS. Cellular immunity in Q fever: modulation of responsiveness by a suppressor T cell-monocyte circuit. J Immunol 1985; 135(2):1067–1072.
35. Capo C, Zaffran Y, Zugun F, et al. Production of interleukin-10 and transforming growth factor beta by peripheral blood mononuclear cells in Q fever endocarditis. Infect Immun 1996; 64(10):4143–4147.
36. Honstettre A, Imbert G, Ghigo E, et al. Dysregulation of cytokines in acute Q fever: role of interleukin-10 and tumor necrosis factor in chronic evolution of Q fever. J Infect Dis 2003; 187(6):956–962.
36a. Meghari S, Capo C, Raoult D, et al. Deficient transendotheliel migration of leukocytes in Q fever: the role played by interleukin-10. J Infect Dis 2006; 194(3):365–369.
37. Dellacasagrande J, Moulin PA, Guilianelli C, et al. Reduced transendothelial migration of monocytes infected by *Coxiella burnetii*. Infect Immun 2000; 68(6):3784–3786.

38. Capo C, Amirayan N, Ghigo E, et al. Circulating cytokine balance and activation markers of leucocytes in Q fever. Clin Exp Immunol 1999; 115(1):120–123.
39. Capo C, Zugun F, Stein A, et al. Upregulation of tumor necrosis factor alpha and interleukin-1 beta in Q fever endocarditis. Infect Immun 1996; 64(5):1638–1642.
40. Dellacasagrande J, Ghigo E, Capo C, et al. *Coxiella burnetii* survives in monocytes from patients with Q fever endocarditis: involvement of tumor necrosis factor. Infect Immun 2000; 68(1):160–164.
40a. Meghari S, Desnues B, Capo C, Grau GE, Raoult D, Mege JL. *Coxiella burnetii* stimulates production of RANTES and MCP-1 by mononuclear cells: modulation by adhesion to endothelial cells and its implication in Q fever. Eur Cytokine Netw 2006; 17:1–7.
41. Penttila IA, Harris RJ, Storm P, et al. Cytokine dysregulation in the post-Q-fever fatigue syndrome. Q J Med 1998; 91(8):549–560.
42. Capo C, Lindberg FP, Meconi S, et al. Subversion of monocyte functions by *Coxiella burnetii*: impairment of the cross-talk between $\alpha v \beta 3$ integrin and CR3. J Immunol 1999; 163(11):6078–6085.
43. Meconi S, Jacomo V, Boquet P, et al. *Coxiella burnetii* induces reorganization of the actin cytoskeleton in human monocytes. Infect Immun 1998; 66(11):5527–5533.
44. Meconi S, Capo C, Remacle-Bonnet M, et al. Activation of protein tyrosine kinases by *Coxiella burnetii*: role in actin cytoskeleton reorganization and bacterial phagocytosis. Infect Immun 2001; 69(4):2520–2526.
45. Goosney DL, Gruenheid S, Finaly BB. Gut feelings: enteropathogenic *E. coli* (EPEC) interactions with the host. Annu Rev Cell Dev Biol 2000; 16:173–189.
46. Capo C, Moynault A, Collette Y, et al. *Coxiella burnetii* avoids macrophage phagocytosis by interfering with spatial distribution of complement receptor 3. J Immunol 2003; 170(8):4217–4225.
47. Baca OG, Paretsky D. Q fever and *Coxiella burnetii*: a model for host–parasite interactions. Microbiol Rev 1983; 47(2):127–149.
48. Russell DG. Where to stay inside the cell: a homesteader's guide to intracellular parsitism. In: Cossart P, Normark S, Rappuoli R, eds. Cellular Microbiology. Washington, DC: ASM Press, 2000:131–152.
49. Hackstadt T, Williams JC. Biochemical stratagem for obligate parasitism of eukaryotic cells by *Coxiella burnetii*. Proc Natl Acad Sci USA 1981; 78(5):3240–3244.
50. Maurin M, Benoliel AM, Bongrand P, et al. Phagolysosomal alkalinization and the bactericidal effect of antibiotics: the *Coxiella burnetii* paradigm. J Infect Dis 1992; 166(5):1097–1102.
51. Akporiaye ET, Rowatt JD, Aragon AA, et al. Lysosomal response of a murine macrophage-like cell line persistently infected with *Coxiella burnetii*. Infect Immun 1983; 40(3):1155–1162.
52. Veras PS, de Chastellier C, Moreau MF, et al. Fusion between large phagocytic vesicles: targeting of yeast and other particulates to phagolysosomes that shelter the bacterium *Coxiella burnetii* or the protozoan *Leishmania amazonensis* in Chinese hamster ovary cells. J Cell Sci 1994; 107(11):3065–3076.
53. de Chastellier C, Thibon M, Rabinovitch M. Construction of chimeric phagosomes that shelter *Mycobacterium avium* and *Coxiella burnetii* (phase II) in doubly infected mouse macrophages: an ultrastructural study. Eur J Cell Biol 1999; 78(8):580–592.
54. Heinzen RA, Scidmore MA, Rockey DD, et al. Differential interaction with endocytic and exocytic pathways distinguish parasitophorous vacuoles of *Coxiella burnetii* and *Chlamydia trachomatis*. Infect Immun 1996; 64(3):796–809.
55. Lem L, Riethof DA, Scidmore-Carlson M, et al. Enhanced interaction of HLA-DM with HLA-DR in enlarged vacuoles of hereditary and infectious lysosomal diseases. J Immunol 1999; 162(1):523–532.
56. Baca OG, Akporiaye ET, Aragon AS, et al. Fate of phase I and phase II *Coxiella burnetii* in several macrophage-like tumor cell lines. Infect Immun 1981; 33(1):258–266.
57. Ghigo E, Capo C, Tung CH, et al. *Coxiella burnetii* survival in THP-1 monocytes involves the impairment of phagosome maturation: IFN-γ mediates its restoration and bacterial killing. J Immunol 2002; 169(8):4488–4495.
58. Ghigo E, Honstettre A, Capo C, et al. Link between impaired maturation of phagosomes and defective *Coxiella burnetii* killing in patients with chronic Q fever. J Infect Dis 2004; 190(10):1767–1772.
59. Feldman M, Zusman T, Hagag S, et al. Coevolution between nonhomologous but functionally similar proteins and their conserved partners in the *Legionella* pathogenesis system. Proc Natl Acad Sci USA 2005; 102(34):12206–12211.
60. Yerushalmi G, Zusman T, Segal G. Additive effect on intracellular growth by *Legionella pneumophila* Icm/Dot proteins containing a lipobox motif. Infect Immun 2005; 73(11):7578–7587.
61. Sauer JD, Shannon JG, Howe D, et al. Specificity of *Legionella pneumophila* and *Coxiella burnetii* vacuoles and versatility of *Legionella pneumophila* revealed by coinfection. Infect Immun 2005; 73(8):4494–4504.
62. Sauer JD, Bachman MA, Swanson MS. The phagosomal transporter A couples threonine acquisition to differentiation and replication of *Legionella pneumophila* in macrophages. Proc Natl Acad Sci USA 2005; 102(28):9924–9929.
63. Takeda K, Kaisho T, Akira S. Toll-like receptors. Annu Rev Immunol 2003; 21:335–376.
64. Bafica A, Scanga CA, Feng CG, et al. TLR9 regulates Th1 responses and cooperates with TLR2 in mediating optimal resistance to *Mycobacterium tuberculosis*. J Exp Med 2005; 202(12):1715–1724.
65. Honstettre A, Ghigo E, Moynault A, et al. Lipopolysaccharide from *Coxiella burnetii* is involved in bacterial phagocytosis, filamentous actin reorganization, and inflammatory responses through toll-like receptor 4. J Immunol 2004; 172(6):3695–3703.

66. Zamboni DS, Campos MA, Torrecilhas AC, et al. Stimulation of toll-like receptor 2 by *Coxiella burnetii* is required for macrophage production of pro-inflammatory cytokines and resistance to infection. J Biol Chem 2004; 279(52):54405–54415.
67. Meghari S, Honstettre A, Lepidi H, et al. TLR2 is necessary to inflammatory response in *Coxiella burnetii* infection. Ann NY Acad Sci 2006; 1063:161–166.
68. Steiman RM, Hawiger D, Nussenzweig MC. Tolerogenic dendritic cells. Annu Rev Immunol 2003; 21:685–711.
69. Colonna M, Pulendran B, Iwasaki A. Dendritic cells at the host–pathogen interface. Nat Immunol 2006; 7(2):117–120.
70. Shannon JG, Howe D, Heinzen RA. Virulent *Coxiella burnetii* does not activate human dendritic cells: role of lipopolysaccharide as a shielding molecule. Proc Natl Acad Sci USA 2005; 102(24):8722–8727.
71. Boehm U, Klamp T, Groot M, et al. Cellular responses to interferon-γ. Annu Rev Immunol 1997; 15:749–795.
72. Dellacasagrande J, Capo C, Raoult D, et al. IFN-γ-mediated control of *Coxiella burnetii* survival in monocytes: the role of cell apoptosis and TNF. J Immunol 1999; 162(4):2259–2265.
73. Akporiaye ET, Baca OG. Superoxide anion production and superoxide dismutase and catalase activities in *Coxiella burnetii*. J Bacteriol 1983; 154(1):520–523.
74. Baca OG, Roman MJ, Glew RH, et al. Acid phosphatase activity in *Coxiella burnetii*: a possible virulence factor. Infect Immun 1993; 61(10):4232–4239.
75. Baca OG, Li YP, Kumar H. Survival of the Q fever agent *Coxiella burnetii* in the phagolysosome. Trends Microbiol 1994; 2(12):476–480.
76. Akporiaye ET, Stefanovich D, Tsosie V, et al. *Coxiella burnetii* fails to stimulate human neutrophil superoxide anion production. Acta Virol 1990; 34(1):64–70.
77. Yoshiie K, Matayoshi S, Fujimura T, et al. Induced production of nitric oxide and sensitivity of alveolar macrophages derived from mice with different sensitivity to *Coxiella burnetii*. Acta Virol 1999; 43(5):273–278.
78. Zamboni DS, Rabinovitch M. Nitric oxide partially controls *Coxiella burnetii* phase II infection in mouse primary macrophages. Infect Immun 2003; 71(3):1225–1233.
79. Brennan RE, Russell K, Zhang G, et al. Both inducible nitric oxide synthase and NADPH oxidase contribute to the control of virulent phase I *Coxiella burnetii* infections. Infect Immun 2004; 72(11):6666–6675.
80. Clifton DR, Goss RA, Sahni SK, et al. NF-κB-dependent inhibition of apoptosis is essential for host cell survival during *Rickettsia rickettsii* infection. Proc Natl Acad Sci USA 1998; 95(8):4646–4651.
81. Wahl C, Oswald F, Simnacher U, et al. Survival of *Chlamydia pneumoniae*-infected Mono Mac 6 cells is dependent on NF-κB binding activity. Infect Immun 2001; 69(11):7039–7045.
82. Dellacasagrande J, Ghigo E, Raoult D, et al. IFN-γ-induced apoptosis and microbicidal activity in monocytes harboring the intracellular bacterium *Coxiella burnetii* require membrane TNF and homotypic cell adherence. J Immunol 2002; 169(11):6309–6315.
83. Dellacasagrande J, Ghigo E, Hammami SM, et al. αvβ3 integrin and bacterial lipopolysaccharide are involved in *Coxiella burnetii*-stimulated production of tumor necrosis factor by human monocytes. Infect Immun 2000; 68(10):5673–5678.
84. Weinberg ED. Modulation of intramacrophage iron metabolism during microbial cell invasion. Microbes Infect 2000; 2(1):85–89.
85. Howe D, Mallavia LP. *Coxiella burnetii* infection increases transferrin receptors on J774A.1 cells. Infect Immun 1999; 67(7):3236–3241.
86. Moore KW, de Waal Malefyt R, Coffman RL, et al. Interleukin-10 and the interleukin-10 receptor. Annu Rev Immunol 2001; 19:683–765.
87. Yang X, Gartner J, Zhu L, et al. IL-10 gene knockout mice show enhanced Th1-like protective immunity and absent granuloma formation following *Chlamydia trachomatis* lung infection. J Immunol 1999; 162(2):1010–1017.
88. Ghigo E, Capo C, Raoult D, et al. Interleukin-10 stimulates *Coxiella burnetii* replication in human monocytes through tumor necrosis factor down-modulation: role in microbicidal defect of Q fever. Infect Immun 2001; 69(4):2345–2352.
89. Honstettre A, Meghari S, Nunès JA, et al. Role for the CD28 molecule in the control of *Coxiella burnetii* infection. Infect Immun 2006; 74(3):1800–1808.

20 | Epidemiology of Q Fever

Thomas J. Marrie
Faculty of Medicine and Dentistry, University of Alberta, Edmonton, Alberta, Canada

INTRODUCTION

Q fever is a zoonosis, and as such, the epidemiology of this infection is very much intertwined with that of the animal reservoirs of the causative organism, *Coxiella burnetii*. Once physicians make a diagnosis of Q fever, they should try to determine the source of the infection. The subsequent investigation often represents field epidemiology at its best. In many health regions, Q fever is a notifiable disease.

HISTORICAL ASPECTS

Q fever was described in 1935 as an outbreak of febrile illness among abattoir workers in Brisbane, Australia (1). Derrick, a pathologist who also functioned as a medical officer of health, was asked to investigate this outbreak. He examined all those who were affected and could not arrive at a diagnosis from the patients' history, physical examination, and a few investigations. As a result, he termed the illness "Q" for query fever. Later, some workers suggested that the Q stood for Queensland, the Australian state in which the disease was first described (2). However, once the epidemiology of the disease became known and its status as a zoonosis established, this designation lost favor.

Derrick obtained urine samples from his febrile patients and injected the urine into guinea pigs (2). The guinea pigs became febrile and developed splenomegaly. He was unable to isolate any conventional pathogens from the spleen of these animals but fortunately the eminent scientist, Sir McFarlane Burnet, lived nearby. He consulted Dr. Burnet and sent the guinea pig spleens to him. Burnet was able to isolate a filterable agent from the spleens (2).

At about the same time that these events were happening in Australia, Cox, and Davis were trying to isolate the agent of Rocky Mountain spotted fever at the NIH Laboratory in Hamilton, Montana (3). They collected ticks from the Nine Mile Creek region of Montana and were able to isolate an agent. In May of 1938, Dr. Dyer, Director of NIH, visited the Rocky Mountain Laboratory in Montana to try to confirm the findings of Cox and Davis. Ten days later, on the train ride back to Washington, DC, he became ill with fever. A sample of his blood obtained at the time of his illness resulted in fever in guinea pigs. The "Nine Mile Agent" was isolated from these guinea pigs.

In April 1938, Burnet sent spleens from the guinea pigs infected with the Q fever agent to Dyer, who was able to show that the Q fever agent and the Nine Mile agent were identical. Cox named the organism *Rickettsia diaporica*—diaporica is derived from the Greek word meaning having the property or ability to pass through (4). This property referred to the ability of the agent to pass through a filter and hence is a reflection of its size. Later it was renamed *R. burnetii* in honor of Burnet and still later *C. burnetii* in honor of both Cox and Burnet (5).

EPIDEMIOLOGY OF Q FEVER IN HUMANS

From its very beginnings in an abattoir in Australia, Q fever has spread worldwide. The only areas currently not reporting cases are Antarctica and New Zealand (6,7). The predominant manifestations of Q fever, however, vary from country to country and sometimes even within a country. In Nova Scotia, Canada, and in the Basque region of Spain, pneumonia is the predominant manifestation of Q fever (8,9), whereas in the Canary Islands and elsewhere in southern Spain the dominant features are fever and hepatitis (10,11). In contrast, in the south of France both hepatitis and pneumonia are observed, but hepatitis is more frequent than pneumonia (12). It is noteworthy that in Canada, the features of an outbreak of Q fever in Newfoundland were confined to a self-limited febrile illness; in Alberta, sporadic cases consist mostly of hepatitis or a self-limited febrile illness. Interestingly, in this province many of the patients with Q fever have an urticarial rash. Thus, one might ask why pneumonia is a dominant manifestation of Q fever in Nova Scotia and not elsewhere in Canada. Furthermore, Q fever in a geographic area may be endemic or epidemic and shift back and forth between these two entities.

In the late 1940s and early 1950s, there were a considerable number of cases of Q fever in California. Careful studies by Lennette et al. and by Huebner et al. led to the conclusion that Q fever was associated with exposure to sheep and goats (13–16). During the course of these studies, *C. burnetii* was recovered from the air of premises housing infected goats (14), from raw milk (15), and from the placentas of infected cow's (16).

The epidemiology of Q fever can best be illustrated by considering detailed studies in two areas: the province of Nova Scotia, Canada, and in Germany, and by considering the valuable lessons that have been learned from selected outbreaks around the world.

Q fever was first recognized in Nova Scotia in 1979 during a study of atypical pneumonia (17). It soon became apparent that the epidemiology of Q fever in Nova Scotia was unique—it was associated with exposure to infected parturient cats and stillborn kittens (18–22). Nova Scotia is a small province on the east coast of Canada with a population of about 900,000 people. Despite less than comprehensive surveillance, in one year 50 cases of Q fever were identified for an incidence of 55 per million, or 5.5 per 100,000. In contrast, recent data from Germany shows an incidence ranging from 0.1 in the northern states to 3.1 per million in Baden-Wurttemberg in the south (23). The prevalence of Q fever was 14.1/100,000 in 1989 in Barcelona, Spain (24). In 1994, 667 cases of Q fever were reported from Australia for an incidence of 3.7/100,000 and in 1998, there were 571 cases, with an incidence of 3.0/100,000 (25). In another study, the annual notification rates per 100,000 population for Q fever in Australia have ranged from 3.11 to 4.99 (26). The prevalence of Q fever in Marseille, France has been estimated at 50/100,000 (27). In Australia, 85% to 90% of the cases are from Queensland and New South Wales and the male to female ratio of those affected is 5.1:1 (25).

The major manifestation of acute Q fever in Nova Scotia is pneumonia. This is differs from what occurs almost everywhere else in the world. It is noteworthy that in Nova Scotia only a few cases have been associated with exposure to cattle and none with exposure to sheep and goats. Cases in this province have also been associated with exposure to infected deer, dogs (28), and wild rabbits (22). In all instances, these epidemiological associations have been supported by isolation of the organism from the implicated animal or positive serology for *C. burnetii* from the implicated animal (22). Cases of Q fever declined in Nova Scotia during the late 1990s and the first few years of the twenty-first century, probably due to decreased surveillance after the departure of one of the investigators who was very interested in Q fever. Indeed from 1999 to 2002, only seven cases of Q fever were identified in Nova Scotia. However, in 2004–2005, almost 30 years after the first cases were described, a new study of Q fever began in Nova Scotia, which made showed that cases are still occurring at a relatively lower rate of 0.5/100,000. There are five species of ticks in Nova Scotia, but the dominant one is the American dog tick, *Dermacentor variabilis* var. Say. This tick was introduced to the Yarmouth area of Nova Scotia by the dogs of American hunters. Over time, these ticks spread over a considerable portion of this province. In 1994, 193 ticks were examined, 24 (12%) of which were found positive for *C. burnetii* DNA by polymerase chain reaction (PCR; Marrie and Raoult, unpublished observations). This is an incredibly high positivity rate. It is likely that the ticks bite and infect a number of wild and domestic animals and these contaminate the environment with *C. burnetti*. Cats can become infected in several ways, including hunting infected rabbits or from the contaminated environment. In any event, it is very likely that infected ticks are at the top of the chain of *C. burnetii* infection in Nova Scotia.

In a remarkable study, Hellenbrand et al. (23) chronicled Q fever in Germany from 1947 to 1999. The incidence of Q fever in Germany is increasing—from 1979 to 1989 it was 0.8 per million and from 1990 to 1999 it was 1.4 per million. The seasonality of community outbreaks in this country has shifted from winter–summer to spring–summer, possibly because of changes in sheep husbandry. The location of recent outbreaks suggests that urbanization of rural areas may be contributing to the increase in Q fever. Forty outbreaks have been identified in Germany since 1947. Sheep were the source in 24 outbreaks, whereas cattle were implicated in four community outbreaks and two abattoir outbreaks.

France is a country where considerable Q fever activity has been documented. A number of investigators with a major interest in this disease reside in France and a World Health Organization laboratory for the study of rickettsial diseases is located in Marseille. These combined factors have led to studies that have provided new insights into the epidemiology of Q fever. Two studies (one from the Marseille area) have documented that high winds can result in infection with *C. burnetii* up to 11 miles (18.3 km) from the source of contamination (29,30). Other unique insights from studies in Marseille have included an outbreak due to infected pigeons (31) and studies of risk factors for Q fever among the homeless population in Marseille (32). The investigators studied individuals in homeless shelters in Marseille and found that 10.8% of those in shelter A were seropositive at a much higher rate than in the other shelters. This shelter was close to an abandoned slaughterhouse that was used to kill sheep at the time of the Muslim Aid El Khebir sacrifice. Investigators postulated that this, combined with prevailing winds from an area outside Marseille where there are many sheep, was the source (32). Another study by these investigators from Marseille involved an outbreak of 29 cases of Q fever in a town of 12,000 in the French Alps. The source was likely airborne transmission from contaminated sheep waste left uncovered in a slaughterhouse area. Helicopter landings in a nearby area created winds and probably facilitated the airborne spread of *C. burnetii* (33).

A recent outbreak of Q fever in Newfoundland and Labrador, Canada, indicates just how easily Q fever can be introduced into a community. An investigation of an outbreak of abortions among goats in 1999 revealed that 66 of 179 (37%) goat farmers, their family members, and farm workers had acute Q fever (34). About one year previously, the community of Bonavista imported goats from Ontario, Prince Edward Island, and Maine to start a goat farming cooperative. At the time of the investigation, most of the goats were infected.

ROUTES OF TRANSMISSION OF *C. BURNETII* TO HUMANS
Inhalation of Contaminated Aerosols

From experimental and epidemiological evidence, there is no doubt that contaminated aerosols are the major mechanism whereby *C. burnetii* is transmitted to humans (35–39). Volunteers who inhaled a single infectious dose of this organism had an incubation period of 16 days, whereas those who were exposed to 1500 infectious doses had an incubation period of 10 days (35). This experiment indicates that there is a dose–response effect and is direct evidence that inhalation of the organism causes disease. Indirect exposure to contaminated material may also lead to Q fever, such as when contaminated clothing from the Rocky Mountain Laboratory in Montana led to cases of Q fever among laundry workers who processed this clothing (40). Ninety-five persons at a local pub who had contact with animal attendants who were assisting abortions and births of goats developed Q fever (41). The authors postulated that aerosols from the contaminated garments of these animal attendants led to this outbreak of Q fever. Even a game of poker may result in Q fever if your infected cat delivers kittens during the game (42). There have been several outbreaks of Q fever in research institutions when infected pregnant animals, especially sheep, have been transported through the building to the laboratory (43–46). In order to avoid such events, most research institutions have regulations for the use of such animals and invariably only animals seronegative for *C. burnetti* can be used. A traveling petting zoo in two shopping malls in Quebec, Canada, with 13 goats and five sheep on exhibit between March 25 and April 3, 1999, was the source of 95 cases of Q fever (Millford et al., personal communication).

Oral Route

Epidemiological studies have suggested that ingestion of contaminated milk is a risk factor for Q fever infection (47,48). However, evidence from experiments in which contaminated milk was fed to volunteers is contradictory (49–51). In a case–control study, Hatchette et al. (34) found that both ingestion of pasteurized cheese and tobacco smoking were risk factors for acquisition of

Q fever during an outbreak of Q fever on a caprine cooperative in Newfoundland. From direct observations, it was evident that workers smoked cigarettes without washing their hands. Kim et al (52) tested 316 bulk milk tanks in the United States using PCR to amplify *C. burnetii* DNA. The milk was collected from January 2001 to December 2002 and 94.3% of the samples were positive. If even some of the organisms are not killed by pasteurization and infection can occur by the oral route, there is a chance for large numbers of cases of Q fever to occur. However, one can also argue that infection via the oral route must not be very efficient or there would be many cases of Q fever given this degree of contamination of milk.

The route of infection may explain the difference in the manifestations of Q fever in some countries, for example, pneumonia in Nova Scotia, Canada, versus hepatitis in Marseille, France. Five different strains of *C. burnetii* were used to infect mice via the intraperitoneal or intranasal route. Pneumonia developed in those infected via the nasal route, whereas those infected intraperitoneally developed hepatitis, splenomegaly, and pneumonia (53). Similar findings were reported when similar experiments were carried out in guinea pigs (54).

Percutaneous Route

Crushing an infected tick between the fingers has resulted in Q fever (55), as has intradermal inoculation (55) and transfusion of contaminated blood (56). However, the percutaneous route is a very uncommon route for Q fever transmission.

Vertical Transmission

This rarely occurs (57,58), but increased surveillance may reveal additional cases of vertical transmission. Indeed, in the town of Martigues in southern France, Q fever complicated at least one in 540 pregnancies (59). In Nova Scotia, a serosurvey of 7658 pregnant women found that 4% were positive for antibodies to *C. burnetti*. (60). In another study, a similar percentage of 200 pregnant Japanese women were seropositive (61). Thus, the potential at least exists for vertical transmission.

Person-to-Person Transmission

Despite the fact that pneumonia (and hence the potential for spread via aerosols) is a common manifestation of Q fever in some areas of the world, there have been only a few cases of person-to-person transmission (62–64). The intracellular location of the organism is the likely explanation for the rarity of such transmission. There are two reports of transmission of Q fever to attendants during autopsies (62,63), and one report of transmission of infection from a patient to hospital staff (64). One wonders why more cases of Q fever do not develop in obstetrical staff who assist at the delivery of infected pregnant women since infected parturient cats, sheep, and cattle readily spread infection to people. Raoult and Stein (58) have documented Q fever in an obstetrician who attended the delivery of a woman with Q fever during pregnancy. No serosurveys of obstetricians have been carried out to determine if they have a higher rate of antibodies to *C. burnetii* than do other physicians.

Sexual Transmission

Sexual transmission of Q fever has been demonstrated in mice (65), and viable *C. burnetii* has been found in bull semen (66). It has been suggested that Q fever can be transmitted sexually in humans (67). The case reported by Milazzo et al. (68) supports this. They reported the case of a 53-year-old man who developed orchitis as a complication of Q fever. The orchitis had its onset three days after he had intercourse with his spouse (29 days after onset of his illness). Fifteen days later, his spouse developed Q fever. *C. burnetii* DNA was identified by PCR in the semen of the index case 4 and 15 months after onset of the acute illness.

EFFECTS OF AGE AND GENDER

There are several studies in which young age seems to be protective of infection with *C. burnetii*. In a large outbreak of Q fever in Switzerland, symptomatic infection was five times more likely to occur in those over 15 years of age compared with those younger than 15 (69). In a study of

Q fever among children in Greece, increasing age seemed to be associated with increasing rates of infection (70). Twenty children with Q fever were reported in Darling Downs and southwest Queensland during 2001 and 2002. The authors noted that the number of infections among children was increasing (71).

In many outbreaks of Q fever, men are affected more commonly than women. It has been assumed that this is due to the fact that certain occupations in which males predominate are more likely to be associated with Q fever. However, in France, despite similar exposures, the male to female ratio is 2.45:1 (72). It is noteworthy that this gender difference does not occur in children (73). The explanation for the gender difference is that female sex hormones are protective against Q fever infection (74).

Q FEVER IN WARTIME

Christopher et al. (75) reviewed the literature of the importance of Q fever during wartime. They infer that Q fever may have been a significant factor during the American Civil War. During World War II, outbreaks of Q fever occurred among American and British soldiers in Greece and Italy, and among American soldiers in Panama. The Axis troops in Bulgaria, Greece, Crimea, and the Ukraine also suffered from Q fever during this war. Seven outbreaks among U.S. troops in the Mediterranean theater resulted in more than 1000 serologically confirmed cases. Cases were epidemiologically linked to occupancy of barns and two-story dwellings where the bottom story served as a barn. After World War II, an explosive outbreak occurred among troops in Libya, and most recently cases were acquired during Operation Desert Storm. Q fever cases were diagnosed at four United Nations stabilization bases in Bosnia and Herzegovina in 1997.

Q FEVER AS A BIOTERRORISM AGENT

Biological agents that might be used for bioterrorism have been categorized as A, B, or C (76). Class A agents are easily disseminated or transmitted from person to person, cause high mortality, might cause public panic and social disruption, and require special action for public preparedness. Category B agents are moderately easy to disseminate, cause moderate morbidity and low mortality, and require special enhancement of Centers for Disease Control's diagnostic capacity and disease surveillance activity. Category C agents are those that could be used because of their availability, ease of production, and potentially high morbidity and mortality. Category A agents include *Bacillus anthracis*, *Franciscella tularensis*, *Yersinia pestis*. Category B agents are *C. burnetii*, *Brucella* spp., *Burkholderia mallei*. Category C currently consists of multidrug-resistant *Mycobacterium tuberculosis*, Nipha virus, Hantavirus, Yellow fever virus, and tick-borne hemorrhagic fever viruses (76).

Q fever is the ideal biological warfare agent in that it is easily dispersed as an aerosol, and there is a very high infectivity rate with pneumonia as the major manifestation. The resulting infection results in incapacitation with very rare mortality. The agent forms spores, and secondary wind-borne spread of the spores can occur. There is no damage to the environment.

Q FEVER IN ANIMALS

Cattle, sheep, and goats are the primary reservoirs of Q fever for humans. *C. burnetii* localizes to the uterus and mammary glands of infected animals (77). However, *C. burnetii* is able to infect many species including mammals, birds, and arthropods (77,78). The importance of the various animal reservoirs can be emphasized by reviewing the outbreaks that have been reported (78). From 1999 to 2004, there were 18 reported outbreaks of Q fever from 12 different countries involving two to 289 people. Six outbreaks involved sheep; three involved goats; one resulted from exposure to goat manure; one from exposure to ovine manure; one involved exposure to wild animals; one involved exposure to cats and dogs, and in two outbreaks the source was unknown (78).

In animals, Q fever infection is generally asymptomatic but abortion and stillbirth can occur. Low birth-weight animals can also occur (53). Aborted fetuses usually appear normal (78). The abortion rates can range from 3% to 80%. The highest rates are observed in caprine herds. Infected placentas exhibit exudates and intracotyledonary fibrous thickening. A severe inflammatory response is noted in the myometrium of goats. Metris is frequently a unique manifestation of the disease in cattle (78). Milk shedding is more frequent and lasts longer in cows and goats than in ewes. Ewes shed more and longer in vaginal discharges than goats and can shed bacteria at subsequent pregnancies. Goats shed *C. burnetii* in feces before and after kidding, and the mean duration of excretion is 20 days. Infected cows can shed *C. burnetii* in milk for up to 32 months (79). Large concentrations of *C. burnetii* are present in the infected placenta, and aerosols are created during parturition (80). Inhalation of these contaminated aerosols by a susceptible human results in Q fever.

Sanford et al. (81) described abortions that occurred in five goat herds that were exposed to three goats from another herd that kidded prematurely during a fair. All of the goats were housed in the same barn. Twenty-one days after exposure, abortions began and affected 20% to 46% of the pregnant animals in each herd. Immunohistochemistry methods have shown that organisms are present on both surfaces of the chorioallantoic membrane (82,83). The placentas of infected sheep can contain 10^9 guinea pig infective doses of *C. burnetii* per gram of tissue (84). The stillbirth rate among infected cats is about 70% compared with the usual rate of 10% for uninfected cats (85). Dairy cows are important in the spread of Q fever, whereas beef cows are rarely infected (86). Once *C. burnetii* is introduced into a herd, rapid spread occurs so that 80% of the cows are positive within a few months (86). Infected wildlife may be important in infecting cattle, as a source of infection is not found in a large portion of newly infected herds (86,87).

Hares and rabbits in many areas have the highest rate of infection among wild animals (87,88). In a study in Oxfordshire, Webster et al. (89) found that 7% to 53% of wild brown rats (*Rattus norvegius*) were seropositive for *C. burnetii*. These workers postulated that since cats are frequent predators of rats, cats become infected.

Infected ticks are probably most important in maintaining the whole cycle of *C. burnetii* (90). Infected ticks have been found on rabbits, goats, cattle, sheep, and many other animals (90). It is likely that birds are also important in the spread of *C. burnetii* by transporting infected ticks from one area to another. Birds may also be involved directly in the spread of Q fever to humans as evidenced by a recent outbreak of Q fever among family members in southern France due to aerosols from *C. burnetii*-infected pigeon feces (31). In some countries, infection among domestic or wild animals results in considerable infection among humans in contact with these animals, whereas in other areas little if any transmission to humans occurs (91).

REFERENCES

1. Derrick EH. "Q" fever, new fever entity: clinical features, diagnosis and laboratory investigation. Med J Aust 1937; 2:281–299.
2. McDade JE. Historical aspects of Q fever. In: Marrie TJ, ed. Q Fever: The Disease. Vol. I. Boca Raton, FL: CRC Press, 1990:1–21.
3. Parker RR. A filter passing infectious agent isolated from ticks. II. Transmission by *Dermacentor andersoni*. Public Health Rep 1938; 53:2267–2271.
4. Cox HR. Studies of a filter-passing infectious agent isolated from ticks. V. Further attempts to cultivated in cell-free medium. Suggested classification. Public Health Rep 1939; 54:1822–1826.
5. Philip CB. Comments on the name of the Q fever organism. Public Health Rep 1948; 63:58–60.
6. Kaplan MM, Bertagna P. The geographical distribution of Q fever. Bull WHO 1955; 13:829–860.
7. Hilbink F, Penrose M, Kovacova E, Kazar J. Q fever is absent from New Zealand. Intern J Epidemiol 1993; 22:945–949.
8. Marrie TJ, Haldane EV, Faulkner RS, et al. The importance of *Coxiella burnetii* as a cause of pneumonia in Nova Scotia. Can J Public Hlth 1985; 76:233–236.
9. Montejo M, Corral J, Aguirre C. Q fever in the Basque Country: 1981–1984. Rev Infect Dis 1985; 7:700–701.
10. Velasco FP, Enciso MVB, Lama ZG, et al. Clinical presentation of acute Q fever in Lanzarote (Canary Islands): a 2-year prospective study. Scand J Infect Dis 1996; 28:533–534.
11. De Alarcon A, Villanueva JL, Viciana P, et al. Q fever: epidemiology, clinical features and prognosis. A study from 1983 to 1999 in the South of Spain. J Infect 2003; 47:110–116.

12. Maurin M, Raoult D. Q fever. Clin Microbiol Rev 1999; 12:518–533.
13. Lennette EH, Clark WH, Dean BH. Sheep and goats and the epidemiology of Q fever in Northern California. Am J Trop Med 1949; 29:527–541.
14. Lennette EH, Welsh HH. Q fever in California. X. Recovery of *Coxiella burnetii* from the air of premises harbouring infected goats. Am J Hyg 1951; 54:44–49.
15. Huebner RJ, Jellison WL, Beck MD, et al. Q fever studies in Southern California. I. Recovery of *Rickettsia burnetii* from raw milk. Public Health Rep 1948; 63:214–222.
16. Luoto L, Huebner RJ. Q fever studies in Southern California. IX. Isolation of Q fever organisms from parturient placentas of naturally infected cows. Public Health Rep 1950; 65:541–544.
17. Marrie TJ, Haldane EV, Noble MA, et al. Causes of atypical pneumonia: results of a 1-year prospective study. Can Med Assoc J 1981; 125:1118–1123.
18. Embil J, Williams JC, Marrie TJ. The immune response in a cat-related outbreak of Q fever as measured by the indirect immunofluorescence test and the enzyme-linked immunosorbent assay. Can J Microbiol 1990; 36:292–296.
19. Marrie TJ, Fraser J. Prevalence of antibodies to *Coxiella burnetii* among veterinarians and slaughterhouse workers in Nova Scotia. Can Vet J 1985; 26:181–184.
20. Kosatsky T. Household outbreak of Q fever pneumonia related to a parturient cat. Lancet 1984; II:1447–1449.
21. Marrie TJ, Durant H, Williams JC, et al. Exposure to parturient cats: a risk factor for acquisition of Q fever in Maritime Canada. J Infect Dis 1988; 158:101–108.
22. Marrie TJ. Epidemiology of Q fever. In: Marrie TJ, ed. Q fever—The Disease. Vol. 1. Boca Raton, FL: CRC Press, 1990:49–70.
23. Hellenbrand W, Breuer T, Petersen L. Changing epidemiology of Q fever in Germany, 1947–1999. Emerg Infect Dis 2001; 7:789–796.
24. Domingo P, Munoz C, Franquet T, et al. Acute Q fever in adult patients: report on 63 sporadic cases in an urban area. Clin Infect Dis 1999; 29:874–879.
25. Bella F, Espejo E, Mauri M, et al. Clinical presentation of acute Australian Q fever. Am J Med 1994; 96:397–398.
26. Garner MG, Longbottom HM, Cannon RM, et al. A review of Q fever in Australia 1991–1994. Aust NZ J Public Health 1997; 21:722–730.
27. Raoult D. Reply to Bella et al. Am J Med 1994; 96:398.
28. Buhariwalli F, Cann B, Marrie TJ. A dog related outbreak of Q fever. Clin Infect Dis 1996; 23:753–755.
29. Tissot-Dupont H, Torres S, Nezri M, et al. Hyperendemic focus of Q fever related to sheep and wind. Am J Epidemiol 1999; 150:67–74.
30. Hawker JI, Ayres JG, Blair MR, et al. A large outbreak of Q fever in the West Midlands: windborne spread into a metropolitan area. Commun Dis Public Health 1998; 1:180–187.
31. Stein A, Raoult D. Pigeon pneumonia in province: a bird-borne Q fever outbreak. Clin Infect Dis 1999; 29:617–620.
32. Brouqui P, Badiaga S, Raoult D. Q fever outbreaks in homeless shelter. Emerg Infect Dis 2004; 10:1297–1299.
33. Carrieri MP, Tissot-Dupont H, Rey D, et al. Investigation of a slaughterhouse-related outbreak of Q fever in the French Alps. Eur J Clin Microbiol Infect Dis 2002; 21:17–21.
34. Hatchette T, Hudson R, Schlech W, et al. Caprine-associated Q fever in Newfoundland. Can Dis Wkly Rep 2000; 26:17–19.
35. Tiggert WD, Benenson AS. Studies on Q fever in man. Trans Assoc Am Phys 1956; 69:98–104.
36. Gonder JC, Kishimoto RA, Kastello MD, et al. Cynomolgus monkey model for experimental Q fever infection. J Infect Dis 1979; 139:191–196.
37. Laughlin T, Waag D, Williams J, Marrie TJ. Q fever: from deer to dog to man. Lancet 1991; 337:676–677.
38. Marrie TJ, Langille D, Papukna V, et al. Truckin' pneumonia—an outbreak of Q fever in a truck repair plant probably due to aerosols from clothing contaminated by contact with newborn kittens. Epidemiol Infect 1989; 102:119–127.
39. Abinanti FR, Welsh HH, Lennette EH, et al. Q fever studies. XVI. Some aspects of experimental infection induced in sheep by the intratracheal route of inoculation. Am J Hyg 1953; 57:170–184.
40. Oliphant JW, Gordon DA, Meis A, et al. Q fever in laundry workers, presumably transmitted from contaminated clothing. Am J Hyg 1949; 49:76–82.
41. Varga V. An explosive outbreak of Q-fever in Jedl'ove Kostol'any, Slovakia. Cent Eur J Public Health 1997; 4:180–182.
42. Langley JM, Marrie TJ, Covert AA, et al. Poker players pneumonia—an urban outbreak of Q fever following exposure to a parturient cat. N Engl J Med 1988; 319:354–356.
43. Schachter J, Sung M, Meyer KF. Potential danger of Q fever in a university environment. J Infect Dis 1971; 123:301–304.
44. Meiklejohn G, Reimer LG, Graves PS, et al. Cryptic epidemic of Q fever in a medical school. J Infect Dis 1981; 144:107–114.
45. Hall CJ, Richmond SJ, Caul EO, et al. Laboratory outbreak of Q fever acquired from sheep. Lancet 1992; 1:1004–1006.

46. Curet LB, Paust JC. Transmission of Q fever from experimental sheep to laboratory personnel. Am J Obstet Gynecol 1972; 114:566–568.
47. Marmion BP, Stoker MGP, Walker CBV, et al. Q fever in Great Britain—epidemiological information from a serological survey of healthy adults in Kent and East Anglia. J Hyg 1956; 54:118–140.
48. Fishbein DB, Raoult D. A cluster of *Coxiella burnetii* infections associated with exposure to vaccinated goats and their unpasteurized dairy products. Am J Trop Med Hyg 1992; 47:35–40.
49. Benson WW, Brock DW, Mather J. Serologic analysis of a penitentiary group using raw milk from a Q fever infected herd. Public Health Rep 1963; 78:707–710.
50. Editorial. Experimental Q fever in man. Br Med J 1950; 1:1000.
51. Krumbiegel ER, Wisniewski HJ. Q fever in Milwaukee. II. Consumption of infected raw milk by human volunteers. Arch Environ Health 1970; 21:63–65.
52. Kim SG, Kim EH, Lafferty CJ, et al. *Coxiella burnetii* in bulk tank milk samples, United States. Emerg Infect Dis 2005; 11:619–621.
53. Marrie TJ, Stein A, Janigan D, et al. Route of infection determines clinical manifestations of acute Q fever. J Infect Dis 1996; 173:484–487.
54. La Scola B, Lepidi H, Raoult D. Pathologic changes during acute Q fever: influence of the route of infection and inoculum size in infected guinea pigs. Infect Immun 1997; 65:2443–2447.
55. Eklund CM, Parker RR, Lackman DB. Case of Q fever probably contracted by exposure to ticks in nature. Public Health Rep 1947; 62:1413–1416.
56. Editorial Comment on Q fever transmitted by blood transfusion—United States. Can Dis Wkly Rep 1977; 3:210.
57. Fiset P, Wisseman CL Jr, El-Bataine Y. Immunologic evidence of human fetal infection with *Coxiella burnetii*. Am J Epidemiol 1975; 101:65–69.
58. Raoult D, Stein A. Q fever during pregnancy: a risk factor for women, fetuses and obstetricians. N Engl J Med 1994; 330:371 (letter).
59. Stein A, Raoult D. Q fever during pregnancy: a public health problem in Southern France. Clin Infect Dis 1988; 27:592–596.
60. Langley JM, Marrie TJ, Leblanc JC, et al. *Coxiella burnetii* seropositivity in parturient women is associated with adverse pregnancy outcomes. Am J Obstet Gynecol 2003; 189:228–232.
61. Numazaki K, Ueno H, Yokoo K, et al. Detection of serum antibodies to *Bartonella henselae* and *Coxiella burnetii* from Japanese children and pregnant women. Microbes Infect 2000; 2:1431–1434.
62. Harman JB. Q fever in Great Britain: clinical account of eight cases. Lancet 1949; 2:1028–1030.
63. Gerth H-J, Leidig U, Reimenschneider Th. Q-fieber-epidemie in einem Institut fur Humanpathologie. Dtsch Med Wochenschr 1982; 107:1391–1395.
64. Deutch DL, Peterson ET. Q fever: transmission from one human being to others. J Am Med Assoc 1950; 143:348–350.
65. Kruszewska D, Tylewska-Wierzbanowska S. *Coxiella burnetii* penetration into the reproductive system of male mice, promoting sexual transmission of infection. Infect Immun 1993; 61:4188–4195.
66. Kruszewska D, Tylewska-Wierzbanowska S. Isolation of *Coxiella burnetii* from bull semen. Res Vet Sci 1997; 62:299–300.
67. Kruszewska D, Tylewska-Wierzbanowska S. Possibility of sexual transmission of Q fever among humans. J Infect Dis 1996; 22:1087–1088.
68. Milazzo A, Hall R, Storm PA, Harris RJ, Winslow W, Marmion BP. Sexually-transmitted Q fever. Clin Infect Dis 2001; 33:399–402.
69. Dupuis G, Vouilloz M, Peter O, et al. Incidence of Q fever in Valais. Rev Med Suisse Romande 1985; 105:949–954.
70. Maltezou HC, Constantopoulou I, Kallergi C, et al. Q fever in children in Greece. Am J Trop Med Hyg 2004; 70:540–544.
71. Barralet JH, Parker NR. Q fever in children: an emerging public health issue in Queensland. Med J Aust 2004; 180:596–597.
72. Raoult D, Tissot-Dupont H, Foucault C, et al. Q fever 1985–1998—clinical and epidemiological features of 1,383 infections. Medicine 2000; 79:109–123.
73. Maltezou HC, Raoult D. Q fever in children. Lancet Infect Dis 2002; 2:686–691.
74. Leone M, Honstettre A, Lepidi H, et al. Effect of sex on *Coxiella burnetii* infection: protective role of 17 beta-estradiol. J Infect Dis 2004; 189:339–345.
75. Christopher GW, Agan BK, Cieslak TJ, et al. History of US military contributions to the study of bacterial zoonoses. Mil Med 2005; 170:39–48.
76. Karwa M, Currie B, Kvetan V. Bioterrorism: preparing for the impossible or the improbable. Crit Care Med 2005; 33(suppl):S75–S95.
77. Babudieri B. Q fever: a zoonosis. Adv Vet Sci 1959; 5:81–182.
78. Arricau-Bouvery N, Rololakis A. Is Q fever an emerging or re-emerging zoonosis? Vet Res 2005; 36:327–349.
79. Grist NR. The persistence of Q fever infection in a dairy herd. Vet Rec 1959; 71:839–841.
80. Welsh HH, Lennette EH, Abinanti RF, et al. Air-borne transmission of Q fever: the role of parturition in the generation of infective aerosols. Ann NY Acad Sci 1958; 70:528–540.

81. Sanford SE, Josephson GKA, MacDonald A. *Coxiella burnetii* (Q fever) abortion storms in goats after attendance at an annual fair. Can Vet J 1994; 35:376–378.
82. Palmer NC, Kierstead M, Key DW, et al. Placentitis and abortion in sheep and goats in Ontario caused by *Coxiella burnetii*. Can Vet J 1983; 24:60–61.
83. Dilbeck PM, McElwain TF. Immunohistochemical detection of *Coxiella burnetii* in formalin-fixed placenta. J Vet Diagn Invest 1994; 6:125–127.
84. Raju NR, Collings DF, Svaille PH. Abortion in black belly sheep in Fiji caused by *Coxiella burnetii*. Aust Vet J 1988; 65:225–226.
85. Pratt PW. Feline Medicine. 1st ed. Santa Barbara, CA. American Veterinary Publications, 1983:521–526.
86. Luoto L, Pickens EG. A résumé of recent research seeking to define the Q fever problem. Am J Hyg 1961; 74:43–49.
87. Enright JB, Franti CE, Behymer DE, Longhurst WM, Dutson VJ, Wright ME. *Coxiella burnetii* in a wildlife–livestock environment: distribution of Q fever in wild mammals. Am J Epidemiol 1971; 94:79–90.
88. Marrie TJ, Embil J, Yates L. Seroepidemiology of *Coxiella burnetii* among wildlife in Nova Scotia. Am J Trop Med Hyg 1993; 49:613–615.
89. Webster JP, Lloyd G, MacDonald DW. Q fever (*Coxiella burnetii*) reservoir in wild brown rat (*Rattus norvegicus*) populations in the UK. Parasitology 1995; 110:31–35.
90. Stoker MG, Marmion BP. The spread of Q fever from animals to man: the natural history of a rickettsial disease. Bull WHO 1995; 13:781–806.
91. Marmion BP, Stoker MGP. The epidemiology of Q fever in Great Britain: an analysis of the findings and some conclusions. Br Med J 1958; II:809–816.

21 | Clinical Aspects, Diagnosis, and Treatment of Q Fever

Hervé Tissot-Dupont
Faculté de Médecine, Unité des Rickettsies, Centre National de Référence, Marseille, France

Didier Raoult
Faculté de Médecine, Unité des Rickettsies, Université de la Méditerranée, Marseille, France

INTRODUCTION

Q fever is a worldwide zoonosis (1). *Coxiella burnetii*, its etiologic agent, is an obligate intracellular organism. The usual reservoirs for *C. burnetii* are cattle, sheep, and goats that shed the bacterium in urine, feces, milk, and birth products. Infected pets such as cats, rabbits, and dogs can transmit *C. burnetii* to humans, and have been sources of human outbreaks. Human infection mainly occurs following inhalation of contaminated aerosols. The organism is highly infectious and is currently considered as a potential bioterrorism agent, classified as a category B biological agent by the Center for Disease Control and Prevention (2,3).

Because of its varied clinical presentations, the prevalence of *C. burnetii* infections in humans is largely unknown and largely depends on either a local physician's interest in the disease or on the presence of a reliable diagnostic laboratory.

The natural history of Q fever begins with a contact between a nonimmune individual and the bacterium *C. burnetii*. After two to three weeks of incubation, the primary infection can be asymptomatic (60%) or symptomatic, that is, acute Q fever. In healthy subjects, the spontaneous evolution leads to a complete cure. In some people, *C. burnetii* is able to multiply despite the immune response activated by the primary infection (symptomatic or not). These at-risk subjects are pregnant women, people with cardiac valve damages, blood vessel abnormalities, or immunocompromised patients [HIV-infected, splenectomy, diabetes, cancer (lymphoma), immunosuppressive therapy]. After an acute Q fever, symptomatic or not, when the immune system is unable to control the infection, a chronic disease can develop. This theory is strengthened by all studies, in both humans and animals (1).

CLINICAL ASPECTS OF Q FEVER

The main characteristic of Q fever is its clinical polymorphism, so that diagnosis can only be made by systematic tests. Therefore, it has been said that the geographical distribution of Q fever follows that of rickettsiologists (4). After a primary infection, 60% of the patients will exhibit a symptomatic seroconversion, and only 4% of the symptomatic patients will be admitted to hospitals. A chronic disease will develop in at-risk patients, that is, less than 1% of the acute cases. However, due to more frequent hospital admissions, the proportion of diagnosed chronic cases is usually higher than that of acute cases (recruitment bias).

Acute Q Fever

From our large series of acute Q fever cases, we have been able to stress the following facts: the onset of the disease is generally sudden, which associates elevated fever (91%), headaches (51%), myalgias (37%), arthralgias (27%), and cough (34%). Less frequent are rashes (11%) and meningitis (leading to lumbar puncture) (4%). Nonspecific biological findings are a thrombocytopenia (35%), elevated liver enzymes (62%), and an elevated erythrocyte sedimentation rate (ESR) (55%). Abnormal chest X rays can be found in 27% of the patients. Clinical presentation varies according to the country of origin, and one of the three main presentations predominates: isolated fever, hepatitis, or pneumonia. Four hypotheses have been proposed to explain these variations: a specific physician's interest for a clinical presentation, strain variability, way of inoculation (aerosol vs. digestive), and host specificity. We have been able to demonstrate the last hypothesis in our series (5): the patients with an isolated fever were more frequently males, whereas those with a hepatitis were younger, had more frequent contact with animals, and were less frequently immunocompromised. Those presenting as a pneumonia were older, and more often immunocompromised. To our knowledge, this was the first report demonstrating a relationship between clinical presentations of acute infection and host factors.

Isolated fever (without hepatitis or pneumonia) is usually associated with severe headaches, and may last long enough to be considered a prolonged fever of unknown origin. The duration of the fever is longer among elderly patients (6). A rash is more frequent (20%) than in the other presentations.

Pneumonia is the most frequent presentation in Nova Scotia (Canada), in the Spanish Basque Country, and in the United Kingdom. In our series, these patients are less febrile, have less headaches, less thrombocytopenia, and a lower ESR than in the other clinical presentations (5).

Hepatitis is the most common presentation worldwide, particularly in France and Australia. In this presentation, the patients complain more often with pain (headaches, myalgias, arthralgias). Thrombocytopenia and elevated ESR are more often reported than in the other presentations. Hepatitis is generally defined by elevated liver enzymes. However, some patients present with jaundice and/or hepatomegaly. When a liver biopsy is carried out, it reveals a granulomatous hepatitis. The typical pathology finding for the Q fever granulomas is the doughnut image, made of a lipidic vacuola surrounded by a fibrinoid inflammation (1). Those patients with hepatitis often exhibit autoantibodies: antismooth muscle, antinuclear, and antiphospholipids (7).

Neurologic signs occur in 1% of the cases, presenting as meningitis, meningoencephalitis, and peripheral neuropathies (8). In our experience (5), neurologic symptoms were more frequently associated with occupational exposure and direct contacts with animals. Several patients were shepherds, and we hypothesized that they were exposed to heavier inoculums or to repeated infections.

Cardiac involvement is found in 2% of the acute Q fever cases and myocarditis is the leading cause of death (9). The pathophysiology of the heart damage is still not clear, although a relationship has been demonstrated between the onset of a myocarditis and the inoculum size (10). Pericarditis is generally unspecific. However, *C. burnetii* is the main cause of pericarditis in southern France (11), and a frequent one in Spain and in the United Kingdom. Among the patients who present with a pericarditis, 10% will develop a chronic or recurrent pericarditis.

Long-term cardiovascular complications have been studied in Switzerland, 12 years after a major outbreak (12). The authors report an excessively high death rate due to cardiac ischemia, and they hypothesize that *C. burnetii* could be a new infectious cause of atherosclerosis, much like *Chlamydia pneumoniae*. However, usual cardiovascular risk factors, mainly cigarette smoking, should not be neglected as potential biases (13).

Evolutive Risks

Considering the risk of evolution to a chronic disease in people with risk factors, when a patient is diagnosed with acute Q fever, symptomatic or not, these risk factors must be systematically investigated: *pregnancy test* in women, *cardiac ultrasound* (asking the cardiologist to look for any valvular abnormality, even minor ones such as mitral prolapsus, aortic bicuspidy, mitral leak), and a search for a cause of *immune suppression* (HIV, cancer, lymphoma, splenectomy, treatment).

Patients with previous valvular lesions, aneurisms, or vascular grafts, who present with an acute Q fever, have a high risk of chronic Q fever evolution (5). It has been shown that 38% of patients with valvular abnormalities will develop an endocarditis within two years after an acute Q fever (14). This evolution can be prevented by an antibiotic treatment. This study (5) enhances the importance of detecting valvular abnormalities, even minor ones, in a patient with an acute Q fever, and also of diagnosing Q fever in patients with valvular abnormalities. In the general population, between 1% and 2% show valvular abnormalities (14). If one-third of them develop an endocarditis, it means that 0.3% to 0.6% of the patients with an acute

Q fever (symptomatic or not) will have an endocarditis. These figures explain the lack of power of the Swiss cohort (12), which could not show an increase in the risk of endocarditis 12 years after the outbreak (one to two endocarditis cases among 412 Q fever cases during the outbreak).

The evolution of acute Q fever to chronic fatigue syndrome has been described in Australia (15) and in the United Kingdom (16). Ayres et al. (15) interviewed 71 patients five years after the acute phase, and compared them with controls. The patients reported more frequently sweat, dyspnea, blurred vision, and abnormal tiredness. Penttila et al. have demonstrated that the patients with a chronic fatigue syndrome (20%) show moderate abnormalities of their cytokines regulation (16). A geographical variation seems to exist, since none of the 80 patients followed-up in Martigues (southern France) after an acute Q fever developed chronique fatigue syndrome, versus 37% in an English study (17).

Chronic Q Fever
Endocarditis
The most frequent and studied presentation of chronic Q fever is endocarditis. More than 800 cases were reported in various studies between 1949 and 2005 (5,18–23). The main series were studied in the United Kingdom and in Ireland (227 cases), in France (264 cases), in Spain (62 cases), in Israel (35 cases), in Switzerland (21 cases), in Australia (18 cases), and in Canada (10 cases). In France, *C. burnetii* is the etiologic agent of 5% of the endocarditis cases, with an estimated prevalence of one case per million inhabitants per year, which is close to that reported in Switzerland and Israel. Compared with the other causes of endocarditis, *C. burnetii* endocarditis occurs among younger people (mean age 48 years), more often on abnormal native valves or on prosthetic valves (24). In Marseille, France, *C. burnetii* is the first cause or endocarditis on valvular grafts.

The clinical presentation varies with the diagnostic delay. The visceral involvement increases with time: in our former series of 15 patients, published in 1978, with an estimated delay of 18 months, 12 patients had liver enlargement, seven had spleen enlargement, seven had elevated liver enzymes, and seven had thrombocytopenia (23). Among our 13 more recent patients (estimated mean diagnostic delay: 3 months), only one had liver enlargement, one had spleen enlargement, three had elevated liver enzymes, and three had thrombocytopenia (25).

The main clinical and biological signs of Q fever endocarditis are summarized in Table 1.

Establishing a diagnosis of Q fever endocarditis is not very difficult. Patients without fever, or with sporadic or low-grade fever, are often misdiagnosed. Q fever should be systematically suspected in a patient with valvular abnormalities, presenting with evocative clinical signs (fever, hepatitis, tiredness, clubbed fingers, weight loss, renal failure), or laboratory findings (elevated ESR, elevated liver enzymes, thrombocytopenia). A Q- fever serology must be carried out in such patients, and the diagnosis can be assessed using modified Duke's criteria (26).

The prognosis of chronic Q fever was dramatically improved over the course of just a few years. The mortality rate was 37% in our series of 76 patients reported in 1987 (23), whereas it was only 15% in more recent series of 116 patients, between 1997 and 2000. Among the most recently diagnosed patients, the death rate was under 5% (27), an improvement that is probably related to earlier diagnoses, an efficient long-term treatment, and a better follow-up (21).

An interleukin (IL)-10 hypersecretion is found in patients with Q fever endocarditis (28). Thus, IL-10 can be considered as a marker of relapse, and can be used for treatment follow-up.

Other Presentations of Chronic Q Fever
Vascular infection (aneurisms or vascular grafts) is the second most frequent presentation. We have reported 25 cases (5,29), and six other cases have been reported in other countries—the U.K., U.S.A., Switzerland, and Australia (19,30–32). An aortic aneurism can be infected by *C. burnetii*, leading to an intestinal fistula or a spondylitis, as well as a vascular graft. The prognosis is poor in the absence of treatment. The medical treatment is the same as that of endocarditis, but necessarily associated to surgery (Fig. 1).

Other manifestations of chronic Q fever have been described: osteomyelitis (33), chronic hepatitis in alcohol addicts (5), pseudotumors of the spleen or the lung (34), infection of a ventriculo-peritoneal drain (35). A case of vascularitis with pulmonary amylosis has been described, after an acute Q fever, leading to the patient's death (36).

TABLE 1 Clinical and Biological Signs in Chronic Q Fever Endocarditis

Clinical signs	%
Sex male	76
Aortic valve	33
Mitral valve	50
Aortic and mitral valve	17
Fever	68
Cardiac failure	67
Hepatomegaly	56
Splenomegaly	55
Clubbed fingers	37
Purpuric rash	19
Artery embolism	21
Death	57
Laboratory findings	
Elevated leucocytes	25
Leucopenia	15
Elevated liver enzymes	40–83
Thrombocytopenia	26–56
Anemia	40–55
Elevated creatinine	65–73
Elevated ESR	88
Elevated gammaglobulines	94
Circulating immune complexes	90
Antinuclear antibodies	35
Rheumatoid factor	60
Antismooth muscle antibodies	40

Abbreviation: ESR, erythrocyte sedimentation rate.

Variations in Q Fever Clinical Presentation

Again, the main characteristic of Q fever is its variations in clinical presentations, which are related to numerous factors. The main factor is the host itself, in terms of predisposition, geographic distribution, and occupational exposure.

During the Swiss outbreak in the valley of Bagnes in 1983, among the 415 serologically confirmed cases, 224 (54%) were asymptomatic, and only eight patients (4%) were admitted to hospital (37). The same proportions are reported in other studies on outbreaks (38).

We had the opportunity to compare the two main presentations (189 hepatitis, 79 pneumonia): the patients with hepatitis were younger, less frequently immunocompromised, had more often fever, headaches, myalgia, thrombocytopenia, and elevated ESR. Those with pneumonia more often had EKG abnormalities. Also, patients who presented without hepatitis or pneumonia were more frequently females.

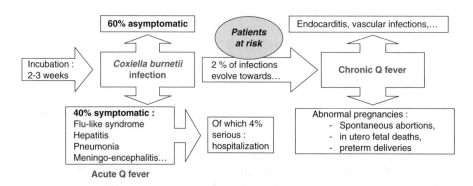

FIGURE 1 Q fever: natural history in the absence of treatment.

Age
Few pediatric cases are reported: the most recent review has compiled 46 cases (39). However, seroepidemiological studies show frequent exposure in children: a Dutch study reports a seroprevalence of 37% among boys and 70% among girls (40). Dupuis et al. report a seroprevalence of 23.3% in the Valais (41), 18.5% of positive children in a Spanish study (42), and 18.6% in Greece (43). Thus, children are more likely to be asymptomatic than adults, and show more attenuated clinical presentations. In Dupuis et al. study, children under 14 years represented 19% of positive sera, but only 5% of the 191 symptomatic people, and none of them had been admitted to a hospital (37). Among the 80 children involved in the survey, 70 (87.5%) were asymptomatic, versus 121 (36%) among those older than 14 years ($p < 0.001$). In an epidemic in an English secondary school, one out of 30 children with a positive serology was symptomatic (44). In a recent study, the multivariate analysis shows a relationship between clinical expression and age: children in the age group 11 to 14 years are 12 times more often symptomatic than the younger ones, and present more often as pneumonia (45).

Sex
Large series in adults usually report a male/female ratio of 2.5, whereas the seroprevalence is the same in both sexes (5,46). In children, the sex ratio of clinical cases as well as that of infections is 1:1. The change in sex ratio at puberty can be explained by the protective role of 17beta-estradiol in clinical expression, which has been demonstrated in mice (47).

According to these data regarding age and sex influence, it becomes clear that most of the symptomatic cases and hospital admissions are among men between 30 and 70 years, with the highest relative risk (1.8) in the 50- to 59-year age group (5).

Pregnant Women: Specific Risks
When a woman is infected by *C. burnetii* during pregnancy, the bacteria settle down in the uterus and in the mammary glands. The consequences are of great importance: (*i*) there is an immediate risk for the mother; (*ii*) there is an immediate risk to the fetus: 100% of fetuses abort when the infection occurs during the first trimester and there is a risk of preterm delivery, or low birth-weight if infection occurs during the second or third trimester; (*iii*) there is a long-term risk of chronic Q fever in the mother, related to the duration of the disease during the pregnancy, which is not prevented by treatment during pregnancy.

We have reported 23 Q fever cases during pregnancy (48), the majority of which showed complications: 11 fetal deaths and seven preterm births. Only five patients had a normal pregnancy. One-half of the patients show a chronic infection serological profile. As in other mammals, *C. burnetii* could be isolated from milk, placenta, and vaginal secretions. Without treatment, repeated abortions or preterm births are observed during later pregnancies. In mice, endocarditis cases have been reported as a Q-fever complication after repeated pregnancies (49), but this has not been reported in humans. However, in cases of acute Q fever outside pregnancy, there is no risk of relapse during later pregnancies.

General Status
General status, and mainly immunodeficiency, is a risk factor for seriousness and relapses (50): in HIV-infected patients, the Q fever seroprevalence is threefold higher than among blood donors, whereas the yearly incidence of hospitalized cases is 13 times higher than among HIV-negative patients (51). Moreover, immunocompromised patients (HIV-infected or with lymphomas) show a high risk of relapse or evolution to chronic Q fever (52). They are also the only patients able to develop a *C. burnetii* endocarditis without previous valvular abnormality (5,50).

Geographic Variations
Without logical explanation, mainly in terms of contamination, the clinical presentation of acute Q fever varies from country to country, and even from region to region: hepatitis (fever and elevated liver enzymes) is the most common presentation in France (46), in Australia (53), in Ontario (Canada) (54), in Andalusia (Spain) (55), and in California (6), whereas pneumonia is more prevalent in Nova Scotia (Canada) (56), in the Basque Country (Spain) (57), and in Switzerland (58).

Occupational Exposure

All studies stress a higher exposure in the subjects with occupations that require contact with animals, birth products, or slaughtering products. An occupational exposure has been markedly emphasized in a study on neurologic presentations of acute Q fever (29 cases out of 1269 diagnosed in the laboratory) (59).

Inoculum

The role of the *inoculum size* has been demonstrated in animals: only heavy inoculums are able to cause myocarditis or endocarditis in the guinea pig (10). The same role is hypothesized in the intensity of the clinical expression, mainly in myocarditis cases (9).

It seems logical to associate the *route of inoculation* with the variations in clinical presentation. This has been demonstrated in mice (60) and guinea pigs (10), but not in humans: this factor cannot explain the geographic variations.

DIAGNOSTIC TOOLS
Handling of Samples

C. burnetii virulence is particularly high, and numerous cases of laboratory-acquired infections have been reported. Thus, potentially *C. burnetii*-infected biological samples should be handled and processed only by experienced laboratory technicians, in biohazard conditions (P3). The same precautions should be taken for the handling of cell cultures and infected animals.

Serology

C. burnetii exhibits an antigenic variation, due to modifications of the surface lipopolysaccharide. Phase I is the natural, virulent phase, found in infected humans, animals, and arthropods. The less virulent phase II is found only in laboratories, after passages on cell cultures or embryonated eggs.

The diagnosis of Q fever is based on serology, which allows for differentiation between acute and chronic cases. Various techniques have been tested. The most commonly used are complement fixation (61–63), indirect immunofluorescence (64,65), enzyme-linked immunosorbent serologic assay (66–69), and microagglutination (63,70,71).

In our laboratory, indirect immunofluorescence is the reference technique, which is simple and reliable. All the sera are screened, using antigens prepared from the Nine Mile reference *C. burnetii* strain, cultured on L929 mice fibroblasts. For the sera positive at screening IgG, IgM, and IgA are quantified in both phases I and II. These tests allow diagnosis of Q fever and differentiation between acute and chronic Q fever in most cases on a single serum (72). A second serum, two weeks later, is systematically required, in order to observe an increase in antibody titers or a seroconversion. This seroconversion generally occurs between 7 and 30 days after the onset of clinical symptoms. The other techniques lack sensitivity and specificity. The interpretation of the titers and the determination of cut-offs depend on the technique used, and thus on the laboratory, but also on the prevalence of the disease.

Molecular Biology

Direct polymerase chain reaction (PCR) amplification from various biopsy samples [cardiac valve, placenta, aneurism, cerebra spinal fluid (CSF), etc.], from blood or serum, is now the most specific technique used to diagnose *C. burnetii* infections, before seroconversion (73,74). Various genes have been used. In our laboratory, two specific genes (IS1111 and IS30a) are amplified by real-time PCR, using hydrolysis probes. Whatever the amplified gene, the specificity of the amplified fragments must be checked, either by sequencing or by specific hybridation.

Kinetics of the Diagnostic Tests
Acute Q Fever

A diagnosis of acute Q fever is assessed if the phase II IgM titer is greater or equal to 50 and the phase II IgG titer is greater or equal to 200 (72). Figure 2 shows the kinetics of antibodies and other diagnostic tests in acute cases. In acute Q fever, PCR is generally negative when the antibody titer is high (74).

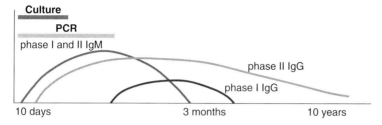

FIGURE 2 Kinetics of antibodies and diagnostic techniques in acute Q fever. *Abbreviation*: PCR, polymerase chain reaction.

Chronic Q Fever

Diagnose chronic Q fever is assessed when the phase I IgG titer is greater than or equal to 1600. However, a titer of 800, associated with phase I IgA can be found in some chronic cases. These results must be interpreted by a specialist, according to clinical criteria (72). Figure 3 shows the kinetics of antibodies and other diagnostic tests in chronic cases. PCR and culture are less frequently positive in endocarditis cases when phase I IgG titer is very high: the association of an elevated IgG titer with positive PCR must evoke chronicity (74).

Culture

C. burnetii isolation from biological samples is carried out on HEL cells, using the shell-vial centrifugation technique (75). The samples must be handled in a laminar flow hood, under P3 biohazard conditions. After inoculation and centrifugation ($700 \times g$ for one hour), the inoculum is withdrawn and replaced by fresh culture medium. The bacterial growth is detected in the shell vial. The presence of *C. burnetii* is carried out on cells using immunofluorescence. Species identification requires molecular biology techniques.

Immunohistochemistry

C. burnetii can be detected on pathology samples (mainly cardiac valves), fresh or formaldehyde fixed. Immunodetection is carried out using immunoperoxidase techniques (76) or immunofluorescence with polyclonal or monoclonal antibodies (77–79). Only this last technique can be used on paraffin-embedded samples (80).

TREATMENT OF Q FEVER

The reference treatment associates doxycycline to hydroxychloroquine, which alkalinizes the phagolysosome in which *C. burnetii* multiplies. Cotrimoxazole and rifampin can be used in case of allergy or contraindication (81,82). The effectiveness of fluoroquinolones is variable (83,84), whereas that of erythromycin is inconsistent, around 30%. *C. burnetii* isolates are susceptible to macrolides in vitro (85–87).

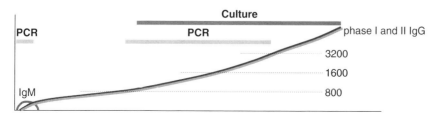

FIGURE 3 Kinetics of antibodies and diagnostic techniques in chronic Q fever. *Abbreviation*: PCR, polymerase chain reaction.

Treatment of Acute Q Fever

Acute Q Fever, Symptomatic at the Time of Diagnosis
Bi Dayly/Ozally Dayly doxycycline prescribed, until one week after apyrexia (81).

Acute Q Fever in Children
It has now been admitted that age is not a contraindication to doxycycline, when this antibiotic is specific of the disease. It has been demonstrated that three treatments lasting 21 days do not cause dental side effects (88).

Acute Q Fever During Pregnancy
Specific treatment using cotrimoxazole (800/160) BID, until delivery, associated to folinic acid (25 mg OD). Hematologic side effects should be monitored every other week (89).

After delivery, if the woman shows a chronic serologic profile, she should be treated as a chronic case, in order to prevent endocarditis and relapsing abortions. Breast feeding is contraindicated (89).

Treatment of Chronic Q Fever

Association of doxycycline and hydroxychloroquine should be prescribed, between 1.5 and 3 years (27). The initial dosing for doxycycline is 100 mg BID and 200 mg TID for hydroxychloroquine. These dosages should be adapted according to Tree day monitoring: doxycycline plasmatic level must remain over 5 µg/ml (90). When available, the *C. burnetii* strain should be cultured from blood or valves in order to evaluate the doxycycline minimal inhibitory concentration (MIC) (which takes three months): the doxycycline plasmatic level should be adjusted between 1.5 and 2 MICs (91). Hydroxychloroquine dosing should also be adapted according to plasmatic levels (1 ± 0.2 mg/L). The usual dosing decreases to 200 mg BID after three to six months, and 200 to 300 mg a day after six months.

The efficiency of this antibiotic treatment is monitored by serological follow-up: a twofold decrease in phase I IgA and phase I IgG is expected after one year of treatment (27).

Treatment of Acute Q Fever in Patients at Risk of Chronic Evolution

An acute Q fever in any patient presenting a risk factor for chronic evolution, valvular damage (even minimal), vascular or valvular graft, aneurism, immunodeficiency (mainly lymphoma), should be treated according to the same protocol as chronic cases. The duration of this treatment is one year (14).

Vaccination

Immunization is the most logical strategy for preventing Q fever in exposed humans, and in animals.

A formaldehyde-inactivated live vaccine (Q-Vax, Commonwealth Serum Laboratories), prepared with phase I *C. burnetii*, Henzerling strain, was approved in Australia in 1989. A preimmunization test is essential. Local reactions are common and important. A single dose of 30 µg confers immunity after 10 to 15 days, lasting at least five years. In endemic zones, people with an occupational exposure might benefit from such a vaccine: abattoir workers, occupational contacts with ruminants (cattle, sheep, goats), and dairy industry.

REFERENCES

1. Maurin M, Raoult D. Q fever. Clin Microbiol Rev 1999; 12(4):518–553.
2. Madariaga MG, Rezai K, Trenholme GM, et al. Q fever: a biological weapon in your backyard. Lancet Infect Dis 2003; 3(11):709–721.
3. Bellamy RJ, Freedman AR. Bioterrorism. Q J Med 2001; 94(4):227–234.
4. Raoult D. Q fever: still a query after all these years. J Med Microbiol 1996; 44(2):77–78.
5. Raoult D, Tissot-Dupont H, Foucault C, et al. Q fever 1985–1998: clinical and epidemiologic features of 1,383 infections. Medicine (Baltimore) 2000; 79(2):109–123.

6. Clark WH, Lennette EH, Railsback OC, et al. Q fever in California. VII. Clinical features in one hundred eighty cases. Arch Intern Med 1951; 88(2):155–167.
7. Ordi-Ros J, Selva-O'Callaghan A, Monegal-Ferran F, et al. Prevalence, significance, and specificity of antibodies to phospholipids in Q fever. Clin Infect Dis 1994; 18(2):213–218.
8. Derrick EH. The course of infection with *Coxiella burnetii*. Med J Aust 1973; 1(21):1051–1057.
9. Fournier PE, Etienne J, Harle JR, et al. Myocarditis, a rare but severe manifestation of Q fever: report of 8 cases and review of the literature. Clin Infect Dis 2001; 32(10):1440–1447.
10. La SB, Lepidi H, Raoult D. Pathologic changes during acute Q fever: influence of the route of infection and inoculum size in infected guinea pigs. Infect Immun 1997; 65(6):2443–2447.
11. Levy PY, Carrieri P, Raoult D. *Coxiella burnetii* pericarditis: report of 15 cases and review. Clin Infect Dis 1999; 29(2):393–397.
12. Lovey PY, Morabia A, Bleed D, et al. Long term vascular complications of *Coxiella burnetii* infection in Switzerland: cohort study. Br Med J 1999; 319(7205):284–286.
13. Wildman M, Ayres JG. Long term vascular complications of *Coxiella burnetii* infection: cardiovascular risk factors cannot be ignored. Br Med J 2000; 320(7226):58–59.
14. Fenollar F, Fournier PE, Carrieri MP, et al. Risks factors and prevention of Q fever endocarditis. Clin Infect Dis 2001; 33(3):312–316.
15. Ayres JG, Flint N, Smith EG, et al. Post-infection fatigue syndrome following Q fever. Q J Med 1998; 91(2):105–123.
16. Penttila IA, Harris RJ, Storm P, et al. Cytokine dysregulation in the post-Q-fever fatigue syndrome. Q J Med 1998; 91(8):549–560.
17. Smith DL, Ayres JG, Blair I, et al. A large Q fever outbreak in the West Midlands: clinical aspects. Respir Med 1993; 87(7):509–516.
18. Boyle B, Hone R. Q fever endocarditis revisited. Ir J Med Sci 1999; 168(1):53–54.
19. Duroux-Vouilloz C, Praz G, Francioli P, et al. Q fever with endocarditis: clinical presentation and serologic follow-up of 21 patients. Schweiz Med Wochenschr 1998; 128(14):521–527.
20. Sanchez-Recalde A, Mate I, Lopez E, et al. *Coxiella burnetii* endocarditis: long-term clinical course in 20 patients. Rev Esp Cardiol 2000; 53(7):940–946.
21. Siegman-Igra Y, Kaufman O, Keysary A, et al. Q fever endocarditis in Israel and a worldwide review. Scand J Infect Dis 1997; 29(1):41–49.
22. Brouqui P, Tissot-Dupont H, Drancourt M, et al. Chronic Q fever: ninety-two cases from France, including 27 cases without endocarditis. Arch Intern Med 1993; 153(5):642–648.
23. Raoult D, Etienne J, Massip P, et al. Q fever endocarditis in the south of France. J Infect Dis 1987; 155(3):570–573.
24. Brouqui P, Raoult D. Endocarditis due to rare and fastidious bacteria. Clin Microbiol Rev 2001; 14(1):177–207.
25. Raoult D, Mege JL, Marrie TJ. Q fever: queries remaining after decades of research. In: Scheld WM, Craig WA, Hugues JM, eds. Emerging Infections. Washington, DC: ASM Press, 2001:29–56.
26. Fournier PE, Casalta JP, Habib G, et al. Modification of the diagnostic criteria proposed by the Duke Endocarditis Service to permit improved diagnosis of Q fever endocarditis. Am J Med 1996; 100(6):629–633.
27. Raoult D, Houpikian P, Tissot-Dupont H, et al. Treatment of Q fever endocarditis: comparison of 2 regimens containing doxycycline and ofloxacin or hydroxychloroquine. Arch Intern Med 1999; 159(2):167–173.
28. Capo C, Zaffran Y, Zugun F, et al. Production of interleukin-10 and transforming growth factor beta by peripheral blood mononuclear cells in Q fever endocarditis. Infect Immun 1996; 64(10):4143–4147.
29. Fournier PE, Casalta JP, Piquet P, et al. *Coxiella burnetii* infection of aneurysms or vascular grafts: report of seven cases and review. Clin Infect Dis 1998; 26(1):116–121.
30. Ellis ME, Smith CC, Moffat MA. Chronic or fatal Q-fever infection: a review of 16 patients seen in North-East Scotland (1967–1980). Q J Med 1983; 52(205):54–66.
31. Fergusson RJ, Shaw TR, Kitchin AH, et al. Subclinical chronic Q fever. Q J Med 1985; 57(222):669–676.
32. Mejia A, Toursarkissian B, Hagino RT, et al. Primary aortoduodenal fistula and Q fever: an underrecognized association? Ann Vasc Surg 2000; 14(3):271–273.
33. Cottalorda J, Jouve JL, Bollini G, et al. Osteoarticular infection due to *Coxiella burnetii* in children. J Pediatr Orthop B 1995; 4(2):219–221.
34. Lipton JH, Fong TC, Gill MJ, et al. Q fever inflammatory pseudotumor of the lung. Chest 1987; 92(4):756–757.
35. Lohuis PJ, Ligtenberg PC, Diepersloot RJ, et al. Q-fever in a patient with a ventriculo-peritoneal drain: case report and short review of the literature. Neth J Med 1994; 44(2):60–64.
36. Kayser K, Wiebel M, Schulz V, et al. Necrotizing bronchitis, angiitis, and amyloidosis associated with chronic Q fever. Respiration 1995; 62(2):114–116.
37. Dupuis G, Peter O, Pedroni J, et al. Clinical aspects observed during an epidemic of 415 cases of Q fever. Schweiz Med Wochenschr 1985; 115(24):814–818.
38. Carrieri MP, Tissot-Dupont H, Rey D, et al. Investigation of a slaughterhouse-related outbreak of Q fever in the French Alps. Eur J Clin Microbiol Infect Dis 2002; 21(1):17–21.

39. Maltezou HC, Raoult D. Q fever in children. Lancet Infect Dis 2002; 2(11):686–691.
40. Richardus JH, Donkers A, Dumas AM, et al. Q fever in the Netherlands: a sero-epidemiological survey among human population groups from 1968 to 1983. Epidemiol Infect 1987; 98(2):211–219.
41. Dupuis G, Vouilloz M, Peter O, et al. Incidence of Q fever in Valais. Rev Med Suisse Romande 1985; 105(10):949–954.
42. Ruiz-Beltran R, Herrero-Herrero JI, Martin-Sanchez AM, et al. Prevalence of antibodies to *Rickettsia conorii*, *Coxiella burnetii* and *Rickettsia typhi* in Salamanca Province (Spain): serosurvey in the human population. Eur J Epidemiol 1990; 6(3):293–299.
43. Antoniou M, Tselentis Y, Babalis T, et al. The seroprevalence of ten zoonoses in two villages of Crete, Greece. Eur J Epidemiol 1995; 11(4):415–423.
44. Jorm LR, Lightfoot NF, Morgan KL. An epidemiological study of an outbreak of Q fever in a secondary school. Epidemiol Infect 1990; 104(3):467–477.
45. Maltezou HC, Constantopoulou I, Kallergi C, et al. Q fever in children in Greece. Am J Trop Med Hyg 2004; 70(5):540–544.
46. Tissot-Dupont H, Raoult D, Brouqui P, et al. Epidemiologic features and clinical presentation of acute Q fever in hospitalized patients: 323 French cases. Am J Med 1992; 93(4):427–434.
47. Leone M, Honstettre A, Lepidi H, et al. Effect of sex on *Coxiella burnetii* infection: protective role of 17beta-estradiol. J Infect Dis 2004; 189(2):339–345.
48. Stein A, Raoult D. Q fever during pregnancy: a public health problem in southern France. Clin Infect Dis 1998; 27(3):592–596.
49. Stein A, Lepidi H, Mege JL, et al. Repeated pregnancies in BALB/c mice infected with *Coxiella burnetii* cause disseminated infection, resulting in stillbirth and endocarditis. J Infect Dis 2000; 181(1):188–194.
50. Raoult D. Host factors in the severity of Q fever. Ann NY Acad Sci 1990; 590:33–38.
51. Raoult D, Levy PY, Tissot-Dupont H, et al. Q fever and HIV infection. AIDS 1993; 7(1):81–86.
52. Raoult D, Brouqui P, Marchou B, et al. Acute and chronic Q fever in patients with cancer. Clin Infect Dis 1992; 14(1):127–130.
53. Bella F, Espejo E, Mauri M, et al. Clinical presentation of acute Australian Q fever. Am J Med 1994; 96(4):397–398.
54. Vellend H, Salit IE, Spence LP. Q fever—Ontario. Can Dis Wkly Rep 1982; 8:170–171.
55. Raoult D, Marrie T. Q fever. Clin Infect Dis 1995; 20(3):489–495.
56. Marrie TJ, Pollak PT. Seroepidemiology of Q fever in Nova Scotia: evidence for age dependent cohorts and geographical distribution. Eur J Epidemiol 1995; 11(1):47–54.
57. Montejo BM, Corral CJ, Aguirre EC. Q fever in the Basque Country: 1981–1984. Rev Infect Dis 1985; 7(5):700–701.
58. Dupuis G, Petite J, Peter O, et al. An important outbreak of human Q fever in a Swiss Alpine valley. Int J Epidemiol 1987; 16(2):282–287.
59. Bernit E, Pouget J, Janbon F, et al. Neurological involvement in acute Q fever: a report of 29 cases and review of the literature. Arch Intern Med 2002; 162(6):693–700.
60. Marrie TJ, Stein A, Janigan D, et al. Route of infection determines the clinical manifestations of acute Q fever. J Infect Dis 1996; 173(2):484–487.
61. Herr S, Huchzermeyer HF, Te Brugge LA, et al. The use of a single complement fixation test technique in bovine brucellosis, Johne's disease, dourine, equine piroplasmosis and Q fever serology. Onderstepoort J Vet Res 1985; 52(4):279–282.
62. Kovacova E, Kazar J, Spanelova D. Suitability of various *Coxiella burnetii* antigen preparations for detection of serum antibodies by various tests. Acta Virol 1998; 42(6):365–368.
63. Nguyen SV, Otsuka H, Zhang GQ, et al. Rapid method for detection of *Coxiella burnetii* antibodies using high-density particle agglutination. J Clin Microbiol 1996; 34(12):2947–2951.
64. Field PR, Hunt JG, Murphy AM. Detection and persistence of specific IgM antibody to *Coxiella burnetii* by enzyme-linked immunosorbent assay: a comparison with immunofluorescence and complement fixation tests. J Infect Dis 1983; 148(3):477–487.
65. Peter O, Dupuis G, Burgdorfer W, et al. Evaluation of the complement fixation and indirect immunofluorescence tests in the early diagnosis of primary Q fever. Eur J Clin Microbiol 1985; 4(4):394–396.
66. Kovacova E, Gallo J, Schramek S, et al. *Coxiella burnetii* antigens for detection of Q fever antibodies by ELISA in human sera. Acta Virol 1987; 31(3):254–259.
67. Peter O, Dupuis G, Peacock MG, et al. Comparison of enzyme-linked immunosorbent assay and complement fixation and indirect fluorescent-antibody tests for detection of *Coxiella burnetii* antibody. J Clin Microbiol 1987; 25(6):1063–1067.
68. Uhaa IJ, Fishbein DB, Olson JG, et al. Evaluation of specificity of indirect enzyme-linked immunosorbent assay for diagnosis of human Q fever. J Clin Microbiol 1994; 32(6):1560–1565.
69. Waag D, Chulay J, Marrie T, et al. Validation of an enzyme immunoassay for serodiagnosis of acute Q fever. Eur J Clin Microbiol Infect Dis 1995; 14(5):421–427.
70. Fiset P, Ormsbee RA, Silberman R, et al. A microagglutination technique for detection and measurement of rickettsial antibodies. Acta Virol 1969; 13(1):60–66.
71. Kazar J, Brezina R, Schramek S, et al. Suitability of the microagglutination test for detection of post-infection and post-vaccination Q fever antibodies in human sera. Acta Virol 1981; 25(4):235–240.

72. Tissot-Dupont H, Thirion X, Raoult D. Q fever serology: cutoff determination for microimmunofluorescence. Clin Diagn Lab Immunol 1994; 1(2):189–196.
73. Fenollar F, Fournier PE, Raoult D. Molecular detection of *Coxiella burnetii* in the sera of patients with Q fever endocarditis or vascular infection. J Clin Microbiol 2004; 42(11):4919–4924.
74. Fournier PE, Raoult D. Comparison of PCR and serology assays for early diagnosis of acute Q fever. J Clin Microbiol 2003; 41(11):5094–5098.
75. Marrero M, Raoult D. Centrifugation-shell vial technique for rapid detection of Mediterranean spotted fever rickettsia in blood culture. Am J Trop Med Hyg 1989; 40(2):197–199.
76. Brouqui P, Dumler JS, Raoult D. Immunohistologic demonstration of *Coxiella burnetii* in the valves of patients with Q fever endocarditis. Am J Med 1994; 97(5):451–458.
77. McCaul TF, Williams JC. Localization of DNA in *Coxiella burnetii* by post-embedding immunoelectron microscopy. Ann NY Acad Sci 1990; 590:136–147.
78. Muhlemann K, Matter L, Meyer B, et al. Isolation of *Coxiella burnetii* from heart valves of patients treated for Q fever endocarditis. J Clin Microbiol 1995; 33(2):428–431.
79. Thiele D, Karo M, Krauss H. Monoclonal antibody based capture ELISA/ELIFA for detection of *Coxiella burnetii* in clinical specimens. Eur J Epidemiol 1992; 8(4):568–574.
80. Raoult D, Laurent JC, Mutillod M. Monoclonal antibodies to *Coxiella burnetii* for antigenic detection in cell cultures and in paraffin-embedded tissues. Am J Clin Pathol 1994; 101(3):318–320.
81. Raoult D. Treatment of Q fever. Antimicrob Agents Chemother 1993; 37(9):1733–1736.
82. Boulos A, Rolain JM, Maurin M, et al. Measurement of the antibiotic susceptibility of *Coxiella burnetii* using real time PCR. Int J Antimicrob Agents 2004; 23(2):169–174.
83. Jabarit-Aldighieri N, Torres H, Raoult D. Susceptibility of *Rickettsia conorii*, *R. rickettsii*, and *Coxiella burnetii* to PD 127,391, PD 131,628, pefloxacin, ofloxacin, and ciprofloxacin. Antimicrob Agents Chemother 1992; 36(11):2529–2532.
84. Raoult D, Bres P, Drancourt M, et al. In vitro susceptibilities of *Coxiella burnetii*, *Rickettsia rickettsii*, and *Rickettsia conorii* to the fluoroquinolone sparfloxacin. Antimicrob Agents Chemother 1991; 35(1):88–91.
85. Rolain JM, Maurin M, Raoult D. Bacteriostatic and bactericidal activities of moxifloxacin against *Coxiella burnetii*. Antimicrob Agents Chemother 2001; 45(1):301–302.
86. Maurin M, Raoult D. Bacteriostatic and bactericidal activity of levofloxacin against *Rickettsia rickettsii*, *Rickettsia conorii*, 'Israeli spotted fever group rickettsia' and *Coxiella burnetii*. J Antimicrob Chemother 1997; 39(6):725–730.
87. Raoult D. Use of macrolides for Q fever. Antimicrob Agents Chemother 2003; 47(1):446.
88. Herz G, Gfeller J. Vibramycin in paediatrics: an evaluation of the onset of action and efficacy. Chemotherapy 1975; 21(suppl 1):58–67.
89. Raoult D, Fenollar F, Stein A. Q fever during pregnancy: diagnosis, treatment, and follow-up. Arch Intern Med 2002; 162(6):701–704.
90. Rolain JM, Mallet MN, Raoult D. Correlation between serum doxycycline concentrations and serologic evolution in patients with *Coxiella burnetii* endocarditis. J Infect Dis 2003; 188(9):1322–1325.
91. Rolain JM, Boulos A, Mallet MN, et al. Correlation between ratio of serum doxycycline concentration to MIC and rapid decline of antibody levels during treatment of Q fever endocarditis. Antimicrob Agents Chemother 2005; 49(7):2673–2676.

Section VI: *WOLBACHIA*

22 | *Wolbachia* and Filarial Nematode Diseases in Humans

Kelly L. Johnston and Mark J. Taylor
Filariasis Research Laboratory, Molecular and Biochemical Parasitology, Liverpool School of Tropical Medicine, Pembroke Place, U.K.

INTRODUCTION

Filariasis is a leading cause of global disability, affecting approximately 138 million individuals throughout the tropics (1,2). Filarial diseases are chronic infections, each with a range of disease manifestations. The reason for the inclusion of a chapter on filarial nematodes in a book on rickettsial diseases is the discovery that many of these parasites have evolved a symbiotic relationship with *Wolbachia* bacteria. Recent research has highlighted the role of this symbiosis in the development and fertility of these nematodes. The bacteria have also been shown to contribute to inflammatory activity associated with disease pathogenesis and adverse reactions to antifilarial drugs and most importantly have provided a novel target for the treatment of filariasis with antibiotics.

FILARIAL NEMATODE PARASITES

Filariasis encompasses two major diseases caused by infection with parasitic filarial nematodes: lymphatic filariasis and onchocerciasis. Although there are eight main species of filarial nematodes that infect humans (*Wuchereria bancrofti*, *Brugia malayi*, *B. timori*, *Onchocerca volvulus*, *Mansonella perstans*, *M. streptocerca*, *M. ozzardi*, and *Loa loa*), only four species are responsible for the majority of morbidity associated with filariasis. These are *W. bancrofti*, *B. malayi*, and *B. timori*, the causative agents of lymphatic filariasis, and *O. volvulus*, which causes onchocerciasis. Evidence so far shows that all of these pathogenic species are dependent on a symbiosis with *Wolbachia* bacteria. Of the remaining species that infect man only *M. ozzardi* has been shown to be infected with *Wolbachia* (3).

Lymphatic Filariasis

The nematodes *W. bancrofti*, *B. malayi*, and *B. timori* are vascular-dwelling parasites transmitted by mosquitoes of the genera *Anopheles*, *Aedes*, *Culex*, and *Mansonia*. The infective stage of the parasite is the third-stage larva (L3). These L3s escape from the mosquito labium or proboscis during feeding and enter the human host through the wound made by the mosquitoes. Following entry, the L3s migrate to the lymphatics and undergo two molts to attain sexual maturity. The adult lymphatic filariae thereafter reside exclusively in the lymphatics. Highly motile adults of both sexes lie coiled within the nodular dilations of the vessels and have an estimated lifespan of 8 to 16 years. The females are ovoviviparous and produce thousands to millions of microfilariae that enter the bloodstream. A mosquito, on taking a blood meal, ingests these forms that migrate through the gut wall. They then penetrate the thoracic muscles and molt to form the second-stage larvae (L2). Following a second molt to the filariform L3, the infective stage moves to the head of the insect in preparation for transmission to a new host.

Lymphatic filariasis is responsible for a disease burden of approximately 5.8 million disability adjusted life years (DALYs). In other words, lymphatic filariasis accounts for a loss of 5.8 million years of productive life due to disability. However, the disabling symptoms of lymphatic filariasis are varied and, importantly, are not present in every infected individual.

The traditional classification of individuals within an endemic area consists of three groups of subjects: endemic normals, asymptomatic microfilaremics, and those with chronic pathology, as reviewed recently by Ravindran (4).

A major risk factor to the development of chronic disease is the occurrence of recurrent episodes of acute filarial lymphangitis, associated with the death of adult worms. These attacks involve an inflammatory response, and repeated episodes of these attacks predispose the individual to developing chronic pathology. One factor is the host immune response. Inflammatory responses are associated with chronic pathology. Another factor associated with the development of elephantiasis is the occurrence of secondary bacterial infections. These bacterial infections occur as a result of the lymphatic dysfunction and can lead to episodes of acute adenolymphangitis. These attacks can be reduced or prevented through the implementation of local hygiene methods of the affected limbs (5).

Onchocerciasis

O. volvulus infects approximately 18 million people worldwide and is transmitted by blackflies (*Simulium* species). The intermediate hosts' requirement for fast-flowing water during larval development leads to a focus of infection around major river systems. Onchocerciasis is endemic in 28 countries in Africa, six countries in the Americas, and in Yemen. In addition, 99% of the 18 million people infected reside in Africa (2).

Like lymphatic filariasis, onchocerciasis is a cause of high levels of morbidity, being responsible for 484,000 DALYs (6). Moreover, a recent study has also shown an increase in host mortality associated with onchocerciasis (7). However, unlike lymphatic filariasis where the pathology is initiated by the adult worms, the microfilariae of *O. volvulus* are responsible for the pathology observed. The pathology consists of cutaneous and ocular manifestations, with the cutaneous symptoms accounting for the majority of pathology observed. Three main groups of individuals exist in endemic areas: (*i*) endemic normals, (*ii*) those with generalized onchocerciasis, and (*iii*) those with a hyperreactive form of onchocerciasis (8,9).

The most severe effect of infection with *O. volvulus* is blindness, which accounts for the name "river blindness." The microfilariae invade the conjunctiva from the skin, and subsequently the cornea. A punctate keratitis develops as a result of an inflammatory response around dead microfilaria. Following years of exposure, a sclerosing keratitis, a hardening inflammation of the cornea can form, causing permanent visual impairment or blindness (10). There are two separate disease patterns in sub-Saharan Africa. The savannah form exhibits a much higher prevalence of blindness in comparison to the disease found in rain-forest regions, even in forest communities where there is a high intensity of infection (11,12).

WOLBACHIA
Discovery and General Characteristics

The first description of *Wolbachia* was made following the discovery of intracellular bacteria within the ovaries of the mosquito *Culex pipiens* (13). At this point, the bacterium was classified as an unnamed *Rickettsia*, although it was subsequently named *Wolbachia pipientis* (14). Since then, *Wolbachia* have been demonstrated in numerous arthropods, including insects, mites, spiders, and crustaceans, and also in filarial nematodes (15–19).

Wolbachia are maternally inherited through the cytoplasm of the egg, and are members of the α-subdivision of proteobacteria. These obligate intracellular bacteria are surrounded by a double-membrane and are found within host-derived membrane-bound vacuoles in the cytoplasm of the cell (20–27). Figure 1 illustrates their ultrastructural characteristics, including the pleomorphic nature of the bacterial cells that range in size from 0.2 to 4 μm in length (28). *Wolbachia* are thought to multiply primarily by binary fission, although a more complex *Chlamydia*-like reproductive cycle may be involved (28). In terms of movement, the lack of flagellar, fimbrial, or pili genes in the *B. malayi Wolbachia* genome suggests that *Wolbachia* are immotile, although actin polymerization may be employed for cell-to-cell spread (29).

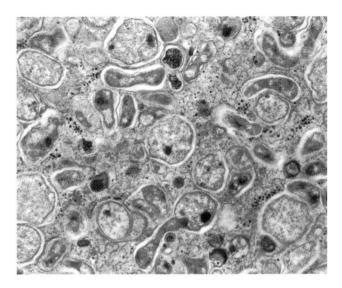

FIGURE 1 Ultrastructural characteristics of *Wolbachia*. Electron micrograph showing *Wolbachia* within vacuoles in a hypodermal lateral cord of an adult female *O. ochengi* nematode. Different forms of *Wolbachia*, including spherical and elongate, can be observed, demonstrating the pleomorphic nature of these bacteria.

Taxonomy and Phylogeny

The genus *Wolbachia* consists of only one valid species, *W. pipientis*, as other members previously assigned to this genus (*W. persica* and *W. melophagi*) do not belong to the α-proteobacteria (30). *W. pipientis*, therefore, is the type species of the genus *Wolbachia*, which, in turn, is a member of the family Anaplasmataceae within the order Rickettsiales. The Anaplasmataceae replicate within host cell membrane–derived vacuoles, whereas all species in the family Rickettsiaceae grow freely in the cytoplasm of their eukaryotic host cells. The phylogenetic relationship between these species is shown in Figure 2 (31).

Although only a single species of *Wolbachia* exists, there is great diversity within the genus. Genetic analysis has allowed the formation of six taxonomic supergroups within the genus, known as supergroups A to F (32,33). Supergroups A and B are found only in arthropods, whereas supergroups C and D are found only in filarial nematodes. The members of supergroups E and F are less well-defined, although supergroup E includes the *Wolbachia* of the springtail *Folsomia candida* and supergroup F encompasses termite wolbachiae and those of the nematode *M. ozzardi* (32,33). Separation between the main lineages of *Wolbachia* may have occurred 50 to 100 million years ago (34,35). C and D (nematode) supergroups of *Wolbachia* have congruent phylogenies with their hosts, but the A and B (arthropod) supergroups do not (34,36). This phylogenetic congruence exhibited by filarial nematodes and their *Wolbachia* endosymbionts is indicative of a strict dependent association, which is further supported by more direct evidence (see below). This also indicates that horizontal transmission occurs between arthropod hosts (34), but not between nematodes.

Wolbachia in Filarial Nematodes
Localization of Wolbachia *Within the Nematode Host*

Unlike arthropod bacteria, which can infect a range of host cells, nematode *Wolbachia* are more restricted, being predominantly found within the lateral hypodermal cord (HC) cells, as shown in Figure 3. The HC cells are syncitial cells that extend throughout the length of the nematode and the bacteria are unevenly distributed throughout the length of this hypodermal tissue (20,23,24,27). *Wolbachia* are also found within the female reproductive tissue, infecting the cell layer surrounding the basal lamina of the oviduct shortly after the molt to adult (23,27). *Wolbachia* are found in all stages of the life cycle of the nematode, although variation in the levels of infection occurs between individual worms and different developmental stages (20,21,27). The bacteria are maternally transmitted through the cytoplasm of the egg. Although the precise mechanisms of bacterial growth and transmission within the nematode are still unknown, recent studies have investigated, using quantitative polymerase chain reaction (qPCR), the population dynamics of the bacterium–nematode association (27,37).

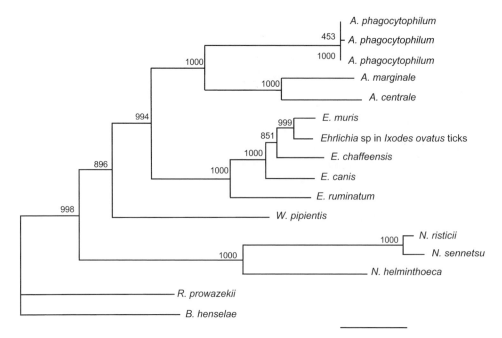

FIGURE 2 Phylogenetic relationship of *W. pipientis* with other rickettsia. Phylogram is based on the deduced amino acid sequences of the citrate synthase gene and was constructed using the neighbor-joining method and the ClustalW program. The scale bar represents 1% divergence, and the numbers at the nodes are the proportions of 1000 bootstrap resamplings. *B. henselae* is *Bartonella henselae*. *Source*: From Ref. 31.

Replication and Population Dynamics

In *B. malayi*, an increase in bacterial numbers coincides with infection of the mammalian host (27). The lowest ratios of *Wolbachia*/nematode DNA are observed in microfilariae and the mosquito-borne larval stages (L2 and L3), but a dramatic increase in division occurs following entry into the mammalian host. A 600-fold increase in bacterial numbers occurs during the first seven days, around the time of the L3-to-L4 molt. The major period of bacterial growth occurs

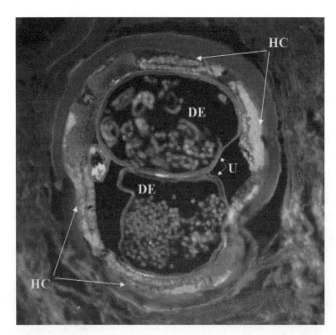

FIGURE 3 *Wolbachia* in a female *O. volvulus* nematode. Anti-*Wolbachia* surface protein immunofluorescence staining of *Wolbachia* in the HC cells of a female *O. volvulus* worm within a nodule. The uteri (U) are also shown, and on close observation *Wolbachia* can be observed in the developing embryos (DEs). *Abbreviations*: HC, hypodermal cord; DE, developing embryo.

during L4 development, within the first month of infection. On maturation, the bacterial numbers were maintained in filaria up to 15 months of age. In female worms, a further increase in numbers occurs due to the presence of *Wolbachia* in the female reproductive organs and DEs (27).

Distribution of Wolbachia in Filarial Nematodes

Nineteen species of the 31 examined are positive for the presence of *Wolbachia*. These include the species responsible for major human disease (including *B. malayi*, *B. timori*, *W. bancrofti*, and *O. volvulus*) in addition to species of veterinary importance, such as *Dirofilaria immitis*, the agent of canine/feline heartworm disease. However, the less pathogenic species have been found to be *Wolbachia*-negative. The most notable of these are the species *L. loa* and *M. perstans* (38–42). Given that the phylogenies of *Wolbachia* and their host nematodes are congruent, the absence of the bacteria in these species implies that there have been events of symbiont loss during evolution (42). Overall, the symbiosis of *Wolbachia* with their nematode hosts appears stable, as *Wolbachia*-positive species are present along the main branches of filarial evolution (36). Of those nematode species that harbor *Wolbachia*, the prevalence appears to be 100%, indicating that the relationship between the nematode and *Wolbachia* is obligatory in those species.

Role of Wolbachia in Filarial Biology

The bacterium and its host, the filarial nematode, appear to have evolved a mutualistic symbiosis. The precise nature of this symbiosis has yet to be elucidated, although many studies using antibiotics have shed some light on the involvement of *Wolbachia* in important aspects of filarial biology, such as in embryogenesis and molting. In addition to these processes, *Wolbachia* may also play a role in maintaining the general health of the nematode both metabolically and through protection from the host's immune response.

A number of antibiotic-based studies have been conducted, which emphasize the dependency of the filarial nematode on its bacterial symbiont. Antibiotic treatments of *Wolbachia*-containing nematodes have demonstrated a range of deleterious effects. These include the inhibition of larval development, the inhibition of embryogenesis, infertility, and the stunting of adult worm growth. It is notable that larval and embryonic development are especially prone to disruption through the action of bacteriostatic drugs, as in these stages of development the *Wolbachia* divide most rapidly (41). This may also explain the prolonged effects on other stages of the parasite, such as the adult, in which the bacteria are more slowly dividing. It has been demonstrated that the macrofilaricidal activity of an antibiotic may only become evident after one year following treatment (43).

Nematode Metabolism and Survival: Genomic Analysis

Despite the evidence that exists regarding the involvement of *Wolbachia* in the reproduction and development of the parasite, the precise mechanisms by which *Wolbachia* contributes to these events are still unknown. However, the recent sequencing and annotation of the *Wolbachia* genome (29) has implicated one such possible mechanism in the form of the metabolite heme, which appears to be absent from the nematode genome in *B. malayi*. The involvement of heme-containing ecdysteroid-like hormones in filarial molting and reproduction (44) may be dependent on *Wolbachia* as a source of heme (29,45). In addition, *Wolbachia* have complete pathways for de novo biosynthesis of purines and pyrimidines. These are thought to supplement the nucleotide pool of the nematode and, therefore, the need for this resource may be especially important at times of DNA synthesis, such as at embryogenesis.

The localization of *Wolbachia* may allude to its role in the nutrition and metabolism of the nematode. The high concentration of bacteria within the lateral HCs suggests that they may be involved in the transcuticular uptake and processing of nutrients (46,47). *Wolbachia* has all genes for biosynthesis of fatty acids and contains all enzymes for the biosynthesis of riboflavin and flavin adenine dinucleotide. However, on the other side of this relationship, *Wolbachia* must receive factors from the nematode in return. *Wolbachia*, for example, lack the capability to synthesize amino acids, with the exception of *meso*-diaminopimelate, which must therefore be supplied by the host nematode. Indeed, the bacteria are thought to use amino acids as growth substrates obtained through the proteolysis of host proteins by *Wolbachia* proteases. Other examples of components supplied by the nematode include the precursors required for biosynthesis of vitamins and cofactors such as coenzyme A, biotin, and folate.

Aside from providing metabolites, it has also been suggested that *Wolbachia* may contribute to the long-term survival of the nematode within the immunocompetent host (48). *Wolbachia* possess the genes for the biosynthesis of glutathione (29), a compound known to protect against oxidative stress.

Role of *Wolbachia* in Filarial Pathogenesis
Inflammatory Activity of Wolbachia

Soluble extracts of *B. malayi* have been demonstrated to induce the production of proinflammatory cytokines by macrophages in vitro. In contrast, soluble extracts of the aposymbiotic species *Acanthocheilonema viteae* did not stimulate macrophages, and furthermore, only *Wolbachia*-containing extracts from insect cell lines induced an inflammatory response, strongly suggesting a role for *Wolbachia* in this response (49). Similarly, another study demonstrated that soluble extracts of *O. volvulus* and *O. ochengi* induced the production of pro- and antiinflammatory cytokines from isolated monocytes in vitro (50).

Extracts prepared from *O. volvulus* extirpated from doxycycline-treated and untreated patients were compared in terms of neutrophil chemotactic activity and in the stimulation of human monocytes (51). It was demonstrated that extracts from untreated patients had neutrophil chemotactic activity and induced strong tumor necrosis factor (TNF) and interleukin-8 (IL-8) production from monocytes, in contrast to the extracts from antibiotic-treated nematodes. This chemotactic activity was also demonstrated in vivo in these patients, as nodules from drug-treated patients contained a much reduced neutrophil accumulation around the worms (51). Indeed, a similar study also demonstrated that *B. malayi* extracts activated murine neutrophils in vitro to produce the neutrophil chemotactic factors, macrophage inflammatory protein-2, and keratinocyte-derived chemokine, which was greatly reduced when extracts from doxycycline-treated worms were used to stimulate cells (52). The role for *Wolbachia* in this neutrophil activation was clearly demonstrated by the fact that whole, purified *Wolbachia* were also able to activate neutrophils in vitro (52).

Together with other members of the Anaplasmataceae, *Wolbachia* lack the genes required for lipopolysaccharide biosynthesis (29,53) and, therefore, other *Wolbachia*-derived molecules must be involved. One such molecule that has been a subject of investigation is the major surface protein (WSP) of *Wolbachia*.

Recombinant WSP (rWSP) from *D. immitis* has been shown to activate IL-8 transcription in canine neutrophils and was also found to stimulate chemokinesis of these cells (54). In another study, proinflammatory cytokines, including TNF, IL-12, and IL-8, were produced in response to *D. immitis* rWSP by cells of the innate immune system (55). This stimulation by rWSP was also found to involve toll-like receptors (TLRs), TLR2 and TLR4, but not any other TLRs. This work suggests that WSP has major involvement in the innate, and adaptive, responses to *Wolbachia*, although further investigation is required to determine whether this is the dominant or exclusive inflammatory molecule of *Wolbachia*.

A murine model of onchocerciasis has highlighted the involvement of *Wolbachia* in the corneal pathology associated with onchocerciasis. Extracts from doxycycline-treated *O. volvulus* and the aposymbiotic species *A. viteae* produced minimal stromal thickness, stromal haze, and neutrophil infiltration than extracts from *B. malayi* and *O. volvulus*, thereby indicating a role for *Wolbachia* (56). In a further study, in which *B. malayi* microfilariae were injected directly into the cornea, it was demonstrated that neutrophils associated directly with the microfilariae and, furthermore, that the WSP was present within neutrophil phagolysosomes (52). This work was conducted in conjunction with in vitro neutrophil stimulation assays using whole *Wolbachia* and suggested that the death of microfilariae in the eye promotes the release of chemokines in response to *Wolbachia*. This results in the recruitment of neutrophils that subsequently ingest *Wolbachia*, stimulating the production of proinflammatory cytokines and chemokines and thereby leading to further neutrophil recruitment. This process ultimately results in a cytotoxic effect on resident cells thus contributing to visual impairment (52). Furthermore, two different epidemiological patterns of disease caused by *O. volvulus* in sub-Saharan Africa exist. The savannah form is typically more severe, with a high prevalence of blindness and, interestingly, the savannah strains of *O. volvulus* were found to have a significantly higher *Wolbachia* DNA to nematode DNA ratio than the milder forest strains (57), thereby supporting a role for these bacteria in onchocercal pathogenesis.

The release of *Wolbachia* or *Wolbachia* products throughout the life span of the adult worms may occur through the release of uterine debris with the microfilariae (28) or alternatively from developing larval stages that fail to reach maturity. The repeated exposure of innate immune cells to *Wolbachia* may result in the desensitization of these cells and therefore increase the susceptibility to opportunistic pathogens, as is often observed in patients with lymphoedema and elephantiasis (58).

Wolbachia *and Adverse Post-Treatment Reactions*

Adverse post-treatment reactions to filarial chemotherapy occur as a result of a systemic inflammatory response. In lymphatic filariasis, the severity of these adverse reactions is associated with increasing proinflammatory cytokine production and high pretreatment parasite burdens (59). These reactions, characterized by headache, fever, and myalgia, are similar to the acute inflammatory responses observed with bacterial infections (59). Analysis of plasma samples by PCR and immunoelectron microscopy demonstrated the persistence of *Wolbachia* in the blood of patients with severe systemic inflammatory reactions (60). A similar observation was made in patients with onchocerciasis. An increased peripheral neutrophil count was accompanied by increased levels of TNF and antibacterial peptides, demonstrating that *Wolbachia* played a prominent role in these post-treatment reactions (61).

Wolbachia *and the Adaptive Immune Response: Serology*

Although antibody responses to a number of *Wolbachia* antigens, such as an aspartate aminotransferase and HtrA-type serine protease (62,63) have been reported, the antibody responses to the major surface protein, WSP, are the most well characterized. Anti-WSP antibody responses have been demonstrated in filarial infections of cats (64,65), dogs (66), rhesus monkeys (67), mice (68), and humans (55,68–70).

Anti-WSP antibody responses have been associated with disease. In rhesus monkeys experimentally infected with *B. malayi*, only two out of 12 monkeys exhibited IgG responses to WSP and both the WSP-positive monkeys developed lymphoedema after becoming amicrofilaremic (67). This association between WSP reactivity and disease has also been demonstrated in humans. Human subjects with chronic disease, such as lymphoedema and hydrocele, were more likely to be seropositive for anti-WSP IgG (68,69). Also, in *D. immitis* infection of humans, in which the human is a dead-end host, an IgG response against WSP was only detectable in patients with pulmonary nodules and not in healthy donors from endemic areas, again suggesting that exposure of *Wolbachia* to the immune system is related to clinical disease (70).

The death of adult worms is a significant factor involved in the development of chronic disease in filariasis (71) and this maybe associated with the release of *Wolbachia* and the activation of WSP-specific immune responses. The evidence that *Wolbachia* bacteria play a significant role in the pathogenesis of filariasis, in addition to the vital roles played in the biology of the parasites, offers a new target for the control of filarial disease.

Wolbachia *as a Drug Target for Filariasis*

Soon after the "rediscovery" of *Wolbachia* in filarial nematodes, the targeting of *Wolbachia* was identified as a novel strategy to develop better antifilarial chemotherapy (72). Mass drug administration programs are currently ongoing, with a view to eliminating human filariasis (73). These programs are predominantly transmission control programs, in that the drugs used [ivermectin, albendazole, and diethylcarbamazine (DEC)] have limited adulticidal effects, and the adult worms are long-lived. In addition, to interrupt transmission the mass drug administration has to be repeated annually and for several years (74), although annual treatment may not be sufficient to prevent the transmission of onchocerciasis (75,76). The drugs currently used do not affect early microfilariae production and therefore a reemergence of microfilariae occurs. Treatments with permanent sterilization or macrofilaricidal activity have been a long sought-after goal in filariasis research.

Anti-Wolbachia *Chemotherapy in Humans*

A number of studies have been conducted in order to investigate the effects of depletion of *Wolbachia* on their filarial hosts. Initial experiments conducted in animals and in vitro prompted the consideration of *Wolbachia* as a target for control of human filariasis (72,77).

Clinical trials of anti-*Wolbachia* treatment have been conducted using doxycycline treatment. Initial trials involved a six-week course of this drug at 100 mg/day as a treatment against *O. volvulus*, and it was established that this treatment led to the depletion of *Wolbachia* and the long-term sterility of adult female worms. This block in embryogenesis resulted in a sustained reduction in skin microfilariae—the agents of disease in onchocerciasis (77–79). Similarly, an almost complete elimination of microfilaremia was observed following doxycycline treatment of *W. bancrofti* infection (80).

Macrofilaricidal activity of a filarial drug would be extremely advantageous and such activity is observed after sustained antibiotic treatment in animal models (46). A randomized, placebo-controlled trial demonstrated such macrofilaricidal activity in *W. bancrofti* infection (43). In this study, a treatment regimen of 200 mg doxycycline/day was administered for a period of eight weeks. An almost complete elimination of microfilaremia was observed with macrofilaricidal effects demonstrated by a lack of scrotal worm nests detectable by ultrasonography and a decrease in circulating filarial antigen levels in doxycycline-treated individuals compared to the placebo group (43). The macrofilaricidal activity was observed at 14 months post-treatment, suggesting that macrofilaricidal activity of antibiotic treatment may take more than one year following the onset of treatment to become evident. This slow death of filariae, however, offers a potential benefit in the avoidance of adverse post-treatment reactions.

Anti-*Wolbachia* chemotherapy, therefore, offers a sustained, and possibly permanent, block of embryogenesis and the destruction of adult worms with superior efficacy in lymphatic filariasis and onchocerciasis compared with standard treatments. Also, the anti-*Wolbachia* drugs are already licensed and available in endemic areas and, therefore, preclude the restrictive costs of developing new compounds. However, at present, antibiotic therapy for use in mass drug administration cannot be implemented due to logistic difficulties of long-term treatments together with known contraindications of doxycycline in children under nine years of age, as well as in pregnant and breastfeeding women. Current research is aimed at identifying alternative antibiotics effective at eliminating *Wolbachia* suitable for mass treatment strategies.

REFERENCES

1. WHO. Lymphatic filariae fact sheet No. 102. www.who.int/inf-fs/en/fact102.html, 2000.
2. WHO. Onchocerciasis: strategic direction for research. www.who.int/tdr/diseases/oncho/direction.htm, 2002.
3. Taylor MJ, Bandi C, Hoerauf A. *Wolbachia* bacterial endosymbionts of filarial nematodes. Adv Parasitol 2005; 60:245–284.
4. Ravindran B. Aping Jane Goodall: insights into human lymphatic filariasis. Trends Parasitol 2003; 19(3):105–109.
5. Shenoy RK. Management of disability in lymphatic filariasis—an update. J Commun Dis 2002; 34(1):1–14.
6. WHO. The world health report 2004. www.who.int/whr/2004/en/index.html, 2004.
7. Little MP, Breitling LP, Basanez MG, et al. Association between microfilarial load and excess mortality in onchocerciasis: an epidemiological study. Lancet 2004; 363(9420):1514–1521.
8. Hoerauf A, Brattig N. Resistance and susceptibility in human onchocerciasis—beyond Th1 vs. Th2. Trends Parasitol 2002; 18(1):25–31.
9. Brattig NW. Pathogenesis and host responses in human onchocerciasis: impact of *Onchocerca* filariae and *Wolbachia* endobacteria. Microbes Infect 2004; 6(1):113–128.
10. Burnham G. Onchocerciasis. Lancet 1998; 351(9112):1341–1346.
11. Remme J, Dadzie KY, Rolland A, et al. Ocular onchocerciasis and intensity of infection in the community. I. West African savanna. Trop Med Parasitol 1989; 40(3):340–347.
12. Dadzie KY, Remme J, Rolland A, et al. Ocular onchocerciasis and intensity of infection in the community. II. West African rainforest foci of the vector *Simulium yahense*. Trop Med Parasitol 1989; 40(3):348–354.
13. Hertig M, Wolbach S. Studies on rickettsia-like microorganisms in insects. J Med Res 1924; 44:329–374.
14. Hertig M. The Rickettsia, *Wolbachia pipientis* (gen. et sp. n.) and associated inclusions of the Mosquito, *Culex pipiens*. Parasitology 1936; 28:453–486.
15. Werren JH. Biology of *Wolbachia*. Annu Rev Entomol 1997; 42:587–609.

16. Taylor MJ, Hoerauf A. *Wolbachia* bacteria of filarial nematodes. Parasitol Today 1999; 15(11):437–442.
17. Bandi C, Anderson TJ, Genchi C, et al. The *Wolbachia* endosymbionts of filarial nematodes. In: Kennedy MW, Harnett W, eds. Parasitic Nematodes: Molecular Biology, Biochemistry and Immunology. Oxford: CAB International, 2001:25–43.
18. Bandi C, Dunn AM, Hurst GD, et al. Inherited microorganisms, sex-specific virulence and reproductive parasitism. Trends Parasitol 2001; 17(2):88–94.
19. Stevens L, Giordano R, Fialho RF. Male-killing, nematode infections, bacteriophage infection, and virulence of cytoplasmic bacteria in the genus *Wolbachia*. Annu Rev Ecol Syst 2001; 32:519–545.
20. Kozek WJ, Marroquin HF. Intracytoplasmic bacteria in *Onchocerca volvulus*. Am J Trop Med Hyg 1977; 26(4):663–678.
21. Kozek WJ. Transovarially-transmitted intracellular microorganisms in adult and larval stages of *Brugia malayi*. J Parasitol 1977; 63(6):992–1000.
22. O'Neill SL, Pettigrew MM, Sinkins SP, et al. In vitro cultivation of *Wolbachia pipientis* in an *Aedes albopictus* cell line. Insect Mol Biol 1997; 6(1):33–39.
23. Taylor MJ, Bilo K, Cross HF, et al. 16S rDNA phylogeny and ultrastructural characterization of *Wolbachia* intracellular bacteria of the filarial nematodes *Brugia malayi*, *B. pahangi*, and *Wuchereria bancrofti*. Exp Parasitol 1999; 91(4):356–361.
24. Egyed Z, Sreter T, Szell Z, et al. Electron microscopic and molecular identification of *Wolbachia* endosymbionts from *Onchocerca lupi*: implications for therapy. Vet Parasitol 2002; 106(1):75–82.
25. Fischer P, Schmetz C, Bandi C, et al. *Tunga penetrans*: molecular identification of *Wolbachia* endobacteria and their recognition by antibodies against proteins of endobacteria from filarial parasites. Exp Parasitol 2002; 102(3–4):201–211.
26. Noda H, Miyoshi T, Koizumi Y. In vitro cultivation of *Wolbachia* in insect and mammalian cell lines. In Vitro Cell Dev Biol Anim 2002; 38(7):423–427.
27. McGarry HF, Egerton GL, Taylor MJ. Population dynamics of *Wolbachia* bacterial endosymbionts in *Brugia malayi*. Mol Biochem Parasitol 2004; 135(1):57–67.
28. Kozek WJ. What is new in the *Wolbachia*/*Dirofilaria* interaction? Vet Parasitol 2005; 133(2–3):127–132.
29. Foster J, Ganatra M, Kamal I, et al. The *Wolbachia* genome of *Brugia malayi*: endosymbiont evolution within a human pathogenic nematode. PLoS Biol 2005; 3(4):e121.
30. Dumler JS, Barbet AF, Bekker CP, et al. Reorganization of genera in the families Rickettsiaceae and Anaplasmataceae in the order *Rickettsiales*: unification of some species of *Ehrlichia* with *Anaplasma*, *Cowdria* with *Ehrlichia* and *Ehrlichia* with *Neorickettsia*, descriptions of six new species combinations and designation of *Ehrlichia equi* and 'HGE agent' as subjective synonyms of *Ehrlichia phagocytophila*. Int J Syst Evol Microbiol 2001; 51(pt 6):2145–2165.
31. Fenollar F, La Scola B, Inokuma H, et al. Culture and phenotypic characterization of a *Wolbachia pipientis* isolate. J Clin Microbiol 2003; 41(12):5434–5441.
32. Lo N, Casiraghi M, Salati E, et al. How many *Wolbachia* supergroups exist? Mol Biol Evol 2002; 19(3):341–346.
33. Casiraghi M, Werren JH, Bazzocchi C, et al. dnaA gene sequences from *Wolbachia pipientis* support subdivision into supergroups and provide no evidence for recombination in the lineages infecting nematodes. Parassitologia 2003; 45(1):13–18.
34. Werren JH, Zhang W, Guo LR. Evolution and phylogeny of *Wolbachia*: reproductive parasites of arthropods. Proc R Soc Lond B Biol Sci 1995; 261(1360):55–63.
35. Bandi C, Anderson TJ, Genchi C, et al. Phylogeny of *Wolbachia* in filarial nematodes. Proc R Soc Lond B Biol Sci 1998; 265(1413):2407–2413.
36. Casiraghi M, Anderson TJ, Bandi C, et al. A phylogenetic analysis of filarial nematodes: comparison with the phylogeny of *Wolbachia* endosymbionts. Parasitology 2001; 122(1):93–103.
37. Fenn K, Blaxter M. Quantification of *Wolbachia* bacteria in *Brugia malayi* through the nematode lifecycle. Mol Biochem Parasitol 2004; 137(2):361–364.
38. Brouqui P, Fournier PE, Raoult D. Doxycycline and eradication of microfilaremia in patients with loiasis. Emerg Infect Dis 2001; 7(suppl 3):604–605.
39. Grobusch MP, Kombila M, Autenrieth I, et al. No evidence of *Wolbachia* endosymbiosis with *Loa loa* and *Mansonella perstans*. Parasitol Res 2003; 90(5):405–408.
40. Buttner DW, Wanji S, Bazzocchi C, et al. Obligatory symbiotic *Wolbachia* endobacteria are absent from *Loa loa*. Filaria J 2003; 2(1):10.
41. McGarry HF, Pfarr K, Egerton G, et al. Evidence against *Wolbachia* symbiosis in *Loa loa*. Filaria J 2003; 2(1):9.
42. Casiraghi M, Bain O, Guerrero R, et al. Mapping the presence of *Wolbachia pipientis* on the phylogeny of filarial nematodes: evidence for symbiont loss during evolution. Int J Parasitol 2004; 34(2):191–203.
43. Taylor MJ, Makunde WH, McGarry HF, et al. Macrofilaricidal activity after doxycycline treatment of *Wuchereria bancrofti*: a double-blind, randomised placebo-controlled trial. Lancet 2005; 365(9477):2116–2121.
44. Warbrick EV, Barker GC, Rees HH, et al. The effect of invertebrate hormones and potential hormone inhibitors on the third larval moult of the filarial nematode, *Dirofilaria immitis*, in vitro. Parasitology 1993; 107(4):459–463.

45. Pfarr K, Hoerauf A. The annotated genome of *Wolbachia* from the filarial nematode *Brugia malayi*: what it means for progress in antifilarial medicine. PLoS Med 2005; 2(4):e110.
46. Langworthy NG, Renz A, Mackenstedt U, et al. Macrofilaricidal activity of tetracycline against the filarial nematode *Onchocerca ochengi*: elimination of *Wolbachia* precedes worm death and suggests a dependent relationship. Proc R Soc Lond B Biol Sci 2000; 267(1448):1063–1069.
47. Sacchi L, Corona S, Kramer L, et al. Ultrastructural evidence of the degenerative events occurring during embryogenesis of the filarial nematode *Brugia pahangi* after tetracycline treatment. Parassitologia 2003; 45(2):89–96.
48. Townson S, Hutton D, Siemienska J, et al. Antibiotics and *Wolbachia* in filarial nematodes: antifilarial activity of rifampicin, oxytetracycline and chloramphenicol against *Onchocerca gutturosa*, *Onchocerca lienalis* and *Brugia pahangi*. Ann Trop Med Parasitol 2000; 94(8):801–816.
49. Taylor MJ, Cross HF, Bilo K. Inflammatory responses induced by the filarial nematode *Brugia malayi* are mediated by lipopolysaccharide-like activity from endosymbiotic *Wolbachia* bacteria. J Exp Med 2000; 191(8):1429–1436.
50. Brattig NW, Rathjens U, Ernst M, et al. Lipopolysaccharide-like molecules derived from *Wolbachia* endobacteria of the filaria *Onchocerca volvulus* are candidate mediators in the sequence of inflammatory and antiinflammatory responses of human monocytes. Microbes Infect 2000; 2(10):1147–1157.
51. Brattig NW, Buttner DW, Hoerauf A. Neutrophil accumulation around *Onchocerca* worms and chemotaxis of neutrophils are dependent on *Wolbachia* endobacteria. Microbes Infect 2001; 3(6):439–446.
52. Gillette-Ferguson I, Hise AG, McGarry HF, et al. *Wolbachia*-induced neutrophil activation in a mouse model of ocular onchocerciasis (river blindness). Infect Immun 2004; 72(10):5687–5692.
53. Wu M, Sun LV, Vamathevan J, et al. Phylogenomics of the reproductive parasite *Wolbachia pipientis* wMel: a streamlined genome overrun by mobile genetic elements. PLoS Biol 2004; 2(3):E69.
54. Bazzocchi C, Genchi C, Paltrinieri S, et al. Immunological role of the endosymbionts of *Dirofilaria immitis*: the *Wolbachia* surface protein activates canine neutrophils with production of IL-8. Vet Parasitol 2003; 117(1–2):73–83.
55. Brattig NW, Bazzocchi C, Kirschning CJ, et al. The major surface protein of *Wolbachia* endosymbionts in filarial nematodes elicits immune responses through TLR2 and TLR4. J Immunol 2004; 173(1):437–445.
56. Saint Andre A, Blackwell NM, Hall LR, et al. The role of endosymbiotic *Wolbachia* bacteria in the pathogenesis of river blindness. Science 2002; 295(5561):1892–1895.
57. Higazi TB, Filiano A, Katholi CR, et al. *Wolbachia* endosymbiont levels in severe and mild strains of *Onchocerca volvulus*. Mol Biochem Parasitol 2005; 141(1):109–112.
58. Taylor MJ, Cross HF, Ford L, et al. *Wolbachia* bacteria in filarial immunity and disease. Parasite Immunol 2001; 23(7):401–409.
59. Haarbrink M, Abadi GK, Buurman WA, et al. Strong association of interleukin-6 and lipopolysaccharide-binding protein with severity of adverse reactions after diethylcarbamazine treatment of microfilaremic patients. J Infect Dis 2000; 182(2):564–569.
60. Cross HF, Haarbrink M, Egerton G, et al. Severe reactions to filarial chemotherapy and release of *Wolbachia* endosymbionts into blood. Lancet 2001; 358(9296):1873–1875.
61. Keiser PB, Reynolds SM, Awadzi K, et al. Bacterial endosymbionts of *Onchocerca volvulus* in the pathogenesis of posttreatment reactions. J Infect Dis 2002; 185(6):805–811.
62. Fischer P, Bonow I, Buttner DW, et al. An aspartate aminotransferase of *Wolbachia* endobacteria from *Onchocerca volvulus* is recognized by IgG1 antibodies from residents of endemic areas. Parasitol Res 2003; 90(1):38–47.
63. Jolodar A, Fischer P, Buttner DW, et al. *Wolbachia* endosymbionts of *Onchocerca volvulus* express a putative periplasmic HtrA-type serine protease. Microbes Infect 2004; 6(2):141–149.
64. Bazzocchi C, Ceciliani F, McCall JW, et al. Antigenic role of the endosymbionts of filarial nematodes: IgG response against the *Wolbachia* surface protein in cats infected with *Dirofilaria immitis*. Proc R Soc Lond B Biol Sci 2000; 267(1461):2511–2516.
65. Morchon R, Ferreira AC, Martin-Pacho JR, et al. Specific IgG antibody response against antigens of *Dirofilaria immitis* and its *Wolbachia* endosymbiont bacterium in cats with natural and experimental infections. Vet Parasitol 2004; 125(3–4):313–321.
66. Kramer LH, Tamarozzi F, Morchon R, et al. Immune response to and tissue localization of the *Wolbachia* surface protein (WSP) in dogs with natural heartworm (*Dirofilaria immitis*) infection. Vet Immunol Immunopathol 2005; 106(3–4):303–308.
67. Punkosdy GA, Dennis VA, Lasater BL, et al. Detection of serum IgG antibodies specific for *Wolbachia* surface protein in rhesus monkeys infected with *Brugia malayi*. J Infect Dis 2001; 184(3):385–389.
68. Lamb TJ, Le Goff L, Kurniawan A, et al. Most of the response elicited against *Wolbachia* surface protein in filarial nematode infection is due to the infective larval stage. J Infect Dis 2004; 189(1):120–127.
69. Punkosdy GA, Addiss DG, Lammie PJ. Characterization of antibody responses to *Wolbachia* surface protein in humans with lymphatic filariasis. Infect Immun 2003; 71(9):5104–5114.
70. Simon F, Prieto G, Morchon R, et al. Immunoglobulin G antibodies against the endosymbionts of filarial nematodes (*Wolbachia*) in patients with pulmonary dirofilariasis. Clin Diagn Lab Immunol 2003; 10(1):180–181.

71. Dreyer G, Noroes J, Figueredo-Silva J, et al. Pathogenesis of lymphatic disease in bancroftian filariasis: a clinical perspective. Parasitol Today 2000; 16(12):544–548.
72. Taylor MJ, Bandi C, Hoerauf A, et al. *Wolbachia* bacteria of filarial nematodes: a target for control? Parasitol Today 2000; 16(5):179–180.
73. Molyneux DH, Bradley M, Hoerauf A, et al. Mass drug treatment for lymphatic filariasis and onchocerciasis. Trends Parasitol 2003; 19(11):516–522.
74. Ottesen EA. The global programme to eliminate lymphatic filariasis. Trop Med Int Health 2000; 5(9):591–594.
75. Richards F, Hopkins D, Cupp E. Programmatic goals and approaches to onchocerciasis. Lancet 2000; 355(9216):1663–1664.
76. Abiose A, Homeida M, Liese B, et al. Onchocerciasis control strategies. Lancet 2000; 356(9240):1523–1524.
77. Hoerauf A, Volkmann L, Hamelmann C, et al. Endosymbiotic bacteria in worms as targets for a novel chemotherapy in filariasis. Lancet 2000; 355(9211):1242–1243.
78. Hoerauf A, Mand S, Adjei O, et al. Depletion of *Wolbachia* endobacteria in *Onchocerca volvulus* by doxycycline and microfilaridermia after ivermectin treatment. Lancet 2001; 357(9266):1415–1416.
79. Hoerauf A, Mand S, Volkmann L, et al. Doxycycline in the treatment of human onchocerciasis: kinetics of *Wolbachia* endobacteria reduction and of inhibition of embryogenesis in female *Onchocerca* worms. Microbes Infect 2003; 5(4):261–273.
80. Hoerauf A, Mand S, Fischer K, et al. Doxycycline as a novel strategy against bancroftian filariasis-depletion of *Wolbachia* endosymbionts from *Wuchereria bancrofti* and stop of microfilaria production. Med Microbiol Immunol (Berl) 2003; 192(4):211–216.

Section VII: DIAGNOSTIC STRATEGY OF RICKETTSIAL DISEASES IN HUMANS

23 | Diagnostic Strategy of Rickettsioses and Ehrlichioses

Florence Fenollar, Pierre-Edouard Fournier, and Didier Raoult
Faculté de Médecine, Unité des Rickettsies, Université de la Méditerranée, Marseille, France

INTRODUCTION

Traditional identification methods used in bacteriology are hardly applicable to rickettsiae because of the few phenotypic characters expressed by these strictly intracellular organisms. As a consequence, "rickettsia" has long been used as a generic term for many small bacteria that could not be cultivated. However, the taxonomy of bacteria within the order Rickettsiales has been reorganized over recent years and continues to be modified as new data become available (1–3). Currently, this order contains the family Rickettsiaceae, which includes the genera *Rickettsia* and *Orientia*, and the family Anaplasmataceae, which groups the genera *Ehrlichia*, *Anaplasma*, *Neorickettsia*, and *Wolbachia*.

Rickettsial diseases are among the oldest known arthropod-borne diseases (4). Until 1984, few rickettsioses had been reported, including Rocky Mountain spotted fever (RMSF), Mediterranean spotted fever (MSF), rickettsialpox, epidemic typhus, murine typhus, Siberian tick typhus, Israeli spotted fever, and Queensland tick typhus. Over the last 12 years, another 11 of these infections have been characterized, including Astrakhan fever, Flinders Island spotted fever, African tick-bite fever (ATBF), Japanese spotted fever, tick-borne lymphadenitis (TIBOLA), lymphangitis-associated rickettsiosis, Far Eastern rickettsiosis, and unnamed infections caused by *Rickettsia helvetica*, *R. aeschlimannii*, *R. massiliae*, and *R. parkeri* (5–10). Thus, many of the currently known tick-borne rickettsial diseases are considered to be emerging infections. Various circumstances have played a role in the recent description of new rickettsioses, including: (*i*) clinician curiosity; (*ii*) modification of human behavior, as seen in ATBF with the development of tourism to sub-Saharan Africa (11); and (*iii*) development of new diagnostic tools, including new cell-culture systems (12) or new serology and molecular methods (13).

In this chapter, we will consider various aspects of the diagnosis of rickettsioses and ehrlichioses including modern diagnostic tools.

CLINICAL SUSPICION

Although the advent of novel diagnostic tools, such as cell culture and molecular amplification, has dramatically improved the efficiency of diagnosing rickettsioses and ehrlichioses, it is important to consider that diseases such as RMSF caused by *R. rickettsii* and MSF caused by *R. conorii* have been initially described solely on the basis of clinical evidence. Careful clinical examination and epidemiologic investigation of patients with potential rickettsioses and ehrlichioses is critical. Clinically, the mainstay of the diagnosis has been the presence of a characteristic rash, eventually associated to high fever and headache. The disease can be mild or severe but will usually last for two to three weeks. This very basic knowledge should always be considered.

ASPECIFIC DIAGNOSIS

Routine, nonspecific laboratory tests may aid in the diagnostic process. Most of the knowledge on aspecific biological variations for rickettsioses has been collected from MSF and RMSF. In MSF, anemia may occur in 12% of patients (14). The leucocyte count is usually normal but leucocytosis is observed in 11% to 28% of cases and leucopenia in 12% to 20% of cases. Thrombocytopenia occurs in 12.5% to 30% of cases. Inflammatory proteins from the acute-phase response such as C-reactive protein and fibrinogen are often increased. Hypoprotidemia is observed in up to 3% of cases for MSF and in 18% for RMSF (14,15). There is a striking elevation of transaminases. Serum glutamic pyruvate transaminase (SGPT) and serum glutamic oxaloacetic transaminase (SGOT) levels could be increased in 37% to 39% of patients with MSF (14,16). Elevated levels of creatine phosphokinase, lactic dehydrogenase, and bilirubinemia may be present in 18% and in 44% of cases, respectively (14). Increased levels of creatinine and urea occur in 17% and 25% of patients, respectively (14). In severe cases, coagulopathy marked by decreased clotting factors may cause bleeding or thrombosis, hypocalcaemia is frequent, and hyponatremia caused by increased secretion of antidiuretic hormone is common (14,17).

Most frequent abnormalities in patients with murine typhus and epidemic typhus are mildly elevated transaminases, elevated lactate dehydrogenase levels, mild hyponatremia and hypocalcemia, elevated levels of alkaline phosphates, and hypoalbuminamia (18). Thrombocytopenia is observed (18). The leucocyte count is usually normal but leucocytosis is observed (18).

For human monocytic ehrlichiosis (HME) and human granulocytic anaplasmosis (HGA), the most common abnormalities are thrombocytopenia and leucopenia, usually accompanied by abnormal liver function, manifesting as mild increases in serum concentrations of SGPT, SGOT, and most frequently, lactate dehydrogenase (19,20). An elevated concentration of C-reactive protein has been observed in almost all patients. Other less common laboratory findings are anemia and elevated serum creatinine and blood urea nitrogen levels.

COLLECTION AND STORAGE OF SAMPLES

Ideally, the specimens should be sampled before antibiotic therapy. Five milliliters of blood should be collected in either heparin- or citrate-containing tubes (leucocyte buffy coat) for culture or ethylene diamine tetraacetic acid (EDTA) tubes for molecular diagnosis. EDTA anticoagulant should be avoided for culture, as it is harmful to the cell monolayer used for the recovery of rickettsiae. Heparinized blood can also be used for immunodetection of rickettsiae in circulating endothelial cells (21). When culture or molecular diagnosis is delayed, samples should be frozen at −70°C for isolation procedures or at −20°C for molecular diagnosis. For serological diagnosis, 10 mL of blood should be collected early and late in the course of the disease. Sera can be preserved at/or below −20°C for several months without degradation of the antibodies. An alternative, inexpensive, and convenient method for collecting, storing, and transporting blood samples for serological testing is to collect few drops of blood on a blotting paper (22). Thus, the blotting paper can be sent to a reference laboratory. Skin biopsy specimens, collected preferably from the site of tick attachment (i.e., eschar inoculation), are particularly valuable samples that can be used for culture, immunodetection, and polymerase chain reaction (PCR) (23–25). If processing of biopsy material is delayed, the sample should be preserved frozen at −70°C for culture and PCR, or formalin for immunodetection. Diagnosis of HME and HGA by observation of bacteria in blood smears or other tissues is best achieved if smears are prepared immediately after collection. Smears should be air-dried and preserved at room temperature. Finally, lice (26–28), ticks (29,30), and fleas (31) could also be used for PCR and culture. Collection of samples and diagnostic tools for the diagnosis of rickettsioses and ehrlichioses are summarized in Figure 1.

DIRECT DIAGNOSIS
Xenodiagnostic

Ticks may be collected after they have bitten human. Ideally, they should be kept alive before being tested. If they need to be transported or kept for long periods, a humidifier box is useful. While the ticks are still alive, the hemolymph test should be performed following surface sterilization (32). In this procedure, one tick leg is broken, allowing the collection of a drop of hemolymph, which can be spread onto a slide and then subjected either to Gimenez staining or to immunodetection methods (30,33,34). Molecular methods based on PCR could also be performed on ticks, lice, and fleas (26–31).

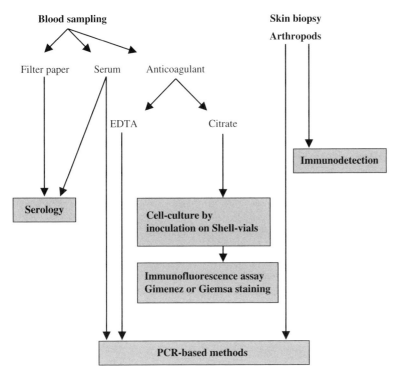

FIGURE 1 Strategy for the diagnosis of rickettsial diseases: collection of samples and diagnostic tools. *Abbreviations*: EDTA, ethylene diamine tetraacetic acid; PCR, polymerase chain reaction.

Nonimmunological Staining Methods

The diagnosis of HME and HGA could be performed on peripheral blood smears or other tissues by detection of a typical cluster of bacteria called morula, stained by Romanowsky methods (19,35–39).

Immunodetection

The use of immunodetection incorporating specific polyclonal or monoclonal antibodies, the latter of which can be used to determine the infecting species, allows the detection of rickettsiae in blood or other tissues such as inoculation eschar (40–43). This technique allows rickettsiae to be recovered with relative ease, even in patients receiving antibiotic therapy before their seroconversion. Samples can be tested fresh, frozen, or after fixation and paraffin embedding allowing a retrospective diagnosis on fixed tissues. Immunofluorescent labels have been widely used in conjunction with these antibodies, but immunoperoxidase labels and detection systems appear to allow a better microscopic definition of cells around the detected rickettsiae (44). Detection of rickettsiae in skin biopsy specimens using magnetic beads has also proven to be useful (45,46). This technique has been adapted to allow the immunodetection of *R. conorii* in circulating endothelial cells, which are isolated from whole blood with immunomagnetic beads coated with an endothelial cell-specific monoclonal antibody (47). Bacteria are detected by immunofluorescence with polyclonal *R. conorii* antiserum. The sensitivity of this method is estimated to be 50% for acutely ill patients (48). Moreover, it has a prognostic value, because the number of circulating endothelial cells detected is directly proportional to the severity of the infection (49). The main limitation of this diagnostic approach is that the antibodies have been developed in selected specialized laboratories but are not available commercially.

SEROLOGICAL METHODS

Serological assays are the easiest methods for the diagnosis of rickettsial diseases. The Weil–Felix test, which was the first serological assay to be developed, involves antigens from three *Proteus* strains: *P. vulgaris* 0X2, *P. vulgaris* 0X19, and *P. mirabilis* OXK. It is used to diagnose rickettsioses based on serological cross-reactions (50). Antibody reaction to 0X19 identifies typhus group (TG) rickettsiae (*R. prowazekii* and *R. typhi*) and *R. rickettsii*, whereas reaction to 0X2 identifies spotted fever group (SFG) rickettsiae and reaction to OXK identifies *Orientia tsutsugamushi*. This test lacks sensitivity and specificity. It is also simple to carry out. It continues to be used in some areas as a first-line test such as Asia. Techniques such as complement fixation tests, which lack both sensitivity and specificity, are not recommended (13). The enzyme-linked immunosorbent assay was first introduced for detection of antibodies against *R. typhi* and *R. prowazekii* (51). This technique is highly sensitive and reproducible, allowing differentiation of IgG and IgM antibodies. The method was later adapted to the diagnosis of RMSF (52).

Presently, the most commonly used technique for the diagnosis of rickettsioses, anaplasmosis, and ehrlichioses is the indirect immunofluorescence assay, which is widely accepted as the reference serological test (13,35,36,38,53–56). The indirect immunoperoxidase assay (IFA) has been widely used in Asia and is of comparable efficiency. IFA is commercially available. This assay has been improved as a micro-method called microimmunofluorescence (MIF), which can simultaneously detect antibodies to several antigens with the same drop of serum in a single well containing multiple dots. Its main limitation is the titer variations linked to reader subjectivity. This assay allows determination of both IgG and IgM antibodies. The early-phase serum (<15 days following onset of symptoms) is often negative. Thus, a late or convalescence phase serum (>15 days) is frequently required. A seroconversion marked by a fourfold or greater increase in antibody titers has a great value for the diagnosis of a rickettsiosis. Cut-off values of 1:64 for IgG and 1:32 for IgM are usually used for the diagnosis of rickettsioses in the Unité des Rickettsies in Marseille, but cut-off value may be different in other laboratories. For ATBF due to *R. africae*, it has been demonstrated that seroconversion is often delayed by comparison with other tick-transmitted rickettsioses and therefore the convalescence-phase serum should be sampled a minimum of four weeks following the onset of symptoms (57). In TIBOLA due to *R. slovaca*, the serological response is most often weak. This is possibly linked to the lack of generalized infection. Thus, other diagnostic methods, such as culture or PCR from skin or lymph node biopsies for this disease, should be preferred (58).

IFA is highly sensitive but may lack specificity. Indeed, cross-reactions can occur between rickettsiae and *Proteus*, *Legionella*, *Bartonella*, and *Ehrlichia* infections (50). These cross-reacting antibodies appear to be directed against the lipopolysaccharide. Additional false-positive IgM antibodies are observed with the rheumatoid factor and in viral and parasitic infections generating unspecific lymphocyte B proliferation (cytomegalovirus, Epstein–Barr virus, malaria). Cross-reactions occur also within the TG (41,59) and within the SFG. Thus, it is important to consider that tests for a single antigen do not allow a definitive conclusion regarding the causative agent (60). Tests for several antigens on the same slide may allow the causative agent to be identified from its comparatively higher antibody level (10,61). The panel of tested antigens at the Unité des Rickettsies for the patients with an history of arthropod exposure and depending on their geographical origin is developed in Figure 2 (8,62,63). In case of cross-reactions, Western blot (WB) immunoassay associated to cross-adsorption techniques of sera are done to perform a specific diagnosis (59,61). Cross-reactions have also been observed between the TG and the SFG (31). This cross-reaction has been mainly observed in patients with rickettsioses due to *R. felis* (31). Cross-reactions could also be observed between HME and HGA. At the Unité des Rickettsies, when cross-reactions are noted between several rickettsial antigens using IFA, the standard procedure comprises three steps:

1. A rickettsial antigen is considered to represent the agent of infection when titers of IgG and/or IgM antibody against this antigen are at least two serial dilutions higher than titers of IgG and/or IgM antibody against other rickettsial antigens.

2. When differences in titers between several antigens are lower than two dilutions, WB immunoassays are performed. Then, a rickettsial antigen is considered to represent the agent of the infection when acute or convalescent sera show an exclusive reactivity with the specific proteins antigens of this antigen only.
3. When WB immunoassays are not diagnostic, cross-absorption studies are performed. IgG/IgM titers must be greater than or equal to 128:32. Specific diagnosis criteria after cross-absorption studies include (*i*) IF serology positive for a single antigen or (*ii*) WB immunoassay showing an exclusive reactivity with specific proteins of a sole agent.

Cross-Adsorption Assay

In order to identify the infecting rickettsiae by discriminating cross-reacting antibodies between two or more antigens, cross-adsorption assay has been successfully developed to patients with rickettsioses (11,61). A schema of this procedure is presented in Figure 3. First, the serum of the patient is mixed separately with the bacteria involved in the cross-reaction, and then tested against each of these antigens. Cross-adsorption results in the disappearance of both homologous and heterologous antibodies when adsorption is performed with the bacterium responsible for the disease, whereas only heterologous antibodies are removed when adsorption is performed with the bacterium responsible for the cross-reaction. These could be showed using either MIF or WB immunoassay (Fig. 4). Although this technique is accurate, it is limited. Indeed, this assay is very expensive and time-consuming because a large number of rickettsiae are required for each absorption step.

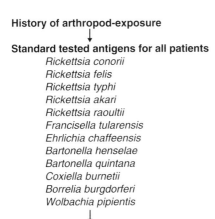

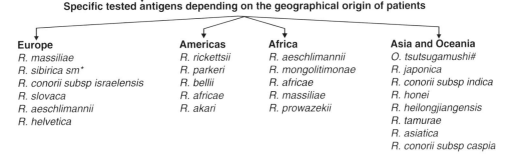

*R. sibirica subsp mongolitimonae
#O. tsutsugamushi: 2 serotypes are tested: Kato and Kuroki

FIGURE 2 Panel of tested antigens at the Unité des Rickettsies for the patients with a history of arthropod exposure and depending on their geographical origin.

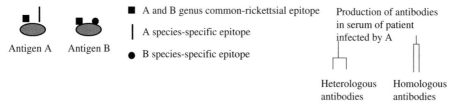

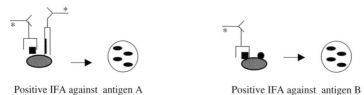

I. Indirect immunofluorescence assay (IFA) with patient's serum

Positive IFA against antigen A   Positive IFA against antigen B

II. Adsorption of patient's serum by specific antigen A followed by IFA

1. Adsorption of heterologous and homologous antibodies

→ Centrifugation

No remaining antibodies in supernatant

2. IFA using adsorbed serum and antigen A and antigen B

Negative IFA against antigen A   Negative IFA against antigen B

III. Adsorption of patient's serum by nonspecific antigen B followed by IFA

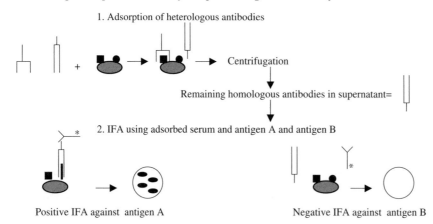

FIGURE 3 Schematic presentation of cross-adsorption assay. *Abbreviation*: IFA, immunofluorescence antibody.

The WB immunoassays employing sodium dodecyl sulfate gel-electrophoresed and electroblotted antigens are available in research laboratories. This test is able to detect early antibodies when other tests are still negative. WB detects two types of antigens for rickettsioses, lipopolysaccharide and high-molecular-weight proteins (rOmpA, rOmpB, and

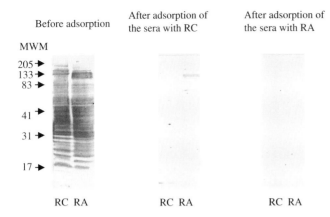

FIGURE 4 Western blot (WB) immunoassay for the diagnosis of rickettsioses: WB immunoassay and cross-adsorption study to differentiate *R. conorii* (RC) and *R. aeschlimanii* (RA) infection. Once adsorbed with *R. conorii*, the antibodies that remain are those directed against *R. aeschlimanii*; all antibodies disappeared following adsorption with *R. aeschlimanii*, indicating that antibodies contained in the sera were directed specifically against *R. aeschlimanii*. *Abbreviations*: MWM, molecular size marker; WB, Western blot.

surface cell antigen 4). These proteins are species-specific (50), and provide the basis for rickettsial serotyping (64). However, although inoculated mice produce a predominance of antibodies against these proteins, human do not, and cross-reactions between rickettsial proteins make it difficult to identify the infecting rickettsiae to the species level (65). If sera are collected very early in infection, strong homologous reactions are often observed, making a specific diagnosis possible. However, as this rarely occurs, more specific methods such as cross-adsorption are needed (11,23). Moreover, WB is time-consuming. Differentiation between HME and HGA, which sometimes can induce formation of cross-reactive antibodies, is possible by WB. Antibodies reactive with one or more of the 22, 28, 29, 49, 54, 120, or 200 kDa proteins confirm the presence of HME (66,67). A recombinant 120-kDa protein used in a dot blot format proved to be both sensitive and specific as a confirmation tool (68).

Finally, serological methods such as IFA are the most widely used method for confirmation of rickettsioses, HME, and HGA. However, the diagnosis is usually made on a retrospective basis because patients may lack antibodies at the time of the first visit during the acute phase.

POLYMERASE CHAIN REACTION–BASED DETECTION

Molecular methods based on PCR have enabled the development of sensitive, specific, and rapid tools for both detection and identification of rickettsiae from various samples. Specific sample management must be used prior the tests. Blood must be held at ambient temperature until cells are sedimented and rickettsiae are sought in the leucocytes cell buffy coat. Fresh tissues are preferred for PCR. However, paraffin-embedded tissues and even slide-fixed specimens may be used (69). PCR assays can be very useful because infection can be detected before seroconversion or positive culture occurred.

For rickettsioses, detection strategies based on recognition of sequences within the genes encoding the 16S rRNA gene (2), a 17-kDa protein (70–72), the citrate synthase (73–76), the outer membrane proteins rOmpA (77,78), the rOmpB (79), the surface cell antigen 4 (80), and the surface cell antigen 1 (81) have been developed (Table 1). For ehrlichioses, several PCRs have been reported targeting the 16S rRNA gene, the *groESL* operon, the 120-kDa antigen e-gene (coding for a surface-exposed glycoprotein with variable tandem-repeats units), the *nadA* gene, and the *p28* multigene (20,39,82–86). For HGA, several targets have also been used for PCR such as the 16S rRNA gene, the epank1 gene, and the operon *groESL* (Table 2) (87–96). The complete sequences of *R. conorii*, *R. rickettsii*, *R. prowazekii*, *R. typhi*, *R. felis*, *R. africae*,

TABLE 1 DNA Targets and Nucleotide Sequences of Primers Exploited for Polymerase Chain Reaction Detection of Rickettsioses

DNA target	Forward (f) and reverse (r) primers (5'–3')	References
16S RNA	fD1 f AGAGTI'I'GATCCTGGCTCAG	(2)
	rp 2 r ACGGCTACCTTGTrACGACTT	
Citrate synthase (*gltA*)	CS1d f ATGACTAATGGCAATAATAA	(73)
	CS890 r GCTTTAGCTACATATTTAGG	
	Rp877p f GGGGACCTGCTCACGGCGG	
	Rp1258n r ATTGCAAAAAGTACAGTGAACA	
Outer-membrane protein A (*ompA*)	190-70p f ATGGCGAATATTTCTCCAAAA	(77)
	190-701 r GTTCCGTTAATGGCAGCATCT	
Outer-membrane protein B (*ompB*)	120-M59 f CCGCAGGGTTGGTAACTGC	(79)
	120-807 r CCTTTTAGATTACCGCCTAA	
Surface cell antigen 4 (*Sca4*)	D1 f ATGAGTAAAGACGGTAACCT	(80)
	D928 r AAGCTATTGCGTCATCTCCG	
	D767 f CGATGGTAGCATTAAAAGCT	
	D1390 r CTTGCTTTTCAGCAATATCAC	
Surface cell antigen 1 (*Sca1*)	s1.cono.f TGAGGGTATGGCGATGAGT	(81)
	s1.cono.r CAGTAGGCGAAGACGCTG	

R. slovaca, R. akari, R. massiliae, R. belli, R. canadensis, R. siberica, Anaplasma phagocytophilum, Ehrlichia chaffeensis, and *Neorickettsia sennetsu* genomes have provided an important source of gene sequences for PCR-based assays (97–102) (http://www.genomesonline.org/).

Several PCR techniques have been used for the diagnosis of rickettsioses and ehrlichioses. Nested-PCR techniques have been described in order to increase the analytical sensitivity of the test but the risk of DNA-amplicon contamination could not be neglected using this approach (103). Recently, quantitative real-time PCR assays have been developed for the diagnosis of infections caused by *A. phagocytophilum, E. chaffeensis, O. tsutsugamushi*, SFG, and TG rickettsiae (75,96,104–108). The main advantages of this approach include speed and low risk of contamination. Real-time quantitative PCR assays using species-specific probes targeting *R. prowazekii, R. typhi,* and *R. felis* are also available (109,110). To validate PCR assays, it is important to include positive controls (such as *R. montaniensis* and *A. phagocytophilum*) and

TABLE 2 DNA Targets and Nucleotide Sequences of Primers Exploited for Polymerase Chain Reaction Detection of *A. phagocytophilum* in Samples from Infected Patients

DNA target	Forward (f) and reverse (r) primers (5'–3')	Method	References
16S rRNA	GE9 f AACGGATTATTCTTTATAGCTTGCT	Regular PCR	(87–89)
	GE10 r GGAGATTAGATCCTTCTTAACGGAA		
16S rRNA	EC9 f AAGGATCCTACCTTGTTACGACTT	Nested PCR	(90,91)
	EC12 r AATCTAGATTAGATACCCT(A/T/G)GTAGTCC		
	Ge9 f AACGGATTATTCTTTATAGCTTGCT		
	Ge10 r GGAGATTAGATCCTTCTTAACGGAA'		
Epank1	LA6 f GAGAGATGCTTATGGTAAGAC	Regular PCR	(92)
	LA1 r CGTTCAGCCATCATTGTGAC		
HGE 44	Not published	Regular PCR	(93)
P44 (*msp2*) paralog sequence	P44f1 TTGATCTTGAGATTGGTTACG	Nested PCR	(94)
	P44r1 GGCAGATCATCATAAACRCC		
	P44f2 CAAGGGTATTAGAGATAGT		
	P44r2 AAACTGAACAATATCCTTAC		
GroESL	HS1 f TGGGCTGGTA(A/C)TGAAAT	Nested PCR	(95,86)
	HS6 r CCICCIGGIACIA(C/T)ACCTTC		
	HS43 f AT(A/T)GC(A/T)AA(G/A)GAAGCATAGTC		
	HS45 r ACTTCACG(C/T)(C/T)TCATAGAC		

negative controls (water, mix run, and arthropod free of infection) in each PCR run. Negative controls were tested after every seven samples. All the controls must be correct to interpret the results.

A PCR assay with increased sensitivity, named "suicide-PCR," exists also (10,58,111–113). This test was mainly designed to detect DNA from blood samples as regular PCR has a poor sensitivity when applied to blood. This technique is a nested-PCR using single-use primers targeting a gene never amplified previously in the laboratory. Such a procedure avoids "vertical" contamination by amplicons from previous assays. All positive PCR products are sequenced to identify the causative agent. Suicide-PCR has been successful with EDTA-blood, serum, and skin and lymph node specimens.

CULTIVATION

Isolation of rickettsiae is of great importance, as the ultimate goal is recovery of the bacterial agent from a patient or an arthropod vector. However, this approach is reserved to specialized laboratories with cell-culture facilities and equipped with biohazard facilities. Currently, *R. rickettsii* and *R. prowazekii* have been recognized as potential agents of bioterrorism. Thus, their isolation must be performed only in Biosafety Level 3 laboratories. Rickettsiae have been isolated using different methods. For a long time, animal inoculation has been performed with guinea pigs. Embryonated eggs have also been used. Presently, cell culture is the most frequent system used for the primary isolation. The shell-vial cell culture is a microculture system which has been shown to be highly efficient for obtaining rickettsial isolates from various specimens (12,114,115). Each sample is assayed in cell culture in triplicate. This method comprises a centrifugation step, which is critical as it increases the ratio of rickettsiae to cells. Another advancement for the successful isolation of rickettsiae has been the use of various cell lines such as tick or mammalian cells (114,116). One of the most useful cell lines for the isolation of tick-borne rickettsiae is the human embryonic lung (HEL) cells (114). The multiplication of cell lines and variation of culture temperature allow a variety of culture conditions. For example, optimal temperature growth of the TG of Rickettsiae is 35°C and of the SFG is 32°C. For *R. felis*, XTC-2 cells were used to grow the bacterium at 28°C (117).

Rickettsiae could be detected within cells by Gimenez staining and immunofluorescence staining followed by microscopic examination. For immunofluorescence staining, after fixation with acetone, the coverslips are incubated with the patient's serum and various monoclonal antibodies directed against rickettsiae. The culture is kept for two weeks with examination of one shell-vial each week. After this time, if immunofluorescence is negative, the culture is considered to be negative. If immunofluorescence is positive, parallel shell vials are inoculated onto confluent monolayer of HEL cells in culture flasks in an attempt to obtain isolates, and PCR assays are performed in parallel to allow specific identification. Usually, culture of rickettsiae takes three to seven days. Many rickettsiae, including *R. conorii*, *R. rickettsii*, *R. massiliae*, *R. aeschlimannii*, *R. slovaca*, *R. helvetica*, *R. sibirica* subsp. *mongolitimonae*, *R. africae*, and *R. prowazekii* have been isolated using this approach (114,115,118). Although this assay is useful, about one-third of the isolates are lost on passage for unknown reasons.

Isolation of *A. phagocytophylum* should be only attempted in a Biohazard Level 3 laboratory. The promyelotic HL-60 leukemia cell line is the most widely used cell line for growing *A. phagocytophylum* (119). Infection can be assessed by Giemsa staining. Infection is usually detectable as observable morulae at days three to seven postinoculation (120). The isolation takes several days to two or more weeks, thus limiting the utility of this method (121). PCR assays are performed to allow specific identification.

The most widely used cell type for isolation of *E. chaffeensis* is the canine histiocytic cell line DH82. Successful isolation has also been reported using THP-1 (a human monocytic leukemia cell line), HEL-22 cells (fibroblast-like cells), Vero cells, and HL-60. Cultures are maintained for four to six weeks and examined every five to seven days by scraping monolayers or cytocentrifugation flowed by immunofluorescent staining or Romanowsky stains to detect intracytoplasmic morulae. Confirmation is done with PCR. Cultivation of *E. ewingii* is presently elusive.

The cultivation is reserved to specialized laboratories and is not a practical tool for the routine diagnosis. However, the importance of culture cannot be underestimated, as obtaining an isolate from a patient or an arthropod vector is a clue for rickettsial disease description.

IDENTIFICATION AND DIFFERENTIATION OF RICKETTSIAE

For many years, the differentiation of rickettsiae has been based solely on a few phenotypic criteria and on immunodetection. Initially, the toxin neutralization test in mice was used (122,123). This was followed by complement fixation (124) and later by MIF serotyping in mice, which has long been the reference method for the taxonomic classification of rickettsial isolates (64). The main problems with these techniques are that reference sera are needed and that each time a new isolate is tested, the test sample and all other antigens need to be screened against all antisera.

Over the last 20 years, several new identification techniques have successively been introduced, including use of monoclonal antibodies, protein electrophoresis, DNA restriction-based techniques, and DNA sequencing. Monoclonal antibodies against *R. rickettsii* (125), *R. akari* (126,127), *R. conorii* (127), *R. japonica* (128), *R. massiliae* (129), *R. africae* (127), *R. sibirica* (127), and *R. slovaca* (127) have been developed. Although these are useful tools for species identification, a complete collection, organized in pools, is required to identify all rickettsiae.

Protein analysis by sodium dodecyl sulfate–polyacrylamide gel electrophoresis (SDS–PAGE) has also been used to differentiate rickettsial species (130). The molecular masses of the major protein antigens, that is, rOmpA, PS 120, and rOmpB, which are members of the surface cell antigen family of autotransporter proteins (131), are estimated to be 115, 120, and 155 kDa for *R. rickettsii*, respectively, although their sizes vary among rickettsial species, and these proteins determine the serospecificity in mice (132). However, as the reproducibility of SDS–PAGE is never perfect and depends on gel conditions and solubilization temperature, it is usually necessary to include all species when attempting to identify a new isolate. Furthermore, as comparison with other species or strains is needed, it is necessary to introduce all purified rickettsiae; the technique is time-consuming and laborious.

Macrorestriction analysis of rickettsiae by pulsed-field gel electrophoresis is also a sensitive method for differentiating species (78). It has been a useful approach for identifying rickettsiae, but much biomass is required and it is necessary to include other rickettsiae on the gel to obtain a precise comparison of profiles. In addition, results may not easily be comparable among laboratories. Thus, applying this approach each time a strain is isolated is almost impossible. PCR amplification of a gene fragment coupled with restriction fragment length polymorphism (PCR–RFLP) has proven to be sensitive and practical, especially when applied to the *ompA* and *ompB* genes (78,133), or to the 17-kDa protein-encoding gene (134). However, PCR–RFLP also suffers lack of reproducibility and interlaboratory reproducibility.

The most recent and efficient identification method for rickettsiae has been gene sequencing. Indeed, sequencing a PCR amplification product allows a precise identification of a new isolate by comparison with international computerized databases. Such a method is reproducible, its results are reliably comparable among laboratories, and it has the advantage of being applicable both to isolates and directly to clinical specimens. The first gene sequenced for rickettsiae has been 16S rRNA, which could be amplified from all species but lacked discriminatory power at the species level (2). Then the *gltA* gene, encoding the citrate synthase, was used but also lacked discriminatory power (73). However, the most useful identification genes have undoubtfully been the *sca*-family genes, encoding autotransporter proteins. Of these, the 52-end of the *ompA* gene is the most discriminant for the identification of SFG rickettsial isolates (77), and the *sca*1 gene is the only gene present in all species, with a 488-bp fragment amplifiable with a single primer pair allowing amplification, sequencing, and thus identification of all *Rickettsia* species (81). Finally, a method based on the amplification and sequencing of rationally selected intergenic spacer sequences named multispacer typing has been developed to identify rickettsiae at the strain level (135,136). This method is especially useful for

TABLE 3 Diagnostic Criteria for African Tick-Bite Fever

A. Direct evidence of *R. africae* infection by culture and/or PCR
Or
B. Clinical and epidemiological features highly suggestive of ATBF, such as multiple inoculation eschars and/or regional lymphadenitis and/or a vesicular rash and/or regional lymphadenitis and/or a vesicular rash and/or similar symptoms among other members of the same group of travelers coming back from and endemic area (sub-Saharan Africa or French West Indies)
And
Positive serology against SFG rickettsiae
Or
C. Clinical and epidemiological features consistent with an SFG rickettsiosis such as fever and/or any cutaneous rash and/or single inoculation eschar after travel to sub-Saharan Africa or French West Indies
And
Serology specific for a recent *R. africae* infection (seroconversion or presence of IgM 1:32), with antibodies to *R. africae* greater than those to *R. conorii* by at least two dilutions, and/or a WB or cross-adsorption showing antibodies specific for *R. africae*

A patient is considered to have ATBF when criteria A, B, or C are met.
Abbreviations: PCR, polymerase chain reaction; SFG, spotted fever group; WB, Western blot.

tracing outbreaks of infection caused by rickettsiae considered as putative bioterrorism agents such as *R. prowazekii*.

CONCLUSIONS

Rickettsial diseases could be suspected in front of various clinical manifestations. Besides, even if fever, rash, and eschar inoculation are the classical clinical manifestations, they can lack. Thus, etiological diagnosis of rickettsial diseases is often difficult and relies on specialized laboratories using very specific tools. Interpretation of laboratory data is very important in order to establish the diagnosis. Diagnostic criteria have also been proposed to help physicians in diagnosing ATBF, MSF, and HGA (Tables 3–5) (54) (137).

TABLE 4 Diagnostic Criteria for Mediterranean Spotted Fever

Criteria	Score[a]
Epidemiological criteria	
Stay in endemic criteria	2
Occurrence in May–October	2
Contact (certain or possible) with dog ticks	2
Clinical criteria	
Fever >39°C	5
Eschar	5
Maculopapular or purpuric rash	5
Two of the above criteria	3
All three of the above criteria	
Nonspecific laboratory findings	
Platelets <150 g/L	1
SGOT or SGPT >50 U/L	1
Bacteriological criteria	
Blood culture positive for *R. conorii*	25
Detection of *R. conorii* in a skin biopsy	25
Serological criteria	
Single serum and IgG >1:128	5
Single serum and IgG >1:128 and IgM >1:64	10
Fourfold increase in two sera obtained within a 2-wk interval	20

[a] A positive diagnosis is made when the overall score is ≥25.
Abbreviations: IG, immunoglobulin; SGOT, serum glutamate-oxaloacetate transaminase; SGPT, serum glutamate-pyruvate transaminases.

TABLE 5 Diagnostic Criteria for Human Granulocytic Anaplasmosis

Confirmed human anaplasmosis
1. Febrile illness with a history of tick bite or tick exposure
And
2. Demonstration of *A. phagocytophilum* infection by seroconversion or ≥4-fold Change in antibody titer (IFA)
Or
3. Positive-PCR result with subsequent sequencing of the amplicons demonstrating *Anaplasma*-specific DNA in blood
Or
4. Isolation of *A. phagocytophilum* in blood culture

Probable human anaplasmosis
1. Febrile illness with a history of tick bite or tick exposure
And
2. Presence of stable titer of *A. phagocytophilum* antibodies in acute and convalescent sera titer >4-fold above the cut-off value (IFA)
Or
3. Positive-PCR result without sequencing confirmation
Or
4. Presence of intracytoplasmic morulae in a blood smear diagnostic criteria for HGA

Abbreviations: IFA, immunofluorescence antibody; PCR, polymerase chain reaction.

REFERENCES

1. Dumler J, Barbet A, Bekker C, et al. Reorganization of genera in the families Rickettsiaceae and Anaplasmataceae in the order *Rickettsiales*: unification of some species of *Ehrlichia* with *Anaplasma*, *Cowdria* with *Ehrlichia* and *Ehrlichia* with *Neorickettsia*, descriptions of six new species combinations and designation of *Ehrlichia equi* and "HGE agent" as subjective synonyms of *Ehrlichia phagocytophila*. Int J Syst Evol Microbiol 2001; 51:2145–2165.
2. Roux V, Raoult D. Phylogenetic analysis of the genus *Rickettsia* by 16S rDNA sequencing. Res Microbiol 1995; 146:385–396.
3. Tamura A, Ohashi N, Urakami H, Miyamura S. Classification of *Rickettsia tsutsugamushi* in a new genus, *Orientia* gen. nov., as *Orientia tsutsugamushi* comb. nov. Int J Syst Bacteriol 1995; 45:589–591.
4. Raoult D, Roux V. Rickettsioses as paradigms of new or emerging infectious diseases. Clin Microbiol Rev 1997; 10:694–719.
5. Fournier PE, Gouriet F, Brouqui P, Lutch F, Raoult D. Lymphagitis-associated rickettsiosis, a new rickettsiosis caused by *Rickettsia sibirica mongolotimonae*: seven new cases and review of the literature. Clin Infect Dis 2005; 40:1435–1444.
6. Fournier P, Grunnenberger F, Jaulhac B, Gastinger G, Raoult D. Evidence of *Rickettsia helvetica* infection in humans, in Eastern France. Emerg Infect Dis 2000; 6:389–392.
7. Mediannikov OY, Sidelnikov Y, Ivanov L, et al. Acute tick-borne rickettsiosis caused by *Rickettsia heilongjiangensis* in Russian Far East. Emerg Infect Dis 2004; 10:810–817.
8. Parola P, Paddock CD, Raoult D. Tick-borne rickettsioses around the world: emerging diseases challenging old concepts. Clin Microbiol Rev 2005; 18:719–756.
9. Raoult D, Fournier P, Abboud P, Caron F. The first documented *Rickettsia aeschlimannii* infection in human. Emerg Infect Dis 2002; 8:748–749.
10. Raoult D, Fournier P, Fenollar F, et al. *Rickettsia africae*, a tick-borne pathogen in travellers to sub-Saharan Africa. N Engl J Med 2001; 344:1504–1510.
11. Fournier PE, Roux V, Caumes E, Donzel M, Raoult D. Outbreak of *Rickettsia africae* infections in participants of an adventure race in South Africa. Clin Infect Dis 1998; 27:316–323.
12. Marrero M, Raoult D. Centrifugation-shell vial technique for rapid detection of Mediterranean spotted fever rickettsia in blood culture. Am J Trop Med Hyg 1989; 40:197–199.
13. Lakos A. Tick-borne lymphadenopathy—a new rickettsial disease? Lancet 1997; 350:1006.
14. Drancourt M, Raoult D, Harle JR, et al. Biological variations in 412 patients with Mediterranean spotted fever. Ann NY Acad Sci 1990; 590:39–50.
15. Helmick CG, Bernard KW, D'Angelo LJ. Rocky Mountain spotted fever: clinical, laboratory, and epidemiological features of 262 cases. J Infect Dis 1984; 150:480–488.
16. Guardia J, Martinez-Vazquez JM, Moragas A, et al. The liver in boutonneuse fever. Gut 1974; 15:549–551.
17. Raoult DA, Weiller PJ, Juhan-Vague I, Finaud M, Mongin M. Platelet antibodies in Mediterranean tick typhus. Trans R Soc Trop Med Hyg 1985; 79:699.
18. Dumler JS, Taylor JP, Walker DH. Clinical and laboratory features of murine typhus in south Texas, 1980 through 1987. J Am Med Assoc 1991; 266:1365–1370.

19. Dumler JS, Choi KS, Garcia-Garcia JC, et al. Human granulocytic anaplasmosis and *Anaplasma phagocytophilum*. Emerg Infect Dis 2005; 11:1828–1834.
20. Olano JP, Masters E, Hogrefe W, Walker DH. Human monocytotropic ehrlichiosis, Missouri. Emerg Infect Dis 2003; 9:1579–1586.
21. La Scola B, Raoult D. Diagnosis of Mediterranean spotted fever by cultivation of *Rickettsia conorii* from blood and skin samples using the centrifugation-shell vial technique and by detection and *R. conorii* in circulating endothelial cells: a 6-year follow-up. J Clin Microbiol 1996; 34:2722–2727.
22. Fenollar F, Raoult D. Diagnosis of rickettsial diseases using samples dried on blotting paper. Clin Diag Lab Immunol 1999; 6:483–488.
23. Brouqui P, Harle JR, Delmont J, Frances C, Weiller PJ, Raoult D. African tick-bite fever: an imported spotless rickettsiosis. Arch Intern Med 1997; 157:119–124.
24. Raoult D, Brouqui P, Roux V. A new spotted fever-group rickettsiosis. Lancet 1996; 348:412.
25. Williams WJ, Radulovic S, Dasch GA, et al. Identification of *Rickettsia conorii* infection by polymerase chain reaction in a soldier returning from Somalia. Clin Infect Dis 1994; 19:93–99.
26. Fournier PE, Ndihokubwayo JB, Guidran J, Kelly PJ, Raoult D. Human pathogens in body and head lice. Emerg Infect Dis 2002; 8:1515–1518.
27. Higgins JA, Azad AF. Use of polymerase chain reaction to detect bacteria in arthropods: a review. J Med Entomol 1995; 32:213–222.
28. Roux V, Raoult D. Body lice as tools for diagnosis and surveillance of reemerging diseases. J Clin Microbiol 1999; 37:596–599.
29. Gage KL, Schrumpf ME, Karstens RH, Burgdorfer W, Schwan TG. DNA typing of rickettsiae in naturally infected ticks using a polymerase chain reaction/restriction fragment length polymorphism system. Am J Trop Med Hyg 1994; 50:247–260.
30. Kelly PJ, Raoult D, Mason PR. Isolation of spotted fever group rickettsias from triturated ticks using a modification of the centrifugation-shell vial technique. Trans R Soc Trop Med Hyg 1991; 85:397–398.
31. Perez-Arellano JL, Fenollar F, Angel-Moreno A, et al. Human *Rickettsia felis* infection, Canary Islands, Spain. Emerg Infect Dis 2005; 11:1961–1964.
32. Burgdorfer W. Hemolymph test: a technique for detection of rickettsiae in ticks. Am J Trop Med Hyg 1970; 19:1010–1014.
33. Gimenez D. Staining rickettsiae in yolk-sac cultures. Stain Technol 1964; 39:135–130.
34. Peter O, Raoult D, Gilot B. Isolation by a sensitive centrifugation cell culture system of 52 strains of spotted fever group rickettsiae from ticks collected in France. J Clin Microbiol 1990; 28:1597–1599.
35. Aguero-Rosenfeld ME, Horowitz HW, Wormser GP, et al. Human granulocytic ehrlichiosis: a case series from a medical center in New York State. Ann Intern Med 1996; 125:904–908.
36. Bakken JS, Krueth J, Wilson-Nordskog C, Tilden RL, Asanovich K, Dumler JS. Clinical and laboratory characteristics of human granulocytic ehrlichiosis. J Am Med Assoc 1996; 275:199–205.
37. Blanco JR, Oteo JA. Human granulocytic ehrlichiosis in Europe. Clin Microbiol Infect 2002; 8:763–772.
38. Dumler J, Walker D. Tick borne ehrlichioses. Lancet Infect Dis 2001; 1:21–28.
39. Standaert SM, Yu T, Scott MA, et al. Primary isolation of *Ehrlichia chaffeensis* from patients with febrile illnesses: clinical and molecular characteristics. J Infect Dis 2000; 181:1082–1088.
40. Dumler JS, Dawson JE, Walker DH. Human ehrlichiosis: hematopathology and immunohistologic detection of *Ehrlichia chaffeensis*. Hum Pathol 1993; 24:391–396.
41. La Scola B, Raoult D. Laboratory diagnosis of Rickettsioses: current approaches to diagnosis of old and new rickettsial diseases. J Clin Microbiol 1997; 35:2715–2727.
42. Lepidi H, Fournier PE, Raoult D. Histologic features and immunodetection of African tick-bite fever eschar. Emerg Infect Dis 2006; 12:1332–1337.
43. Yu X, Brouqui P, Dumler JS, Raoult D. Detection of *Ehrlichia chaffeensis* in human tissue by using a species-specific monoclonal antibody. J Clin Microbiol 1993; 31:3284–3288.
44. Dumler JS, Gage WR, Pettis GL, Azad AF, Kuhadja FP. Rapid immunoperoxidase demonstration of *Rickettsia rickettsii* in fixed cutaneous specimens from patients with Rocky Mountain spotted fever. Am J Clin Pathol 1990; 93:410–414.
45. Walker DH, Cain BG. A method for specific diagnosis of Rocky Mountain spotted fever on fixed, paraffin-embedded tissue by immunofluorescence. J Infect Dis 1978; 137:206–209.
46. Walker DH, Gay RM, Valdes-Dapena M. The occurrence of eschars in Rocky Mountain spotted fever. J Am Acad Dermatol 1981; 4:571–576.
47. George F, Brisson C, Poncelet P, et al. Rapid isolation of human endothelial cells from whole blood using S-Endo1 monoclonal antibody coupled to immuno-magnetic beads: demonstration of endothelial injury after angioplasty. Thromb Haemost 1992; 67:147–153.
48. Lackman DB, Bell EJ, Stoenner HG, Pickens EG. The Rocky Mountain spotted fever group of *Rickettsiae*. Health Lab Sci 1965; 74:135–141.
49. George F, Brouqui P, Boffa MC, et al. Demonstration of *Rickettsia conorii*-induced endothelial injury in vivo by measuring circulating endothelial cells, thrombomodulin, and von Willebrand factor in patients with Mediterranean spotted fever. Blood 1993; 82:2109–2116.
50. Raoult D, Dasch GA. Immunoblot cross-reactions among *Rickettsia*, *Proteus* spp. and *Legionella* spp. in patients with Mediterranean spotted fever. FEMS Immunol Med Microbiol 1995; 11:13–18.

51. Halle S, Dasch GA, Weiss E. Sensitive enzyme-linked immunosorbent assay for detection of antibodies against typhus rickettsiae, *Rickettsia prowazekii* and *Rickettsia typhi*. J Clin Microbiol 1977; 6:101–110.
52. Walker DH. Rocky Mountain spotted fever: a disease in need of microbiological concern. Clin Microbiol Rev 1989; 2:227–240.
53. Bakken JS, Haller I, Riddell D, Walls JJ, Dumler JS. The serological response of patients infected with the agent of human granulocytic ehrlichiosis. Clin Infect Dis 2002; 34:22–27.
54. Brouqui P, Bacellar F, Baranton G, et al. Guidelines for the diagnosis of tick-borne bacterial diseases in Europe. Clin Microbiol Infect 2004; 10:1108–1132.
55. Brouqui P, Salvo E, Dumler JS, Raoult D. Diagnosis of granulocytic ehrlichiosis in humans by immunofluorescence assay. Clin Diagn Lab Immunol 2001; 8:199–202.
56. Childs JE, Sumner JW, Nicholson WL, Massung RF, Standaert SM, Paddock CD. Outcome of diagnostic tests using samples from patients with culture-proven human monocytic ehrlichiosis: implications for surveillance. J Clin Microbiol 1999; 37:2997–3000.
57. Fournier P, Jensenius M, Laferl H, Vene S, Raoult D. Kinetics of antibody responses in *Rickettsia africae* and *Rickettsia conorii* infections. Clin Diag Lab Immunol 2002; 9:324–308.
58. Raoult D, Lakos A, Fenollar F, Beytout J, Brouqui P, Fournier P. Spotless rickettsiosis caused by *Rickettsia slovaca* and associated with *Dermacentor* ticks. Clin Infect Dis 2002; 34:1331–1336.
59. Raoult D, Ndihokubwayo JB, Tissot-Dupont H, et al. Outbreak of epidemic typhus associated with trench fever in Burundi. Lancet 1998; 352:353–358.
60. Rolain JM, Shpynov S, Raoult D. Spotted-fever-group rickettsioses in north Asia. Lancet 2003; 362:1939.
61. La Scola B, Rydkina L, Ndihokubwayo JB, Vene S, Raoult D. Serological differentiation of murine typhus and epidemic typhus using cross-adsorption and Western blotting. Clin Diagn Lab Immunol 2000; 7:612–616.
62. Fournier PE, Takada N, Fujita H, Raoult D. *Rickettsia tamurae* sp. nov., isolated from *Amblyomma testudinarium* ticks. Int J Syst Evol Microbiol 2006; 56:1673–1675.
63. Zhang JZ, Fan MY, Wu YM, Fournier PE, Roux V, Raoult D. Genetic classification of "*Rickettsia heilongjiangii*" and "*Rickettsia hulinii*," two Chinese spotted fever group rickettsiae. J Clin Microbiol 2000; 38:3498–3501.
64. Philip RN, Casper EA, Burgdorfer W, Gerloff RK, Hughes LE, Bell EJ. Serologic typing of rickettsiae of the spotted fever group by microimmunofluorescence. J Immunol 1978; 121:1961–1968.
65. Hechemy KE, Raoult D, Fox J, Han Y, Elliott LB, Rawlings J. Cross-reaction of immune sera from patients with rickettsial diseases. J Med Microbiol 1989; 29:199–202.
66. Brouqui P, Dumler JS, Raoult D, Walker DH. Antigenic characterization of ehrlichiae: protein immunoblotting of *Ehrlichia canis*, *Ehrlichia sennetsu*, and *Ehrlichia risticii*. J Clin Microbiol 1992; 30:1062–1066.
67. Wong SJ, Brady GS, Dumler JS. Serological responses to *Ehrlichia equi*, *Ehrlichia chaffeensis*, and *Borrelia burgdorferi* in patients from New York State. J Clin Microbiol 1997; 35:2198–2205.
68. Yu XJ, Crocquet-Valdes P, Cullman LC, Walker DH. The recombinant 120-kilodalton protein of *Ehrlichia chaffeensis*, a potential diagnostic tool. J Clin Microbiol 1996; 34:2853–2855.
69. Stein A, Raoult D. A simple method for amplification of DNA from paraffin-embedded tissues. Nucleic Acids Res 1992; 20:5237–5238.
70. Anderson BE, Tzianabos T. Comparative sequence analysis of a genus—common rickettsial antigen gene. J Bacteriol 1989; 171:5199–5201.
71. Baird RW, Stenos J, Stewart R, et al. Genetic variation in Australian spotted fever group rickettsiae. J Clin Microbiol 1996; 34:1526–1530.
72. Balayeva NM, Eremeeva ME, Tissot-Dupont H, Zakharov IA, Raoult D. Genotype characterization of the bacterium expressing the male-killing trait in the ladybird beetle *Adalia bipunctata* with specific rickettsial molecular tools. Appl Environ Microbiol 1995; 61:1431–1437.
73. Roux V, Rydkina E, Eremeeva M, Raoult D. Citrate synthase gene comparison, a new tool for phylogenetic analysis, and its application for the rickettsiae. Int J Syst Bacteriol 1997; 47:252–261.
74. Shpynov SN, Fournier PE, Rudakov NV, et al. Molecular identification of a collection of spotted fever group rickettsiae obtained from patients and ticks from Russia. Am J Trop Med Hyg 2006; 74:440–443.
75. Stenos J, Graves SR, Unsworth NB. A highly sensitive and specific real-time PCR assay for the detection of spotted fever and typhus group rickettsiae. Am J Trop Med Hyg 2005; 73:1083–1085.
76. Wood DO, Williamson LR, Winkler HH, Krause DC. Nucleotide sequence of the *Rickettsia prowazekii* citrate synthase gene. J Bacteriol 1987; 169:3564–3572.
77. Fournier PE, Roux V, Raoult D. Phylogenetic analysis of spotted fever group rickettsiae by study of the outer surface protein rOmpA. Int J Syst Bacteriol 1998; 48:839–849.
78. Roux V, Fournier PE, Raoult D. Differentiation of spotted fever group rickettsiae by sequencing and analysis of restriction fragment length polymorphism of PCR-amplified DNA of the gene encoding the protein rOmpA. J Clin Microbiol 1996; 34:2058–2065.
79. Roux V, Raoult D. Phylogenetic analysis of members of the genus *Rickettsia* using the gene encoding the outer-membrane protein rOmpB (ompB). Int J Syst Evol Microbiol 2000; 50(pt 4):1449–1455.
80. Sekeyova Z, Roux V, Raoult D. Phylogeny of *Rickettsia* spp. inferred by comparing sequences of 'gene D', which encodes an intracytoplasmic protein. Int J Syst Evol Microbiol 2001; 51:1353–1360.

81. Ngwamidiba M, Blanc G, Raoult D, Fournier PE. Sca1, a previously undescribed paralog from autotransporter protein-encoding genes in *Rickettsia* species. BMC Microbiol 2006; 6:12.
82. Anderson BE, Sumner JW, Dawson JE, et al. Detection of the etiologic agent of human ehrlichiosis by polymerase chain reaction. J Clin Microbiol 1992; 30:775–780.
83. Everett ED, Evans KA, Henry RB, McDonald G. Human ehrlichiosis in adults after tick exposure: diagnosis using polymerase chain reaction. Ann Intern Med 1994; 120:730–735.
84. Paddock CD, Folk SM, Shore GM, et al. Infections with *Ehrlichia chaffeensis* and *Ehrlichia ewingii* in persons coinfected with human immunodeficiency virus. Clin Infect Dis 2001; 33:1586–1594.
85. Standaert SM, Dawson JE, Schaffner W, et al. Ehrlichiosis in a golf-oriented retirement community. N Engl J Med 1995; 333:420–425.
86. Sumner JW, Nicholson WL, Massung RF. PCR amplification and comparison of nucleotide sequences from the *groESL* heat shock operon of *Ehrlichia* species. J Clin Microbiol 1997; 35:2087–2092.
87. Bakken JS, Dumler JS, Chen SM, Eckman MR, Van Etta LL, Walker DH. Human granulocytic ehrlichiosis in the upper Midwest United States: a new species emerging? J Am Med Assoc 1994; 272:212–218.
88. Edelman DC, Dumler JS. Evaluation of an improved PCR diagnostic assay for human granulocytic ehrlichiosis. Mol Diagn 1996; 1:41–49.
89. Petrovec M, Lotric FS, Zupanc TA, et al. Human disease in Europe caused by a granulocytic *Ehrlichia* species. J Clin Microbiol 1997; 35:1556–1559.
90. Anderson BE, Dawson JE, Jones DC, Wilson KH. *Ehrlichia chaffeensis*, a new species associated with human ehrlichiosis. J Clin Microbiol 1991; 29:2838–2842.
91. Comer JA, Nicholson WL, Sumner JW, Olson JG, Childs JE. Diagnosis of human ehrlichiosis by PCR assay of acute-phase serum. J Clin Microbiol 1999; 37:31–34.
92. Walls JJ, Caturegli P, Bakken JS, Asanovich KM, Dumler JS. Improved sensitivity of PCR for diagnosis of human granulocytic ehrlichiosis using epank1 genes of *Ehrlichia phagocytophila*-group ehrlichiae. J Clin Microbiol 2000; 38:354–356.
93. van Dobbenburgh A, van Dam AP, Fikrig E. Human granulocytic ehrlichiosis in western Europe. N Engl J Med 1999; 340:1214–1216.
94. Remy V, Hansmann Y, De Martino S, Christmann D, Brouqui P. Human anaplasmosis presenting as atypical pneumonitis in France. Clin Infect Dis 2003; 37:846–848.
95. Lotric-Furlan S, Petrovec M, Zupanc TA, et al. Human granulocytic ehrlichiosis in Europe: clinical and laboratory findings for four patients from Slovenia. Clin Infect Dis 1998; 27:424–428.
96. Bell CA, Patel R. A real-time combined polymerase chain reaction assay for the rapid detection and differentiation of *Anaplasma phagocytophilum*, *Ehrlichia chaffeensis*, and *Ehrlichia ewingii*. Diagn Microbiol Infect Dis 2005; 53:301–306.
97. Andersson SG, Zomorodipour A, Andersson JO, et al. The genome sequence of *Rickettsia prowazekii* and the origin of mitochondria. Nature 1998; 396:133–140.
98. Hotopp JC, Lin M, Madupu R, et al. Comparative genomics of emerging human ehrlichiosis agents. PLoS Genet 2006; 2:e21.
99. Malek JA, Wierzbowski JM, Tao W, et al. Protein interaction mapping on a functional shotgun sequence of *Rickettsia sibirica*. Nucleic Acids Res 2004; 32:1059–1064.
100. McLeod MP, Qin X, Karpathy SE, et al. Complete genome sequence of *Rickettsia typhi* and comparison with sequences of other rickettsiae. J Bacteriol 2004; 186:5842–5855.
101. Ogata H, Audic S, Renesto-Audiffren P, et al. Mechanisms of evolution in *Rickettsia conorii* and *R. prowazekii*. Science 2001; 293:2093–2098.
102. Ogata H, Renesto P, Audic S, et al. The genome sequence of *Rickettsia felis* identifies the first putative conjugative plasmid in an obligate intracellular parasite. PLoS Biol 2005; 3:e248.
103. Apfalter P, Reischl U, Hammerschlag MR. In-house nucleic acid amplification assays in research: how much quality control is needed before one can rely upon the results? J Clin Microbiol 2005; 43:5835–5841.
104. Courtney JW, Kostelnik LM, Zeidner NS, Massung RF. Multiplex real-time PCR for detection of *Anaplasma phagocytophilum* and *Borrelia burgdorferi*. J Clin Microbiol 2004; 42:3164–3168.
105. Doyle CK, Labruna MB, Breitschwerdt EB, et al. Detection of medically important *Ehrlichia* by quantitative multicolor TaqMan real-time polymerase chain reaction of the dsb gene. J Mol Diagn 2005; 7:504–510.
106. Jiang J, Chan TC, Temenak JJ, Dasch GA, Ching WM, Richards AL. Development of a quantitative real-time polymerase chain reaction assay specific for *Orientia tsutsugamushi*. Am J Trop Med Hyg 2004; 70:351–356.
107. Singhsilarak T, Leowattana W, Looareesuwan S, et al. Short report: detection of *Orientia tsutsugamushi* in clinical samples by quantitative real-time polymerase chain reaction. Am J Trop Med Hyg 2005; 72:640–641.
108. Sirigireddy KR, Ganta RR. Multiplex detection of *Ehrlichia* and *Anaplasma* species pathogens in peripheral blood by real-time reverse transcriptase-polymerase chain reaction. J Mol Diagn 2005; 7:308–316.
109. Henry KM, Jiang J, Rozmajzl PJ, Azad AF, Macaluso KR, Richards AL. Development of quantitative real-time PCR assays to detect *Rickettsia typhi* and *Rickettsia felis*, the causative agents of murine typhus and flea-borne spotted fever. Mol Cell Probes 2007; 21:17–23.

110. Svraka S, Rolain JM, Bechah Y, Gatabazi J, Raoult D. *Rickettsia prowazekii* and real-time polymerase chain reaction. Emerg Infect Dis 2006; 12:428–432.
111. Fournier PE, Raoult D. "Suicide" PCR on skin biopsies for the diagnoses of rickettsioses. J Clin Microbiol 2004; 42:3428–3434.
112. Raoult D, Aboudharam G, Crubezy E, Larrouy G, Ludes B, Drancourt M. Molecular identification by "suicide PCR" of *Yersinia pestis* as the agent of Medieval Black Death. Proc Natl Acad Sci USA 2000; 97:12800–12803.
113. Cichter J, Fournier P, Petridou J, Häussinger D, Raoult D. *Rickettsia felis* infection acquired in Europe and documented by polymerase chain reaction. Emerg Infect Dis 2002; 8:207–208.
114. Gouriet F, Fenollar F, Patrice JY, Drancourt M, Raoult D. Use of shell-vial cell culture assay for isolation of bacteria from clinical specimens: 13 years of experience. J Clin Microbiol 2005; 43:4993–5002.
115. Vestris G, Rolain JM, Fournier PE, et al. Seven years' experience of isolation of *Rickettsia* spp. from clinical specimens using the shell vial cell culture assay. Ann NY Acad Sci 2003; 990:371–374.
116. Raoult D, La Scola B, Enea M, et al. Isolation and characterization of a flea-associated rickettsia pathogenic for humans. Emerg Infect Dis 2001; 7:73–81.
117. La Scola B, Meconi S, Fenollar F, Rolain JM, Roux V, Raoult D. Emended description of *Rickettsia felis* (Bouyer et al. 2001), a temperature-dependent cultured bacterium. Int J Syst Evol Microbiol 2002; 52:2035–2041.
118. Birg ML, La Scola B, Roux V, Brouqui P, Raoult D. Isolation of *Rickettsia prowazekii* from blood by shell vial cell culture. J Clin Microbiol 1999; 37:3722–3724.
119. Goodman JL, Nelson C, Vitale B, Madigan JE, Dumler JS, Kurtti TJ. Munderloh UG. Direct cultivation of the causative agent of human granulocytic ehrlichiosis. N Engl J Med 1996; 334:209–215.
120. Bjoersdorff A, Bagert B, Massung RF, Gusa A, Eliasson I. Isolation and characterization of two European strains of *Ehrlichia phagocytophila* of equine origin. Clin Diagn Lab Immunol 2002; 9:341–343.
121. Bakken JS, Dumler JS. Human granulocytic ehrlichiosis. Clin Infect Dis 2000; 31:554–560.
122. Bell EJ, Stoenner HG. Immunologic relationships among the spotted fever group of rickettsias determined by toxin neutralization tests in mice with convalescent animal serums. J Immunol 1960; 84:171–182.
123. Robertson RG, Wisseman CL Jr. Tick-borne rickettsiae of the spotted fever group in West Pakistan. II. Serological classification of isolates from West Pakistan and Thailand: evidence for two new species. Am J Epidemiol 1973; 97:55–64.
124. Plotz H, Reagan RL, Wertman K. Differentiation between "Fièvre boutonneuse" and Rocky Mountain spotted fever by means of complement fixation. Proc Soc Exp Biol Med 1944; 55:173–176.
125. Anacker RL, McDonald GA, List RH, Mann RE. Neutralizing activity of monoclonal antibodies to heat-sensitive and heat-resistant epitopes of *Rickettsia rickettsii* surface proteins. Infect Immun 1987; 55:825–827.
126. McDade JE, Black CM, Roumillat LF, Redus MA, Spruill CL. Addition of monoclonal antibodies specific for *Rickettsia akari* to the rickettsial diagnostic panel. J Clin Microbiol 1988; 26:2221–2223.
127. Xu WB, Raoult D. Taxonomic relationships among spotted fever group rickettsiae as revealed by antigenic analysis with monoclonal antibodies. J Clin Microbiol 1998; 36:887–896.
128. Uchida T. *Rickettsia japonica*, the etiologic agent of Oriental spotted fever. Microbiol Immunol 1993; 37:91–102.
129. Xu WB, Raoult D. Production of monoclonal antibodies against *Rickettsia massiliae* and their use in antigenic and epidemiological studies. J Clin Microbiol 1997; 35:1715–1721.
130. Pedersen CE Jr, Walters VD. Comparative electrophoresis of spotted fever group rickettsial proteins. Life Sci 1978; 22:583–587.
131. Blanc G, Ngwamidiba M, Ogata H, Fournier PE, Claverie JM, Raoult D. Molecular evolution of rickettsia surface antigens: evidence of positive selection. Mol Biol Evol 2005; 22:2073–2083.
132. Beati L, Kelly PJ, Mason PR, Raoult D. Species-specific BALB/c mouse antibodies to rickettsiae studied by Western blotting. FEMS Microbiol Lett 1994; 119:339–344.
133. Eremeeva M, Yu X, Raoult D. Differentiation among spotted fever group rickettsiae species by analysis of restriction fragment length polymorphism of PCR-amplified DNA. J Clin Microbiol 1994; 32:803–810.
134. Radulovic S, Higgins JA, Jaworski DC, Dasch GA, Azad AF. Isolation, cultivation, and partial characterization of the ELB agent associated with cat fleas. Infect Immun 1995; 63:4826–4829.
135. Fournier PE, Zhu Y, Ogata H, Raoult D. Use of highly variable intergenic spacer sequences for multispacer typing of *Rickettsia conorii* strains. J Clin Microbiol 2004; 42:5757–5766.
136. Zhu Y, Fournier PE, Ogata H, Raoult D. Multispacer typing of *Rickettsia prowazekii* enabling epidemiological studies of epidemic typhus. J Clin Microbiol 2005; 43:4708–4712.
137. http://www.cdc;gov/epo/dphsi/casedef/ case_definitions.htm

Section VIII: RICKETTSIAL DISEASES OF DOMESTIC ANIMALS

24 | Rickettsial Diseases of Domestic Animals

Patrick J. Kelly
Ross University School of Veterinary Medicine, Basseterre, St. Kitts, West Indies

INTRODUCTION

Ticks are the natural hosts and vectors of most rickettsias, and domestic and wild animals that ticks feed on are commonly infected with the organisms. Some rickettsias are highly pathogenic in animals with two of the most important diseases of livestock, bovine anaplasmosis and heartwater, being caused by rickettsias. These diseases result in considerable direct and indirect economic losses to the livestock industry worldwide, from morbidity and mortality, decreased productivity, and the development and implementation of control strategies such as disease monitoring, use of acaricides, chemoprophylaxis, and vaccinations. Rickettsias also cause disease in companion animals, dogs, cats, and horses, causing animal suffering and mental and emotional distress to the owners. There are also substantial financial costs to owners, for veterinary treatments and also for tick-prevention programs.

Although much is known about the more severe and economically important rickettsias of livestock and companion animals, there are still many poorly characterized organisms and diseases. The recent discovery of new human rickettsioses has attracted considerable interest and funding and promoted research on rickettsias, organisms that are notoriously difficult to study. As a result, techniques used by rickettsiologists have advanced considerably and enabled studies that have increased our understanding of animal rickettsioses. In this chapter, the major rickettsial diseases of livestock and companion animals are reviewed in the order in which they are summarized in Table 1.

NOFEL

A. bovis, formerly *E. bovis* (1), has been seen in monocytes of cattle from South America, Africa, and the Indian subcontinent and has now been found in cottontail rabbits in the United States (2). There are few phylogenetic data on the organism and it seems likely that more than one species is involved, as multiple ticks, including *Amblyomma*, *Hyalomma*, and *Rhipicephalus* transmit infections and there are widely divergent accounts of the pathogenicity of the organism (3). Although only mild or subclinical disease is reported in most countries, a distinct disease, *Nofel* (ear in local language), occurs in West Africa with mortalities approaching 50%. The disease is particularly severe in cattle stressed by rain, emaciation, or high tick burdens and is characterized by fever, depression, lymph node enlargement, nasal and ocular discharge, severe lung edema, and renal necrosis. Neurological signs develop that are similar to those of heartwater, but without convulsions. Animals frequently shake their heads and one or both ears are held downward over the parotid salivary gland which is markedly inflamed, swollen, and painful. Treatment with tetracyclines is reported effective, and the only prevention is tick control.

BOVINE ANAPLASMOSIS/GALLSICKNESS

Of the *Anaplasma* that infect cattle, *A. marginale* is the most important, causing almost all clinical outbreaks of bovine anaplasmosis (4). The closely related *A. centrale* is of limited pathogenicity and seldom causes disease; a South African isolate has been used extensively as a live vaccine against *A. marginale*.

Bovine anaplasmosis due to *A. marginale* occurs in all six continents and is especially prevalent in tropical areas where vectors, ticks, and biting insects are common. The disease is of great economic importance because of losses from mortalities, decreased production, and costs of prevention and treatment. Also, the disease limits the introduction of superior breeding stock into endemic areas to increase productivity of local animals. *A. marginale* can be transmitted by a range of ticks with *Rhipicephalus* (*Boophilus*) species being particularly important in Africa and Australia, and *Dermacentor* species in the US. Intrastadial and trans-stadial transmission occurs, and males may be particularly important vectors. Various biting insects (horseflies, mosquitoes, stable flies) have been implicated as mechanical vectors, particularly in the United States, but their importance is unknown and probably varies geographically. Iatrogenic

TABLE 1 Major Rickettsial Diseases of Livestock and Companion Animals

Species	Animal	Disease	Vector	Distribution
Anaplasma bovis	Cattle	Nofel	*Amblyomma* spp., *Hyalomma* spp., *Rhipicephalus* spp.	South America, Africa, Iran, India
A. marginale	Cattle	Bovine anaplasmosis/gallsickness	Various ticks; biting insects	Worldwide
A. ondiri	Cattle	Bovine petechial fever/Ondiri disease	Unknown	Africa
A. ovis	Sheep, goats	Ovine/caprine anaplasmosis	Various ticks	Worldwide
A. phagocytophilum[a]	Horses	Equine ehrlichiosis/equine granulocytic anaplasmosis	*Ixodes* spp.	Americas, Europe
	Dogs	Canine granulocytic ehrlichiosis/anaplasmosis		
	Cats	Feline granulocytic ehrlichiosis/anaplasmosis		
	Ruminants	Pasture fever/tick-borne fever		
A. platys	Dogs	Canine infectious cyclic thrombocytopenia/canine thrombocytotrophic anaplasmosis	Unknown	Worldwide
Ehrlichia canis[a]	Dogs	Canine monocytic ehrlichiosis	*Rhipicephalus sanguineus*	Worldwide
	Cats	Feline monocytic ehrlichiosis	Unknown	Americas, Europe, Asia
E. chaffeensis[a]	Dogs	Canine monocytic ehrlichiosis	*Amblyomma americanum*	North America
E. ewingii[a]	Dogs	Canine granulocytic ehrlichiosis	*A. americanum*	North America, Africa
E. ovina	Sheep, goats	Ovine/caprine ehrlichiosis	*Rhipicephalus* spp.	Africa, Turkey
E. ruminantium	Cattle, sheep, goats	Heartwater	*Amblyomma* spp.	Africa, Caribbean
Neorickettsia helminthoeca	Dogs	Salmon poisoning disease	*Nanophyetes salmincola*	Pacific Northwest U.S.A.
N. risticii	Horses	Potomac horse fever/equine monocytic neorickettsiosis	Digenic trematodes	North America
	Dogs	Canine monocytic neorickettsiosis		
Rickettsia rickettsii[a]	Dogs	Rocky Mountain spotted fever	*Dermacentor* spp.	Americas
A. platys	Dogs	Canine infectious cyclic thrombocytopenia/canine thrombocytotrophic anaplasmosis	Unknown	Worldwide

[a]Also infects people.

transmission has been described with veterinary instruments and syringe needles. Cattle that survive infection become persistently infected for life and are the main reservoirs of infection. A number of wild ruminants may also be reservoirs in Africa and the United States (5).

A. marginale organisms are only found in erythrocytes where they divide by binary fission to form up to eight initial bodies that are released by exocytosis and infect other erythrocytes. Cells containing parasites are removed by the mononuclear phagocytic system, resulting in fever and anemia, which are the hallmarks of bovine anaplasmosis.

Clinical disease is common when susceptible animals are introduced into endemic areas or the vector distribution expands; mortality rates can be over 50%. The incubation period is around three to four weeks and clinical signs depend largely on age (4). Cattle of all ages can be infected, but in enzootic areas animals are exposed at a young age. Calves under six months of age have a nonspecific resistance to infection, irrespective of their dams' immune status; they usually develop only mild anemia and show few, if any, clinical signs. In cattle up to three years of age, signs are usually only seen with parasitemias of over 15%. They include steady or fluctuating fever for up to two weeks, partial anorexia, weight loss, and jaundice that develops later in the course of the disease. There is no hemoglobinuria or hemoglobinemia and convalescence is slow, over one to two months. Pregnant cows frequently abort and there is decreased milk production in lactating animals. Young bulls might have reduced fertility for some months after infection. Animals over three years of age commonly have acute and sometimes even peracute infections. With the latter, animals usually die in 24 hours with high fever, severe anemia, dyspnea, and hyperexcitability. Recovered cattle become chronic carriers and have periodic subclinical parasitemias; the percentage of parasitized erythrocytes decreases as an animal ages.

INFECTIONS IN SHEEP AND GOATS

Diagnosis of clinical cases is usually made by identifying organisms near the margin of erythrocytes in Giemsa- or Diff-Quik-stained venous blood smears. The organisms must be differentiated from those of *A. centrale*, which appear to be similar but are situated away from the margin of the erythrocyte. The number of visible *A. marginale* varies with the stage and severity of disease. They are usually detectable when clinical signs first appear, and the parasitemia approximately doubles each day for about 10 days with levels peaking at up to 70%. Thereafter, parasitemias decrease at a similar rate.

Various serological tests are available to detect infections in chronic carriers and animals in the late stages of infection when parasitemia is low. Although the complement fixation test has been widely used, it has poor sensitivity (20%) in identifying chronic carriers (6). A card agglutination test, which is cheap and rapid, has been widely used, but it also lacks sensitivity as well as specificity. Other tests include the indirect enzyme-linked immunosorbent serologic assay (ELISA), dot ELISA, and indirect fluorescent antibody assay (IFA). Cross-reactions with *A. phagocytophilum* have recently been reported (7). A commercially available competitive enzyme-linked immunosorbent assay (C-ELISA) has high sensitivity (96%) and specificity (95%) relative to a nested polymerase chain reaction (PCR) procedure (8).

Nucleic-acid-based tests for *A. marginale* have been developed and include RNA and DNA probes, and PCR-based methods including a nested PCR and a reverse-line blot hybridization assay that can identify as few as 50 infected erythrocytes per milliliter of blood, well below the lowest levels in carriers (9).

Eradication of bovine anaplasmosis is impractical in endemic areas because of the wide range of vectors and the large number of carriers. In these areas, it is probably best to ensure endemic stability by limiting acaricide use and allowing sufficient tick numbers to ensure calves will be infected while they have nonspecific resistance to disease. For naïve animals that will be introduced to endemic areas, and for animals living in epidemic areas, various vaccines are available (10). A live vaccine containing *A. centrale* is used widely, but not in the United States or areas where there is reluctance to introduce *A. centrale*. It gives partial protection against challenge with virulent *A. marginale* after six to eight weeks and immunity lasts for several years. The vaccine must be kept chilled or frozen, which limits its use. Also, it is not entirely safe and can cause clinical disease and death, especially in older animals. The vaccine is best used on calves because their nonspecific immunity minimizes the risk of serious vaccine reactions. All vaccinates, however, should be monitored for reactions after four to six weeks and responders treated with tetracycline or imidocarb dipropionate.

An attenuated vaccine was developed that contained *A. marginale* passaged through non-bovine hosts, such as deer or sheep. Killed vaccines are available, but two initial doses and yearly boosters are required, which is often impractical. Their efficacy is also limited because of antigenic strain diversity. The vaccine does not prevent infections but does reduce severity of signs. Recently, four novel antigens of *A. marginale* have been recognized that have shown promise in preliminary vaccine trials (11).

Treatment of clinical cases is with oxytetracycline (6–10 mg/kg IM q24 hours for three days) or long-acting chlortetracycline (20 mg/kg IM once) (4). Imidocarb dipropionate (3 mg/kg SC once) can also be used. Treatments do not interfere with immunity, and most animals will become chronic carriers. Although there are reports that tetracyclines and imidocarb dipropionate can eliminate infections, recent experiments have shown the currently recommended regimens for tetracyclines are not effective (12).

BOVINE PETECHIAL FEVER/ONDIRI DISEASE

This disease was common in the highlands of Kenya and East Africa, in the 1960s and 1970s, but now occurs sporadically (13). The etiological agent occurs mainly in neutrophils and was named *Cytoecetes ondiri* in 1972; at this time, *Cytoecetes* was the name given to *Ehrlichia*-like organisms that did not occur in monocytes. Recent serological studies, however, have shown that the organism is closely related to *A. phagocytophilum* and the agent is tentatively thought to be *A. ondiri* (3). A vector has not been identified but cattle that graze near the edges of forests or in thick scrub are predisposed, and bushbucks (*Tragelaphus scriptus*) appear to be reservoirs of infection. Other domestic and wild ruminants can be infected experimentally, but only cattle introduced to endemic areas show clinical signs.

There is usually high fever for three to four days and hemorrhagic diathesis over 10 days. Anemia can be marked and there is severe leucopenia and thrombocytopenia. Affected animals have sudden agalactia and may abort. Diagnosis is made by detecting organisms in blood smears, but parasitemia declines later in the disease and serology for *A. phagocytophilum* might be useful. The mortality rate can reach 50% but tetracyclines are effective if given at onset of illness. Cattle surviving infections become carriers for many months or years.

OVINE AND CAPRINE ANAPLASMOSIS

A. ovis is seen in erythrocytes of sheep and goats in most tropical and subtropical areas of the world where it can be transmitted by a number of species of ticks (14). Most infections are subclinical and the organism is of comparatively little economic importance. Goats are more susceptible than sheep. In animals that are immunosuppressed from heavy helminth or tick burdens or other arthropod-borne diseases, there might be listlessness, mild fever, and anemia. Recovered animals have solid immunity but remain chronic carriers. *A. marginale* can induce subclinical infections in small ruminants.

EQUINE EHRLICHIOSIS/EQUINE GRANULOCYTIC ANAPLASMOSIS

The etiological agent was first named *E. equi*, but is now recognized as a strain of *A. phagocytophilum* (1). The disease is common in northern California but has been reported across the United States and in Europe and South America. The vectors are *Ixodes* spp., in particular *I . pacificus* (black-legged tick) in California (15) and *I. ricinus* in Europe. Most infections are subclinical but in horses that develop a more severe vasculitis, clinical signs evolve over a number of days and include fluctuating fever, depression, partial anorexia, ataxia, reluctance to move, limb edema, and icterus (16). Deaths are uncommon and animals gradually improve after one to two weeks. Laboratory abnormalities include anemia, leucopenia, thrombocytopenia, and increased bilirubin. After a few days of clinical signs, morulae are readily seen in neutrophils or eosinophils, but infections can also be diagnosed using an IFA or by identification of the organism in blood using PCR. Although oxytetracycline (7 mg/kg IV q24 hours) causes rapid defervescence, treatment should continue for a week to prevent reoccurrence of signs. There is no vaccine, and infections are best prevented by tick control.

CANINE GRANULOCYTIC EHRLICHIOSIS/ANAPLASMOSIS

Dogs naturally and experimentally infected with equine or human strains of *A. phagocytophilum* show no clinical signs or have acute disease with mild pyrexia, lethargy, anorexia and musculoskeletal pain/discomfort with lameness, and reluctance to move (17). There might be transient thrombocytopenia and mild anemia. Diagnosis is usually made by detecting morulae that can be seen in neutrophils (3–35%) for up to nine days. Analysis by PCR is needed to differentiate *A. phagocytophilum* from the other granulocytic organism, *E. ewingii*. The recommended treatment is doxycycline (10 mg/kg PO q24 hours for 10 days).

FELINE GRANULOCYTIC EHRLICHIOSIS/ANAPLASMOSIS

Experimental infections of cats with *A. phagocytophilum* cause no clinical signs but animals seroconvert, and morulae are seen in the neutrophils. There are seropositive cats in Europe and the United States (18), and animals with clinical signs attributable to *A. phagocytophilum* have been reported (19). Major signs include fever, anorexia, and muscle and joint pain. Treatment with tetracycline appears to be effective.

PASTURE FEVER AND TICK-BORNE FEVER

In Europe, *A. phagocytophilum* transmitted transstadially by *I. ricinus* (castor-bean tick) causes pasture fever and tick-borne fever in domestic ruminants (20). Although *A. phagocytophilum* also occurs in the United States, clinical cases have not been reported in cattle and it seems these strains are of low pathogenicity in ruminants (21).

Pasture fever occurs in dairy cattle that have over-wintered in barns and are turned out onto tick-infested pastures in spring. There is a severe drop in milk yield, high fever, mild depression, anorexia, and occasional coughing.

Tick-borne fever occurs in sheep, cattle, and very occasionally in goats that are moved from tick-free to tick-infested areas. Infections are usually subclinical but there may be fever, anorexia, coughing, and mild weight loss. Infected lambs may have reduced weight gain (22). Although clinical signs in lambs are usually mild, there are marked hematological changes including high parasitemias (80%) of neutrophils and lymphopenia, neutropenia, and thrombocytopenia. Up to 50% of pregnant animals abort or give birth to weak premature offspring, whereas the leucopenia predisposes to a variety of severe concurrent bacterial (lamb pyemia due to *Staphylococcus aureus*, pasteurellosis, and listeriosis) and viral infections (louping ill). Affected animals, especially sheep, usually become carriers for months to years, and relapses can occur with sudden leucopenia, parasitemia, and transient fever.

Deer can also be infected and might also be reservoirs of infection.

Diagnosis usually depends on the observation of inclusion in granulocytes and may be supported by serology. Tetracyclines reduce parasitemias and clinical signs and may lessen losses from decreased milk production, weight gain, and secondary infections. Disease is best prevented by avoiding tick-infested areas. If this is not possible, animals should be treated with appropriate acaricides, and long-acting tetracyclines can be given prophylactically. Abortions may be prevented by exposing animals to infected ticks before they are bred.

CANINE INFECTIOUS CYCLIC THROMBOCYTOPENIA/CANINE THROMBOCYTOTROPHIC ANAPLASMOSIS

The etiological agent is *A. platys* which occurs in the United States, Western Europe, Africa, the Middle and Far East, and Australia (23). The pathogenicity of strains varies, with those in the United States generally causing minimal clinical signs. The organism is thought to be transmitted by ticks, and high percentages of platelets are infected in the initial parasitemic episode. Clinical signs include fever, anorexia, lymphadenomegaly, pallor, and petechial hemorrhages of the mucous membranes and skin. There is a precipitous decline in platelet numbers until the parasites disappear and, within three to four days, platelet numbers return to normal levels. Parasitemias and subsequent thrombocytopenias recur at one- to two-week intervals but their intensity diminishes with time. Finally, there is a slowly resolving thrombocytopenia, with parasites occurring only sporadically. Infections can be diagnosed if parasites are seen in stained blood smears but serology with a commercially available IFA is usually necessary. Specific and sensitive PCR primers for *A. platys* have been developed (24). Tetracyclines appear to be effective in treatment, and tick control is recommended for prevention of infections.

CANINE MONOCYTIC EHRLICHIOSES

E. canis is the more important of the two agents causing canine monocytic ehrlichiosis. Previously, the disease caused by *E. canis* was known as canine tropical pancytopenia, with infections reported worldwide, apart from Australia and New Zealand (25). *E. canis* is transmitted transstadially, but not transovarially, by *Rh. sanguineus*, the brown dog tick, and transstadially by *D. variabilis* (the American dog tick). *E. canis* infects monocytes attracted to the site of tick attachment that spread in the blood and lymph to tissues throughout the body. The organism persists in the different organs in macrophages resulting in plasmacytosis and generalized perivascular lymphoid and plasma cell accumulation. Persistence of *E. canis* in the body stimulates production of reactive antibodies, but these are not protective. Dogs only become susceptible to reinfection with *E. canis* once existing infections are cleared by appropriate therapy or self-cure (26), even if high antibody titers are still present.

Classically there are three phases of infection:

1. The acute phase may be subclinical or there may be depression, lethargy, anorexia, mild weight loss, fever, lymph node enlargement, and splenomegaly. Thrombocytopenia is common but there might also be anemia and leucopenia; the bone marrow is usually hypercellular. Most dogs recover in one to four weeks and enter the subclinical phase.
2. In the subclinical phase, dogs appear healthy but remain infected with *E. canis*, commonly with hyperglobulinemia (90%) and thrombocytopenia (50%). Polyclonal gammopathies are most common, but monoclonal gammopathies may occur. The subclinical phase may last between four months and 10 years and during this time dogs may spontaneously eliminate the organism (26).
3. In some dogs, a severe, life-threatening chronic phase of the disease develops (27). Animals have weight loss and emaciation, fever, pallor, weakness, hemorrhage, and peripheral edema, particularly of the hind limbs and scrotum. There is usually a pronounced nonregenerative anemia, severe leucopenia, and thrombocytopenia. The bone marrow is hyperplastic initially, but later it is hypoplastic. Death is usually from extensive hemorrhage or secondary bacterial infections.

In naturally infected dogs, in which the stage of infection is unknown, depression (67%), weight loss (59%), anorexia (56%), hemorrhagic tendencies, in particular, epistaxis (46%), pyrexia (40%), and lymphadenomegaly (30%) are the most commonly reported clinical signs in the United States (28). Rarely, there might be polymyositis, paresis, meningoencephalitis, cranial nerve deficits, seizures, abortions and infertility, corneal opacity, anterior uveitis, hyphema, focal chorioretinal lesions, retinal detachment, coughing, and exercise intolerance.

German Shepherd dogs and their crosses are particularly likely to show more severe signs of disease, and infections in this breed are associated with a poorer prognosis.

Accurate diagnosis of *E. canis* infection is important as it enables appropriate treatment, particularly in the subclinical phase before the severe life-threatening chronic form develops. As there are no pathognomonic clinical or laboratory signs, special tests are needed for definitive diagnoses. Morulae of *E. canis* are seldom seen, and isolation of organisms is impractical, taking as long as two months. The IFA and commercial "cage-side" ELISAs have become the most widely used tests for the diagnosis of *E. canis* infections. Positive results show exposure to *E. canis*, whereas rising IFA titers indicate recent infection. Decreasing IFA titers show successful treatment or elimination of the infection. Unfortunately, antibody titers often remain elevated for months after the organism has been eliminated and serology cannot reliably detect ongoing infection. Usefulness of tests is also limited by serological cross-reactivity between *E. canis* and other ehrlichias that might give false-positive results (29).

PCR performed on blood or splenic aspirates is a sensitive test for detecting experimental infections (30) and enables differentiation between *E. canis* and *E. chaffeensis*. There is poor correlation, however, between PCR and serology results in naturally infected dogs, which could be due to poor sensitivity of the PCR or positive serology persisting despite clearance of infections (31).

Doxycycline (10 mg/kg PO q24 hours for two to six weeks) is the recommended treatment but, although this antibiotic has a marked bactericidal effect against *E. canis* in vivo (32), a complete response to treatment is seen in only 45% of dogs and inadequate response to treatment is seen in up to 41% of dogs (33). Possible reasons include lack of owner compliance, reinfection, and lack of penetration of drug into all infected organs.

There are anecdotal reports that imidocarb dipropionate is effective against *E. canis*, but in vivo and clinical data indicate that the drug is ineffective (32).

There are no vaccines available against canine ehrlichioses but a preliminary study has shown killed *E. canis* stimulate a humoral and cell-mediated immune response and animals may be protected against challenge (34). Chemoprophylaxis is effective (doxycycline 100 mg PO q24 hours) but the best prevention at the moment involves strict control of the tick vectors.

It is now recognized that concurrent infections of dogs with *Ehrlichia* and other tick-borne pathogens is common (35,36). Further studies are indicated to determine the relative contributions these agents make to the overall clinical and laboratory abnormalities that may be detected in dogs with concurrent infections. Studies are also indicated to determine the effects of concurrent infections on the diagnosis, treatment, and prognosis of affected dogs.

E. chaffeensis is the agent of human monocytic ehrlichiosis, which can also infect dogs and cause canine monocytic ehrlichiosis. The organism was first found in the United States where it is transmitted mainly by *A. americanum* and perhaps by *D. variabilis*; more recently, it (or a very similar organism) has been shown to also occur in other parts of the world (37). High prevalences of natural infections of dogs have been reported with some showing signs similar to those caused by *E. canis* (35). Experimental infections of dogs, however, result in minimal clinical and hematological abnormalities although dogs become carriers for two to four months and may be important reservoirs of infection (38). Certain data suggests that infection with *E. chaffeensis* does not protect against subsequent infection with *E. canis*.

FELINE MONOCYTIC EHRLICHIOSIS

Bodies resembling morulae have been detected in mononuclear cells of cats from the United States, Kenya, Brazil, France, and Thailand (39). DNA studies in the United States and in France have indicated that the organism is most consistent with *E. canis*. Infected cats have had a wide variety of clinical signs including fever, anorexia, weight loss, hyperesthesia, and joint pain. Doxycycline is the recommended treatment.

CANINE GRANULOCYTIC EHRLICHIOSIS

E. ewingii, the agent of canine granulocytic ehrlichiosis, is common in the southeastern and south-central areas of the United States and has recently been described in Africa (40). It is transmitted by *A. americanum* (41) and has been found in *D. variabilis* and *R. sanguineus*. White-tailed deer may be important reservoirs of infection (42). In naturally infected dogs, *E. ewingii* is commonly seen in circulating neutrophils in the first week of clinical signs that are generally mild and include suppurative polyarthritis in one or more limbs, acute lameness, mild fever, and thrombocytopenia (43). The organism has not been grown in tissue culture and there are no specific serological assays. There is variable cross-reactivity with antigens of *E. canis*, which might facilitate diagnosis. Currently, definitive diagnoses are usually obtained with a species-specific PCR assay.

OVINE/CAPRINE EHRLICHIOSIS

Organisms named *E. ovina* (sometimes incorrectly written as *E. ovis*) have been observed in monocytes of sheep and goats in Africa and Turkey (3). Infections are transmitted by

Rhipicephalus spp. and appear to be of little clinical significance. There are no isolates, and the phylogenetic status of the organism requires investigation (1).

HEARTWATER

Heartwater is a severe disease of African and Caribbean cattle, sheep, and goats caused by *E. ruminantium* (44), previously *Cowdria ruminantium* (1). Infections in African wild ruminants are usually not apparent, but these animals may be reservoirs of infection. Guinea fowl, leopard tortoises, and scrub hare can also be infected and remain carriers; whether they constitute reservoirs in nature is unknown. Although *E. ruminantium* can be transmitted transstadially by many *Amblyomma* spp., *A. variegatum* (the tropical bont tick) is the most widespread and important vector. *E. ruminantium* occurs widely in sub-Saharan Africa and spread to the Caribbean in the 1700s or 1800s with *A. variegatum* on cattle imported from Senegal. The presence of the organism in the Caribbean poses a threat to livestock on the American mainland where there is a fully susceptible domestic ruminant population, a competent vector (*A. maculatum*), and potential wildlife reservoirs of infection (such as white-tailed deer) (45).

After injection in tick saliva, *E. ruminantium* multiplies in the local lymph nodes before entering the circulation and infecting vascular endothelial cells throughout the body. The resulting increased vascular permeability often leads to hydropericardium (hence the name *heartwater*), ascites, hydrothorax, mediastinal edema, and marked edema of the lungs. There is also degeneration of the vital organs, and petechiae and larger hemorrhages.

The incubation period is about two weeks in the field and four clinical forms of heartwater may be distinguished, depending on the susceptibility of the host and the virulence of the strain of *E. ruminantium* (44). The peracute form lasts for a day or so and is seen mainly in European breeds that are introduced into endemic areas. Animals have fever, severe respiratory distress and diarrhea, and terminal convulsions. The mortality rate is 100%.

In the acute form, up to 90% of animals die, usually within six days. It is the most common form of the disease, occurring in local and exotic breeds. There is acute fever, anorexia, depression, tachypnea, and classic neurological signs including high-stepping gait, circling, chewing movements, exaggerated blink reflexes, tongue protrusion, and occasionally aggression and apparent blindness. Later, animals become recumbent, make paddling movements with their legs, and have opisthotonus, nystagmus, hyperesthesia, frothing at the mouth and nostrils, and convulsions. There can also be profuse diarrhea.

Subacute disease is uncommon with animals having prolonged fever, coughing, and mild ataxia over one to two weeks. In the mild or subclinical form of the disease, there is a transient fever, called heartwater fever. It is usually seen in wild ruminants, calves under three weeks, indigenous breeds with high natural resistance, and partially immune animals. Animals that recover become carriers and remain infective for ticks for at least a year (44).

Postmortem diagnoses are traditionally made by observing organisms in endothelial cells of capillaries in brain smears. A variety of serological tests have been used for surveys and to detect carrier animals that might spread *E. ruminantium* when transported from endemic areas (44). The IFA, ELISA, and competitive ELISA are all of limited use as they give false-positive reactions with animals exposed to other *Ehrlichia* species. More recently, an indirect ELISA has been developed that detects antibodies to a fragment of the major outer membrane protein of *E. ruminantium*, designated MAP 1B (46). Although this test is more specific, it can give false negatives in chronically infected cattle that down-regulate production of antibodies to the MAP 1 protein (47). Infections are probably best diagnosed using one of the recently developed molecular techniques utilizing probes targeting the pCS20, 16S RNA, and MAP 1 genes (44).

Although several drugs can be used to treat heartwater, oxytetracycline (10–20 mg/kg IM repeated after 24 hours) is most widely used. It is very effective if given very early in the course of the disease. Animals that recover, even with treatment, develop a solid immunity against homologous strains which is mainly T-cell-mediated. This immunity persists if there is continual challenge.

Heartwater can be prevented by tick control, chemoprophylaxis, and/or vaccination (44). Unfortunately, eradication of *Amblyomma* using acaricides is not possible as the tick has a high rate of reproduction and will also feed on many species of wildlife. Calves (<3 weeks) and lambs (<1 weeks) are very resistant to *E. ruminantium* and exposure at this time results in solid immunity with very mild or no clinical signs. To obtain a stable disease situation, acaricides should be used to maintain numbers of *Amblyomma* at levels that ensure exposure of animals when they are young and also enable reinfection of immune animals to maintain protective immunity. Chemoprophylaxis with tetracyclines can be used to protect animals being moved into heartwater endemic areas if the infection pressure is sufficiently great.

The current vaccination system was developed 50 years ago in South Africa and involves infection of animals with cryopreserved sheep blood containing virulent *E. ruminantium* (44). When there is a febrile response, the infection is treated with tetracyclines. Some mortality is common with this procedure, which is labor-intensive. To help overcome the labor problem, a block method of immunization has been devised where animals are all vaccinated on day 0 and then all treated 11 to 16 days later, depending on the species and breed. A method using vaccination and doxycycline implants to prevent clinical disease has proven unreliable (48).

Attempts are being made to develop vaccines with attenuated strains (49) but there is considerable genetic variability between stocks, which can result in poor cross-protection. Also, not all strains can be attenuated. Killed vaccines have been tested, but they have so far proved disappointing in the field where multiple genotypes occur (50). Subunit and DNA vaccines have also been developed and tested with variable results.

SALMON POISONING DISEASE

This is a highly fatal disease of dogs in the Pacific Northwestern region of the United States caused by *N. helminthoeca*, which is transmitted by *N. salmincola*, a small intestinal trematode of dogs (51). Its life cycle involves the dog, a freshwater snail, and a salmonid fish. Coyotes also show clinical signs but cats do not.

The incubation period is about a week and signs include fever, anorexia, lymph node enlargement, and severe hemorrhagic enteritis that may be fatal in 7 to 10 days if untreated. Diagnosis is based on the presence of intracellular pleomorphic rods that fill the cytoplasm of the mononuclear phagocytic cells in lymph node aspirates. Finding ova of *N. salmincola* in the animal's feces supports the diagnosis.

N. salmincola can be treated with praziquantel (5 mg/kg sc) and *N. helminthoeca* with oxytetracycline (7 mg/kg q8h for five days) which should be given intravenously because of the vomiting and diarrhea. There are no vaccines, and infections are best controlled by preventing dogs eating uncooked salmonid fish.

POTOMAC HORSE FEVER/EQUINE MONOCYTIC NEORICKETTSIOSIS

This is an acute enterocolitis of horses in North America that is caused by *N. helminthoeca* and closely related species (52). The vectors are digenetic trematodes that use freshwater snails and aquatic insects, such as caddisflies, as intermediate hosts. It is not known how infections are transmitted from the aquatic insects to horses, but insectivores, such as bats and swallows, may be natural reservoirs (53).

N. risticii circulates in monocytes and has a predilection for the mucosa of the cecum and large colon. Most infections are subclinical and when signs appear they are very inconsistent, including combinations of fever, depression, anorexia, colic, and ileus. Diarrhea occurs in under 60% of horses and laminitis in up to 40% of cases (54). The mortality rate can reach 30%; signs in horses that survive without treatment usually resolve over 5 to 10 days. Organisms are seldom seen in blood smears, serology is unreliable, and diagnosis is best based on PCR detection of organisms (54).

Oxytetracycline (6.6 mg/kg IV q24 hours for five days) is the treatment of choice and a response is usually seen within 12 hours. Inactivated, partially purified, whole-cell vaccines are available but protection is short-lived (around four months) and vaccine failures occur, possibly because of lack of cross-protection between strains of *N. risticii* (55).

CANINE MONOCYTIC NEORICKETTSIOSIS

Dogs experimentally infected with *N. risticii* show no clinical signs (56) but naturally acquired infections have been described with signs of fever, bleeding tendencies, edema, neurological signs, polyarthritis, anemia, and thrombocytopenia. It is not certain whether the agent is *N. risticii* or a caninotropic strain of the organism (57).

CANINE ROCKY MOUNTAIN SPOTTED FEVER

R. rickettsii is the agent of Rocky Mountain spotted fever (RMSF) in people. The organism occurs in Central and South America but is most widely reported in North America where it is transmitted principally by *D. andersoni* (the woodtick) and *D. variabilis*. In dogs, the organism multiplies in endothelial cells causing vasculitis and activation of platelets and the coagulation system (58). Many infections are subclinical and high percentages of apparently healthy dogs are seropositive in endemic areas. Other nonpathogenic spotted fever group (SFG) rickettsias including *R. rhipicephali*, *R. montana*, and *R. belli* may stimulate immune responses in dogs, which protect them from infections with *R. rickettsii*.

Dogs with clinical signs often have fever, depression, anorexia, lymph node enlargement, subcutaneous edema, muscle and joint pain, and petechiation of the skin and mucous membranes (58). There might also be epistaxis, melena, hematuria, focal neurological signs, necrosis of the extremities, and death from hemorrhagic diathesis, failure of vital organs, or vascular collapse and shock. Dogs seropositive due to previous exposure are common but rising titers in serial samples are diagnostic for RMSF. Direct fluorescent antibody tests on skin samples may be diagnostic, and PCR is available for blood and skin samples. Isolation is possible in specialized laboratories but may take many weeks.

Early treatment with doxycycline (20 mg/kg PO or IV q12 hours for one week) improves the prognosis, and there is usually a rapid response in one to two days. There are no commercial vaccines and prevention depends on tick control.

OTHER SPOTTED FEVER GROUP RICKETTSIAL INFECTIONS

There is little information on the effects of the numerous other SFG rickettsiae on domestic animals. In limited studies, SFG rickettsiae that are nonpathogenic in people have also been found to not cause signs in animals. Similarly, dogs experimentally infected with *R. conorii*, the agent of Mediterranean spotted fever in people, show no clinical or laboratory abnormalities although they seroconvert and become rickettsemic for up to 10 days (59). Also, dogs infected with *R. australis* show no signs and do not become rickettsemic although seroconversion occurs (60). Cattle and goats infected with *R. africae*, the agent of African tick-bite fever, show no systemic signs but are rickettsemic for up to 30 days and might be important reservoirs of infection (61,62). *R. felis* is the recently described agent of flea-borne spotted fever in people. The organism is maintained in nature by the cat flea, *Ctenocephalides felis*. Cats show no clinical signs when infected but they become rickettsemic for short periods (under a month) before reactive antibodies develop and clear the infection (63).

PUBLIC HEALTH CONSIDERATIONS

A number of the animal rickettsioses are also zoonoses (Table 1) and domestic animals and livestock are important sentinels for human infections. A recent report describes a fatal case of RMSF a few weeks after two of the patient's dogs died, probably of the same disease (64). This case emphasizes the importance of direct communication between veterinarians and physicians when zoonoses are diagnosed or suspected. Around the world, animal serology has been shown to be a reliable means of determining the distribution of human exposure to rickettsiae and predicting changes in the incidence of human infections. As examples, surveys of horses for antibodies to *R. rickettsii* have been recommended for Brazilian spotted fever surveillance (65), seroprevalences against SFG rickettsia in dogs are significantly higher in areas of Japan were Japanese spotted fever caused by *R. japonica* is endemic (66), and in Africa, seroprevalences in domestic ruminants have been shown to correlate with human exposure to SFG rickettsiae (61,62).

Although direct infections from animals are unlikely, animals play important roles in human infections by increasing the numbers of infected ticks in the environment and bringing ticks into the household and into contact with people. Ticks on livestock are most readily controlled by regular application of acaricides; however, new environment-friendly strategies are being developed (67). Control of ticks on wildlife is more problematic, but application of pour-on acaricides with devices such as the Duncan Self Medicating Applicator® has been very successful (68). Appropriate fencing will prevent larger wildlife species entering and bringing ticks into gardens and recreational areas where survival of ticks is decreased if vegetation is kept well trimmed. Various acaricides are available that can be applied to vegetation to decrease tick numbers, and people venturing into the countryside can use tick repellants such as DEET (69).

Dogs and cats play a particularly important role in bringing infected ticks into the household and into contact with people. There are, however, a number of very effective acaricides (70) for control of ticks and fleas on dogs and cats, and veterinarians actively promote their use. Where such products are not used, ticks will occur on pets, in which case owners remove the parasites. Ticks have high levels of SFG rickettsias in their hemolymph and feces, and people have been infected by inoculation of skin lesions or the conjunctiva. Ideally, gloves should be worn and ticks removed by grasping the head with tweezers. Excessive pressure on the body can cause the tick to rupture, which might lead to conjunctival exposure. This is prevented by covering ticks with a facial tissue during removal. Ticks that are removed are best killed by placing them in alcohol or bleach, or by applying an insecticide. At the end of the procedure, hands should be washed thoroughly.

REFERENCES

1. Dumler JS, Barbet AF, Bekker CP, et al. Reorganization of genera in the families Rickettsiaceae and Anaplasmataceae in the order *Rickettsiales*: unification of some species of *Ehrlichia* with *Anaplasma*, *Cowdria* with *Ehrlichia*, and *Ehrlichia* with *Neorickettsia*, descriptions of five new species combinations and designation of *Ehrlichia equi* and 'HGE agent' as subjective synonyms of *Ehrlichia phagocytophila*. Int J Syst Evol Microbiol 2001; 51:2145–2165.
2. Goethert H, Telford S. Enzootic transmission of *Anaplasma bovis* in Nantucket cottontail rabbits. J Clin Microbiol 2003; 41(8):3744–3747.
3. Sumption KJ, Scott GR. Lesser-known rickettsias infecting livestock. In: Coetzer JAW, Tustin RC, eds. Infectious Diseases of Livestock. 2nd ed. Vol. 1. Cape Town: Oxford University Press, 2005:536–549.
4. Potgieter F, Stoltsz W. Bovine anaplasmosis. In: Coetzer JAW, Tustin R, eds. Infectious Diseases of Livestock. 2nd ed. Vol. 1. Cape Town: Oxford University Press, 2004:594–616.
5. Kuttler KL. *Anaplasma* infections in wild and domestic ruminants: a review. J Wildl Dis 1984; 20(1):12–20.
6. Bradway DS, Torioni de Echaide S, Knowles DP, et al. Sensitivity and specificity of the complement fixation test for detection of cattle persistently infected with *Anaplasma marginale*. J Vet Diagn Invest 2001; 13:79–81.
7. Dreher UM, de la Fuente J, Hofmann-Lehmann R, et al. Serologic cross-reactivity between *Anaplasma marginale* and *Anaplasma phagocytophilum*. Clin Diagn Lab Immunol 2005; 12:1177–1183.
8. Torioni de Echaide S, Knowles DP, McGuire TC, et al. Detection of cattle naturally infected with *Anaplasma marginale* in a region of endemicity by nested PCR and a competitive enzyme-linked immunosorbent assay using recombinant major surface protein 5. J Clin Microbiol 1998; 36:777–782.
9. Molad T, Mazuz ML, Fleiderovitz L, et al. Molecular and serological detection of *A. centrale*- and *A. marginale*-infected cattle grazing within an endemic area. Vet Microbiol 2005; 113(1–2):55–62.
10. Kocan K, de la Fuente J, Guglielmone A, et al. Antigens and alternatives for control of *Anaplasma marginale* infection in cattle. Clin Microbiol Rev 2003; 16(4):698–712.
11. Riding G, Hope M, Waltisbuhl D, et al. Identification of novel protective antigens from *Anaplasma marginale*. Vaccine 2003; 21(17–18):1874–1883.
12. Coetzee JF, Apley MD, Kocan KM, et al. Comparison of three oxytetracycline regimes for the treatment of persistent *Anaplasma marginale* infections in beef cattle. Vet Parasitol 2005; 127(1):61–73.
13. Davies G. Bovine petechial fever (Ondiri disease). Vet Microbiol 1993; 34(2):103–121.
14. Stoltsz WH. Ovine and caprine anaplasmosis. In: Coetzer JAW, Tustin R, eds. Infectious Diseases of Livestock. 2nd ed. Vol. 1. Cape Town: Oxford University Press, 2004:617–624.
15. Richter PJ Jr, Kimsey RB, Madigan JE, et al. *Ixodes pacificus* (Acari: Ixodidae) as a vector of *Ehrlichia equi* (Rickettsiales: Ehrlichieae). J Med Entomol 1996; 33(1):1–5.
16. Madigan JE, Gribble DH. Equine ehrlichiosis in northern California: 49 cases (1968–1981). J Am Vet Med Assoc 1987; 190:445–448.

17. Greig B, Armstrong PJ. Canine granulocytotrophic anaplasmosis (*A. phagocytophilum* infection). In: Greene CE, ed. Infectious Diseases of the Dog and Cat. 3rd ed. St Louis: Saunders Elsevier, 2006:219–224.
18. Magnarelli LA, Bushmich SL, Ijdo JW, et al. Seroprevalence of antibodies against *Borrelia burgdorferi* and *Anaplasma phagocytophilum* in cats. Am J Vet Res 2005; 66(11):1895–1899.
19. Tarello W. Microscopic and clinical evidence for *Anaplasma* (*Ehrlichia*) *phagocytophilum* infection in Italian cats. Vet Rec 2005; 156(24):772–774.
20. Woldehiwet Z, Scott G. Tick-borne (pasture) fever. In: Woldehiwet Z, Ristic M, eds. Rickettsial and Chlamydial Diseases of Domestic Animals. 1st ed. Oxford: Pergamon Press, 1993:427–432.
21. Pusterla N, Anderson RJ, House JK, et al. Susceptibility of cattle to infection with *Ehrlichia equi* and the agent of human granulocytic ehrlichiosis. J Am Vet Med Assoc 2001; 218(7):1160–1162.
22. Stuen S, Bergström K, Palmér E. Reduced weight gain due to subclinical *Anaplasma phagocytophilum* (formerly *Ehrlichia phagocytophila*) infection. Exp Appl Acarol 2002; 28:209–215.
23. Harvey JW. Thrombocytotrophic anaplasmosis (*A. platys* [*E. platys*] infection). In: Green CE, ed. Infectious Diseases of the Dog and the Cat. 3rd ed. St Louis: Saunders Elsevier, 2006:229–232.
24. Martin AR, Brown GK, Dunstan RH, et al. *Anaplasma platys*: an improved PCR for its detection in dogs. Exp Parasitol 2005; 109(3):176–180.
25. Kelly PJ. Canine ehrlichioses: an update. J S Afr Vet Assoc 2000; 71(2):77–86.
26. Breitschwerdt EB, Hegarty BC, Hancock SI. Doxycycline hyclate treatment of experimental canine ehrlichiosis followed by challenge inoculation with two *Ehrlichia canis* strain. J Clin Microbiol 1998; 36:362–368.
27. Mylonakis ME, Koutinas AF, Breitschwerdt EB, et al. Chronic canine ehrlichiosis (*Ehrlichia canis*): a retrospective study of 19 natural cases. J Am Anim Hosp Assoc 2004; 40(3):174–184.
28. Woody BJ, Hoskins JD. Ehrlichial diseases of dogs. Vet Clin North Am Small Anim Pract 1991; 21:75–98.
29. Neer TM, Harrus S. Canine monocytotrophic ehrlichiosi and neorickettsiosis (*E. canis*, *E. chaffeensis*, *E. ruminantium*, *N. sennetsu* and *N. risticii* infections). In: Greene CE, ed. Infectious Diseases of the Dog and the Cat. 3rd ed. Vol. St Louis: Saunders Elsevier, 2006:203–217.
30. Harrus S, Kenny M, Miara L, et al. Comparison of simultaneous splenic sample PCR with blood sample PCR for diagnosis and treatment of experimental *Ehrlichia canis* infection. Antimicrob Agents Chemother 2004; 48(11):4488–4490.
31. Seaman R, Kania S, Hegarty B, et al. Comparison of results for serologic testing and a polymerase chain reaction assay to determine the prevalence of stray dogs in eastern Tennessee seropositive to *Ehrlichia canis*. Am J Trop Med Hyg 2004; 65(9):1200–1203.
32. Kelly PJ, Matthewman LA, Broqui P, et al. Lack of efficacy of imidocarb dipropionate against *Ehrlichia canis*. J S Afr Vet Assoc 1998; 69:55–56.
33. Frank JR, Breitschwerdt EB. A retrospective study of ehrlichiosis in 62 dogs from North Carolina and Virginia. J Vet Intern Med 1999; 13:194–201.
34. Mahan S, Kelly PJ, Mahan SM. A preliminary study to evaluate the immune responses induced by immunization of dogs with inactivated *Ehrlichia canis* organisms. Onderstepoort J Vet Res 2005; 72(2):119–128.
35. Kordick SK, Breitschwerdt EB, Hegarty BC, et al. Coinfection with multiple tick-borne pathogens in a Walker Hound kennel in North Carolina. J Clin Microbiol 1999; 37(8):2631–2638.
36. Matthewman LA, Kelly PJ, Bobade PB, et al. Infections with *Babesia canis* and *Ehrlichia canis* in dogs in Zimbabwe. Vet Rec 1993; 133:344–346.
37. Lee SO, Na DK, Kim CM, et al. Identification and prevalence of *Ehrlichia chaffeensis* infection in *Haemaphysalis longicornis* ticks from Korea by PCR, sequencing and phylogenetic analysis based on 16S rRNA gene. J Vet Sci 2005; 6(2):151–155.
38. Zhang X, Zhang J, Long S, et al. Experimental *Ehrlichia chaffeensis* infection in beagles. J Med Microbiol 2003; 52(pt 11):1021–1026.
39. Lappin MR, Breitschwerdt EB. Feline mononuclear ehrlichiosis. In: Greene CE, ed. Infectious Diseases of the Dog and the Cat. 3rd ed. Vol. St Louis: Saunders Elsevier, 2006:224–227.
40. Ndip LM, Ndip RN, Esemu SN, et al. Ehrlichial infection in Cameroonian canines by *Ehrlichia canis* and *Ehrlichia ewingii*. Vet Microbiol 2005; 111(1–2):59–66.
41. Anziani OS, Ewing SA, Barker RW. Experimental transmission of a granulocytic form of the tribe Ehrlichieae by *Dermacentor variabilis* and *Amblyomma americanum* to dogs. Am J Vet Res 1990; 51(6):929–931.
42. Yabsley MJ, Varela AS, Tate CM, et al. *Ehrlichia ewingii* infection in white-tailed deer (*Odocoileus virginianus*). Emerg Infect Dis 2002; 8(7):668–671.
43. Goodman RA, Hawkins EC, Olby NJ, et al. Molecular identification of *Ehrlichia ewingii* infection in dogs: 15 cases (1997–2001). J Am Vet Med Assoc 2003; 222(8):1102–1107.
44. Allsopp BA, Bezuidenhout JD, Prozesky L. Heartwater. In: Coetzer JAW, Tustin R, eds. Infectious Diseases of Livestock. 2nd ed. Vol. 1. Cape Town: Oxford University Press, 2004:507–535.
45. Burridge MJ, Simmons LA, Peter TF, et al. Increasing risks of introduction of heartwater onto the American mainland associated with animal movements. Ann NY Acad Sci 2002; 969:269–274.

46. van Vliet AH, van der Zeijst BA, Camus E, et al. Use of a specific immunogenic region on the *Cowdria ruminantium* MAP1 protein in a serological assay. J Clin Microbiol 1995; 33(9):2405–2410.
47. Semu SM, Peter TF, Mukwedeya D, et al. Antibody responses to MAP 1B and other *Cowdria ruminantium* antigens are downregulated in cattle challenged with tick-transmitted heartwater. Clin Diagn Lab Immunol 2001; 8(2):388–396.
48. Lawrence JA, Tjornehoj K, Whiteland AP, et al. The serological response to heartwater immunization in cattle is an indicator of protective immunity. Rev Elev Med Vet Pays Trop 1995; 48(1):63–65.
49. Zweygarth E, Josemans AI, Van Strijp MF, et al. An attenuated *Ehrlichia ruminantium* (Welgevonden stock) vaccine protects small ruminants against virulent heartwater challenge. Vaccine 2005; 23(14):1695–1702.
50. Mahan S, Barbet A, Burridge M. Development of improved vaccines for heartwater. Devel Biol (Basel) 2003; 114:137–145.
51. Graham J, Foreyt W. Salmon poisoning disease. In: Greene CE, ed. Infectious Diseases of the Dog and Cat. 3rd ed. St Louis: Saunders Elsevier, 2006:198–203.
52. Wen B, Rikihisa Y, Fuerst P, et al. Diversity of 16S rRNA genes of new *Ehrlichia* strains isolated from horses with clinical signs of Potomac horse fever. Int J Syst Evol Microbiol 1995; 45(2):315–318.
53. Pusterla N, Johnson E, Chae J, et al. Digenetic trematodes, *Acanthatrium* sp. and *Lecithodendrium* sp., as vectors of *Neorickettsia risticii*, the agent of Potomac horse fever. J Helminthol 2003; 77(4):335–339.
54. Palmer JE. Potomac horse fever. In: Coetzer JAW, Tustin R, eds. Infectious Diseases of Livestock. 2nd ed. Vol. 1. Cape Town: Oxford University Press, 2004:583–591.
55. Dutta SK, Vemulapalli R, Biswas B. Association of deficiency in antibody response to vaccine and heterogeneity of *Ehrlichia risticii* strains with Potomac horse fever vaccine failure in horses. J Clin Microbiol 1998; 36(2):506–512.
56. Ristic M, Dawson J, Holland CJ, et al. Susceptibility of dogs to infection with *Ehrlichia risticii*, causative agent of equine monocytic ehrlichiosis (Potomac horse fever). Am J Vet Res 1988; 49(9):1497–1500.
57. Kakoma I, Hansen RD, Anderson BE, et al. Cultural, molecular, and immunological characterization of the etiologic agent for atypical canine ehrlichiosis. J Clin Microbiol 1994; 32(1):170–175.
58. Greene CE, Breitschwerdt EB. Rocky Mountain spotted fever, murine typhus-like disease, rickettsialpox, typhus, and Q fever. In: Greene CE, ed. Infectious Diseases of the Dog and Cat. 3rd ed. St Louis: Saunders Elsevier, 2006:232–245.
59. Kelly PJ, Matthewman LA, Mason PR, et al. Experimental infection of dogs with a Zimbabwean strain of *Rickettsia conorii*. J Trop Med Hyg 1992; 95(5):322–326.
60. Sexton DJ, Banks J, Graves S, et al. Prevalence of antibodies to spotted fever group rickettsiae in dogs from southeastern Australia. Am J Trop Med Hyg 1991; 45(2):243–248.
61. Kelly PJ, Mason PR, Manning T, et al. Role of cattle in the epidemiology of tick-bite fever in Zimbabwe. J Clin Microbiol 1991; 29(2):256–259.
62. Kelly PJ, Mason PR, Rhode C, et al. Transient infections of goats with a novel spotted fever group rickettsia from Zimbabwe. Res Vet Sci 1991; 51(3):268–271.
63. Wedincamp J, Foil L. Infection and seroconversion of cats exposed to cat fleas (*Ctenocephalides felis* Bouche) infected with *Rickettsia felis*. J Vector Ecol 2000; 25(1):123–126.
64. Elchos BN, Goddard J. Implications of presumptive fatal Rocky Mountain spotted fever in two dogs and their owner. J Am Vet Med Assoc 2003; 223(10):1450–1452.
65. Sangioni LA, Horta MC, Vianna MC, et al. Rickettsial infection in animals and Brazilian spotted fever endemicity. Emerg Infect Dis 2005; 11(2):265–270.
66. Morita C, Tsuboi Y, Iida A, et al. Spotted fever group rickettsia in dogs in Japan. Jpn J Med Sci Biol 1989; 42(4):143–147.
67. George JE. Present and future technologies for tick control. Ann NY Acad Sci 2000; 916:583–588.
68. Duncan IM, Monks N. Tick control on eland (*Taurotragus oryx*) and buffalo (*Syncerus caffer*) with flumethrin 1% pour-on through a Duncan applicator. J S Afr Vet Assoc 1992; 63(1):7–10.
69. Jensenius M, Pretorius AM, Clarke F, et al. Repellent efficacy of four commercial DEET lotions against *Amblyomma hebraeum* (Acari: Ixodidae), the principal vector of *Rickettsia africae* in southern Africa. Trans R Soc Trop Med Hyg 2005; 99(9):708–711.
70. Davoust B, Marie JL, Mercier S, et al. Assay of fipronil efficacy to prevent canine monocytic ehrlichiosis in endemic areas. Vet Parasitol 2003; 112(1–2):91–100.

Section IX: GENOMICS OF RICKETTSIAL AGENTS

25 | Genomics of Rickettsial Agents

Hiroyuki Ogata
Structural and Genomic Information Laboratory, Parc Scientifique de Luminy, Marseille, France

Patricia Renesto
Faculté de Médecine, Unité des Rickettsies, Marseille, France

INTRODUCTION

In the last decade, we have experienced a major revolution in the biological sciences resulting from a tremendous flux of genome sequence information. Availability of complete microbial genome sequences has greatly benefited our knowledge of microorganisms with regard to their evolutionary history, the metabolic processes they catalyze, as well as their antigenic proteins and virulence factors. Obtaining a whole bacterial sequence is not a trivial undertaking. Therefore, technical progress in sequencing and data processing continue to reduce both the time and expenses involved (1,2). According to the genome project database of the National Center for Biotechnology Information at the National Institutes of Health, over 300 genomes have been completely sequenced and another 573 are in progress. Here, we review insights gained from genome sequences of bacteria of the order Rickettsiales (the genera *Rickettsia*, *Ehrlichia*, *Anaplasma*, *Neorickettsia*, and *Wolbachia*) (Table 1, Fig. 1). These bacteria are obligate intracellular parasites of eukaryotes, and many of them are pathogens. Based on their similar lifestyles and parasitic strategies, they were historically considered "Rickettsia-like." Their phylogenic diversity was highlighted from 16S rRNA gene sequence analysis (14). Because of the intrinsic difficulty in working with these intracellular bacteria and the lack of adequate methods for their genetic manipulation, their biology is still poorly understood. To better grasp the molecular mechanisms underlying their evolution and pathogenicity, genome sequencing efforts have targeted these parasites/pathogens. While obtained genomic data revealed marked similarities between them, each genome exhibited specific features, reflecting a large diversity in their parasitic and infectious strategies. A number of genes emerging from these genomic studies provided a remarkable opportunity to enhance our understanding of these bacteria.

GENERAL GENOMIC FEATURES
Genome Size

Bacteria species display an incredible amount of variation in the size, composition, and architecture of their genomes. A common trait of bacteria from the genera *Rickettsia*, *Ehrlichia*, *Anaplasma*, *Neorickettsia*, and *Wolbachia* is their small genome size, ranging from 0.86 to 1.56 Mb (Table 1). It is clear that habitat is a major factor contributing to genome reduction. Indeed, loss of genes is not a random event but it is rather thought to be related to adaptations to a parasitic and pathogenic lifestyle in which certain functions are no longer required (15). Accordingly, these bacteria have become completely dependent on their hosts and are no longer capable of surviving outside the host cell. Although these bacteria show consistently small genomes, variations in chromosome length is evident. This is particularly true when considering the genus *Rickettsia*, with a number of putative proteins of 834 for *R. prowazekii* (3) and 1562 for *R. bellii* (8). Such variations could result from lateral gene transfer between distantly related intracellular pathogens (16). In rickettsial genomes, while the occurrence of recent gene transfers was not found, traces of ancient gene acquisitions were evidenced, especially from bacteria living in amoeba (8). The duplication of existing genes can also take place during genome evolution as observed for the homologous genes on the plasmids and chromosome of *R. felis*. In contrast, genome size is relatively constant across genetically diverse isolates of *Ehrlichia* spp.

TABLE 1 Characteristics of the Sequenced Genomes of *Rickettsiales*

Bacteria	Genome	G + C%	Proteins	Reference/GenBank
Rickettsia prowazekii Madrid E	One chromosome (1.12 Mb)	29	835	(3)
R. typhi Wilmington	One chromosome (1.11 Mb)	28	838	(4)
R. conorii Malish 7	One chromosome (1.27 Mb)	32	1374	(5)
R. rickettsii	One chromosome (1.23 Mb)	32	1217	AADJ00000000
R. siberica 246	One chromosome (1.25 Mb)	32	1234	AABW00000000 (6)
R. felis URRWXCal2	One chromosome (1.485 Mb)	32	1400	(7)
	One plasmid pRF (62.9 Kb)	33	68	
	One plasmid pRFδ (39.3 Kb)	33	44	
R. akari Hartford	One chromosome (1.23 Mb)	32	1217	AAFE00000000
R. bellii RML369-C	One chromosome (1.56 Mb)	32	1562	(8)
Anaplasma marginale St. Maries	One chromosome (1.2 Mb)	49	949	(9)
A. phagocytophilum HZ	One chromosome (1.47 Mb)	42	1369	(10)
Ehrlichia canis Jake	One chromosome (1.32 Mb)	28	925	CP000107
E. ruminantium Gardel	One chromosome (1.5 Mb)	27	950	CR925677
E. ruminantium Welgevonden	One chromosome (1.52 Mb)	27	958	CR925678
E. ruminantium Welgevonden	One chromosome (1.52 Mb)	27	888	(11)
E. chaffeensis Arkansas	One chromosome (1.2 Mb)	30	1115	(10)
Wolbachia pipentis (*w*Mel)	One chromosome (1.27 Mb)	35	11195	(12)
Wolbachia strain TRS (*w*Bm)	One chromosome (1.08 Mb)	34	805	(13)
Neorickettsia sennetsu Miyayama	One chromosome (0.86 Mb)	41	935	(10)

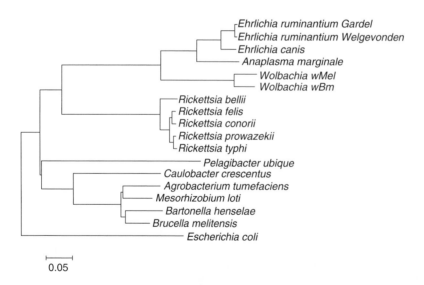

FIGURE 1 Phylogeny of *Rickettsiales* and other α-proteobacteria. The phylogenetic tree was built using the neighbor-joining method with JTT model, based on the concatenated protein sequences of RNA polymerase β (RpoB) and β' (RpoC) chains. *Escherichia coli* sequences are used as an outgroup. *Abbreviations*: JTT, Jones-Taylor-Thornton.

Plasmids

Although all sequenced *Anaplasma*, *Ehrlichia*, *Neorickettsia*, and *Wolbachia* strains possess a single circular chromosome, plasmids have been found in *R. felis* (7). *R. felis* exhibits two circular plasmids of 63 and 39 kb, named pRF and pRFδ, respectively. The sequence of the smaller pRFδ is identical to a part of the larger pRF. In general, plasmids carry genes that are nonessential to bacterial replication but confer selective advantages in special circumstances. Predicted proteins encoded in the *R. felis* plasmids include ankyrin-repeat-containing proteins, thymidylate kinase, hyaluronidase, small heat shock proteins, and several homologs for conjugative DNA transfer machinery.

G+C Composition

Sequencing of complete bacterial genome gives the exact proportion and distribution of each of the four bases in the genome. The relative amount of each base, reported as the G + C content, is characteristic of a genus (17). Localized variations in the G + C content along the genome have significant implications for understanding the potential routes of genetic exchange between organisms. The pathogenicity islands, which are clusters of genes encoding virulence traits, correspond to such distinct regions with unusual nucleotide composition that were acquired through lateral gene transfer (18). Although the presence of pathogenicity islands is a common feature in many pathogens, they were not found in these intracellular bacteria.

Repeats

Repeated DNA sequences are abundant in some Rickettsiales genomes but can be rare in closely related species. For example, typhus group rickettsiae exhibit a small fraction of repeated sequences, while spotted fever group rickettsiae exhibit many short palindromic elements (19) and insertion sequences (7). Of sequenced *Rickettsia*, *R. felis* and *R. bellii* exhibit the highest proportions (about 4%) of repeats, mostly originating in duplication of transposases. The two sequenced *Wolbachia* genomes (wMel and wBm) also exhibit a marked difference in the proportions of repeats. About 14% of the wMel genome corresponds to repeated sequences, while only 5.4% for wBm (13). In *E. ruminantium*, 8.3% of the genome corresponds to repeated sequences, which are divided into simple sequence repeats (2–5 bp unit), large tandem repeats (six to hundreds bp), and dispersed repeats (11). The abundance of repeated sequences in *E. ruminantium* appears to correlate with frequent gene-duplication events in this genome. Although the nature of repeated sequences are variable and dependent on the repeat types (i.e., insertion sequences, palindromic sequences, short tandem repeats, etc.), contraction and expansion of repeat-sequence moiety of the genome appears to be a frequent theme in *Rickettsiales*. This contrasts with the genomes of other obligate symbionts such as *Buchnera* spp. (20,21) and *Wigglesworthia glossinidia* (22) that exhibit small proportions of repeated DNA sequences.

GENOME STREAMLINING
Reductive Evolution

Genome reduction process was probably initiated very early in the evolution of Rickettsiales. By comparative genome analysis, Boussau et al. (23) reconstructed the evolutionary history of gene loss and gain process for α-proteobacterial genomes. Their estimate points out a massive reduction in the lineage from the α-proteobacterial ancestor (3000–5000 genes) to the last common ancestor of Rickettsiales (1000–2000 genes). Lost gene functions cover a wide spectrum of cellular activities including transport systems, energy metabolism, biosynthesis of small molecules, and DNA metabolism. A major loss of transcriptional regulators also appears to have occurred in the common ancestor of Rickettsiales, suggesting that most of their genes are likely constitutively expressed (12). The sole functional category that has been retained as mostly intact in Rickettsiales is that of genes involved in translation process.

With the determination of various Rickettsiales genomes, it has become apparent that genome reduction has continued independently in different lineages leading to existing species of this group. Consequently, Rickettsiales genomes show substantial variation in their gene content. Different Rickettsiales species might have evolved distinct strategies for intracellular parasitism. For example, complete pathways for the synthesis of purine and pyrimidine nucleotides were identified in the members of Anaplasmataceae (*A. marginale*, *Ehrlichia* spp., and *Wolbachia* spp.), whereas *Rickettsia* spp. lack the ability to synthesize nucleotides (11).

Rickettsia spp. replicate in the host cytoplasm, where host nucleotides are freely available, and exhibit five paralogues for the adenosine triphosphate/adenosine diphosphate (ATP/ADP) translocase for uptaking ATP from hosts (3). In contrast, members of Anaplasmataceae replicate in an intracellular vacuole, and lack the ATP/ADP exchanger protein. These differences in intracellular compartment where they replicate and in gene repertoires for nucleotide transport may reflect the variable capacity of Rickettsiales to synthesize nucleotides.

Genomes belonging to a same Rickettsiales genus exhibit substantial variations in gene content. The genome of R. conorii [1374 open reading frames (ORFs)] exhibits 552 ORFs lacking clear orthologues in the genome of R. prowazekii (834 ORFs). Notably, 229 (41%) of the R. conorii-specific ORFs exhibit a significant sequence similarity in intergenic regions of R. prowazekii genome, suggesting that a substantial part of the difference between the two Rickettsia genomes is due to accelerated genome reduction in R. prowazekii (5) after the separation of the two species. Comparison of two Wolbachia genomes also revealed a substantial difference in the level of genome decay (13). Wolbachia wMel (1270 ORFs) is a parasitic endosymbiont of Drosophila melanogaster, while Wolbachia wBm (806 ORFs) is probably a mutualistic symbiont of the nematode Brugia malayi. The smaller size of the wBm genome may reflect the loss of genes required for infecting host cells and avoiding host defense system.

Genomes of Rickettsiales exhibit various levels of coding capacity (Fig. 2). E. ruminantium exhibits the smallest proportion of coding regions (62%) among sequenced Rickettsiales. The genomes of Wolbachia wBm (67%), E. canis (72%), and R. prowazekii (76%) also exhibit a relatively low level of coding capacity. In contrast, the genomes of A. marginale (86%) and R. bellii (85%) show a coding capacity close to E. coli genome (87%). Apparently, these variations originate in ongoing genome degradation in the species exhibiting a low coding capacity (i.e., a large proportion of intergenic sequences containing pseudogenes) (24), although critical factors that determine the retention/elimination of noncoding DNA sequences remains elusive (25).

Pseudogenes

Many pseudogenes have been identified in Rickettsiales genomes. A pseudogene is an inactive vestige of a gene, usually identified as several short consecutive ORFs exhibiting sequence similarities to functional genes but being interrupted by stop codons. Notably, A. marginale has genomic regions defined as "functional pseudogenes." During its lifelong persistent infection in mammalian hosts, A. marginale continuously generates immune escape variants that are in part due to variations in the expressed major surface protein 2 (MSP2). The underlying mechanism that generates the variability of MSP2 is the recombination between a functional msp2 gene and msp2 pseudogenes (26,27). The genome sequencing of A. marginale revealed 56 members of the msp2 superfamily, including 16 pseudogenes. A. marginale might be explored for a unique way to maximally use its small streamlined genome. Similar functional pseudogenes are known in A. phagocytophilum (28), but have not yet been described in other genera of Rickettsiales.

In some cases, computational analysis gives no clear division between functional genes and pseudogenes. Some pseudogene-like sequences are thus designated as "split genes" to

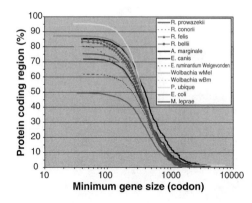

FIGURE 2 Protein coding capacity of Rickettsiales genomes. Percentage of protein coding regions (vertical axis) for a given minimum open reading frame size (horizontal axis) is indicated for each sequenced Rickettsiales

represent their intermediate status, pending experimental validation of their functionality or inactivity (5,9). For instance, *Rickettsia* genomes exhibit several paralogous *spoT* genes. Most of the *spoT* genes are much shorter than known functional homologs in other bacteria, thus were initially annotated pseudogenes based on classical convention (3). However, later accumulation of several *Rickettsia* genomes revealed a high level of sequence conservation, including predicted active site residues, for *spoT* genes (4,7). Transcriptional regulation of different *spoT* genes was also demonstrated in *R. conorii* (29). Thus, most rickettsial *spoT* genes now appear functional. In contrary, Davids et al. (30) argued that most of the split/fragmented genes in *R. conorii*, including those expressing mRNAs, are nonfunctional based on an analysis of substitution frequencies at nonsynonymous sites. In *E. ruminantium*, the generation of pseudogenes appears to be linked with gene-duplication events, rather than the result of the reductive evolution seen in *Rickettsia* and *Wolbachia* (11).

Horizontal Gene Transfer

Horizontal gene transfer is an important source of genome variability in prokaryotes (31–33). However, obligate intracellular bacteria, due to their isolated way of life, appear to have little opportunity to exchange DNA with other microbes, making their genome relatively immune to horizontal gene transfer. Consistently, *Rickettsiales* genome sequences exhibit few traces of recent lateral gene transfer events, except for many insertion sequences and phage-related genes in *Wolbachia* wMel (12), *R. felis* (7), and *R. bellii* (8). Recently acquired genes can be detected by methods based on the bias in nucleotide composition if the statistical property of donor genomes is different from that of recipient ones. Systematic analyses of prokaryotic genomes based on such methods also demonstrated limited levels of gene transfers in *Rickettsia* spp. (34,35). Wu et al. (12) examined horizontal gene transfers between *Wolbachia* wMel and its host, *D. melanogaster*, whose genome sequence has been determined. They identified no clear case of horizontal transfer of genes between the host and parasite.

Genome Impairment

Buchnera spp., the obligate endosymbionts of aphids, exhibit an increase in the rate of sequence evolution. Enhanced mutation rate and relaxation of selection have been suggested as main causes of this accelerated evolutionary rate (36). *Buchnera* spp. lack several important DNA repair enzymes, which might explain the increased mutation rate. Several authors have suggested that small effective populations, due to strict maternal transmission of the microbes, led to the relaxation of the extent of purifying selection, resulting in the increased fixation rate of slightly deleterious mutations (15,37). Higher ratios of nonsynonymous-to-synonymous substitutions in *Buchnera* relative to their free-living relatives, together with the lack of strong relationships between codon usages and expression levels, supports the relaxed-selection hypothesis. In addition, accumulation of slightly deleterious mutations has been suggested for a wide taxonomic range of endosymbiotic bacteria and fungi with small effective population sizes using 16S rRNA genes (38). A similar effect may be expected for Rickettsiales, as its members are all obligate intracellular bacteria, and maternal transmission is known for both *Rickettsia* and *Wolbachia*. Wu et al. (12) indeed marked faster sequence evolution in *Wolbachia* wMel and *Rickettsia* than in their free-living relative *Caulobacter crescentus*. Although further studies are required, this study implies that the genomes of Rickettsiales might have accumulated detrimental mutations in many genes, such as *Buchnera*. It is thought that *R. prowazekii* RNA polymerase-promoter complexes are less stable than those of *E. coli* (39). The *R. prowazekii* S-adenosylmethionine synthetase MetK is less efficient than those of *R. typhi* or *E. coli* (40). On a more global scale, Mira et al. (25) suggested that insufficient purifying selection could lead to the degradation of genes that are beneficial but unnecessary in obligate intracellular bacteria. This invokes the idea that such an impairment of genomic function may lead to inefficient multiplication of obligate intracellular bacteria. Interestingly, Winkler (41) hypothesized that the slow growth of *R. prowazekii* may be needed to provide minimal trauma to the host and to maximize the chance for the bacterium to transmit to another host before killing the host. Disrupted rRNA operons observed in all the sequenced genomes of Rickettsiales, but not in other α-proteobacteria, has been suggested to be linked with the slow growth of these intracellular bacteria (42).

EMERGING GENOMIC PLASTICITY
Genome Rearrangements

Comparison of three *Rickettsia* (*R. prowazekii*, *R. conorii*, and *R. typhi*) has revealed a high level of conservation of gene order in their genomes (4). This parallels the lack of rearrangement in the genomes of obligate endosymbionts *Buchnera* (21). However, subsequent determinations of the genome sequences of other members of Rickettsiales have provided evidence that genome shuffling has occurred in many lineages of Rickettsiales. The first striking figure was obtained by the comparison of two *Wolbachia* genomes (wMel and wBm) (13). There is no genome synteny between these genomes. Among *Rickettsia*, *R. felis* genome appears to have been shuffled many times after the separation from *R. conorii* (7). Genome rearrangements in *R. felis* were probably mediated by recombination through highly conserved transposase genes. More recently, the genome sequence of *R. bellii* provided further evidence for an extensive genome shuffling in this early diverging *Rickettsia* species (8). Overall, some Rickettsiales genomes are not as stable as those of *Buchnera*, pointing to a dynamic genome evolution in this group of obligate intracellular bacteria.

Gene Transfer Between Chromosome and Plasmids

Analysis of the *R. felis* genome provided evidence for gene transfers between the chromosome and plasmids. Ogata et al. listed 11 genes encoded in the pRF plasmid that exhibit close homologs in the chromosome. These genes correspond to seven transposases, patatin-like phospholipase, thymidylate kinase, and two small heat-shock proteins. Among these, patatin-like proteins exhibit the most intriguing phylogeny. All sequenced *Rickettsia* genomes exhibit chromosome-encoded patatin-like phospholipase (*pat1*). Gene organization around *pat1* is similar between different *Rickettsia* (Fig. 3). *R. felis* possesses an additional paralogue *pat2* in the pRF plasmid. Phylogenetic reconstruction shows a close relationship of *pat1* from *R. felis* and *R. akari* with the *R. felis pat2*. This provides a clear case of gene transfer from plasmid to chromosome; the chromosome *pat1* was replaced by the plasmid-encoded *pat2* in the lineage leading to the ancestor of *R. akari* and *R. felis* (Fig. 3).

Intragenome Recombination

Evidence is emerging that intragenome recombination could be a source of genome variability in *Wolbachia* and *Rickettsia*. Intragenic recombination between *Wolbachia* strains has been suggested for the *Wolbachia* surface protein gene (*wsp*) (43) and for *gltA* gene (44), resulting in mosaic nature of those genes. By sequencing four house keeping genes (*gltA*, *dnaA*, *ftsZ*, and *groEL*) in different strains of *Wolbachia*, Baldo et al. (44) also showed evidences that intergenic recombination has occurred frequently between different strains. The recombination occurred within and between the supergroups of *Wolbachia*. More recently, intraspecies recombination was suggested for three rickettsial antigenic protein genes (*rompA*, *rompB*, and *sca4*) (45). In this case as well, intragenic recombination was suggested for *rompB* between *R. felis* and *R. prowazekii*. These studies are focusing on only several genes. Genome-wide analysis is necessary to better understand the impact of intragenome recombination for the evolution of these obligate intracellular bacteria.

Gene Duplication

The genomes of several Rickettsiales species appear to depend on gene duplication to create new genes, despite evident genome reduction. *A. marginale* genome encodes a number of paralogues for two families containing immunodominant proteins (the *msp1* superfamily: nine members; and the *msp2* superfamily: 56 members including 16 pseudogenes) (9). In *E. ruminantium* (11) and *Wolbachia* wMel (12), gene duplication seems to contribute significantly to the increase in gene content. In *Rickettsia*, recent gene duplication appears infrequent, although they exhibit several paralogous gene families. Multiple duplication events for large gene families such as *sca* (7) and *spoT* (46) have been suggested to predate the divergence of *Rickettsia* species.

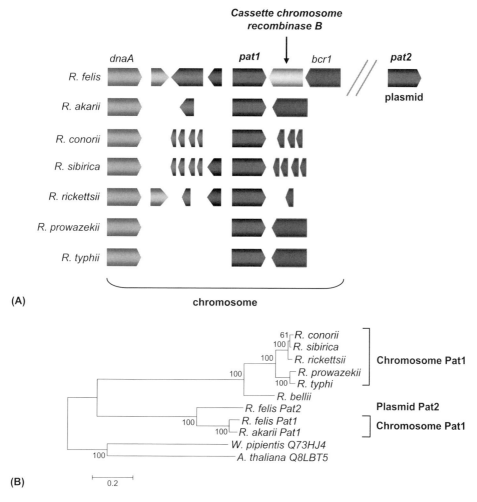

FIGURE 3 Evidence of a plasmid–chromosome gene transfer for patatin-like phospholipase genes. (**A**) Gene organization around chromosomally encoded pat1 in different Rickettsia genomes. R. felis exhibit paralogous pat2 in the plasmids. pat1 of R. bellii is split (not shown). (**B**) A neighbor-joining phylogenetic tree for pat1 and pat2 with JTT model and midpoint rooring. Abbreviation: JTT, Jones-Taylor-Thornton.

Protein-Coding Palindromic Repeats

Rickettsia and *Wolbachia* exhibit mobile palindromic sequences that have a capacity to invade both coding and noncoding regions of the genome: *Rickettsia* palindromic element (RPE-1 to 8) (47,48) and *Wolbachia* palindromic element (49). The size of those repeats is about 100 to 150 bp. By inserting themselves within existing protein-coding genes, these repeats generate a new reading frame as a part of preexisting genes, resulting in an additional peptide segment (30–50 aa) in the final gene products. These mobile elements thus have enhanced sequence diversity in coding regions of *Rickettsia* and *Wolbachia*. Similar phenomenon has been described in an archaebacterium, *Methanocaldococcus jannaschii* (50). Recent study also evidenced remnants of transposable elements in thousands of human proteins (51).

Ancient Gene Exchanges Within Amoebae

Despite the lack of evidence for recent gene transfers, *Rickettsia* genomes exhibit traces of ancient gene acquisitions especially from bacteria living in amoebae (8). Phylogenetic analyses indicate that some of the genes associated with intracellular parasitism have been acquired from bacteria living in amoebae. For instance, the ancestral gene for the ATP/ADP translocase appears to have been transferred from *Parachlamydia* to *Rickettsia* (52,53). The conjugal DNA-transfer genes identified in *R. bellii* and *R. felis* are most similar to those found in *Protochlamydia amoebophila*, an obligate endosymbiont of amoebae (8). Furthermore, comparative genome analyses revealed the abundance of Rickettsiales genes exhibiting a high level of sequence similar to the homologs in intraamoebal bacteria, such as *Legionella pneumophila* and *P. amoebophila* (Fig. 4). The ancestor of Rickettsiales may have lived within amoebae. In fact, amoebal symbionts related to the members of Rickettsiales have been recently identified (54). As many amoeba-associated bacteria or their relatives are pathogens of humans, amoebae have been suggested to act as evolutionary "training grounds" for bacteria, in which they acquire the ability to infect the cells of higher eukaryotes (55,56). Gene exchanges between these bacteria might have significantly contributed to their evolution, by conferring an immediate selective advantage in the adaptation to the intracellular environment of eukaryotic cells.

ADAPTATION TO HOSTS/PATHOGENICITY
Stringent Response in Rickettsiae

Most *Rickettsia* species are stably associated with their arthropod hosts for a long period of time. *Rickettsia* are thus thought to have developed a molecular mechanism to synchronize

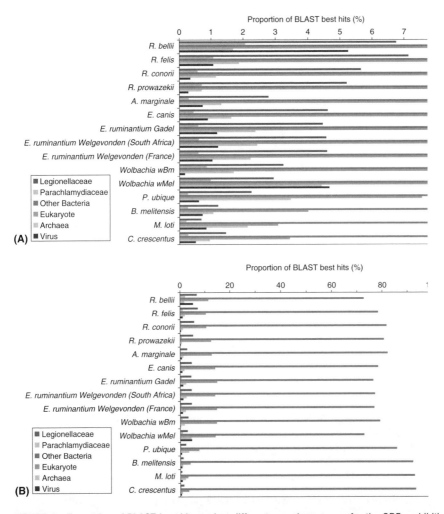

FIGURE 4 Proportion of BLAST best hits against different organism groups for the ORFs exhibiting significant database homology (E-value $< 10^{-5}$). For this analysis, BLAST hits against sequences from α-proteobacteria are discarded. *Abbreviation*: ORF, open reading frame; BLAST, basic local alignment search tool.

their replication with that of the hosts. Genome analyses suggest that *spoT* and toxin–antitoxin (TA) systems could be the major players in this process (7). Despite their reduced genome size, all the sequenced *Rickettsia* possess paralogous *spoT* genes. The *spoT* and *relA* genes control the concentration of alarmone, (p)ppGpp (guanosine tetra- and pentaphosphates), in response to starvation in enterobacteria (57). The alarmone in turn acts as an effector of transcription and changes the global cellular metabolism (i.e., stringent response). Evidence is also accumulating for the role of (p)ppGpp-mediated regulation during the pathogenesis and symbiosis of bacteria (58). *Rickettsia* genomes contain many fragmented *spoT* paralogues (4–14 copies), encoding ppGpp hydrolase and/or synthetase domains. In *R. felis*, all the 14 *spoT* genes were demonstrated to be transcribed (7). In *R. conorii*, the transcription of five *spoT* genes is differentially regulated depending on the stress conditions or the types of infected hosts (29). The chromosomes of SFG *Rickettsia* and *R. bellii* harbor genes for TA systems (7,8). Genes for TA systems were originally identified in bacterial plasmids. TA systems are composed of toxin and antitoxin gene pairs, and ensure stable plasmid inheritance by a mechanism known as "postsegregational killing" when they are encoded in plasmids. Recent genome surveys showed that TA systems could be abundant in the chromosomes of bacteria (59). TA systems encoded in the bacterial chromosomes participate in the cascade of the stringent response pathway (Fig. 5). Thus, the rickettsial TA systems might contribute to the global regulation of metabolism, eventually leading to selective killing (a primitive form of bacterial apoptosis) or reversible stasis of bacterial subpopulations during a period of starvation or other stress (60,61).

Genes Associated with Host Specificity

Species of Rickettsiales exhibit a diverse host range. Comparative genome analysis may help to detect genes and pathways responsible for host specificity. Brayton et al. (9) listed 15 genes present in tick-associated species (*A. marginale*, *E. ruminantium*, *R. conorii*) and absent in the nontick-transmitted *Wolbachia* wMel. Those genes include a conserved cell-surface protein gene, and several genes for nucleotide-processing enzymes such as tRNA pseudouridine 55 synthase, GTP cyclohydrolase I, cytidylate kinase, and exodeoxyribonuclease. The functions of the remaining genes are mostly unknown. To investigate insect-associated rickettsial genes, Ogata et al. listed 10 genes present in flea-associated *Rickettsia* (*R. felis* and *R. typhi*) and absent or degraded in the tick-associated *R. conorii*, including cell-surface antigen (*sca3*) and lipopolysaccharide 1,2-glucosyltransferase (*rfaJ*). This type of comparative approach, which is

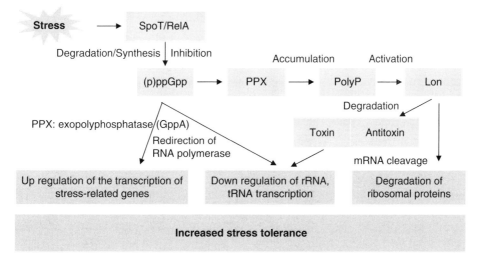

FIGURE 5 A model for the stringent response pathway integrating the role of TA systems. All the enzymes involved in the pathway have been identified in *Rickettsia* genomes. *Abbreviations*: LON, lon protease; PolyP, polyphosphates; PPX, exopolyphosphatase (GppA); TA, toxin–antitoxin. *Source*: Taken From Ref. 59.

potentially powerful with the increased sampling of diverse *Rickettsiales* genomes, should be routinely applied to new genomes.

Cell Surface Proteins

Bacterial cell-surface proteins play a role in host-parasite interactions and adaptive response to host defense systems. Cell-surface proteins also represent candidates for vaccine development and serve as useful markers for discrimination of closely related species or strains. As previously described, the *Wolbachia* surface protein gene exhibits a high level of sequence diversity between species, and has been used as a standard gene for strain identification. Genome sequencing of *Wolbachia* wMel identified two additional paralogues (named *wspB* and *wspC*) in the genome (12). Wu et al. showed that *wspB* evolves faster than *wsp*, and proposed that *wspB* may be an additional marker for discriminating between closely related *Wolbachia* strains. The *A. marginale* genome contains two large superfamilies containing immunodominant proteins (56-member *msp2* superfamily and 9-member *msp1* superfamily). As previously described, recombination between functional genes and pseudogenes contributes to the diversity of the expressed *msp2*-encoded proteins. Analysis of the unfinished genome sequences of *A. phagocytophilum* HZ strain also revealed more than 52 *msp2* paralogues, suggesting an important role of *msp2* in immune evasion for this genus (62). In *E. ruminantium* genome, 16 paralogues of *map1* multigene family of outer-membrane proteins were identified (11). The outer-membrane protein family contains immunodominant proteins, but has not been found to be a good vaccine candidate. The genome encodes two additional membrane protein families (a 14-member family and a 10-member family), for which no homologues have been identified in other genomes.

In *Rickettsia*, the surface-cell antigen (Sca) family represents one of the largest protein families. Several members of the family, such as rOmpA (63), rOmpB (64), and Sca4 (65), are known antigenic determinants. Recently, *R. conorii* rOmpB was shown to be involved in the adhesion to host cells by interacting with membrane-associated Ku70 (66). The analysis of the *Rickettsia* genomes revealed 17 members of the Sca family (67). Interestingly, the genes for the Sca proteins exhibit remarkably diverse patterns of presence/absence across different species. The N-terminal parts of these proteins, which are exported to the cell surface, are highly variable between orthologues. It has been suggested that accelerated amino acid changes and differential gene degradation of Sca paralogues contributed to the intraspecies variation of those cell-surface proteins and adaptation to different environments (7,67). Genome sequence analysis reveals the evolutionary mechanisms that diversify the cell-surface proteins of Rickettsiales. Duplication, fast sequence evolution, and occasional intra- or intergenome rearrangements appear to be major evolutionary themes of these proteins.

Type IV Secretion Systems

Bacterial type IV secretion systems (T4SS) constitute a family of multiprotein complexes, which serves to export effector proteins, virulence factors, or nucleic acids, and is implicated in the pathogenesis of many bacterial species (68). Their role in promoting intracellular survival of several bacteria species has been suggested (68). Despite some discrepancies in genome annotation, most of the genes encoding VirB-type T4SS were found in all sequenced Rickettsiales genomes (7). The chromosomal location of these genes and their conservation in species lacking plasmids suggest a role of these T4SS in excretion of virulence factors to hosts. Genes for a complete T4SS organized in two distinct operons were also found in two *Wolbachia* genomes. Interestingly, a conserved gene order was noticed for these genes between *R. conorii* and *W. pipientis* wMel (12). From this observation, it was hypothesized that the putative membrane-spanning proteins could form a novel and possibly an integral part of a functioning T4SS within these bacteria. Moreover, the close association of one of the T4SS operons with a homologue of the *Wolbachia* surface protein, suggested that this protein could be exported to the vacuole in which the bacterium resides (69). T4SS machinery was also described within *Ehrlichia* (70). A specific feature evidenced in *E. chaffeensis* was the cotranscription of a superoxide dismutase gene (*sodB*) and three *virB* genes (*virB3*, *-B4*, and *-B6*) through *sodB* promoters. Although the precise role of this T4SS remains to be elucidated, a link has been established between the T4SS and ankyrin-repeat proteins, which could thus be transported into host cells (69). Finally, the genome *R. bellii* encodes a complete set of genes for another type of T4SS, which probably functions for conjugative DNA transfer (8). Several homologues of these genes have also been identified in the *R. felis* pRF plasmid (7).

Ankyrin-Repeat Proteins

Although ankyrin domains are a common feature of eukaryotic and viral proteins (71), they are relatively rare in bacteria. Among sequenced bacteria, those exhibiting the highest number of ankyrin repeats are obligate intracellular microorganisms, namely *Orientia tsutsugamushi* and *Wolbachia pipientis* wMel with 42 and 23 candidates respectively (69,72). Although less represented in some other strains, all Rickettsiales exhibit at least two proteins with ankyrin repeats. It is thought that these domains, which can bind the host chromatin, could play a critical role in interactions with host cells (73).

Identification of Other Virulence Factors from Genome Analysis

As other bacterial genomes, Rickettsiales genomes contain many ORFs without homologies with proteins of known function. The identification of functions of these ORFs represents another major challenge of the post-genomic era. Here again, efforts have been aimed at searching for putative virulence factors. This can be exemplified with the finding of a rickettsial phospholipase D, not assigned in the initial genome annotation (5) but later identified using a sequence analysis program dedicated for the search of phospholipase signatures (74). More recently, rickettsial ORFs encoding for patatin-like phospholipase were characterized in rickettsiae (4,75). Comparison of *R. conorii* and *R. prowazekii* also facilitated the identification of *rickA*, the gene encoding for the protein responsible for actin polymerization (76). Indeed, *rickA* is lacking in *R. prowazekii*, as is consistent with the default of motility of typhus group rickettsiae. Analysis of *Ehrlichia* genomes highlighted several families of hypothetical membrane protein (11). Most importantly, one adhesion domain that is necessary and sufficient for infection of tick cells was also characterized (77). Predictions resulting from extensive analysis of *Wolbachia* genomes have been recently reviewed (69).

POSTGENOMICS STUDY OF RICKETTSIALES

Genome sequencing is not an end in itself. In the new millennium, postgenomic research will undoubtedly be a major scientific discipline. This field of investigation includes the comparisons between genomes of various microbial species, as exemplified above. Availability of genomic sequences also opens the way for targeted in-silico analysis, which can be achieved through several convenient Web sites providing information such as phylogenetic relationships, operon organization, functional predictions, three-dimensional structure, or metabolic reconstructions. Genome-based metabolic reconstruction was recently demonstrated as an efficient approach to establishing the first cell-free culture medium for *Tropheryma whipplei* (78), the growth of this fastidious bacterium being initially host-cell-dependent (79). Such an approach should be applied for other obligate intracellular bacteria including the members of Rickettsiales. A knowledge base called Metagrowth thus has been developed to help rationally design a new culture medium for fastidious bacteria (81). In addition to such computer analyses, microbial postgenomic research requires the implementation of high-throughput methods characterizing the expression of RNAs and proteins from a genome. The final goal is to analyze the complete genetic information in a microorganism (genomics), to study global gene expression of many genes (transcriptomics), and to characterize all expressed proteins in an organism (proteomics). Here, the recent achievements and future prospects concerning Rickettsiales are summarized.

Genome-Based Phenotypic Characterization of Rickettsiales

Analysis of a microbial genome sequence offers opportunities to rapidly characterize phenotypic features of a fastidious microorganism. This was the case for *R. felis* (7). Identification of predicted genes for pili biogenesis in the genome of *R. felis* prompted a careful electron microscopic study.

This allowed the observation of two types of surface appendages: a rare and long sex pili-like appendage connecting bacteria and small hairlike projections emerging out from the cell surfaces likely to be involved in bacterial attachment to eukaryotic cells.

Global Transcriptomic Analysis of Rickettsiales: The State of the Art

A characteristic feature of rickettsiae is their ability to survive under a variety of hostile environmental conditions, such as default of nutrients and reduced temperatures. These microorganisms most probably adapt to different conditions in the environment or during interaction with the host by changing their gene-expression program. In a preliminary reverse transcriptase-polymerase chain reaction (RT-PCR) analysis, we demonstrated that, following *R. conorii* exposure to various experimental stresses mimicking starvation, *spoT* genes were differentially regulated (29). Differential expression of bacterial membrane proteins such as *rOmpA*, which vary according to the host, was also observed (82). Undoubtedly, the study of the global transcriptome of rickettsiae would be helpful in characterizing their metabolic adaptations and the manipulation of host cellular processes in the course of infection. Genome-wide transcription analysis can be performed with DNA microarrays (DNA chips), which are powerful tools that have already had a marked impact in many fields, including the understanding of the pathogen side of the host-pathogen interaction (83). However, the use of such a technology has been hindered for obligate intracellular bacteria such as *Rickettsia*, *Ehrlichia*, and *Wolbachia*. Indeed, isolation of bacterial RNA from infected mammalian cells is challenging, because both purity and quality of the prokaryotic RNA are required for subsequent hybridizations. In order to circumvent eukaryotic RNA contaminations, several methods such as a differential lysis or differential centrifugation have been applied (84). The delay of purification procedures, which are mainly performed at 4°C, can induce substantial changes in gene expression. Another limitation is the amount of available RNA required for each experiment. To bypass these obstacles, we recently developed a method based on the total RNA extraction from *R. conorii*-infected Vero cells. Eukaryotic RNA was then removed, and prokaryotic material amplified before labeling and hybridization. In a previous set of experiments, the whole procedure was validated. Thus, estimated changes in gene expression were shown not to be statistically different when a dedicated *R. conorii* microarray was hybridized with amplified material as compared with qRT-PCR measurements using mRNA as template (unpublished data).

Investigation of the global *Rickettsia* transcriptomics is now feasible. Encountered difficulties might explain that up to the present no global transcriptome analysis has been described. To our knowledge, the DNA microarray containing all 834 protein-coding genes of *R. prowazekii* Madrid E strain was only used to investigate the genomic variations between this strain and Breinl, by DNA cohybridization experiments (85). Concerning *E. chaffeensis* pathogeniciy, only the transcriptional profile of the infected human monocytes was investigated by oligonucleotide arrays infection (86).

Proteomics

A complete picture of genome expression implicates proteome analysis. Two-dimensional electrophoresis coupled with high-throughput matrix-assisted laser desorption/ionization time of flight mass spectrometry is a powerful approach to recognize and identify proteins of microbial pathogens. Here again, difficulties encountered with Rickettsiales are mainly based on their close association with host cells. To remove eukaryotic proteins without damaging prokaryotic ones, gentle extensive purification steps are required.

This method permitted the establishment of the preliminary proteome map of both *R. conorii* (87) and *R. prowazekii* (88). Although widely used, this approach is time consuming and shares some limitations mainly based on the physicochemical properties of the proteins analyzed (89). Such a classical proteome analysis is now complemented by capillary chromatography/mass spectrometry combinations (90), which allowed characterization of 252 proteins out of 834 predicted protein-coding genes of *R. prowazekii* (91). In fact, the comprehensive proteome analysis of microorganisms must integrate both approaches. Quantitative comparative analysis and demonstration of isoforms resulting from posttranslational modifications can be highlighted on two-dimensional gels. Another relevant application is immunoproteomics.

In the case of *R. conorii* the antigenic properties of *groEL* were demonstrated (87). In addition, overlay assays on *R. conorii* and *R. prowazekii* two-dimensional gels were shown to be very convenient for the identification of two putative rickettsial adhesins, namely the β-peptide and the protein encoded by RC1281 (92).

A whole proteome analysis of *E. chaffeensis* was also carried out (93). Comparative two-dimensional gel analysis showed significant variations among *E. chaffeensis* proteins when bacteria were grown in macrophages or in tick cells, proteins being mainly resolved within the alkaline or acidic pH ranges, respectively. In contrast, two-dimensional gel profiles were unchanged following temperature variations. This analysis also demonstrated the existence of extensive post-translational modifications, namely glycosylations and phosphorylations. Although glycosylated proteins were previously described for the p120 antigen of *E. chaffeensis*, as well as for the major surface protein 1 of *A. marginale* (94,95), phosphorylation of proteins from *Ehrlichia* strain had never before been reported. Although the significance of such post-translational modification remains to be studied, the possibility that these forms may differ in their function and antigenicity has been hypothesized. Finally, immunoproteomics further supported the existence of host-cell–specific differences. To our knowledge, proteome analysis of *Wolbachia* strains has not yet been investigated. Another promising area in microbial genomics is the prediction of epitopes endowed with antigenic properties and susceptible to be targeted in serological diagnosis.

FUTURE PROSPECTS

The availability of the whole genome sequences will change the way we view microbiology, which has entered the postgenomics era. Genome sequence analysis of Rickettsiales and comparisons to related bacterial genomes have already provided some information about their interactions with hosts and pathogenesis. The ultimate understanding of the molecular mechanisms underlying their adaptation to various conditions requires application of high-throughput approaches, such as global transcriptome analysis by microarray. Such a methodology has not yet been extensively applied for Rickettsiales, but we believe that experimental progress will make such a technology more accessible in a few years. A better knowledge of a microorganism can also be gained by proteomic analysis, a field in full expansion.

ACKNOWLEDGMENTS

This work was partially supported by Marseille-Nice Génopole and the French National Genome Network (R.N.G.). We thank Prof. Jean-Michel Claverie (Head of IGS) and Prof. Didier Raoult (Head of Unité des Rickettsies) for laboratory space and support.

REFERENCES

1. Margulies M, Egholm M, Altman WE, et al. Genome sequencing in microfabricated high-density picolitre reactors. Nature 2005; 437:376–380.
2. Shendure J, Porreca GJ, Reppas NB, et al. Accurate multiplex polony sequencing of an evolved bacterial genome. Science 2005; 309:1728–1732.
3. Andersson SG, Zomorodipour A, Andersson JO, et al. The genome sequence of *Rickettsia prowazekii* and the origin of mitochondria. Nature 1998; 396:133–140.
4. McLeod MP, Qin X, Karpathy SE, et al. Complete genome sequence of *Rickettsia typhi* and comparison with sequences of other rickettsiae. J Bacteriol 2004; 186:5842–5855.
5. Ogata H, Audic S, Renesto-Audiffren P, et al. Mechanisms of evolution in *Rickettsia conorii* and *R. prowazekii*. Science 2001; 293:2093–2098.
6. Malek JA, Wierzbowski JM, Tao W, et al. Protein interaction mapping on a functional shotgun sequence of *Rickettsia sibirica*. Nucleic Acids Res 2004; 32:1059–1064.
7. Ogata H, Renesto P, Audic S, et al. The genome sequence of *Rickettsia felis* identifies the first putative conjugative plasmid in an obligate intracellular parasite. PLoS Biol 2005; 3:e248.
8. Ogata H, La Scola B, Audic S, et al. Genome sequence of *Rickettsia bellii* illuminates the role of amoebae. PLoS Genet 2006; 2:e76.
9. Brayton KA, Kappmeyer LS, Herndon DR, et al. Complete genome sequencing of *Anaplasma marginale* reveals that the surface is skewed to two superfamilies of outer membrane proteins. Proc Natl Acad Sci USA 2005; 102:844–849.

10. Dunning Hotopp JC, Lin M, Madupu R, et al. Comparative genomics of emerging human ehrlichiosis agents. PLoS Genet 2006; 2:e21.
11. Collins NE, Liebenberg J, de Villiers EP, et al. The genome of the heartwater agent *Ehrlichia ruminantium* contains multiple tandem repeats of actively variable copy number. Proc Natl Acad Sci USA 2005; 102:838–843.
12. Wu M, Sun LV, Vamathevan J, et al. Phylogenomics of the reproductive parasite *Wolbachia pipientis* wMel: a streamlined genome overrun by mobile genetic elements. PLoS Biol 2004; 2:E69 [Epub 2004 Mar 16].
13. Foster J, Ganatra M, Kamal I, et al. The *Wolbachia* genome of *Brugia malayi*: endosymbiont evolution within a human pathogenic nematode. PLoS Biol 2005; 3:e121.
14. Weisburg WG, Dobson ME, Samuel JE, et al. Phylogenetic diversity of the Rickettsiae. J Bacteriol 1989; 171:4202–4206.
15. Moran NA. Accelerated evolution and Muller's rachet in endosymbiotic bacteria. Proc Natl Acad Sci USA 1996; 93:2873–2878.
16. Wolf YI, Aravind L, Koonin EV. Rickettsiae and Chlamydiae: evidence of horizontal gene transfer and gene exchange. Trends Genet 1999; 15:173–175.
17. Karlin S, Mrazek J, Campbell AM. Compositional biases of bacterial genomes and evolutionary implications. J Bacteriol 1997; 179:3899–3913.
18. Hacker J, Kaper JB. Pathogenicity islands and the evolution of microbes. Annu Rev Microbiol 2000; 54:641–679.
19. Ogata H, Audic S, Abergel C, et al. Protein coding palindromes are a unique but recurrent feature in Rickettsia. Genome Res 2002; 12:808–816.
20. Shigenobu S, Watanabe H, Hattori M, et al. Genome sequence of the endocellular bacterial symbiont of aphids *Buchnera* sp. APS. Nature 2000; 407:81–86.
21. Tamas I, Klasson L, Canback B, et al. 50 million years of genomic stasis in endosymbiotic bacteria. Science 2002; 296:2376–2379.
22. Akman L, Yamashita A, Watanabe H, et al. Genome sequence of the endocellular obligate symbiont of tsetse flies, *Wigglesworthia glossinidia*. Nat Genet 2002; 32:402–407.
23. Boussau B, Karlberg EO, Frank AC, et al. Computational inference of scenarios for alpha-proteobacterial genome evolution. Proc Natl Acad Sci USA 2004; 101:9722–9727.
24. Andersson JO, Andersson SG. Genome degradation is an ongoing process in Rickettsia. Mol Biol Evol 1999; 16:1178–1191.
25. Mira A, Ochman H, Moran NA. Deletional bias and the evolution of bacterial genomes. Trends Genet 2001; 17:589–596.
26. Brayton KA, Knowles DP, McGuire TC, et al. Efficient use of a small genome to generate antigenic diversity in tick-borne ehrlichial pathogens. Proc Natl Acad Sci USA 2001; 98:4130–4135.
27. Brayton KA, Palmer GH, Lundgren A, et al. Antigenic variation of *Anaplasma marginale* msp2 occurs by combinatorial gene conversion. Mol Microbiol 2002; 43:1151–1159.
28. Barbet AF, Meeus PF, Belanger M, et al. Expression of multiple outer membrane protein sequence variants from a single genomic locus of *Anaplasma phagocytophilum*. Infect Immun 2003; 71:1706–1718.
29. Rovery C, Renesto P, Crapoulet N, et al. Transcriptional response of *Rickettsia conorii* exposed to temperature variation and stress starvation. Res Microbiol 2005; 156:211–218.
30. Davids W, Amiri H, Andersson SG. Small RNAs in Rickettsia: are they functional? Trends Genet 2002; 18:331–334.
31. Tettelin H, Masignani V, Cieslewicz MJ, et al. Genome analysis of multiple pathogenic isolates of *Streptococcus agalactiae*: implications for the microbial "pan-genome." Proc Natl Acad Sci USA 2005; 102:13950–13955.
32. Daubin V, Moran NA, Ochman H. Phylogenetics and the cohesion of bacterial genomes. Science 2003; 301:829–832.
33. Doolittle WF. Phylogenetic classification and the universal tree. Science 1999; 284:2124–2129.
34. Garcia-Vallve S, Romeu A, Palau J. Horizontal gene transfer in bacterial and archaeal complete genomes. Genome Res 2000; 10:1719–1725.
35. Nakamura Y, Itoh T, Matsuda H, et al. Biased biological functions of horizontally transferred genes in prokaryotic genomes. Nat Genet 2004; 36:760–766.
36. Itoh T, Martin W, Nei M. Acceleration of genomic evolution caused by enhanced mutation rate in endocellular symbionts. Proc Natl Acad Sci USA 2002; 99:12944–12948.
37. Wernegreen JJ, Moran NA. Evidence for genetic drift in endosymbionts (Buchnera): analyses of protein-coding genes. Mol Biol Evol 1999; 16:83–97.
38. Woolfit M, Bromham L. Increased rates of sequence evolution in endosymbiotic bacteria and fungi with small effective population sizes. Mol Biol Evol 2003; 20:1545–1555.
39. Aniskovitch LP, Winkler HH. Instability of *Rickettsia prowazekii* RNA polymerase-promoter complexes. J Bacteriol 1995; 177:6301–6303.
40. Driskell LO, Tucker AM, Winkler HH, et al. Rickettsial metK-encoded methionine adenosyltransferase expression in an *Escherichia coli* metK deletion strain. J Bacteriol 2005; 187:5719–5722.
41. Winkler HH. *Rickettsia prowazekii*, ribosomes and slow growth. Trends Microbiol 1995; 3:196–198.

42. Rurangirwa FR, Brayton KA, McGuire TC, et al. Conservation of the unique rickettsial rRNA gene arrangement in *Anaplasma*. Int J Syst Evol Microbiol 2002; 52:1405–1409.
43. Baldo L, Lo N, Werren JH. Mosaic nature of the *Wolbachia* surface protein. J Bacteriol 2005; 187:5406–5418.
44. Baldo L, Bordenstein S, Wernegreen JJ, et al. Widespread recombination throughout *Wolbachia* genomes. Mol Biol Evol 2006; 23:437–449.
45. Jiggins FM. Adaptive evolution and recombination of Rickettsia antigens. J Mol Evol 2006; 62:99–110.
46. Andersson JO, Andersson SG. Pseudogenes, junk DNA, and the dynamics of Rickettsia genomes. Mol Biol Evol 2001; 18:829–839.
47. Ogata H, Audic S, Barbe V, et al. Selfish DNA in protein-coding genes of Rickettsia. Science 2000; 290:347–350.
48. Claverie JM, Ogata H. The insertion of palindromic repeats in the evolution of proteins. Trends Biochem Sci 2003; 28:75–80.
49. Ogata H, Suhre K, Claverie JM. Discovery of protein-coding palindromic repeats in *Wolbachia*. Trends Microbiol 2005; 13:253–255.
50. Suyama M, Lathe WC III, Bork P. Palindromic repetitive DNA elements with coding potential in *Methanocaldococcus jannaschii*. FEBS Lett 2005; 579:5281–5286.
51. Britten R. Transposable elements have contributed to thousands of human proteins. Proc Natl Acad Sci USA 2006; 103:1798–1803.
52. Greub G, Raoult D. History of the ADP/ATP-translocase-encoding gene, a parasitism gene transferred from a Chlamydiales ancestor to plants 1 billion years ago. Appl Environ Microbiol 2003; 69:5530–5535.
53. Schmitz-Esser S, Linka N, Collingro A, et al. ATP/ADP translocases: a common feature of obligate intracellular amoebal symbionts related to Chlamydiae and Rickettsiae. J Bacteriol 2004; 186:683–691.
54. Fritsche TR, Horn M, Seyedirashti S, et al. In situ detection of novel bacterial endosymbionts of *Acanthamoeba* spp. phylogenetically related to members of the order *Rickettsiales*. Appl Environ Microbiol 1999; 65:206–212.
55. Molmeret M, Horn M, Wagner M, et al. Amoebae as training grounds for intracellular bacterial pathogens. Appl Environ Microbiol 2005; 71:20–28.
56. Barker J, Brown MR. Trojan horses of the microbial world: protozoa and the survival of bacterial pathogens in the environment. Microbiology 1994; 140(pt 6):1253–1259.
57. Chatterji D, Ojha AK. Revisiting the stringent response, ppGpp and starvation signaling. Curr Opin Microbiol 2001; 4:160–165.
58. Braeken K, Moris M, Daniels R, et al. New horizons for (p)ppGpp in bacterial and plant physiology. Trends Microbiol 2006; 14:45–54.
59. Gerdes K, Christensen SK, Lobner-Olesen A. Prokaryotic toxin–antitoxin stress response loci. Nat Rev Microbiol 2005; 3:371–382.
60. Gerdes K. Toxin–antitoxin modules may regulate synthesis of macromolecules during nutritional stress. J Bacteriol 2000; 182:561–572.
61. Engelberg-Kulka H, Glaser G. Addiction modules and programmed cell death and antideath in bacterial cultures. Annu Rev Microbiol 1999; 53:43–70.
62. Scorpio DG, Caspersen K, Ogata H, et al. Restricted changes in major surface protein-2 (msp2) transcription after prolonged in vitro passage of *Anaplasma phagocytophilum*. BMC Microbiol 2004; 4:1.
63. Fournier PE, Roux V, Raoult D. Phylogenetic analysis of spotted fever group rickettsiae by study of the outer surface protein rOmpA. Int J Syst Bacteriol 1998; 48(pt 3):839–849.
64. Roux V, Raoult D. Phylogenetic analysis of members of the genus *Rickettsia* using the gene encoding the outer-membrane protein rOmpB (ompB). Int J Syst Evol Microbiol 2000; 50(pt 4):1449–1455.
65. Sekeyova Z, Roux V, Raoult D. Phylogeny of *Rickettsia* spp. inferred by comparing sequences of 'gene D', which encodes an intracytoplasmic protein. Int J Syst Evol Microbiol 2001; 51:1353–1360.
66. Martinez JJ, Seveau S, Veiga E, et al. Ku70, a component of DNA-dependent protein kinase, is a mammalian receptor for *Rickettsia conorii*. Cell 2005; 123:1013–1023.
67. Blanc G, Ngwamidiba M, Ogata H, et al. Molecular evolution of rickettsia surface antigens: evidence of positive selection. Mol Biol Evol 2005; 22:2073–2083.
68. Christie PJ. Type IV secretion: intercellular transfer of macromolecules by systems ancestrally related to conjugation machines. Mol Microbiol 2001; 40:294–305.
69. Fenn K, Blaxter M. *Wolbachia* genomes: revealing the biology of parasitism and mutualism. Trends Parasitol 2006; 22:60–65.
70. Ohashi N, Zhi N, Lin Q, et al. Characterization and transcriptional analysis of gene clusters for a type IV secretion machinery in human granulocytic and monocytic ehrlichiosis agents. Infect Immun 2002; 70:2128–2138.
71. Mosavi LK, Cammett TJ, Desrosiers DC, et al. The ankyrin repeat as molecular architecture for protein recognition. Protein Sci 2004; 13:1435–1448.
72. Eremeeva ME, Madan A, Shaw CD, et al. New perspectives on rickettsial evolution from new genome sequences of *Rickettsia*, particularly *R. canadensis*, and *Orientia tsutsugamuchi*. Ann NY Acad Sci 2005; 1063:47–63.

73. Caturegli P, Asanovich KM, Walls JJ, et al. ankA: an *Ehrlichia phagocytophila* group gene encoding a cytoplasmic protein antigen with ankyrin repeats. Infect Immun 2000; 68:5277–5283.
74. Renesto P, Dehoux P, Gouin E, et al. Identification and characterization of a phospholipase D-superfamily gene in rickettsiae. J Infect Dis 2003; 188:1276–1283.
75. Blanc G, Renesto P, Raoult D. Phylogenic analysis of rickettsial patatin-like protein with conserved phospholipase A2 active sites. Ann NY Acad Sci 2005; 1063:83–86.
76. Gouin E, Egile C, Dehoux P, et al. The RickA protein of *Rickettsia conorii* activates the Arp2/3 complex. Nature 2004; 427:457–461.
77. de la Fuente J, Garcia-Garcia JC, Barbet AF, et al. Adhesion of outer membrane proteins containing tandem repeats of *Anaplasma* and *Ehrlichia* species (Rickettsiales: Anaplasmataceae) to tick cells. Vet Microbiol 2004; 98:313–322.
78. Renesto P, Crapoulet N, Ogata H, et al. Genome-based design of a cell-free culture medium for *Tropheryma whipplei*. Lancet 2003; 362:447–449.
79. Raoult D, Birg ML, La Scola B, et al. Cultivation of the bacillus of Whipple's disease. N Engl J Med 2000; 342:620–625.
80. http://www.igs.cnrs-mrs.fr/axenic/
81. Ogata H, Claverie JM. Metagrowth: a new resource for the building of metabolic hypotheses in microbiology. Nucleic Acids Res 2005; 33:D321–D324.
82. Rovery C, La MV, Robineau S, et al. Preliminary transcriptional analysis of spoT gene family and of membrane proteins in *Rickettsia conorii* and *Rickettsia felis*. Ann NY Acad Sci 2005; 1063:79–82.
83. Bryant PA, Venter D, Robins-Browne R, et al. Chips with everything: DNA microarrays in infectious diseases. Lancet Infect Dis 2004; 4:100–111.
84. Hinton JC, Hautefort I, Eriksson S, et al. Benefits and pitfalls of using microarrays to monitor bacterial gene expression during infection. Curr Opin Microbiol 2004; 7:277–282.
85. Ge H, Chuang YY, Zhao S, et al. Comparative genomics of *Rickettsia prowazekii* Madrid E and Breinl strains. J Bacteriol 2004; 186:556–565.
86. Zhang JZ, Sinha M, Luxon BA, et al. Survival strategy of obligately intracellular *Ehrlichia chaffeensis*: novel modulation of immune response and host cell cycles. Infect Immun 2004; 72:498–507.
87. Renesto P, Azza S, Dolla A, et al. Proteome analysis of *Rickettsia conorii* by two-dimensional gel electrophoresis coupled with mass spectrometry. FEMS Microbiol Lett 2005; 245:231–238.
88. Renesto P, Azza S, Dolla A. *Rickettsia conorii* and *R. prowazekii* proteome analysis by 2DE-MS: a step toward functional analysis of rickettsiales genomes. Ann NY Acad Sci 2005; 1063:90–93.
89. Rabilloud T. Two-dimensional gel electrophoresis in proteomics: old, old fashioned, but it still climbs up the mountains. Proteomics 2002; 2:3–10.
90. Washburn MP, Wolters D, Yates JR III. Large-scale analysis of the yeast proteome by multidimensional protein identification technology. Nat Biotechnol 2001; 19:242–247.
91. Chao CC, Chelius D, Zhang T, et al. Proteome analysis of Madrid E strain of *Rickettsia prowazekii*. Proteomics 2004; 4:1280–1292.
92. Renesto P, Samson L, Ogata H, et al. Identification of two putative rickettsial adhesins by proteomic analysis. Res Microbiol 2006; 157:605–612.
93. Singu V, Liu H, Cheng C, et al. *Ehrlichia chaffeensis* expresses macrophage- and tick cell-specific 28-kilodalton outer membrane proteins. Infect Immun 2005; 73:79–87.
94. Garcia-Garcia JC, de la Fuente J, Bell-Eunice G, et al. Glycosylation of *Anaplasma marginale* major surface protein 1a and its putative role in adhesion to tick cells. Infect Immun 2004; 72:3022–3030.
95. McBride JW, Yu XJ, Walker DH. Glycosylation of homologous immunodominant proteins of *Ehrlichia chaffeensis* and *Ehrlichia canis*. Infect Immun 2000; 68:13–18.

Section X: ANTIMICROBIAL SUSCEPTIBILITY OF RICKETTSIAL AGENTS

26 Antimicrobial Susceptibility of Rickettsial Agents

Jean-Marc Rolain
Faculté de Médecine et de Pharmacie, Unité des Rickettsies, Université de la Méditerranée, Marseille, France

INTRODUCTION

This chapter discusses susceptibility testing for rickettsial agents including *Rickettsia*, *Ehrlichia*, *Anaplasma*, and *Coxiella burnetii*. Because of the intracellular lifestyle of these bacteria, the susceptibility testing that has been carried out has been somewhat limited in terms of both the number of isolates tested and the number of different anti-infective agents evaluated. In an attempt to better understand the susceptibility to antibiotics of these bacteria, several in vitro cell culture methods of evaluation of the susceptibility to antibiotics have been developed. The major drawbacks of these methods were the absence of reproducibility and the subjectivity of enumeration of the bacteria, which made comparison of the results difficult. Thus, the complexity of the methods needed to propagate these organisms argues for an attempt to standardize the methods used for susceptibility testing. This has been recently addressed by the use of molecular methods for quantification of bacteria and in vitro antibiotic susceptibility testing for fastidious and intracellular bacteria (1) that are reviewed in this chapter. This new methodology will allow testing of more isolates. This is important, because resistance will continue to remain unconfirmed if testing is not carried out (2). Resistance to antimicrobials has been infrequent among these organisms, but recent findings regarding molecular support of resistance to antibiotics have been recently reported.

RICKETTSIA

All members of the genus *Rickettsia* are obligate intracellular pathogens and therefore require either animal models, embryonated eggs, or tissue cultures for susceptibility assays (3,4). It would appear that, of the in vitro techniques now available, the plaque assay and a colorimetric assay (3) were the most practical for evaluating anti-infectives for this group of organisms. However, because of the technical difficulties in working with these agents, susceptibility testing would probably be confined to relatively few laboratories. The two assays (plaque assay and colorimetric assay) depend on the induction of cytopathic effects and plaque formation in cell cultures by the rickettsiae, but some rickettsiae do not normally cause cytopathic effects in primary cultures (1,5). Recently, Ives et al. (6,7) described a new assay that uses immunofluorescence (IF) staining, which avoids the problem of a lack of cytopathic effects. Very recently, we have developed a new quantitative polymerase chain reaction (PCR) DNA assay using the Light Cycler system for the evaluation of antibiotic susceptibilities of three rickettsial species including *Rickettsia felis*, a rickettsial species which does not induce plaque in cell cultures (1).

In Vitro Antimicrobial Susceptibility Testing
Reference Method: Plaque Assay

Vero cell monolayers in plastic, tissue-culture Petri dishes are infected with 1 mL of a solution containing 4×10^3 plaque-forming units (PFUs) of the desired rickettsial strain (3). After a one-hour incubation at room temperature, the plates are overlaid with 4 mL of a medium containing Minimum Eagle Medium, 2% newborn calf serum, 2% (*N*-(2-hydroxyethyl) piperazine-*N'*-(2-ethanesulfonic acid)) (HEPES), and 0.5% agar. The antibiotic solutions are

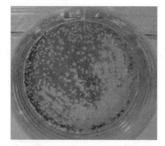 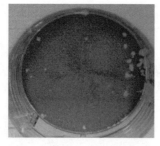 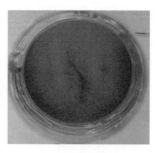

Doxycycline 0.06 µg/mL   **Doxycycline 0.125 µg/mL**   **Control**

FIGURE 1 Plaque assay for *Rickettsia conorii* and doxycycline. The MIC is the lowest concentration of the agent tested, causing complete inhibition of plaque formation compared with the drug-free controls. In this example, MIC is 0.125 µg/mL. *Abbreviation*: MIC, minimal inhibitory concentration.

added to the medium to obtain the desired final concentrations (an antibiotic-free control plate is also included), and the plates are incubated for four to seven days at 35°C in a carbon dioxide incubator. After incubation, the monolayers are then fixed with 4% formaldehyde and stained with 1% crystal violet in 20% ethanol. The minimal inhibitory concentration (MIC) is the lowest concentration of the agent tested, causing complete inhibition of plaque formation compared with drug-free controls (Fig. 1).

Dye-Uptake Assay

Flat-bottomed microdilution plates are seeded with 1.5×10^4 Vero cells (suspended in a solution of Eagle minimum essential medium (MEM), 5% newborn calf serum, and 2 mmol/L L-glutamine) per well and subsequently infected with varying concentrations of a suspension of *Rickettsia* (3). The Vero cell suspension (100 µL) is added to each well. The infectious inoculum is added to individual wells in a final volume of 50 µL. For each 96-well plate, the first horizontal row of eight wells contains no rickettsiae, the second horizontal row is inoculated with 2000 PFUs, the third horizontal row with 200 PFUs, and the fourth with 20 PFUs. Antibiotics are added in 50-µL volumes. Incubation is then carried out at 37°C for four days in a CO_2 incubator.

After this, the medium is removed, 50 µL of neutral red dye is added to each well, and the plate is incubated for 60 minutes at 36°C. Unincorporated dye is then washed three times from the cells using phosphate-buffered saline (pH 6.5). Incorporated dye is removed from the well using 100 µL of phosphate–ethanol buffer (10% ethanol in phosphate-buffered saline, adjusted to pH 4.2).

Finally, the optical density (OD) of the solution is read at 492 nm with a multichannel spectrophotometer designed for use with microdilution plates. The mean OD of the control wells (containing only Vero cells) is assigned a value of 1, and the mean OD of the wells containing 2000 PFUs is assigned a value of 0. The MIC is considered to be any OD value that falls between the mean OD of the wells containing 20 PFUs and the mean OD of the control wells containing only Vero cells. This test is therefore a derivative of the plaque assay but has the advantage of using microdilution technology as well as an automated means of reading the plates.

Other Assays
Immunofluorescence Assay

In this model, Vero cells cultured in wells of chamber culture microscope slides were infected with rickettsiae (6). After incubation of cultures for three hours at 37°C in a 5% CO_2 atmosphere, cell supernatants were replaced by new medium containing various concentrations of the antibiotics to be tested. Drug-free cultures served as controls. Cell culture monolayers were then fixed with methanol and stained using an IF assay to reveal the presence of immunofluorescent foci (clusters of rickettsiae) in 25 random fields for each well. The minimal antibiotic concentration allowing complete inhibition of foci formation as compared to the drug-free control was recorded as the MIC.

Light Cycler Polymerase Chain Reaction Assay

Cells cultured in 24-well plates were infected with rickettsiae and incubated for seven days at 37°C in a 5% carbon dioxide atmosphere with medium containing various concentrations of the antibiotics to be tested (1). Wells were harvested each day for seven days and stored at −20°C before PCR assay. After thawing, harvested tubes were centrifuged at 5000 rpm for 10 minutes, supernatant was discarded, and pellet was washed twice with sterile distilled water and finally resuspended with 200 μL of sterile distilled water. Extraction of the DNA was performed using chelex (Biotechnology-grade chelating resin-Chelex 100, Biorad, Richmond, California) at 20% in sterile water (8). Extraction could also be done using a Qiagen DNA extraction kit (unpublished data). DNA could be stored in sterile tubes at 4°C before use. Master mixes were prepared by following the manufacturer's instructions, using primers of the citrate synthase gene previously described (9). The 20-μL sample volume in each glass capillary contained the following for all single experiments: 2 μL of Light Cycler DNA Master SYBR Green (Roche Biochemicals), 2.4 μL of $MgCl_2$ at 4 mM, 1 μL of each primer at 0.5 μM, 11.6 μL of sterile distilled water, and 2 μL of DNA.

Real-time PCR was performed on Light Cycler instrumentation. The amplification program included an initial denaturation step for one cycle at 95°C for 120 seconds and 40 cycles of denaturation at 95°C for 15 seconds, annealing at 54°C for eight seconds, and extension at 72°C for 15 seconds with fluorescence acquisition at 54° in a single mode. Melting curve analysis was done at 45 to 90°C (temperature transition, 20°C/sec) with stepwise fluorescence acquisition by real-time measurement of fluorescence directly in the clear glass capillary tubes. Sequence-specific standard curves were generated using 10-fold serial dilutions (10^5–10^6 copies) of standard bacterial concentration of *Rickettsia*. The specificity of amplification can be confirmed by melting curve analysis. The number of copies of each sample transcript was then calculated from standard curve using the Light Cycler software. MIC was defined as the first antibiotic concentration allowing the inhibition of growth of bacteria as compared to the number of DNA copies at day 0 (Fig. 2). This technique is specific, reproducible, easy to perform, and rapid. The advantage of this method was to measure the number of DNA copies at any time and we were able to perform for the first time a kinetic of growth of *Rickettsia* even if the bacteria did not lead to plaque in vitro in cell cultures.

Results of Susceptibility Testing

The results of susceptibility testing of *Rickettsia* are summarized in Table 1.

Amoxicillin (MICs from 128 to 256 μg/mL), gentamicin (MICs from 4 to 16 μg/mL), and cotrimoxazole were not effective against rickettsiae (1,5). Doxycycline was the most effective antibiotic against all strains tested, with MICs ranging from 0.06 to 0.25 μg/mL. The MICs of

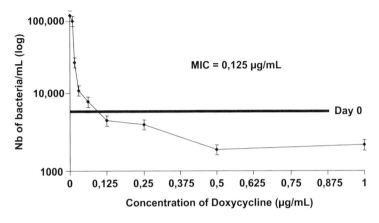

FIGURE 2 Light Cycler assay for *Rickettsia felis* and doxycycline. The MIC is the first antibiotic concentration allowing the inhibition of growth of bacteria as compared to the number of DNA copies at day 0. In this example, MIC is 0.125 μg/mL. *Abbreviation*: MIC, minimal inhibitory concentration.

TABLE 1 Antibiotic Susceptibility of Rickettsial Agents as Determined Using In Vitro Cell Models

Organism	Blm	Dox	Chm	Sxt	Rif	Ery	Tel	Amg	Qui
Rickettsia									
Spotted fever group									
R. conorii subgroup[a]	R	S	S	R	S	R	S	R	S
R. massiliae subgroup	R	S	S	R	R	R	S	R	S
Typhus group[b]	R	S	S	R	S	S	S	R	S
C. burnetii	R	S	R	S	S	V	S	R	S
Ehrlichia									
E. chaffeensis	R	S	R	R	S	R	R	R	R
Anaplasma phagocytophilum	R	S	R	R	S	R	R	R	S

[a]Subgroup including Bar29, *R. massiliae*, *R. aeschlimanii*, *R. montanensis*, and *R. rhipicephali*.
[b]Subgroup including *R. typhi* and *R. prowazekii*.
Abbreviations: Amg, aminoglycosides; Blm, β-lactams; Chm, chloramphenicol; Cla, clarithromycin; Dox, doxycycline; Ery, erythromycin; Qui, quinolones; R, resistant; Rif, rifampin; S, susceptible; Tel, telithromycin; V, variable susceptibility among different strains.

thiamphenicol ranged from 0.5 to 4 µg/mL, whereas the MICs for fluoroquinolone compounds ranged from 0.25 to 2 µg/mL. Among the macrolide compounds, josamycin was the most effective antibiotic, with MICs ranging from 0.5 to 1 µg/mL. Typhus group (TG) rickettsia were susceptible to erythromycin (MICs from 0.125 to 0.5 µg/mL), whereas spotted fever group (SFG) rickettsia were not susceptible to erythromycin (MICs from 2 to 8 µg/mL). Finally, we have demonstrated that the new ketolide compound, telithromycin, was very effective against either TG rickettsia or SFG rickettsiae with MICs ranging from 0.5 to 1 µg/mL (10). Susceptibilities to rifampin varied, with TG rickettsia and most SFG rickettsiae being susceptible (MICs from 0.03 to 1 µg/ml), whereas a cluster including *R. massiliae*, *R. montanensis*, *R. rhipicephali*, *R. aeschlimannii*, and strain Bar 29 were more resistant (MICs from 2 to 4 µg/mL).

Molecular Support of Resistance

The resistance to rifampin found in the *R. massiliae* subgroup was linked to natural mutations in the *rpoB* gene (11). We have reported that TG rickettsiae had a triple amino acid difference in the highly conserved region of the L22 ribosomal protein compared with the SFG rickettsiae (12). We believe that the triple amino acid difference in the L22 ribosomal protein found may explain the difference in susceptibility to erythromycin among the *Rickettsia* genus (12). Finally, we have recently investigated the resistance mechanisms of bacteria of the genus *Rickettsia* to antibiotics by in-silico comparison for the presence of known antibiotic resistance determinants involved in molecular resistance in other bacteria (13). Five specific open reading frames related to antibiotic resistance have been identified in the genome of *R. felis* including a class C β-lactamase, a class D β-lactamase, a penicillin acylase homologue, and an ABC-type multidrug transporter system (14). For the first time, using this approach, it was possible to demonstrate experimentally the presence of a β-lactamase activity for this bacterium (14). Interestingly, we have also found two genes encoding for β-lactamases in the genome of *R. conorii* but without activity (unpublished data) and none in the genome of *R. prowazekii* and *R. typhi*, whereas these three bacteria possess PBPs and *ampG* genes (13). In the genome of *R. conorii*, we have found one gene encoding for a protein similar to an aminoglycoside 3′-phosphotransferase, and a streptomycin-resistant protein homolog in the genome of *R. felis*, whereas genomes of *R. typhi* and *R. prowazekii* do not contain such encoding genes (13). Sulfamethoxazole binds to the enzyme-coding dihydropteroate synthase, which catalyzes this reaction. Trimethoprim is an analog of dihydrofolic acid, an essential component in the synthesis of amino acids and nucleotides that competitively inhibits the enzyme dihydrofolate reductase in the folate pathway. The sequential enzymatic blockade by sulfamethoxazole and trimethoprim is responsible for the very strong synergistic effect observed between these two compounds. For the bacteria of the genus *Rickettsia*, the resistance to these compounds is linked to the absence of such encoding genes (*folA* and/or *folP*) in their genomes (13). Indeed, the genomes of the TG rickettsia (*R. typhi* and *R. prowazekii*) do not contain *folA* and *folP* gene, whereas *R. felis*, *R. conorii*, *R. sibirica* and *R. rickettsii* had *folA* gene only. This is in accordance with the fact that isolation of SFG rickettsiae from ticks by use of cotrimoxazole in the culture medium to prevent overgrowth of bacterial contaminants was possible (15). Moreover, Ruiz Beltran and Herrero-Herrero (16) reported that cotrimoxazole was ineffective in the treatment of rickettsioses.

EHRLICHIA

Ehrlichioses are emerging infectious diseases caused by Gram-negative obligate intracellular bacteria belonging to the α subgroup of proteobacteria (17). The genus *Ehrlichia* is divided into three genogroups: the group *Neorickettsia* with *N. sennetsu*, *N. risticii*, and *N. helminthoeca*; the group *Ehrlichia* with *E. canis*, *E. chaffeensis*, *E. rumitanum*, *E. muris*, and *E. ewingii*; and the group *Anaplasma* with *A. platys*, *A. marginale*, *E. equi*, and *A. phagocytophilum* (17,18).

In vitro and in vivo antibiotic susceptibility studies have been carried out on various species of *Ehrlichia*. All have been found that doxycycline and rifampin are highly effective against ehrlichiae (19), so this is currently the first choice for therapy in animals and in human ehrlichiosis.

In Vitro Antimicrobial Susceptibility Testing
Cell Culture Model

The susceptibility of *Ehrlichia* to various antibiotics has been tested using *Ehrlichia*-infected contact-inhibition-growth cell lines incubated for 48 to 72 hours in the antibiotic concerned (20). Thereafter, the antibiotic-containing media is removed and *Ehrlichia*-infected cells are incubated with antibiotic-free media for at least three more days. The number of *Ehrlichia*-infected cells were counted every day, and an antibiotic was ineffective if the number of *Ehrlichia*-infected cells after exposure to the antibiotic was similar to that of control noninfected cells. Antibiotics are considered bacteriostatic if there is no increase or decrease in *Ehrlichia*-infected cells when the antibiotic is present, but the number of infected cells increases when antibiotic-free media is provided. In vitro tests currently used to assess the antibiotic susceptibilities of the organisms are based on microscopic counting of morulae in cells in tissue cultures before and after exposure to serial dilutions of antibiotics. These tests, however, are not standardized, are not sensitive, are time-consuming, and are not adapted for the screening of new drugs or strains of organisms.

Light Cycler Polymerase Chain Reaction Assay

MICs of antibiotics against *Anaplasma phagocytophilum* (21,22), *Ehrlichia chaffeensis*, and *E. canis* (21) have been recently determined by real-time quantitative PCR with primers of the 16S ribosomal DNA (rDNA). The methodology used and the definition of MICs were similar to those explained for *Rickettsia* (see above) except that target genes and primers were different. In comparison to the reference method for determining sensitivities, which uses Diff-Quick staining, PCR assay was very sensitive and specific (21,22).

Results of Susceptibility Testing

Results of susceptibility testing for *A. phagocytophilum* and *E. chaffeensis* are summarized in Table 1. *E. chaffeensis* was sensitive to 0.5 μg/mL of doxycycline and to 0.125 μg/mL of rifampin (10,20). Chloramphenicol, cotrimoxazole, erythromycin, telithromycin penicillin, gentamicin, and ciprofloxacin were not effective against *E. chaffeensis* (20). The human granulocytic ehrlichiosis (HGE) agent is sensitive to doxycycline, ofloxacin, ciprofloxacin, and trovafloxacin, but is resistant to clindamycin, cotrimoxazole, erythromycin, azithromycin, ampicillin, ceftriaxone, and imipenem (23–25). Chloramphenicol and aminoglycosides only display a poor bacteriostatic activity and are never bactericidal (24). Fluoroquinolones are more active in vitro against *A. phagocytophilum* than against *E. chaffeensis* and *E. canis* (Table 1). Fluoroquinolones might represent a potential therapeutic alternative to tetracycline for HGE, but they have not received

FDA approval for use in children and pregnant women. Using real-time quantitative PCR assay, two reports confirmed that doxycycline and rifampin are highly active against these bacteria and found variable susceptibilities to fluoroquinolones: *A. phagocytophilum* was susceptible (21,22), but *E. canis* and *E. chaffeensis* were only partly susceptible (21). β-Lactam compounds, cotrimoxazole, macrolide compounds, and telithromycin showed no activity against any of the three organisms (21). Thiamphenicol was found to be more active than chloramphenicol.

Molecular Support of Resistance

A *GyrA*-mediated resistance in the related species *E. canis* and *E. chaffeensis* has recently been described and can explain the difference in susceptibility to fluoroquinolones for these species (26). For the first time, we showed that the three species *A. phagocytophilum*, *E. canis*, and *E. chaffeensis* as well as *Wolbachia pipientis* have numerous point mutations in their 23S RNA genes, with those at positions 754, 2057, 2058, 2059, and 2611 (*Escherichia coli* numbering) known to confer resistance to macrolide compounds in other bacteria (21).

COXIELLA BURNETII

Coxiella burnetii, the agent of Q fever, is an obligate, intracellular bacterium that multiplies within acidic vacuoles of eukaryotic cells (27).

Antimicrobial Susceptibility Testing and Results

Antibiotic susceptibility testing of *C. burnetii* is difficult because this organism is an obligate intracellular bacterium. However, three models of infection have been developed: animals, chick embryos, and cell culture. The current method used to test the antibiotic susceptibility of *C. burnetii* is based on cell culture models. Torres and Raoult (28) have developed a shell-vial assay with human embryonic lung (HEL) cells for assessment of the bacteriostatic effect of antibiotics. However, real-time quantitative PCR has been recently developed for antibiotic susceptibility testing of *C. burnetii* that is more reproducible and sensitive than shell-vial assay (29–31).

The Shell-Vial Assay

In this model, HEL fibroblast cells are grown in shell vials at 37°C in a 5% CO_2 atmosphere. Cell monolayers are infected with a *C. burnetii* inoculum previously determined to induce 30% to 50% infection of HEL cells after six days of incubation in the absence of antimicrobial agents, as revealed by an IF technique with anti-*C. burnetii* polyclonal antibodies. The percentage of infected cells in antimicrobial-containing cultures is determined after the same incubation time, using the same IF procedure. MICs correspond to the minimum antimicrobial concentration allowing complete inhibition of growth, that is, 0% infected cells after the six-day incubation period.

Amikacin and amoxicillin were not effective, ceftriaxone and fusidic acid were inconsistently active (28), whereas cotrimoxazole, rifampin, doxycycline, clarithromycin, and the quinolones were bacteriostatic (32,33). There was an heterogeneity of susceptibility of strains tested to erythromycin (28,34). *C. burnetii* can establish a persistent infection in several cell lines, including L929 mouse fibroblasts and J774 or P388D1 murine macrophage-like cells (35). Infected cells can be maintained in continuous cultures for months (36). Raoult et al., using P388D1 and L929 cells, showed that pefloxacin, rifampin, and doxycycline (37) as well as clarithromycin (33) were bacteriostatic against *C. burnetii*. An original model of killing assay has been developed by Maurin et al. (38) to assess the bactericidal activity of antibiotics against *C. burnetii*. The bactericidal activity of antibiotics in this technique is directly evaluated by titration of residual viable bacteria in persistently infected P388D1 cell cultures. On the first day of experiment, P388D1 cells infected with *C. burnetii* were harvested from a 150-cm^2 culture flask and seeded into 25-cm^2 flasks so that each flask received the same primary inoculum. Antibiotics were added to flasks, and flasks with or without antibiotics were incubated for 24 hours at 37°C. Then cells were lysed, and 10-fold serial dilutions of cell lysates were distributed into shell vials containing uninfected HEL cells (39). After six days of incubation, *C. burnetii* were stained by indirect IF in the shell vials. It was demonstrated that doxycycline, pefloxacin, and rifampin did not show any significant bactericidal activity. The lack of bactericidal activity was related to inactivation by the low pH of the phagolysosomes in which *C. burnetii* survives. Maurin et al. (38) demonstrated that the addition of a lysosomotropic alkalinizing agent, chloroquine, to antibiotics improved the activities of doxycycline and pefloxacin, which then became bactericidal. These in vitro results have been corroborated by the demonstration of in vivo efficacy for the combination of doxycycline and hydroxychloroquine (40). This regimen allowed a reduction in the duration of therapy to 18 months for many patients and also reduced the relapse rate to less than 5% (40,41). This regimen is effective clinically, but there is a heterogeneity in the rapidity of the biological response that was correlated with the level of doxycycline in serum (42) as compared to the MIC of the corresponding isolate (43).

Light Cycler Polymerase Chain Reaction Assay

The real-time quantitative PCR for antibiotic susceptibility testing has also been recently adapted to reference isolates of *C. burnetii* by two independent teams (29,30) using methods similar to that of *Rickettsia* described above. These two reports confirm that MICs against doxycycline, fluoroquinolone compounds, and rifampicin were in the range 1 to 4 mg/L (29). Telithromycin was the most effective macrolide compound with MICs of 1 to 2 mg/L (29). The results confirmed previous reports on the accuracy of this new method for the determination of the antibiotic susceptibility of *C. burnetii* and could be used for the screening of new drugs. Interestingly, MICs obtained using this more sensitive method were slightly higher than previous results obtained with reference strains (29). This has been recently confirmed when testing new isolates with MICs against doxycycline ranging from 1 to 8 µg/mL, for which we found a correlation between ratio of doxycycline to MIC and rapid decline of antibody levels during treatment of Q fever endocarditis (43). Especially, we have reported for the first time a human isolate of *C. burnetii* resistant to doxycycline (MIC = 8 µg/mL) in a patient with Q fever endocarditis who died during the course of the treatment (43). More recently, this PCR assay was used for evaluation of susceptibility of 13 new isolates of *C. burnetii* against doxycycline, erythromycin, and telithromycin (31). MICs against doxycycline ranged from 1 to 8 µg/mL, telithromycin from 0.5 to 2 µg/mL, and all strains had MICs $\geq$ 8 µg/mL for erythromycin. There was no difference in MICs for the 13 strains according to their origin (31). In this study, three isolates were considered resistant to doxycycline with MICs at 8 µg/mL. Molecular mechanism of resistance to doxycycline remains unknown at this time.

CONCLUSIONS

All of the organisms considered in this chapter require tissue culture methods for their propagation and susceptibility testing. Because of this, they frequently are not isolated from patients in whom they are causing disease. Thus, it will be important to further simplify and standardize the susceptibility testing procedures to allow additional laboratories to undertake susceptibility testing of their isolates. If emerging resistance is to be detected, it is essential that recent clinical isolates are also tested, particularly those from patients who appear to be failing, or have failed, appropriate therapy. Our new real-time quantitative PCR assay could be useful in the future for the determination of the susceptibility to antibiotics of such fastidious bacteria (1). Moreover, a better understanding of the molecular support of the resistance to antibiotics in these fastidious bacteria may allow the development of new tools for the detection of resistance directly in samples from patients even if the bacteria are not isolated.

REFERENCES

1. Rolain JM, Stuhl L, Maurin M, Raoult D. Evaluation of antibiotic susceptibilities of three rickettsial species including *Rickettsia felis* by a quantitative PCR DNA assay. Antimicrob Agents Chemother 2002; 46:2747–2751.
2. Stapleton JT, Stamm LV, Bassford PJ Jr. Potential for development of antibiotic resistance in pathogenic treponemes. Rev Infect Dis 1985; 7(suppl 2):S314–S317.
3. Raoult D, Roussellier P, Vestris G, Tamalet J. In vitro antibiotic susceptibility of *Rickettsia rickettsii* and *Rickettsia conorii*: plaque assay and microplaque colorimetric assay. J Infect Dis 1987; 155:1059–1062.
4. Tamura A, Ohashi N, Urakami H, Miyamura S. Classification of *Rickettsia tsutsugamushi* in a new genus, *Orientia* gen. nov., as *Orientia tsutsugamushi* comb. nov. Int J Syst Bacteriol 1995; 45:589–591.

5. Rolain JM, Maurin M, Vestris G, Raoult D. In vitro susceptibilities of 27 *Rickettsiae* to 13 antimicrobials. Antimicrob Agents Chemother 1998; 42:1537–1541.
6. Ives TJ, Manzewitsch P, Regnery RL, Butts JD, Kebede M. In vitro susceptibilities of *Bartonella henselae*, *B. quintana*, *B. elizabethae*, *Rickettsia rickettsii*, *R. conorii*, *R. akari*, and *R. prowazekii* to macrolide antibiotics as determined by immunofluorescent-antibody analysis of infected Vero cell monolayers. Antimicrob Agents Chemother 1997; 41:578–582.
7. Ives TJ, Marston EL, Regnery RL, Butts JD. In vitro susceptibilities of *Bartonella* and *Rickettsia* spp. to fluoroquinolone antibiotics as determined by immunofluorescent antibody analysis of infected Vero cell monolayers. Int J Antimicrob Agents 2001; 18:217–222.
8. Stein A, Raoult D. A simple method for amplification of DNA from paraffin-embedded tissues. Nucleic Acids Res 1992; 20:5237–5238.
9. Raoult D, Roux V, Ndihokubwaho JB, Bise G, Baudon D, Martet G,. Birtles RJ. Jail fever (epidemic typhus) outbreak in Burundi. Emerg Infect Dis 1997; 3:357–360.
10. Rolain JM, Maurin M, Bryskier A, Raoult D. In vitro activities of telithromycin (HMR 3647) against *Rickettsia rickettsii*, *Rickettsia conorii*, *Rickettsia africae*, *Rickettsia typhi*, *Rickettsia prowasekii*, *Coxiella burnetii*, *Bartonella henselae*, *Bartonella quintana*, *Bartonella bacilliformis*, and *Ehrlichia chaffeensis*. Antimicrob Agents Chemother 2000; 44:1391–1393.
11. Drancourt M, Raoult D. Characterization of mutations in the *rpoB* gene in naturally rifampin resistant *Rickettsia* species. Antimicrob Agent Chemother 1999; 43(10):2400–2403.
12. Rolain JM, Raoult D. Prediction of resistance to erythromycin in the genus *Rickettsia* by mutations in L22 ribosomal protein. J Antimicrob Chemother 2005; 56:396–398.
13. Rolain JM, Raoult D. Genome comparison analysis of molecular mechanisms of resistance to antibiotics in the *Rickettsia* genus. Ann NY Acad Sci 2006; 1063:222–230.
14. Ogata H, Renesto P, Audic S, Robert C, Blanc G, Fournier PE, Parinello H, Claverie JM, Raoult D. The genome sequence of *Rickettsia felis* identifies the first putative conjugative plasmid in an obligate intracellular parasite. PLoS Biol 2005; 3(8):e248.
15. Kelly PJ, Raoult D, Mason PR. Isolation of spotted fever group rickettsias from triturated ticks using a modification of the centrifugation-shell vial technique. Trans R Soc Trop Med Hyg 1991; 85:397–398.
16. Ruiz Beltran R, Herrero-Herrero JI. Deleterious effect of trimethoprim-sulfamethoxazole in Mediterranean spotted fever (letter). Antimicrob Agents Chemother 1992; 36:1342–1344.
17. Dumler JS, Barbet AF, Bekker CP, et al. Reorganization of genera in the families Rickettsiaceae and Anaplasmataceae in the order Rickettsiales: unification of some species of *Ehrlichia* with *Anaplasma*, *Cowdria* with *Ehrlichia* and *Ehrlichia* with *Neorickettsia*, descriptions of six new species combinations and designation of *Ehrlichia equi* and 'HGE agent' as subjective synonyms of *Ehrlichia phagocytophila*. Int J Syst Evol Microbiol 2001; 51:2145–2165.
18. Dumler JS, Bakken JS. Ehrlichial diseases of humans: emerging tick-borne infections. Clin Infect Dis 1995; 20:1102–1110.
19. Brouqui P, Raoult D. Susceptibilities of *Ehrlichiae* to antibiotics. In: Raoult D, ed. Antimicrobial Agents and Intracellular Pathogens. Boca Raton, FL: CPC Press, Inc., 1993:179–199.
20. Brouqui P, Raoult D. In vitro antibiotic susceptibility of the newly recognized agent of ehrlichiosis in humans, *Ehrlichia chaffeensis*. Antimicrob Agents Chemother 1992; 36:2799–2803.
21. Branger S, Rolain JM, Raoult D. Evaluation of antibiotic susceptibilities of *Ehrlichia canis*, *Ehrlichia chaffensis*, and *Anaplasma phagocytophilum* by real-time PCR. Antimicrob Agents Chemother 2004; 48:4822–4828.
22. Hunfeld KP, Bittner T, Rodel R, Brade V, Cinatl J. New real-time PCR-based method for in vitro susceptibility testing of *Anaplasma phagocytophilum* against antimicrobial agents. Int J Antimicrob Agents 2004; 23:563–571.
23. Horowitz HW, Hsieh TC, Guero-Rosenfeld ME, et al. Antimicrobial susceptibility of *Ehrlichia phagocytophila*. Antimicrob Agents Chemother 2001; 45:786–788.
24. Klein MB, Nelson CM, Goodman JL. Antibiotic susceptibility of the newly cultivated agent of human granulocytic ehrlichiosis: promising activity of quinolones and rifamycins. Antimicrob Agents Chemother 1997; 41:76–79.
25. Maurin M, Bakken JS, Dumler JS. Antibiotic susceptibilities of *Anaplasma* (*Ehrlichia*) *phagocytophilum* strains from various geographic areas in the United States. Antimicrob Agents Chemother 2003; 47:413–415.
26. Maurin M, Abergel C, Raoult D. DNA gyrase-mediated natural resistance to fluoroquinolones in *Ehrlichia* spp. Antimicrob Agents Chemother 2001; 45:2098–2105.
27. Maurin M, Benoliel AM, Bongrand P, Raoult D. Phagolysosomes of *Coxiella burnetii*-infected cell lines maintain an acidic pH during persistent infection. Infect Immun 1992; 60:5013–5016.
28. Torres H, Raoult D. In vitro activities of ceftriaxone and fusidic acid against 13 isolates of *Coxiella burnetii*, determined using the shell vial assay. Antimicrob Agents Chemother 1993; 37:491–494.
29. Boulos A, Rolain JM, Maurin M, Raoult D. Evaluation of antibiotic susceptibilities against *Coxiella burnetii* by real time PCR. Int J Antimicrob Agents 2004; 23:169–174.
30. Brennan RE, Samuel JE. Evaluation of *Coxiella burnetii* antibiotic susceptibilities by real-time PCR assay. J Clin Microbiol 2003; 41:1869–1874.

31. Rolain JM, Lambert F, Raoult D. Activity of telithromycin against thirteen new isolates of *C. burnetii* including three resistant to doxycycline. Ann NY Acad Sci. In press.
32. Rolain JM, Lambert F, Raoult D. Activity of telithromycin against thirteen new isolates of *C. burnetii* including three resistant to doxycycline. Ann NY Acad Sci 2005; 1063:252–256.
33. Maurin M, Raoult D. In vitro susceptibilities of spotted fever group rickettsiae and *Coxiella burnetii* to clarithromycin. Antimicrob Agents Chemother 1993; 37:2633–2637.
34. Raoult D, Torres H, Drancourt M. Shell-vial assay: evaluation of a new technique for determining antibiotic susceptibility, tested in 13 isolates of *Coxiella burnetii*. Antimicrob Agents Chemother 1991; 35:2070–2077.
35. Baca OG, Akporiaye ET, Aragon AS, Martinez IL, Robles MV, Warner NL. Fate of phase I and phase II *Coxiella burnetii* in several macrophage-like tumor cell lines. Infect Immun 1981; 33:258–266.
36. Roman MJ, Coriz PD, Baca OG. A proposed model to explain persistent infection of host cells with *Coxiella burnetii*. J Gen Microbiol 1986; 132:1415–1422.
37. Raoult D, Drancourt M, Vestris G. Bactericidal effect and doxycycline associated with lysosomotropic agents on *Coxiella burnetii* in P388D1 cells. Antimicrob Agents Chemother 1990; 34:1512–1514.
38. Maurin M, Benoliel AM, Bongrand P, Raoult D. Phagolysosomal alkalinization and the bactericidal effect of antibiotics: the *Coxiella burnetii* paradigm. J Infect Dis 1992; 166:1097–1102.
39. Raoult D, Vestris G, Enea M. Isolation of 16 strains and *Coxiella burnetii* from patients by using a sensitive centrifugation cell culture system and establishment of strains in HEL cells. J Clin Microbiol 1990; 28:2482–2484.
40. Raoult D, Houpikian P, Tissot Dupont H, Riss JM, Arditi-Djiane J, Brouqui P. Treatment of Q fever endocarditis: comparison of two regimens containing doxycycline and ofloxacin or hydroxychloroquine. Arch Int Med 1999; 159:167–173.
41. Houpikian P, Habib G, Mesana T, Raoult D. Changing clinical presentation of Q fever endocarditis. Clin Infect Dis 2002; 34:E28–E31.
42. Rolain JM, Mallet MN, Raoult D. Correlation between serum levels of doxycycline and serology evolution in patients treated for *Coxiella burnetii* endocarditis. J Infect Dis 2003; 9:1322–1325.
43. Rolain JM, Boulos A, Mallet MN, Raoult D. Correlation between ratio of serum doxycycline concentration to MIC and rapid decline of antibody levels during treatment of Q fever endocarditis. Antimicrob Agents Chemother 2005; 49:2673–2676.

Index

Acanthocheilonema viteae, 308
Acute Q fever
  clinical aspects, 291–292
  diagnostic tests, 296
  evolutive risks, 292–293
  treatment, 298
    children, 298
    pregnancy, 298
    risk of chronic evolution, 298
    vaccination, 298
Adaptive immunity
  Rickettsia, 18–19
African tick-bite fever, 117–124
  causative organism, 117
  clinical features, 120–121
  diagnostic criteria, 325
  microbiological diagnosis, 121
  pathogenesis, 119
  prevention, 121
  tick vectors, 117–118
  treatment, 121
Amblyomma
  eradication, 338–339
Aminoglycosides
  Ehrlichia, 365
Anaplasma, 224
  antigenic characterization, 183–184
  antigenic variability, 183–184
  host-parasite interaction, 184
  morphology, 183
  target cells, 184
  taxonomy and phylogeny, 182–183
Anaplasma marginale, 202
  nucleic-acid-based tests, 333
Anaplasma phagocytophilum, 199–200, 229
  human seroprevalence rates, 227
  isolation, 323
  PCR
    DNA targets, 322
Anaplasma platys, 202–203
Anaplasmataceae, 179–196, 191–193, 308
  future studies, 206–207
  vectors and reservoir hosts, 199–207
    veterinary importance, 202–206
Anaplasmosis. *See also* Human granulocytic anaplasmosis (HGA)
  bovine, 331–333
  canine granulocytic, 335
  canine thrombocytotrophic, 335–336
  caprine, 332, 333
  clinical features, 226–227
  ecology and epidemiology, 225–226
  equine granulocytic, 334–335
  feline granulocytic, 335
  humans, 223–231

[Anaplasmosis]
  microbiology, pathology and pathogenesis, 223–224
  ovine, 332, 333
  ruminants, 202
  taxonomy and nomenclature, 223–224
  vectors and reservoir hosts, 199–200
Antibodies
  chronic Q fever, 297
  Rickettsia, 20
Antigenic characterization
  Ehrlichia, 185
Antigenic variability
  Anaplasma, 183–184
Antigens
  Orientia tsutsugamushi, 239
  rickettsioses, 319
Antimicrobial susceptibility
  rickettsia, 361–365
  rickettsial agents, 361–367
Antimicrobial susceptibility testing
  Coxiella burnetii, 366
  in vitro
    Ehrlichia, 365–366
Arthropods, 27–36
  rickettsialpox, 67–69
Astrakhan fever rickettsia, 130–131
Autonomous replication sequence
  Coxiella burnetii, 264–265

Bacteriology
  Coxiella, 257–266
  flea-borne spotted fever, 89
  Rickettsia, 1–6
  Rickettsia prowazekii, 51–52
Beta-lactamase, 364
Bleeding, 23–24
Body louse. *See* Human body louse
Bovine anaplasmosis, 331–333
Bovine petechial fever, 333

Candidatus species
  Neoehrlichia mikurensis, 206
  Rickettsia
    amblyommii, 169–170
    andeanae, 170
    kellyi, 156
    marmionii, 156
    midichlorii, 171
    monacensis, 156
    rara, 171
    tarasevichiae, 170
    uilenbergi, 171
Canine
  granulocytic anaplasmosis, 335
  granulocytic ehrlichiosis, 335, 337

[Canine]
    infectious cyclic thrombocytopenia, 335–336
    monocytic ehrlichioses, 336–337
    monocytic ehrlichiosis, 203–204
    monocytic neorickettsiosis, 340
    Rocky Mountain spotted fever (RMSF), 340
    thrombocytotrophic anaplasmosis, 335–336
Caprine anaplasmosis, 332, 333, 334
Caprine ehrlichiosis, 337–338
Cardiopulmonary dynamics, 22
Cattle
    heartwater, 338
CD4 lymphocytes
    Rickettsia, 19
CD8 lymphocytes
    Rickettsia, 19
Cell culture model
    Ehrlichia, 365
Cell surface protein
    rickettsial agents, 354
CGH. *See* Comparative genome hybridization (CGH)
Chiggers, 244
    mites, 240
    Orientia tsutsugamushi, 251
Children
    acute Q fever in, 298
    HGA, 230
    scrub typhus, 244, 249–250
Chloramphenicol
    Ehrlichia, 365
    MSF, 131–132
    rickettsialpox, 78
    scrub typhus, 249
Chronic Q fever
    antibodies, 297
    characteristics, 272
    clinical presentation variations, 294–295
    defective immune response, 272–273
    diagnostic tests, 297
    endocarditis, 293, 294
    prognosis, 293
    treatment, 298
    vascular infection, 293
Ciprofloxacin
    MSF, 133
    rickettsialpox, 78
    scrub typhus, 250
Clarithromycin
    MSF, 133
    rickettsialpox, 78
    scrub typhus, 249
Comparative genome hybridization (CGH)
    Coxiella burnetii, 258
Conjunctival hyperemia
    scrub typhus, 246
Cotrimoxazole
    Q fever, 297
    rickettsia, 363
Cowan, George H., 110
Coxiella
    bacteriology, 257–266
Coxiella burnetii, 271, 291, 366–367
    acidophilic lifestyle, 260
    antimicrobial susceptibility testing, 366
    autonomous replication sequence, 264–265
    CGH, 258
    culture, 297
    cytokine network, 275–277
    death, 275–277

[*Coxiella burnetii*]
    dendritic cells, 275
    developmental life cycle, 261–262
    DNA repair mechanisms, 265
    gender, 284–285
    genetic events, 257
    genome, 264–266, 274
    genomic groups, 259
    immunohistochemistry, 297
    intracellular traffic, 273–274
    lipopolysaccharides, 262–264
    macrophages, 273
    metabolic pathways, 260
    microbiology, 259–264
    phagocytosis, 273
    phase variation, 262–263
    replication, 275–277
    sensors, 274–275
    shell-vial assay, 366–367
    taxonomy, 257–259
    toll-like receptors, 274–275
    transport, 260–261
Cross-adsorption assay
    murine typhus, 43
    rickettsioses, 319–321
    schematic, 320
Cytokines
    macrophage-deactivating
        Q fever, 275–276
    network
        Coxiella burnetii, 275–277

Dendritic cells
    Coxiella burnetii, 275
Dengue fever
    differential diagnosis, 248
Diagnosis
    African tick-bite fever, 121
    flea-borne spotted fever, 92–93
    HGA, 229–230
    human ehrlichioses, 216–218, 218–219
    leptospirosis, 248–249
    louse-borne epidemic typhus, 57
    murine typhus, 41, 45, 248
    MSF, 325
    Orientia tsutsugamushi, 246–247
    Q fever, 291–298
    rickettsialpox, 75
    rickettsioses, 315–326
    scrub typhus, 247–248
Diagnostic tests
    acute Q fever, 296
    chronic Q fever, 297
DNA repair mechanisms
    Coxiella burnetii, 265
Dot blot immunoassay
    scrub typhus, 247
Doxycycline
    acute Q fever, 298
    canine monocytic ehrlichioses, 337
    chronic Q fever, 298
    Coxiella burnetii, 274
    flea-borne spotted fever, 93
    heartwater, 339
    HGA, 227–228, 230
    human ehrlichioses, 219
    MSF, 131
    rickettsia, 362
    rickettsialpox, 78

[Doxycycline]
  RMSF, 102
  scrub typhus, 249, 250
Edema, 22
EDTA. *See* Ethylenediamine tetraacetic acid (EDTA)
Ehrlichia, 365–366
  cell culture model, 365
  in vitro antimicrobial susceptibility testing, 365–366
  light cycler polymerase chain reaction assay, 365
  molecular support of resistance, 366
  susceptibility testing results, 365–366
Ehrlichia
  antigenic characterization, 185
  host-parasite interaction, 185–189
  Ixodes ovatus, 204
  morphology, 185
  species
    canis, 203–204
    chaffeensis, 200–201, 337
    ewingii, 201–202
    muris, 204
    ruminantium, 204
  target cells, 189
  taxonomy and phylogeny, 184–185
Ehrlichial DNA/RNA
  detection, 217
Ehrlichial infections
  serological methods, 217–218
Ehrlichiosis. *See also* Human ehrlichioses; Human monocytotropic ehrlichiosis (HME)
  canine granulocytic, 335, 337
  canine monocytic, 336–337
  diagnostic strategy, 315–326
  equine, 334–335
  feline granulocytic, 335
  feline monocytic, 337
  ovine and caprine, 337–338
  vectors and reservoir hosts, 199–200
Endothelial cells, 18–19
Enzyme-linked immunosorbent assay
  murine typhus, 42
Equine ehrlichiosis, 334–335
Equine granulocytic anaplasmosis, 334–335
Equine monocytic neorickettsiosis, 339
Erythromycin, 364
  rickettsia, 364
  rickettsialpox, 78
Eschars, 245
Ethylenediamine tetraacetic acid (EDTA), 216, 316
Evolutive risks
  acute Q fever, 292–293
Exanthem
  rickettsialpox, 74

Far-Eastern tick-borne rickettsiosis, 144–146
Feline granulocytic anaplasmosis, 335
Feline granulocytic ehrlichiosis, 335
Feline monocytic ehrlichiosis, 337
Ferric-binding protein, 214
Fever. *See also* African tick-bite fever; Flea-borne spotted fever; Mediterranean Spotted Fever (MSF); Rocky Mountain spotted fever (RMSF)
  bovine petechial, 333
  differential diagnosis
    dengue, 248
    typhoid, 248
  Potomac horse, 339
  tick-borne, 335
Filarial nematode disease, 303–310

Filarial nematode parasites, 303–304
Filariasis, 303
  lymphatic, 303–304
Flea-borne spotted fever, 87–96
  bacteriology, 89
  diagnosis features, 92–93
  epidemiology, fleas, and *Rickettsia felis*, 88–89
  history, 87
  molecular characterization, 89–90
  pathogenicity and clinical features, 90–91
  phylogeny and taxonomic position, 87–88
  physiopathology, 91
  prevention, 93
  treatment, 93
Flinders Island spotted fever, 148–149
Fluoroquinolones
  HGA, 230
  rickettsia, 364
Francisella tularensis, 271

Gallsickness, 331–333
Gene expression profile analysis
  Coxiella burnetii, 261–262
Genes
  host specificity
    rickettsial agents, 353–354
Genetic events
  Coxiella burnetii, 257
Genetics
  rickettsialpox, 65–67
Genome
  Coxiella burnetii, 264–266, 274
  rickettsial agents, 345–346, 347–349, 355
  rickettsiales, 346
    ancient gene exchange, 351–352
  RMSF, 99
Genomic groups
  Coxiella burnetii, 259
Gentamicin
  rickettsia, 363
Global transcriptomic analysis
  rickettsiales, 356
Gluconeogenesis, 260
Glycolysis, 260
Granulocytic anaplasmosis
  canine, 335
  equine, 334–335
  feline, 335
Granulocytic ehrlichiosis
  canine, 335, 337
  feline, 335

Heartwater, 338
  African and Caribbean cattle, sheep, and goats, 338
Hemostasis, 21
Heparan sulfate proteoglycans, 242
Hepatic involvement, 23
HGA. *See* Human granulocytic anaplasmosis (HGA)
HIV. *See* Human immunodeficiency virus (HIV)
HME. *See* Human monocytotropic ehrlichiosis (HME)
Horse fever
  Potomac, 339
Host
  genes
    rickettsial agents, 353–354
  reservoir
    anaplasmosis, 199–200
  vertebrate
    rickettsialpox, 69–70

Host cell responses
  rickettsialpox, 76
Host cells
  Rickettsia, 17–18
Host defenses
  Rickettsia, 18–19
Host factors
  illness severity, 24
  Rickettsia, 17–18, 18–19
  rickettsialpox, 76
  RMSF, 102–103
Host-parasite interaction
  Anaplasma, 184
  Ehrlichia, 185–189
  Neorickettsia, 181–182
Host/pathogenicity adaptation
  rickettsial agents, 352–355
Host specificity
  genes associated with
    rickettsial agents, 353–354
Human body louse, 53–55
  anatomy, life cycle, and physiology, 54–55
  epidemiology, 55
  origin and future, 53–54
  Rickettsia prowazekii, 55–56
Human ehrlichioses, 213–219
  case definitions, 218
  clinical features, 215–216
  definition, 213
  differential diagnosis, 218–219
  epidemiology, 213
  laboratory diagnosis, 216–218
  pathogenesis and pathology, 214–215
  treatment and prognosis, 219–220
Human granulocytic anaplasmosis (HGA), 223–224, 316
  case definitions, 229, 230
  case fatality rate, 228
  cases reported, 226
  clinical features, 226–227, 228
  diagnosis, 229–230, 326
  disease course, 227–228
  ecology, 225
  laboratory abnormalities, 228
  Lyme disease, 228
  pediatric antibiotic treatment, 230
  treatment, 230–231
Human granulocytic ehrlichiosis, 199–200
Human immunodeficiency virus (HIV)
  Orientia tsutsugamushi, 251–252
  scrub typhus, 251–252
Human monocytotropic ehrlichiosis (HME), 200–201, 213–219, 316
  laboratory values, 217
  signs and symptoms, 216
Humans
  anaplasmosis, 223–231
  Q fever
    epidemiology, 281–283
    transmission, 283–285
  seroprevalence rates
    A. phagocytophilum, 227
  tick-borne rickettsiae, 163–172
  Wolbachia
    chemotherapy, 310
Hydroxychloroquine
  chronic Q fever, 298

Hyperemia
  conjunctival
    scrub typhus, 246
Hypovolemia, 22

IFA. *See* Immunofluorescence assay (IFA)
Immune clearance
  Rickettsia, 16–17
  RMSF, 102–103
Immune response
  chronic Q fever, 272–273
  down regulation
    Rickettsia, 20
  Neorickettsia, 182
  primary Q fever, 271–272
  Q fever, 271–277
  rickettsialpox, 76–77
Immunity
  adaptive
    Rickettsia, 18–19
    Orientia tsutsugamushi, 241–243, 243–244
    RMSF, 102–103
Immunodetection
  rickettsioses, 317
Immunofluorescence assay (IFA). *See also* Indirect immunofluorescence assay
  rickettsia, 362
Immunohistochemistry
  Coxiella burnetii, 297
Immunoperoxidase assay
  murine typhus, 42
Indian tick typhus fever rickettsia, 131
Indirect hemagglutination test
  murine typhus, 42
Indirect immunofluorescence assay
  antigen A, 320
  antigen B, 320
  cross reactions, 318
  murine typhus, 42
  scrub typhus, 247
  serological methods, 318
Infected ticks
  dogs and cats, 341
Infectious cyclic thrombocytopenia, canine, 335–336
Innate immune system
  Q fever, 273–275
Innate immunity
  Rickettsia, 18
Insect-perpetuated rickettsiae, 31–32
Israeli spotted fever rickettsia, 130

Jail fever, 51
Japanese or Oriental spotted fever, 147
Josamycin
  flea-borne spotted fever, 93
  MSF, 133
  rickettsia, 364
  rickettsialpox, 78

Latex agglutination test
  murine typhus, 42–43
Leptospirosis
  differential diagnosis, 248–249
Life cycle
  developmental
    Coxiella burnetii, 261–262

[Life cycle]
  human body louse, 54–55
  murine typhus, 38–39
Light cycler polymerase chain reaction assay
  Coxiella burnetii, 367
  Ehrlichia, 365
  rickettsia, 363
Line blot assay
  murine typhus, 42
Liponyssoides sanguineus, 67–69
Liponyssus bacoti, 69
Lipopolysaccharides
  Coxiella burnetii, 262–264
Louse. *See* Human body louse
Louse-borne epidemic typhus, 51–62
  biological diagnosis, 57
  clinical manifestations, 57
  control and prevention, 58
  history and epidemiology, 51
  pathophysiology, 56
  treatment, 57–58
  vaccination, 58
  vector, 53–55
Lyme disease
  HGA, 228
Lymphangitis-associated rickettsiosis, 149–151
Lymphatic filariasis, 303–304
Lymphocytes
  Rickettsia, 19

Macrolide compounds
  rickettsia, 364
Macrophage
  Coxiella burnetii, 273
  deactivating cytokines
    Q fever, 275–276
  Rickettsia, 19
McClintic, Thomas, 110
Mediterranean Spotted Fever (MSF), 29, 125–130
  clinical features, 128
  diagnostic criteria, 325
  epidemiology, 127
  pathogenesis, 127–128
  severe forms, 128–130
  treatment, 131–132
  vectors, 126–127
Metabolic pathways
  Coxiella burnetii, 260
Microimmunofluorescence (MIF)
  serological methods, 318
Mites
  chiggers, 240
  rickettsiae, 32–33
Molecular biology
  Q fever, 296
Molecular characterization
  flea-borne spotted fever, 89–90
Monocytic ehrlichioses
  canine, 336–337
  feline, 337
Monocytic neorickettsiosis
  canine, 340
  equine, 339
MSF. *See* Mediterranean Spotted Fever (MSF)
Multi-spacer typing (MST), 10
Murine typhus, 37–51
  clinical manifestations, 43–44
  complications, 45

[Murine typhus]
  cross-adsorption, 43
  differential diagnosis, 45, 248
  enzyme-linked immunosorbent assay, 42
  epidemiology, 38–39
  history, 37–38
  isolation-culture, 41
  laboratory abnormalities, 43–44
  laboratory diagnosis, 40–41
  life cycle, 38–39
  molecular diagnosis, 41
  pathogenesis, 40
  pathologic examination, 41
  pathophysiology, 39–40
  prevention, 46
  serological diagnosis, 42
  specimen collection and storage, 41
  treatment, 45–46

Nematode disease
  filarial, 303–310
Nematode parasites
  filarial, 303–304
Nematodes
  Wolbachia
    genomic analysis, 307–308
Neorickettsia, 179–180, 204
  antigenic characterization, 181
  host-parasite interaction, 182
  metabolism, 181–182
  morphology, 181
  physiopathology and immune response, 182
  taxonomy and phylogeny, 179–180
Neorickettsia helminthoeca, 206
Neorickettsia risticii, 204–206, 339
Neorickettsiosis
  canine monocytic, 340
  equine monocytic, 339
Nomenclature
  anaplasmosis, 223–224
North Asian tick typhus, 139–144
Nucleic-acid-based tests
  Anaplasma marginale, 333

Occupational exposure
  Q fever, 296
Oflaxacin
  rickettsialpox, 78
Onchocerca volvulus, 304
Onchocerciasis, 304
  murine model, 308
Oriental spotted fever, 147
Orientia tsutsugamushi, 237–252
  antigens, 239
  causative organism, 247
  chemoprophylaxis, 250–251
  chigger contract reduction, 251
  diagnosis, 246–247
  differential diagnosis, 247–248
  dual infections, 249
  epidemiology, 239–240
  habitat and ecology, 240–241
  HIV and, 251–252
  immunity, 241–243, 243–244
  intracellular survival
    strategies, 237–238
  laboratory confirmation, 246–247
  pathogenesis, 242–243

[*Orientia tsutsugamushi*]
    perinuclear clusters, 238
    prevention, 250–252
    serodiagnosis, 246–247
    staining, 243
    taxonomy, 237
    treatment, 249–252
Ovine anaplasmosis, 332, 333, 334
Ovine ehrlichiosis, 337–338
Oxytetracycline (Terramycin)
    heartwater, 338
    Potomac horse fever/equine monocytic neorickettsiosis, 339
    rickettsialpox, 78

Parasites. *See also* Host-parasite interaction
    filarial nematode, 303–304
Pasture fever, 335
PCR. *See* Polymerase chain reaction (PCR)
Pefloxacin
    rickettsialpox, 78
Petechial fever
    bovine, 333
Phagocytosis
    Coxiella burnetii, 273
Phagosome
    rickettsial escape, 17
Phase variation
    Coxiella burnetii, 262–263
Phylogeny
    Anaplasma, 182–183
    Ehrlichia, 184–185
    flea-borne spotted fever, 87–88
    Neorickettsia, 179–180
    Orientia tsutsugamushi, 237
    Rickettsia, 6–8, 8–10
    rickettsiae, 164
    rickettsiales, 346
    rickettsialpox, 65–67
    Wolbachia, 190, 305
Plaque assay
    rickettsia, 361–362
Plasmids
    rickettsial agents, 346–347
Polymerase chain reaction (PCR). *See also* Light cycler polymerase chain reaction assay
    Anaplasma phagocytophilum
        DNA targets, 322
    light cycler
        Coxiella burnetii, 367
Potomac horse fever, 339
Pregnancy
    acute Q fever and, 298
    Q fever and, 295
    scrub typhus and, 244–245, 249–250
Primary Q fever
    protective immune response, 271–272
Pristinamycin
    rickettsialpox, 78
Proteomics
    rickettsiales, 356–357
Pseudogenes
    rickettsial agents, 348–349
Public health
    animal rickettsioses, 340–341

Q fever. *See also* Acute Q fever; Chronic Q fever
    age, 284–285, 295
    animals, 285–286

[Q fever]
    bioterrorism agent, 285
    clinical aspects, 291–295
    contaminated aerosols, 283
    diagnostic tools, 296–297
    epidemiology, 281–286
    geographic variations, 295
    historical aspects, 281
    humans
        epidemiology, 281–283
        transmission, 283–285
    immune response, 271–277
    immunological overview, 271–273
    innate immune system, 273–275
    inoculum, 296
    macrophage-deactivating cytokines, 275–276
    molecular biology, 296
    natural history, 291, 294
    occupational exposure, 296
    oral transmission, 283–284
    percutaneous transmission, 284
    person-to-person transmission, 284
    pregnancy and, 295
    primary protective immune response, 271–272
    samples, handling, 296
    serology, 296
    sexual transmission, 284
    treatment, 291–298, 297–298
    vertical transmission, 284
Queensland tick typhus (QTT), 146–147

Rash
    feature of RMSF, 101
    and HGA, 227, 228
    and HME, 215, 216, 219
    macular
        and epidemic typus, 57
        and rickettsioses, 21
        and SFG rickettsioses, 145
    and murine typhus, 38, 43, 44
    scrub typhus, 246
    and Siberian tick typhus, 143
Rats
    mites, 240
Reductive evolution
    rickettsial agents, 347–348
Reservoir hosts
    anaplasmosis, 199–200
Restriction fragment length polymorphism (RFLP)
    Coxiella burnetii, 258
Rickettsia
    antimicrobial susceptibility, 361–365
    dye-uptake assay, 362
    immunofluorescence assay, 362
    in vitro antimicrobial susceptibility testing, 361–362
    light cycler polymerase chain reaction assay, 363
    molecular support of resistance, 364–365
    susceptibility testing results, 363–364
Rickettsia
    adaptive immunity, 18–19
    antibodies, 20
    bacteriology, 1–6
    entry into host cell, 17–18
    features, 2–5
    host defenses against, 18–19
    immune clearance, 16–17

Index

[Rickettsia]
  innate immunity, 18
  lymphocytes, 19
  phylogeny, 6–8
  spread to other cells, 17
  taxonomy, 8–10
  vaccine prospects, 20–21
Rickettsia species
  aeschlimannii, 153–154
  asiatica, 164
  australis, 146–147
  bellii, 164
  canadensis, 166–167
  conorii caspia, 130–131
  conorii indica, 131
  conorii israelensis, 130
  felis
    flea-borne spotted fever, 88–89
    light cycler assay, 363
  heilongjanghensis, 144–146
  helvetica, 167
  honei, 148–149
  japonica, 147
  massiliae, 155
  montanensis, 167–168
  parkeri, 154–155
  peacockii, 168
  prowazekii
    bacteriology, 51–52
    human body louse, 55–56
    origin, 52–53
    reservoir, 53
  raoultii, 155–156
  rhipicephali, 168
  sibirica Mongolitimonae, 149–151
  sibirica sibirica, (North Asian tick typhus), 139–144
  slovaca, 151
  tamurae, 169
Rickettsiae
  identification and differentiation, 324
  insect-perpetuated, 31–32
  isolation, 323
  macrorestriction analysis, 324
  mites, 32–33
  stringent response, 352–353
  taxonomic scheme, 164
  tick-borne, 28–31
  undetermined pathogenicity, 165–166
  validated species, 164
Rickettsial agents
  ankyrin-repeat proteins, 355
  antibiotic susceptibility, 364
  antimicrobial susceptibility, 361–367
  cell surface protein, 354
  G + C composition, 347
  genes associated with host specificity, 353–354
  genome analysis, 355
  genome size, 345
  genome streamlining, 347–348
  genomics, 345–357
  host/pathogenicity adaptation, 352–355
  plasmids, 346–347
  pseudogenes, 348–349
  reductive evolution, 347–348
  repeats, 347
  type IV secretion systems, 354–355
Rickettsial infections
  injury associated with, 16

[Rickettsial infections]
  pathology, 21–22
  pathophysiology, 22–23
  routes of spread in body, 15
  target cells and organs, 15–16
  transmission, 15
Rickettsiales
  future prospects, 357
  genome-based phenotypic characterization, 355–356
  genome characteristics, 346
  global transcriptomic analysis, 356
  phylogeny, 346
  postgenomics study, 355–357
  proteomics, 356–357
Rickettsiales genome
  ancient gene exchange, 351–352
  emerging genomic plasticity, 350–352
  gene duplication, 350
  genome impairment, 349
  genome rearrangements, 350
  genome transfer, 349–350
  intragenome recombination, 350
  protein coding capacity, 349
  protein coding palindromic repeats, 351
Rickettsialpox, 63–86
  animal models, 77–78
  antibiotic susceptibility and therapy, 78
  arthropod transmission, 67–69
  cell culture growth and plaque formation, 65
  cell culture isolation, 79
  cell morphology and staining, 64–65
  clinical disease, 73–74
  cutaneous and mucosal manifestations, 74
  differential diagnosis, 75
  ecology and natural history, 67–68
  entry, intracellular growth and host cell responses, 76
  epidemiology, 70–71
  exanthem, 74
  genetics and phylogenetic position, 65–67
  geographic distribution, 70–71
  histopathology and immunohistochemistry, 79–80
  history, 63–64
  immune response, 76–77
  incubation period, 73
  laboratory diagnosis, 79–80
  microbiology, 64–65
  molecular methods, 81
  pathogenesis, 76–77
  patient demographics, 71–72
  prevention, 73
  primary lesion, 74
  risk factors, 71–72
  seasonality, 71–72
  serology, 79
  systemic manifestations, 74–75
  temporal and spatial characteristics, 72–73
  vertebrate hosts, 69–70
Rickettsioses
  animal
    public health, 340–341
  antigens tested, 319
  clinical suspicion, 315
  cross-adsorption assay, 319–321
  cultivation, 323–324
  diagnostic strategy, 315–326

[Rickettsioses]
- direct diagnosis, 316–319
- immunodetection, 317
- nonimmunological staining methods, 317
- PCR, 321–323
  - DNA targets and nucleotide s, 322
- sample collection and storage, 316
- serological methods, 318–319
- specific diagnosis, 315–316
- xenodiagnostic, 316

Rifampin
- HGA, 230
- human ehrlichioses, 219
- Q fever, 297
- rickettsia, 364
- scrub typhus, 250

Risk factors
- rickettsialpox, 71–72

Risk of chronic evolution
- acute Q fever, 298

Rocky Mountain spotted fever (RMSF), 97–116
- antibiotic therapy, 102
- canine, 340
- case clustering, 105–106
- cell tropism and intracellular pathophysiology, 99–100
- clinical disease, 101–103
- diagnostics, 108–109
- epidemiology, 103–104
- genome, 99
- geographic distribution, 103–104
- history, 97–98
- host factors, immune clearance, immunity, 102–103
- incidence, 104–105
- microbiology, 98
- mortality, 107
- natural history, 99
- persistence, 106
- prevention, 107–108
- seasonality, 104
- transmission, 104

Roxithromycin
- scrub typhus, 249

SCA. *See* Surface cell antigen (SCA)

Scrub typhus, 237–252
- conjunctival hyperemia, 246
- diagnosis, 247
- differential diagnosis, 247–248
- distribution, 239
- dot blot immunoassay, 247
- drug-resistant, 250
- epidemiology, 239–240
- habitats, 240
- HIV and, 251–252
- in children, 244, 249–250
- male vector, 242
- pregnancy and, 244–245, 249–250
- rash, 246
- treatment, 249–252
- vaccine, 251

Seasonality
- rickettsialpox, 71–72
- RMSF, 104

Serology
- ehrlichial infections, 217–218
- Q fever, 296

[Serology]
- rickettsialpox, 79
- *Wolbachia*, 309

Sexual transmission
- Q fever, 284

SFGP. *See* Spotted fever group (SFGP)

Shell-vial assay
- *Coxiella burnetii*, 366–367

Siberian tick typhus (STT), 139–144

Spotted fever group (SFGP), 1–6, 340

Stringent response pathway, 353

STT. *See* Siberian tick typhus (STT)

Sulfamethoxazole, 364

Surface cell antigen (SCA), 6

Susceptibility testing results
- *Ehrlichia*, 365–366

Target cells
- *Ehrlichia*, 190

Taxonomy
- *Anaplasma*, 182–183
- anaplasmosis, 223–224
- *Coxiella burnetii*, 258–259
- *Ehrlichia*, 184–185
- flea-borne spotted fever, 87–88
- *Neorickettsia*, 179–180
- *Orientia tsutsugamushi*, 237
- *Rickettsia*, 8–10
- rickettsiae, 164
- *Wolbachia*, 190, 305

TCA. *See* Tricarboxylic acid cycle (TCA)

Telithromycin
- rickettsia, 364

Terramycin
- heartwater, 338
- Potomac horse fever/equine monocytic neorickettsiosis, 339
- rickettsialpox, 78

Tetracycline
- *Ehrlichia*, 365
- HGA, 230
- scrub typhus, 249

TG. *See* Typhus group (TG)

Thiamphenicol
- rickettsia, 364

Thrombocytotrophic anaplasmosis, canine, 335–336

Thrombosis, 21–22

Tick-bite fever. *See* African tick-bite fever

Tick-borne fever, 335

Tick-borne lymphadenopathy, 151

Tick-borne rickettsiae, 28–31
- human illnesses, 163–172

Tick vectors
- African tick-bite fever, 117–118

Toll-like receptors
- *Coxiella burnetii*, 274–275

Transport
- *Coxiella burnetii*, 260–261

Tricarboxylic acid cycle (TCA), 260

Trimethoprim, 364

Typhoid fever
- differential diagnosis, 248

Typhus. *See* Louse-borne epidemic typhus; Murine typhus; Scrub typhus

Typhus group (TG), 1–6

Vaccine
- acute Q fever, 298

[Vaccine]
    louse-borne epidemic typhus, 58
    Rickettsia, 20–21
    scrub typhus, 251
Validated species
    rickettsiae, 164
Vancomycin
    rickettsialpox, 78
Vascular inflammation, 21
Vectors
    anaplasmosis, 199–200
    louse-borne epidemic typhus, 53–55
    MSF, 126–127
    scrub typhus, 242
    tick
        African tick-bite fever, 117–118
Vertebrate hosts
    rickettsialpox, 69–70

Weil-Felix test
    murine typhus, 42
    scrub typhus, 247
Western blotting
    murine typhus, 42
    rickettsioses, 321

Wolbachia, 303–310
    adaptive immune response, 309
    adverse post-treatment reactions, 309
    characteristics, 304
    chemotherapy
        humans, 310
    distribution in filarial
        nematodes, 307
    drug target for filariasis, 309
    filarial biology, 307
    filarial nematodes, 305
    filarial pathogenesis, 308–309
    host-parasite interaction, 190–191
    immune response, 191
    inflammatory activity, 308–309
    morphology, 190
    nematode metabolism and survival
        genomic analysis, 307–308
    replication and population
        dynamics, 306–307
    serology, 309
    taxonomy and phylogeny, 190, 305
    ultrastructural characteristics, 305
Wolbachia pipientis
    phylogenetic relationships, 306

About the Editors

DIDIER RAOULT, MD, PHD, specializes in infections diseases and clinical microbiology. He is a consultant on infections disease and runs a clinical microbiology laboratory of 2500 beds in Marseille, France. He is director of a research unit on rickettsial diseases, the Unité des Rickettsies, which became a National Reference Center in 1987, WHO Collaborative Center in 1988, and has been associated with CNRS (National Research Agency) since 1994. It is currently the largest laboratory in the world in the field of rickettsial disease. Dr. Raoult has published more than 936 papers in English and 71 in French, and has contributed three chapters in French and 129 in English to such publications as Harrison's *Principles of Internal Medicine* and *Principles and Practices of Infectious Diseases* by Mandell et al. He has made contributions to a total of 14 books on the subject of infectious diseases. Often invited to lecture in various locations around the world, Dr. Raoult holds 18 patents for diagnostic tests and participated in the first isolation of several emerging pathogens from humans, including numerous tick-borne agents, such as *Rickettsia africae* and *R. sibirica mongolitimonae*. He was also involved in the surveys of recent outbreaks of epidemic typhus in Rwanda and Burundi. Dr. Raoult is currently considered one of the main investigators in the field of rickettsial diseases and emerging infections.

PHILIPPE PAROLA MD, PHD, is a clinician specialist in internal medicine, infectious diseases, and tropical medicine. After having obtained both M.D. and Ph.D. degrees at the Medical School of Marseilles, France, he was a post-doctoral fellow at the Harvard School of Public Health, Boston, Massachusetts, U.S.A., in the Laboratory of Public Health Entomology. He spent a total of four years for clinical and/or research activities in tropical settings in Africa and Asia. Besides his clinical activity in an Infectious Diseases and Tropical Medicine Unit, he is now associate professor at the Marseille School of Medicine. His research interest includes medical entomology, particularly tick-, flea-, and louse-borne diseases. He has coauthored more than 100 publications, including the first work in the international literature on various aspects of the epidemiology of vector-borne diseases, particularly in tropical areas. He has also written 10 book chapters in this field.